The Theory and Practice of Psychiatry

THE THEORY AND PRACTICE OF PSYCHIATRY

Fredrick C. Redlich and
Daniel X. Freedman

Basic Books, Inc. Publishers · New York, London

Library of Congress Catalog Card Number: 66–13833
Manufactured in the United States of America
Designed by Sophie Adler

TO

Herta, Mary, Erik, and Peter

PREFACE

◆ As teachers we have learned from our students that they wanted and needed a modern guide to the complex field of psychiatry. We accepted the challenge and wrote this book, which introduces the reader to the essentials of psychiatric theories and practices and their evolution. Because we have quite liberally expressed our own ideas and convictions and tried to point to the frontiers of psychiatric knowledge, this work, we believe, is more than a textbook. It is addressed to students and practitioners of psychiatry, of the medical arts and sciences, and of the various professions working in the area of mental health. We also hope that it will be of interest to community planners and leaders, who have recognized the mental health problem as a significant one of our time.

In giving an overview and a point of view, we express our belief that the specialty of psychiatry, an applied medical science, must and will increasingly rest on the foundation of basic biological and behavioral sciences. The behavioral sciences include psychology, sociology, anthropology, and, last but not least, the biologically oriented behavioral science of psychoanalysis. The bridge to biology is increasingly being built by the basic neurobehavioral sciences in their study of the genetics and evolution of normal and abnormal behavior and its somatic substrates, as well as of neurophysiological and neurochemical correlates of behavior. It is important not to confuse psychiatry either with the cognate disciplines that constitute its basic sciences or with social welfare and education, with which psychiatric practice is closely linked.

Although psychiatry has its own identity, its language and jargon have evolved from many scientific approaches that, according to their emphasis and purpose, differ in questions asked, in methods employed, and in the models and analogies used for explanation. Furthermore, the practices and theories of psychiatry are not only shaped by modern medicine and science, but are historically rooted in theology and philosophy. Psychiatry bears the marks of this diverse and imprecise heritage. This fact of contemporary psychiatric life demands a sturdier response than pity. Clearly, it requires a continuous review of clinical and experimental facts and an ever-increasing precision of the theoretical assumptions in our field and of guidelines for our practices.

In view of the present state of practice and theory, we have not been able or willing to impose an artificial precision or homogeneity that could only misrepresent the current status of the field. Rather, we wish to invite the reader to join us in asking how behavior gets put together or becomes disorganized and in exposing those many junctures where dogma hides our honest ignorance and doubt. We hope that such a stress on unanswered issues and problems will be stimulating, if at times irritating. Our presentation endeavors to be critical and undogmatic. In a field that has grown so rapidly, the textual material as well as the bibliographies cannot be anything but selective and limited. Most of all, we wish to stimulate another generation of scientists and scientific practitioners to find answers to those practical problems that baffle us and to build new theories that are more satisfactory than the current ones.

The future of psychiatry, its proper scope, its emphases, and its directions may be far from certain; this does not mean that there is no set of core problems, issues, facts, and approaches that identifies the body of general psychiatric knowledge. It is this core of theory and practice that we have presented in this book. First, we delineate the field of psychiatry, trace its history, and give a sketch of human behavior as it seems pertinent for psychiatry. A discussion of etiological variables, methods of psychiatric examination and psychological testing (by Dr. Roy Schafer), and of general principles of diagnosis and therapy follows. The first eleven chapters should be read consecutively, so as to establish a basis for the understanding of subsequent chapters. Few approaches in psychiatry can be adequately presented or understood within the confines of a single chapter or heading; therefore, topics (such as psychoanalysis or the neural correlates of behavior) are expanded and illustrated as the text proceeds.

Chapters 12 through 23 consist of a critical review of current knowledge of clinical psychiatry; these chapters are devoted to psychopathology, etiology, and diagnosis and treatment of the main types of behavior disorder, including a chapter on behavior disorders in children by Dr. Seymour L. Lustman and one on mental subnormality by Dr. Seymour S. Sarason. In the final three chapters, we discuss the application of psychiatric principles in law and medicine, ending with a chapter on psychiatry and society.

Many colleagues and friends have helped in the writing of this book. We appreciate the contributions of Prof. Erwin Ackerknecht, Drs. Eugene L. Bliss, Douglas D. Bond, Eugene Brody, Robert N. Butler, Thomas P. Detre, Paul Errera, Robert G. Feldman, Stephen Fleck, John P. Flynn, Gilbert H. Glaser, Jay Katz, Conan Kornetsky, Jules Laffal, Nathanial J. London, and George F. Mahl; Miss Nea Norton; Mr. John F. O'Connor; and Drs. Darius G. Ornston, Henry Payson, Max P. Pepper, James W. Prichard, and Daniel P. Schwartz, who read one or several chapters and contributed to the clinical examples cited in the book. We are particularly indebted for such work to Drs. Arnold J. Benton, John M. Davis, and Edward C. Senay, whose untiring assistance helped us to improve the manuscript. For editorial help we thank Dr. Harvey A. Robinson and Dr. Hulda Flynn, Mrs. Elizabeth Bellis, and Mrs. Janet Turk; for bibliographic assistance, Mrs. Harriette Borsuch, Miss Adriné Kalfayan, and Mr. Stephen Pachl. For their efforts in decoding our handwriting, typing and retyping manuscripts, retrieving lost pages and references, and their patience in coping with the authors' temperaments and predicaments we wish to express our sincere gratitude to Mrs. Eleanor Himel, Mrs. Gail O'Connor, Mrs. Sheila Seligson, particularly to Miss Doris Berndtson and Mrs. Sharon Fanger, and most of all to Miss Marjorie Lacy. Last but not least we thank Mr. Irving Harris and the Social Research Foundation for aiding us with the preparation of this book.

FREDRICK C. REDLICH
DANIEL X. FREEDMAN

New Haven
January 1966

such work to Drs. Arnold I. Levinson, John M. Davis, and Edward C. Senay, whose comments and advice helped us to improve the manuscript. For editorial help we thank Dr. [illegible] A. [illegible] and Dr. [illegible]. Mrs. Elizabeth [illegible] and Mrs. Janet [illegible] for [illegible] assistance. Miss Harriette [illegible], Mrs. Marie [illegible], and Mrs. Stephen [illegible], for their efforts in deciphering our handwriting, preparing typescript manuscripts, retyping lost pages, and rechecking [illegible] with the authors' temperament [illegible] and [illegible] we wish to express our [illegible] gratitude to Mrs. Eleanor [illegible], Mrs. [illegible] O'Connor, Mrs. [illegible], and particularly to [illegible] and most of all to Miss [illegible] and the Social Sciences [illegible] this book.

F[illegible] C. R[illegible]
D[illegible] X. F[illegible]

New Haven
January [illegible]

CONTENTS

The Theory and Practice of Psychiatry

CHAPTER ONE

The Field of Psychiatry

Psychiatry is the medical specialty concerned with the study, diagnosis, treatment, and prevention of behavior disorders. America's most original modern psychiatrist, Harry Stack Sullivan,[44] defined psychiatry as the science of human relations. The scope of psychiatry is admittedly broad; indeed, Alan Gregg[18] once half-seriously remarked that psychiatry is a generality and not a specialty. Nevertheless, Sullivan's definition is too encompassing. It applies overall to the sciences of human behavior but not to psychiatry alone; it is so far-reaching as to invite psychiatrists to assume an absurd sense of omniscience. Psychiatry is an applied science that deals with abnormal human behavior. Psychiatrists are primarily scientifically informed medical practitioners whose task is to help people, not with all, but with certain kinds of difficulties. To accomplish this requires not only psychiatric research but contributions from disciplines that are basic sciences for psychiatry; these explore the spectrum of human or animal behavior largely in an experimental framework and often with systematic and theoretical interest.

The field, today, is in flux. Psychiatry has to some extent become involved in basic research and at the same time enlarged the scope of psychiatric practice beyond the core disorders. A young field, psychiatry has become firmly established as a medical discipline, yet it borrows heavily from the social sciences. What is the field? What are its responsibilities, its major focus and methods, its expanding interests? Who are the patients? What do they present both as practical treatment challenges and as theoretical problems that probe directly at the question of the organization of behavior and the ways and means by which it is disorganized and "repaired"? Some of these questions perhaps are muddled; but all comprise an essential background of the current debate and development that comprise the "field of psychiatry." Throughout this text, some of these questions should become clarified.

What, then, are these difficulties psychiatrists are supposed to treat, the so-called behavior disorders? Defying easy definition, the term refers to the presence of certain behavioral patterns—variously described as abnormal, subnormal, undesirable, inadequate, inappropriate, maladaptive, or maladjusted—that are not compatible with the norms and expectations of the patient's social and cultural system. Persons with behavior disorders are not able to function socially, sexually, and occupationally according to the expectations of their environment. They suffer and make others suffer.

In older texts and in current lay parlance, psychiatry is often defined as the science dealing with mental diseases and illnesses of the mind or psyche. Since these are terms reminiscent of the metaphysical concepts of soul and spirit, we prefer to speak of behavior disorder. Behavior refers to objective data that are accessible to observation, plausible inference, hypothesis-making, and experimentation. The term disorder, although vague, is descriptive of malfunctioning of behavior without specifying etiology or underlying mechanisms. Only some of the behavior disorders are caused by diseases of the brain or are accompanied by somatic reactions. Whereas many cerebral diseases produce a behavior disorder, and while we believe that cerebral processes must be related fundamentally to behavior, *medically* recognizable diseases of the brain cannot, for the most part, be demonstrated in behavior disorders.

The primary subject matter of psychiatry, then, is the disturbed or deviant behavior of the individual. By his behavior we mean his overt conduct—including his verbal behavior. From such behavior we also may infer the subjective life of a person, his private thoughts, reactions, and feelings. Both overt and covert behavior represent, in our view, a systematically related and meaningful series of events. We are concerned less with isolated behavioral fragments than with patterns of behavior. Just how these patterned behavioral events are organized, just how one goes about the task of discovering relationships relevant to the problems of diagnosis, etiology, and treatment—these issues comprise the scientific task of psychiatry.

What constitutes manifest behavior disorders depends on the culture or value system. The culture also sanctions those interventions that are referred to as psychiatric treatment. The expert—as a practitioner—merely carries out highly specialized examinations to determine the type and cause of disorder in the interest of early detection and competent treatment. The expert—as a student of behavior—is concerned with the lawful organization of any instance of behavior, whatever its social significance. Although predominantly guided by the value system of the society, these experts have made discoveries and proposed theories that have changed the prevailing concepts of human nature and thus altered the value system. The concept of unconscious motivation, for example, has influenced the ideas of Western society about individual responsibility. In turn, the development of a new point of view may cause society, for better or for worse, to look differently at behavior disorders.

Instead of describing the overall characteristics of behavior disorders, some pragmatic psychiatrists prefer simply to list a number of broad traditional classes of disorders: (1) The *psychoses* are severe disorders that result in highly idiosyncratic and impaired behavior. They are characterized by an extreme inability to give adequate regard to inner and outer reality and to organize sustained socially adequate response. Some psychoses are associated with brain disease; many are not; and about some we are in doubt. The legal term, insanity, and the obsolete words, madness and lunacy, carry the same general meaning as psychosis. (2) The *neuroses* and *sociopathies,* which we group together, are loose categories of ubiquitous disorders, primarily psychogenic; ironically, they are called minor disorders, although they may cause extreme suffering. They are characterized by an inability to perform optimally and by evidence of internal and external conflict. (3) The *psychosomatic diseases* are a group of organic dysfunctions of unknown etiology, in which psychogenic factors play a prominent role. Some psychosomatic disorders are more closely related to neurosis; others are intimately linked with psychosis. (4) The *mental deficiences* (or mental subnormality) are disorders with primary disturbance of intellectual functions; they are innate or acquired early in life. The psychoses and the severely disabling neuroses and, to a lesser extent, the sociopathies, psychosomatic dysfunctions, and mental deficiencies, comprise the severe "core disorders" for which psychiatry has either the primary or a substantial medical responsibility. It should be stressed at the outset that the major classes of behavior disorders, such as the psychoses and neuroses, cannot always be clearly separated from each other. There is, in fact, no sharp line of demarcation between normal and abnormal behavior; only marked deviations can be clearly recognized. On the whole, the severe deviations are dealt with by psychiatry. Minimal deviations of behavior are usually dealt with by members of the family, teachers, clergy, and associates in work and everyday living. This does not mean, of course, that psychiatrists ignore the fact that major difficulties often grow from minor symptoms and that these may camouflage major disorders; indeed, many psychiatrists—perhaps too many—tend to specialize in treating behavior disorders of any variety only if they are of minimal or moderate severity. Nor does it mean that society refers all major deviations in behavior to the psychiatrist. For instance, most criminal acts are dealt with by other agencies. A large number of behavior deviations that become socially troublesome are, however, defined as psychiatric problems whether or not traditional medical techniques are employed in therapy and management. At present, only psychiatrists and associated mental health workers are equipped by training to deal with these problems; society charges no one else with such responsibility.

Behavior can be seen or structured from a number of different points of view, depending on whether the pertinent questions are asked in theoretical, legal, investigative, or therapeutic frames of reference. To say that in all these viewpoints there is a commitment to an objectively scientific approach sounds almost trite today, but in fact this is quite new and radical in the field of behavior. As scientists we know two simple things about even the most cherished beliefs; first, that patterns of values differ and shift both through time and among cultures; and second, that *some* value is invariably attached to the recurrent features of social life. Since each of us is attached to particular sets of values, we react strongly when our beliefs and conduct are viewed as objects of study. Most people correctly perceive a behavior disorder as a violation of usual norms and values. But even enlightened people tend to react to these deviations with awe, if not with panic and hostility. The day when the deviant with "incorrigible" behavior disorder was mistreated is by no means past. The belief—still encountered—that behavior disorder is equivalent to sin was expressed as doctrine at a time when physics and cellular biology were long since subjects of rational and scientific study. Today, most people—and most experts—are inclined to view behavior disorder as an illness requiring treatment rather than an offense requiring punishment or banishment ("out of mind, out of sight"); in effect, a moratorium on normal social responsibilities and obligations is sanctioned if one is ill. This is what Talcott Parsons termed the social role of being sick—the change of status by which a person in our society can receive treatment rather than censure.[33]

Prevalence and Incidence of Behavior Disorders

Direct knowledge about behavior disorders is derived from three sources: clinical observation, experimentation, and epidemiological studies. Historically, psychiatrists have relied mostly on clinical method and relatively little on experimentation. The epidemiological approach was extended from the study of infectious diseases to the investigation of chronic diseases and only recently to behavior disorders. Epidemiology is concerned both with the prevalence of a disorder, that is, the number of existing cases in a sample population at a given time, and with incidence, or the number of new cases in a sample population in a given period of time. In addition to nose-counting with statistically sophisticated methods, epidemiologists attempt to determine the relationship of the prevalence and incidence of the phenomenon under study to certain interpersonal, environmental, or ecological variables. In seeking answers about etiology or the efficacy of therapy, they may even modify such variables experimentally.

Comprehensive epidemiological information on our own and other cultures is still sparse. Methods of data collection vary widely and prohibit comparisons with results of outstanding studies in Scandinavian countries,[43, 8, 32] in Taiwan,[30] in Africa,[27] in India,[5] and in the United States.[6, 22, 26] To count the number of cases of a particular disorder, one needs not only reliable criteria for identifying the disorder—a thorny problem—but adequate methods for locating the relevant cases. The practical obstacles in the way of finding all psychiatric cases in a given population are more formidable than in general epidemiology. Where, say, estimates of prevalence are based on a census of hospitalized patients, the cross-cultural picture is obscured. For instance, in Nigeria only one in every one hundred thousand persons is in a mental hospital, although, of course, unknown numbers are treated in primitive institutions by so-called native doctors.[27] To be meaningful, epidemiological data would require information about all cases of behavior disorders, treated as well as untreated. A census of all patients under treatment would thus not reflect total prevalence, but instead merely yields a picture of psychiatric practice. In New Haven, Connecticut, in 1950, this figure was 828 per 100,000;[22] in Manhattan, in 1955, based on a sample from the Yorkville section with more patients in ambulatory treatment, it was 1,288 per 100,000.[42] This means that roughly 1 per cent of the population in these metropolitan centers in the United States are visible psychiatric patients at the time of these surveys. In the United States generally, there are approximately 400 patients per 100,000 population. One million psychiatric patients are currently hospitalized; another 400,000 are treated in clinics; and 400,000 are seen in private offices of psychiatrists.[35]

In the Yorkville study the investigators, who did not use conventional psychiatric classifications, found that 19 per cent of the population were well; 36 per cent had mild psychiatric symptoms without impairment of their everyday activities; and 22 per cent were moderately disturbed, with clear-cut symptoms, but functioned adequately in everyday life. Marked disturbances, characterized by definite symptoms and difficulties in functioning, were found in 13 per cent. In more than 7 per cent of the population there was severe disturbance, with pronounced symptoms and appreciable restriction in role functioning. Finally, nearly 3 per cent of the sample was incapacitated. According to Leo Srole, about 10 per cent of the population studied suffers from very definite psychiatric disorders. This figure, it should be noted, is ten times the number of visible patients. It is not unlikely that this estimate is valid for other metropolitan areas in the United States.

We must conclude that the total prevalence of different categories of behavior disorders in different cultures is at present not adequately known. Available figures for *severe* disorders in primitive societies may be lower than those reported elsewhere, not because civilization increases behavior disorders, but because under difficult living conditions the severely ill are less likely to survive. On the other hand, there are value systems and social institutions in some primitive cultures that protect the mentally ill by giving them special status.

Today, we know with certainty only that all major disorders seem to occur in all cultures; probably they have occurred throughout history. If the major disorders are, indeed, distributed more or less equally through space and time, both genetic and environmental points of view would be hard put to suggest factors to account for this relative constancy of distribution. As epidemiological research and correlated advances in the dynamics and genetics of populations develop, the resulting data obviously will be as relevant to problems of etiology as to public control measures.

The Cost of Behavior Disorders

Anyone who has known the disorganized life of a schizophrenic, an alcoholic, or a very neurotic person, and has seen the impact of such behavior on families and the community, can testify to the fact that human misery cannot be appraised in dollars and cents. Yet, not infrequently a prominent—and presumably hard-boiled—citizen will raise the question whether it pays to treat psychiatric patients. It is true that treatment of behavior disorders is not an inexpensive process, but at the same time—because the very existence of behavior disorders is an expensive burden for society—it is the economical approach.

To estimate the cost of behavior disorders to society, economists distinguish between direct costs, which include the costs of institutions, their maintenance and amortization, service personnel, and the expenditures for research and training—and indirect costs, which include loss of manpower and productivity, care of dependents, and such items as damage to property and persons, and legal costs. Rashi Fein estimates that the direct annual cost of mental illness in the United States amounts to the staggering sum of $1.7 billion.[10] This figure does not include capital expenditures for mental health institutions or their amortization, but it does include the cost of training and research in the field. Even in prosperous countries, existing treatment facilities lag behind desirable standards so that even larger sums will be necessary to meet minimal mental health needs. Relatively few people can afford to pay out of their own pockets for the direct costs of hospitalization or for ambulatory treatment; and the fees for private psychotherapy are quite beyond the financial limits of the majority of persons, even in such a wealthy country as the United States. This cannot be explained by the greed of practitioners. It is true that market values (great demand and limited supply) play a role in encouraging high fees of private practitioners whose incomes, nevertheless, are generally within the range of other medical specialists. It is also true that it is expensive to train specialists; but the fact remains that individual psychotherapy is inherently costly. It is time-consuming, requiring fifty to sixty minutes for each patient and must continue over many such fifty-minute "hours," since consolidated, reparative behavior change under any circumstances is rarely rapid. If all psychiatrists in the United States worked a forty-hour week and saw only those alcoholics who belong to Alcoholics Anonymous on a once-a-week basis, there would be no hours left for the remaining populations of alcoholic, neurotic, sociopathic, and psychotic patients. It will be difficult to remedy this situation. Improvement of therapeutic techniques in both individual and group therapy may help. Other means than intensive psychotherapy are needed to expand therapeutic services. Attempts are being made to train a less expensive psychotherapist, available to people who hitherto have been unable to afford this service.[39]

The indirect yearly cost of mental disorders in this country currently is estimated at $2.4 billion. Fein argues rightly that early treatment of patients in the community would reduce the high cost of hospitalization and the enormous concomitant loss in productivity.[10] It should also be mentioned that nowhere is enough skill, time, and money spent on psychiatric training and research. Even the substantial support given in recent years to psychiatric and behavioral science research in the United States must be considered small compared with the sustained investment of moneys for research in other medical areas.

The Mental Health Professions

The mental health professions are composed of experts with special training and skills: psychiatrists, clinical psychologists, psychiatric social workers, psychiatric nurses and occupational therapists. Besides these "clinicians," a large number of basic scientists have lately become interested in behavior disorders: anatomists, physiologists, chemists, geneticists, ethologists, pathologists, pharmacologists, epidemiologists, experimental psychologists, sociologists, anthropologists, and economists. Psychoanalysis is a special basic science that was developed almost singlehandedly by the efforts of one genius apart from the other sciences. It should be kept in mind that lawyers, social and welfare workers, some educators and clergymen, and—most of all—practitioners of medicine and public health also are actively concerned with behavior disorders. Much of the actual daily work in mental hospitals still rests on the shoulders of aides or attendants with minimal training (and often without training). In tackling the hugo problems of mental health, professional mental health workers are expected to cooperate with all these persons, as well as with community leaders.

THE PSYCHIATRIST Psychiatry, the oldest member of the mental health professions, was the first to come to professional maturity. It is astonishing how many people do not know that the psychiatrist, in contrast to other mental health workers, is a physician trained to deal with the entire spectrum of behavior disorders including those that are diseases. He is the only mental health worker with both biological and psychosocial training, the details of which are discussed later in this chapter. In 1963 there were 14,000 psychiatrists in the United States, or one psychiatrist per 17,500 persons. In most countries there are fewer psychiatrists per capita; in the developing countries the shortage is abysmal.

Like most medical specialists, psychiatrists are city dwellers, which creates a serious shortage in non-metropolitan areas. Besides what might be called general psychiatry, a number of subspecialties have developed of which perhaps the best defined is child psychiatry. Other, less circumscribed practical subspecialties, are forensic, occupational, military, and school psychiatry.

Psychiatrists are also classified according to the setting in which they work: for instance, hospital and clinic psychiatrists, psychiatrists in private practice, and academic psychiatrists—teachers and investigators concentrated in academic or other institutional settings. Some psychiatrists have special areas of interest and refer to themselves as biological or social psychiatrists. An important special category consists of psychiatrists who function as administrators, public health officials, and hospital and clinic directors; as mental health work has grown, psychiatric administration has become a challenging field.[1]

Yet with this diversity of special functions, a large percentage of psychiatric talent in the United States is directed toward private practice with a socioeconomically well-situated population of patients. The affluent society has bred an affluent psychiatry. The mark of such affluence is reflected not only in the cost of highly skilled therapists but also in the nature of the disorders that are deemed appropriate for treatment. Of course, it is true in general that, as Jack R. Ewalt has remarked, character problems, "wrist scratchers," and the like, even more than the severe core dysfunctions, increasingly claim psychiatric attention.[9] It may be argued that the best disposition of resources is to focus upon that population for whom remedial efforts will be most successful—persons of talent and potential social influence with disorders of minimal or moderate severity for whom an increment in personal growth is undoubtedly consequential. Indeed, the majority of highly skilled psychiatrists, from the inception of their training to the selection of their pattern of practice, are progressively removed from direct concern with the spectrum of hospitalized severe core disorders; their patients must not only be moderately well to do, but ambulatory. The consequences are a tendency not only to slight the major and minor problems of the less privileged but to divert attention from research in both the therapy and etiology of the severely disabling core disorders.

Counterbalancing this emphasis is the fact that, in the past few decades, talented therapists included severe disorders in their practices, although the patient was selected from an economically privileged group. We can anticipate an inevitable expansion of methods developed in such elite therapeutic practice to a larger population of patients. We are also witnessing attempts to remove patients from remote hospitals to settings in which familial, professional, and community resources can be actively engaged in the acute and rehabilitative phases of treatment. The allocation of public funds linked to social reforms and re-education (and, hence conceivably facilitating prevention as well as rehabilitation) and the advent of effective pharmacotherapies and group therapies may yet allow a larger number of well-trained psychiatrists to focus both on the core disorders generally and on the severe problems of the less economically privileged. They may find ways to translate what is valuable from the inherently costly individual psychotherapies to new and different modes of therapeutic intervention and find personal satisfaction and challenge in so doing. While such developments are clearly in the offing, their success will require sustained sagacity and thoughtful inventiveness, which are always in scarcer supply than sheer enthusiasm.

THE PSYCHOANALYST Psychoanalysis is, variously, a method of clinical observation, a theoretical scientific system, a form of psychological treatment, and also a professional movement. Its originator, Sigmund Freud, felt that the contributions of psychoanalysis as a basic science would be more important than its contributions as a therapy.[14] Most psychoanalysts are psychiatrists. Freud was in favor of training non-medical psychoanalysts, but was opposed in this by many of his students, particularly in the United States, where the most influential psychoanalytic organization, The American Psychoanalytic Association, accepts only psychiatrists for regular training and membership. There are 1,500 psychoanalysts in the United States and not more than 2,000 all over the world.

For psychiatry, the theoretic contributions of psychoanalysis have been particularly important. Psychoanalysts have focused their interest on the unconscious processes that determine behavior. Particularly in the United States, psychoanalysis has exercised a decisive influence on concepts of mental health and on explanations of psychological factors in behavior disorders. While the explanatory power and theoretical interest of Freud's work are widely acknowledged, one of the least-noticed contributions of psychoanalysis derives from its empirical method and focus of observation; that is to say, the sustained, daily observations of a single individual in a special setting over the span of several years. Neither psychiatry nor academic psychology has compiled such an exhaustive body of experience and information about the organization of psychological forces and the nature of mental life in the individual. The significance of psychoanalytic therapy is qualified by the limited spectrum of behavior disorders suitable for treatment, as well as by the length and cost of the treatment.

Many young psychiatrists in the United States are drawn to psychoanalytic theory and practice. The appeal derives from the promise of instructing students in a powerful theory of behavior, to be subjected to a complex and challenging therapy, and to become established in a prestigeful, lucrative, and intellectually gratifying practice. Apart from its notable contributions, psychoanalysis has created certain problems in United States psychiatry because it has attracted to its exclusive practice some of the most gifted psychiatrists. It follows that such men are disinclined to work full time in general psychiatric research and teaching and do not make themselves available to psychiatric patients. This, then, tends to increase the manpower shortage.[13] It has also created a tendency among many psychoanalysts to be satisfied with existing theory and practice, rather than to continue the kind of development and elaboration that Freud himself advocated. The pertinence of psychoanalytic training for psychiatrists will be discussed on page 20.

THE CLINICAL PSYCHOLOGIST This mental health worker receives his basic training in general academic psychology. The undisputed contribution of clinical psychologists is in the area of clinical testing. Their interest and aptitude for conducting research in the psychosocial aspects of behavior disorders are based on intensive training in research methodology and special training in personality theory. A considerable number of clinical psychologists, however, are practitioners, carrying on treatment ranging from counseling (a term that usually means the clarifying of various problems of living, particularly in the realms of education, occupation, and marriage) to psychoanalysis, and, more recently, group therapy. Molly Harrower states that one-half to two-thirds of American clinical psychologists are engaged in some private practice.[20]

Psychiatrists have completely accepted the clinical psychologist, both as a mental health worker who applies psychological tests, and as a research investigator. It was hoped that psychological procedures and methodology, applied to clinical problems in clinical settings, would generate basic research. This hope has not been realized as yet, and there is some danger that as clinical psychologists move more actively into therapeutic work, they will tend to lose touch with experimental approaches and investigations.

It is obvious that progress depends on close and effective cooperation between the two mental health professions, but certain issues have led to feuds that rankle on both sides. Organized psychiatry is opposed to the psychologist's independent practice of psychotherapy. Psychiatrists, with some exceptions, feel that psychologists should not practice psychotherapy, or that they should engage in it only under the supervision of psychiatrists. They hold that the clinical psychologist who has a research degree is not sufficiently trained in the hard facts of clinical life to assume a sustained and socially disciplined responsibility for a wide range of patients, and that in most settings such safeguards as licensure and registration (backed not only by practicing psychologists but also by the universities that train them) are lacking. Clinical psychologists, on the other hand, point to the fact that psychotherapy enables them to make contributions to research; psychotherapy is, as John Dollard remarked, a window on human behavior. They feel that psychotherapy is not essentially a medical but an educational technique, and they stress the great need for more psychotherapists, which psychiatry alone cannot fill. They also feel it is not dignified for an independent profession to work under the supervision of psychiatry. There is little doubt that this ongoing struggle is concerned not only with the needs of the patient population but also with questions of power, prestige, and economic interests.

In the United States, it takes a psychologist three to five years after college graduation to obtain a Ph.D. After this, most clinical psychologists spend one year in an internship before entering research, teaching, or practice. Most graduates work in clinical settings. Among the 20,000 or so psychologists in the United States, there are some 4,000 clinical psychologists; the demand is somewhat greater but the shortage is not excessive. Compared to this, there is a very small number of such workers in other countries. Besides clinical psychologists, a number of psychologists of other specialties—experimental, psychological, developmental, and social psychologists—devote their research talents to problems in mental health; we believe that clinicians in both fields will have to collaborate with these workers for newer research approaches.

THE PSYCHIATRIC SOCIAL WORKER This mental health worker is a social worker who has received specialized training enabling him (or rather her, for most social workers are women) to work in social service agencies, hospitals, and clinics. The worker is trained to handle a great variety of psychosocial problems focused generally, but not exclusively, on the family of the psychiatric patient. The profession has developed almost entirely within the United States.[2] Many aspects of their clinical activities—including psychosocial diagnostic studies, psychotherapy, and rehabilitation—are referred to as "casework." In hospitals, psychiatric social workers have become involved in psychotherapeutic work with families, in order to facilitate the rehabilitation of the patient into the family and community. In psychiatric dispensaries, the caseworker may work not only with families but with patients, and often this work is indistinguishable from the psychotherapeutic work of the psychiatrist and psychologist.

In contrast to clinical psychologists, psychiatric social workers are most often clinically rather than research or theory oriented. Typically, they have a practical know-how of people's behavior and a practical familiarity with the available agencies and facilities in the community, which enables them to assist both patients and psychiatrists to make appropriate use of such facilities. Yet until recently they have been more strongly influenced by psychoanalytic thought than by the thinking and research methods of social scientists. Psychiatric social workers increasingly occupy important executive positions; certain metropolitan mental health agencies are staffed and administered mainly by psychiatric social workers, with psychiatrists employed only as consultants. Like other mental health workers, this group often has difficulty in defining a professional identity. Their most clearly defined traditional role has been casework with parents in child psychiatric clinics. More often than not, the actual utilization of the psychiatric social worker depends on the practice prevailing in a particular clinical setting.

In the United States, training comprises two years after college, leading to a master's degree, and one or two additional years in highly supervised field work. In a few centers, postgraduate training leading to a doctorate is available. Social workers were the first to develop a systematic method of individual case supervision, in which the supervisor not only hears about the progress of the client, but also deals with the junior worker's personal problems as they impinge upon the case. In one form or another this supervisory approach has been adapted as a key training device by other mental health workers engaged in interpersonal professional relations. There is a definite shortage of psychiatric social workers, most of whom work in agencies rather than in private practice. Few psychiatrists use social workers for private patients, since many upper-class patients and their families seem to consider the social worker an "almonry lady," an antiquated and totally unacceptable notion. It is the psychiatrist's responsibility to aid in overcoming such prejudice, which, more often than not, he reinforces out of an unwarranted sense of his own importance.

THE PSYCHIATRIC NURSE This mental health worker is a nurse with postgraduate training and experience in the nursing care of psychiatric patients. The psychiatric nurses are women, but a significant number of men work in the field. The roles of the psychiatric nurse are often less than well defined. In the United States, most schools of nursing teach a bit of psychiatry and also stress psychological points of view in the art of nursing, but beyond this the psychiatric nurse needs specialized postgraduate experience, available only in a few training centers. The task of a psychiatric nurse is much different from that of other nurses.[34] The hospitalized psychiatric patient spends very little time with his therapist, at best one hour a day and usually much less; the remainder of the time is spent with psychiatric nurses and aides. In effect, and implicitly, the psychiatric nurse is a psychotherapist, and relationships of this mental health worker with patients profoundly influence their therapeutic progress. Psychiatric nurses are also often administrators of wards, and their work includes housekeeping, policing, recreational functions, and traditional medical nursing. Although there is no doubt about the world-wide need for such personnel, only clear and hardheaded thinking about the functions and training (in psychotherapy, for example) of psychiatric nurses will dispel the present confusion as to what a psychiatric nurse is and should be.

ANCILLARY MENTAL HEALTH PROFESSIONS Another important professional person, the occupational therapist, organizes meaningful therapeutic activities for patients in mental hospitals and rehabilitation centers. This requires training, not only in arts, crafts, vocational skills, and sports, but also in the principles of psychiatric diagnosis and therapy, and particularly in the psychosocial aspects of work and recreation.[12] Occupational therapists have looked to psychiatrists for leadership, but they have seldom found understanding for their problems and functions. They have protested about this and about their lack of prestige and status in the family of mental health workers. The fact is that the general psychology of work and play in healthy adults is ignored by the behavioral sciences, and sound psychosocial principles of the therapeutic use of work and play in hospitals and rehabilitation centers are being developed only very gradually. Occupational therapy is taught in a number of colleges and professional schools; training involves two years of graduate work followed by an internship in mental hospitals or rehabilitation centers.

The organization of leisure activities for psychiatric patients, referred to as recreational therapy, is usually directed by the occupational therapist, aided by specialists such as the art therapist, the music therapist, and the sports coach. A specially trained social worker, the group worker, has demonstrated his usefulness by a meaningful organization of group activities and the problems of patients living together. More recently, attempts at thoroughgoing vocational and educational rehabilitation have evolved. In some countries, such as the United Kingdom and some Socialist republics, these activities play a crucial role in the treatment of psychiatric patients. With broader concepts, both of what the patient requires for therapy and the community's role in treatment, we can anticipate further expansion of such approaches.

The person with whom the hospitalized psychiatric patient has more contact than with anyone else is the psychiatric aide or attendant. Until a few years ago, these were among the lowest-paid of unskilled jobs, requiring no training and attracting many unreliable people of deprived socioeconomic backgrounds. Although some were intuitive and devoted, the majority often were crudely authoritarian, with a propensity for verbal and physical violence with patients. This had a very undesirable impact on the image, not only of public, but many private institutions. Through Harry Stack Sullivan we learned to appreciate the untutored skill of many aides and the therapeutic power inherent in the job. In the last few decades the general quality and training of aides have been improved.

THE PSYCHIATRIC TEAM In North American settings the notion developed that if, under the explicit or tacit leadership of the psychiatrist, each expert applied his special techniques to the patient, an efficient and smoothly working clinic or hospital would result. Experts have become increasingly aware of the enormous complexities of hospital and clinic organization and of the informal and irrational interactions, as well as administrative arrangements, which influence both patients and staff. In addition, with professional identities also in a state of flux, it has become clear that a strict division of labor, simply according to specialties, produces neither a collaboration of specialists nor an adequate basis for actually operating an efficient psychiatric facility. These facts annoy the bureaucrat and constitute a new challenge for creative public health and psychiatric administrators.

Psychiatric Institutions

In the last few decades therapeutic facilities for ambulatory treatment within the community and psychiatric units in general hospitals have become important, but the bulk of severe behavior disorders are still treated in isolated psychiatric hospitals. In most countries there is a need not only for more psychiatric hospital beds, but also other facilities adapted to the wide range of psychiatric problems; in developing countries such needs are tremendous. Psychiatric hospitals differ from general hospitals in two important respects. First, the majority of psychiatric patients are not physically ill. The psychiatric hospital has been described as a hospital without beds;[40] it requires only to a limited degree the elaborate equipment of the modern general hospital, but it needs other facilities, such as access to therapeutically meaningful occupational and social activities. The second difference lies in the fact that many patients in psychiatric hospitals are—either legally or informally—detained and so deprived of certain of their privileges as citizens. In the traditional psychiatric hospital patients are, generally speaking, considered irresponsible, treated as naughty children, and have to surrender to what Erving Goffman calls a total institution, which differs little from a prison.[16] In such hospitals—whether public or private—there is deep cleavage between patients and hospital personnel.

Responsible mental health workers, civic leaders, and journalists have periodically criticized institutions of this kind.[17] Changes have taken place as the result of humanitarian efforts, the introduction (since the 1930's) of increasingly effective medical therapies and psychotherapies, and, more recently, new concepts about the role of a suitable psychosocial milieu for therapy. Such a milieu requires a balance of meaningful, candid, and intensive interaction between all staff members and patients in the institution, which thus becomes a "therapeutic community."[24] These developments have made patients out of inmates, and the therapeutic community endeavors to make citizens of such patients while converting physicians into collaborative leaders rather than benign despots. Patients are helped to assume responsibility and are prepared to return from a transitional institution to a family setting in their own community.[46] To carry out this role effectively, psychiatric hospitals cannot be isolated but must remain in close contact with the community so that the continuum of care-taking activities may be integrated.

THE PUBLIC MENTAL HOSPITAL The traditional public mental hospital typically is an institution with thousands of patients, located in a rural setting. In the past, these hospitals were run in connection with farms, which provided the food and also certain occupational opportunities for the "inmates"; until a few decades ago, farming occupied hospital administrators as much as the care of patients. The staff includes all types of mental health workers and the needed array of clerical and maintenance workers. Practically all public mental hospitals are woefully understaffed, and if talent is available it must be concentrated on acute rather than chronic treatment units. The functions of the superintendent of the institution are largely administrative, a role not unlike being mayor of a small town. Superintendents are usually responsible to higher administrative functionaries who are in charge of governmental health agencies. The clinical, training, and research responsibilities lie in the hands of directors of professional services. Today it is commonly felt that our public mental hospitals are too large and too impersonal;[41] the bed-capacity of a mental hospital should probably not exceed five hundred. One way to reduce the size of a "metropolis" of insanity—there are institutions in New York State with populations of 13,000 patients—is to break up these oversized establishments into small functional components and also to create satellite hospitals in the community.[4] The caliber of public mental hospitals varies greatly; they range from therapeutically effective and modern institutions to rather miserable asylums. The neglect by urbanized psychiatry and by the public of these hospitals only emphasizes the contribution of those mental health workers who, against odds, continue to work effectively in our public institutions.

PRIVATE MENTAL HOSPITALS Private mental hospitals are found only in those countries where private practice of psychiatry is permitted, although a number are non-profit institutions. In some, care is optimal: staffs are skilled; research and training are advanced; and there is a favorable ratio of therapists to patients. Such hospitals have had a major and beneficial influence on the development of psychiatry as a specialty. Other private institutions offer little more than the worst of public mental hospitals, and the patients overpay to avoid the assumed stigma or "disgrace" of treatment in public institutions. Only a very small segment of the population can afford the prohibitive costs of prolonged private hospitalization—usually from $12,000 to $25,000 yearly. In general, psychiatric care all over the world is increasingly a public rather than a private responsibility.

Geographical, social, and professional isolation of major mental hospitals from communities and medical centers has been traditional. The only exceptions were the psychiatric admission units in metropolitan hospitals and teaching hospitals, usually connected with a university training center. With the increasing emphasis on early diagnosis and treatment in the community, there has been a trend toward establishing treatment units in general hospitals where therapy can be vigorous and attentive as well as medically competent. This not altogether new development has helped to make psychiatry more acceptable to the medical profession and to the public at large. The needs of a psychiatric patient are different from the average patient in a general hospital, and it has required imagination to develop appropriate liaison with the medical staff and the vocational, cultural, and recreational assets of the community. The increasing contact of both the psychiatrist and his patient with the community has led to the development of the day-and-night hospitals, where patients stay according to their needs; the rehabilitation center; and the so-called halfway house where patients, improved after treatment, are taken care of for a brief period before returning to family and job.

Other new approaches of modern community psychiatry are taken up in Chapter 26.

DISPENSARIES AND OFFICE PRACTICE The modern practice is to use psychiatric hospitals selectively. Whenever possible, psychiatry treats patients today in dispensaries, private offices, and increasingly in collaboration with agencies of the community. In most countries, in terms of the spectrum of patients requiring treatment, private practice is not very significant, but in some countries private practitioners enjoy prestige and wealth. Everywhere the social elite is usually treated by a more or less "private arrangement," and nowhere in the world, in or out of hospitals, are the socioeconomically underprivileged psychiatric patients well taken care of.

Dispensaries are ordinarily but not always connected with a hospital. They may serve a total population or a limited one, as in industries, the armed forces, and schools or universities. Some are all-purpose agencies; others specialize, treating only elderly patients or children, or certain diagnostic groups such as alcoholics. In the United States, psychiatric clinics usually offer their services at low cost or without direct cost to indigent patients. In general, dispensaries are now becoming less restricted by social barriers and are of increasing importance as community treatment centers. There is an increasing trend to treat and detect psychological crises promptly.

Psychiatric Organizations

Psychiatric services, training, and research require adequate administrative organization and, in some instances, a vast bureaucratic machinery. Public mental hospitals and clinics in states and large municipalities are usually organized under departments of mental health. These are either separate agencies or part of a department of health; in the latter case, they are often larger and have a bigger budget than the parent organization. In the United States, the National Institute of Mental Health has developed, since World War II, into a mammoth organization. It not only runs its own treatment and research institutions, but also exercises great influence on all public and private services, as well as on the conduct of research and training of mental health workers. Each year the National Institute of Mental Health distributes funds in ever increasing amounts; in 1964, approximately $69 million were being spent for research and $65 million for training. No other public agency has had a greater share in the progress of the field, although the United States Veterans Administration has also been influential in the development of American psychiatry.

In each mental health field, professional workers have formed national and local societies.[3] The bulk of psychiatrists in the United States belong to the American Psychiatric Association, the official professional organization of psychiatrists.[41] The American Orthopsychiatric Association, which unites psychiatrists, clinical psychologists, psychiatric social workers, and some other healthworkers, is particularly concerned with the problems of development and disorders of families and their children. In addition, there are smaller associations with more specific interests, such as the American Psychosomatic Society, the American Association on Mental Deficiency, the Association for Research in Nervous and Mental Disease. An influential organization of vigorous psychiatrists, the Group for the Advancement of Psychiatry, was formed shortly after World War II, first as a reform and later as a study group. Psychoanalysts also have formed a number of societies. There is a world-wide International Psychoanalytic Association. In the United States the largest and most powerful is the American Psychoanalytic Association, consisting almost entirely of medically trained analysts. Other analytic societies, some of them including non-medical analysts, have formed around Karen Horney, Erich Fromm, Theodore Reik, and Harry Stack Sullivan. In England and in South American countries, Melanie Klein has exerted a strong influence. One of the unique American contributions to mental health is the role of citizens' groups, which since late in the nineteenth century have been intermittently active in public-hospital reform and legislation. The National Association of Mental Health has had a sustained and powerful influence in educating the public, lawmakers, administrators, and professional persons to improve and expand services, training, and research. Until now, psychiatry has been a rather parochial discipline; even professional literature, considered highly important in one country, is unknown in another, although this has improved somewhat through translations and reviews and through the creation of international journals. The international counterpart of the National Association of Mental Health is the World Federation of Mental Health, also a non-governmental, voluntary organization; its official counterpart is the Psychiatric Section of the World Health Organization. Both organizations have contributed to a better understanding, appreciation, and solution of world-wide mental health problems.

Training of Psychiatrists

A competent general psychiatrist must master psychosocial and somatic methods of diagnosis and treatment. Who makes a good psychiatrist? So far, research has provided tentative conclusions rather than definite answers to this question.[23] Certainly some of the prerequisites for medical training, such as a degree of intelligence qualifying a student for graduate training, a scientific outlook, a sense of responsibility, compassion and wisdom, are as essential for psychiatry as for medicine in general. It seems that good psychiatrists also tend to have broad cultural interests; they are "psychologically-minded" with an unusual degree of interest in people. It is less important that they themselves be free from neuroses than that they learn to overcome their neurotic traits. Unsolved personal problems, if severe or pervasive, strongly impair the capacity of psychiatrists to help others. It has been said that psychiatry attracts many emotionally disturbed students. Whether this is true, we do not really know; certainly the recognition of emotional difficulties in oneself or in one's family may be a powerful stimulus to study psychiatry. In any case, some of those who have conquered difficulties have become excellent psychiatrists.

Good psychiatrists have overcome some of the cold, authoritarian, and cynical attitudes which are too often inculcated in medical students. They must acquire to an unusual degree the ability to observe themselves and to use their own reactions as a sensitive instrument for diagnosing relevant information in transactions with patients. Nathaniel Hawthorne, portraying a compassionate physician in *The Scarlet Letter*, beautifully describes certain qualities of the psychotherapist:

> If the [physician] possess native sagacity, and a nameless something more—let us call it intuition; if he show no intrusive egotism, nor disagreeably prominent characteristics of his own; if he have the power, which must be born with him, to bring his mind into such affinity with his patient's, that this last shall unawares have spoken what he imagines himself only to have thought; if such revelations be received without tumult, and acknowledged not so often by an uttered sympathy as by silence, an inarticulate breath, and here and there a word, to indicate that all is understood; if to these qualifications of a confidant be joined the advantages afforded by his recognized character as a physician;—then, at some inevitable moment, will the soul of the sufferer be dissolved, and flow forth in a dark, but transparent stream, bringing all its mysteries into the daylight.

The American Psychiatric Association published reports on general psychiatric training of residents, which contain thoughtful reviews of goals, methods, and problems of training.[45] Psychiatric training, as all clinical training, is largely on-the-job training. We believe a good preparation for psychiatry may be had in medical, but especially in pediatric, internships with an emphasis on growth and development. Resident training in a psychiatric hospital emphasizes training in descriptive and diagnostic skills, individual psychotherapy and community psychiatry, with experience in dispensaries and on the wards of general hospitals. The ideal training provides experience in organic and psychosocial techniques with psychotic, neurotic, and psychosomatic patients, adults and children, and their families; and, if possible, also with mentally deficient patients and legal offenders. Furthermore, good training includes the opportunity to acquire knowledge of psychiatry's basic sciences through formal courses, seminars, and laboratory work, but relatively few centers offer formal courses in child development, the biological sciences, psychology, sociology and anthropology, or in fundamentals of psychoanalysis and scientific methodology. The average training center cannot prepare trainees for research, but it should be possible in all good programs to foster a scientific outlook and a spirit of inquiry. Research, it has been said, is the teacher of the mature scholar; and the habits in clinical training of inquiry, exploration, and formulation, disciplined by skills and knowledge, cannot begin too soon.

There are many unsolved problems concerning training and psychotherapy with much room for experimentation.[7] Instruction in psychotherapy is particularly difficult; it must be learned by long and intensive work with patients under careful clinical supervision. Such supervision consists of detailed discussions in hour-by-hour reports of psychopathological material, therapeutic techniques, and those emotional problems within the student that are evoked by the patient. Verbatim detailed reports or recorded interviews of experienced therapists as well as sound recordings of students have been invaluable aids in training.[38] For contemporary students, the importance of psychotherapy is not simply therapeutic; it comprises a continuing method of observation and interaction through which much of contemporary contributions to psychiatric knowledge has been built. In other eras, the psychiatrist generally learned about his patients solely through a formal examination (the "mental status"); however, any psychiatrist who has successfully or unsuccessfully attempted to carry out psychotherapy with a psychotic person has an appreciation of psychotic behavior far beyond what can be gained from formal examinations and textbook descriptions.

Length and content of psychiatric training vary with different countries and according to principles that are considered basic. In general, following medical education and a year's internship, specialty training requires three years, which, however, is not enough for a complex field that has grown and expanded rapidly. In some countries training is regulated by specialty boards. In the United States, the Board of Psychiatry and Neurology sets standards for training by holding examinations for those who want to be considered specialists. There is a critical shortage of psychiatric training centers; this, of course, creates a serious bottleneck in producing the number of psychiatrists required for service, research, and teaching. In terms of quality, current training resources are probably overextended.

At one time neurology and psychiatry were joined as one specialty, but today they are considered two different specialties, a view that has some advantages as well as disadvantages. Clearly, many neurological diseases hold no interest for the psychiatrist, and neurological training does not contribute a great deal to the understanding and therapy of the neuroses. Nevertheless, experience with the management of certain cerebral diseases and the knowledge of anatomy, physiology, pathology of cerebral processes, pharmacology, biochemistry, and genetics—what we call the neurobehavioral sciences—is important for the psychiatrist; as psychiatry moves more into a psychosocial orbit, these subjects are apt to be neglected. In any case, emphasis on clinical neurology has decreased, while there is concomitantly a greater interest in the physiology and chemistry of the nervous system.

Psychoanalytic training and its problems are beyond the scope of this book. It has been aptly described in a recent survey of the training institutes of the American Psychoanalytic Association.[28] The student of psychiatry, however, in considering whether he should enter psychoanalytic training, should know the following in bare outline: analytic training, as given in most American institutes, consists of a didactic analysis of the student by an analyst appointed to conduct training analyses. In addition, there is supervision or "control" of several therapeutic psychoanalyses carried out by the student, four or five years of didactic courses and, in some instances, a thesis. The Institutes of the American Psychoanalytic Association admit regular students only after one year—and sometimes more—of psychiatric training. The didactic analysis usually lasts hundreds of hours over a period of several years. In general, full analytic training takes, at the very least, six years and in the United States costs from $15,000 to $25,000. Obviously, such expenses, which are not underwritten by public funds, are a heavy burden for most young psychiatrists and create serious problems for the leaders and planners of mental health services and training.

Anyone who wishes to become an analyst needs full psychoanalytic training; this assumes a commitment not only to studying behavior as it evolves through the confines of the psychoanalytic method, but also to formulating behavior—as far as is possible—in terms of psychoanalytic theory. Whether a general psychiatrist, one who is impressed with the value of psychoanalytic theory and practice, requires such training is a question that is by no means settled. We believe that a part of the training for those who want to do research in psychotherapy and psychopathology should include an extensive, perhaps modified, course of formal psychoanalytic training. For the general psychiatrist, in addition to residency training, a personal analysis of moderate length is recommended. This will provide him with rich psychopathological material (even if he happens to be a so-called normal person), will give him more direct insight into the patient role than can be obtained in any other way, and will alert him to the personal sources of problems that might interfere with therapeutic work. What is missing in current psychiatric training programs is advanced clinical training, beginning late in residency and extending for several years beyond it. Seminars that scrutinize the experience of psychotherapists in private and community settings can discuss both psychodynamic and behavior theory relevant to the developing activities of the psychiatrist; this would be more pertinent and satisfying for a large number of psychiatrists than formal psychoanalytic training.

Full and formal analytic training has its problems. It is lengthy, costly, and, as such, available to few. As conducted in most institutes, it is apt to indoctrinate students heavily. Edward Glover, for example, pointed to the fact that most professional analysands take over the theoretical and technical idiosyncracies of their analysts.[15] It also seems that many young psychiatrists and psychoanalysts are apt to expect too much both from psychoanalysis and psychoanalytic training; often they will not admit disappointment to themselves or others if their expectations are not fulfilled. The best way to manage problems of this kind is to find a training institute that is self-critical and an analyst who is thoroughly knowledgeable, but not doctrinaire, and who will help the student to analyze such unrealistic attitudes.

Psychiatric Research and the Basic Sciences

Until recent decades much psychiatric research, dominated by schools and cults, was carried on in a rather amateurish and sporadic fashion. Research, of course, is not equivalent to creativity, but as knowledge becomes increasingly specialized and complex, special discipline, special skills, and inventiveness are required. Increasingly, the need for sustained research and research training in advanced centers has been recognized, and the competence of contemporary psychiatry is sufficient to support this development. Students in some countries today can find careers that, based on sound clinical information, are directed toward research rather than practice. In this chapter we cannot review the accomplishments of psychiatric research, nor the achievements of the basic sciences upon which the applied science of psychiatry rests. What has become clear is that behavioral and biological scientists alone cannot do the jobs of research that are required, in part because they are well occupied with problems other than that of severe behavior disorders and in part because they do not know, as do psychiatrists, what the critical problems are in a clinical field. A clinical investigator, of course, must be more than perceptive; he must be sufficiently knowledgeable about the status of both clinical information and psychobiological fact and theory to recognize a finding as significant. Common sense in psychiatry is plainly not enough; it may lead to faulty conclusions as in astronomy when common sense held the earth was flat.

The student of psychiatry has a reasonable degree of familiarity with the biological basic sciences, but the practical relevance of these disciplines has not been very successfully translated, organized, and applied in clinical work. The fact is that an emphasis on behavioral physiology or behavioral chemistry and pharmacology has only recently emerged as a development within the basic sciences, and psychiatrists and psychologists have contributed to this clinically relevant development. Although psychosocial principles are applied in clinical work, the psychiatric student's direct knowledge of the behavioral sciences is usually scant. All psychiatrists have something to learn from their academic colleagues in general methodology, statistics, and experimental design. Special aspects of basic psychology and biology that are of particular interest to the psychiatrist are developmental psychobiology, learning and conditioning theories, personality theory, cognition and perception theory, communications theory, physiological psychology of the nervous system and sensory organs, psychopharmacology, ethology, and psychological testing and measurement.

The general role of the environment in influencing behavior has long been evident to biologists and medical scientists, but "higher order interactions" of organism and environment that are structured specifically around persons, symbols, and values, have been more difficult to convey and have been appreciated in a detailed and scientific way only recently. Social psychologists, sociologists, anthropologists, and, to a lesser degree, economists and political scientists, have taught physicians something about the role of social and cultural factors in behavior and about methods and models for their study. The special impact both of psychoanalysis and of the behavioral sciences on medically trained persons has been the demonstration that an understanding of the lawful organization of bodily functions is insufficient to account adequately for an instance or pattern of behavior. Among the multiple meaningful determinants of behavior, social and psychological factors are inherently related but not simply reducible to the language of bodily functions. The ability to think a thought rather than act it; to prefer an action rather than to be compelled into one; to be moved to thought, feeling, or action by the power of words or memory and in the absence of immediate bodily rewards —these are the activities and capacities of man. The social, psychological, and biological contingencies that influence these human capacities represent special problems for which special orders and integrations of knowledge are required.

In this book, the view is taken that the applied science of psychiatry rests on the tripod of the basic biological sciences, the behavioral sciences, and psychoanalysis. Why, it may be asked, is psychoanalysis mentioned separately? The answer is that psychoanalysis developed apart, both from academic psychology and psychiatry, and so far has not been satisfactorily integrated either in theory or in practice with the other basic sciences. In many respects, psychiatry occupies a "bridge" position both in the medical school curriculum and with respect to the biological and behavioral sciences. The laboratory of disordered human behavior presents a special vantage point from which information is conveyed to other disciplines, and it is clear that accessibility to developments in basic areas will more and more require special effort and skills on the part of the psychiatrist.

Schools of Psychiatry

Beyond any special school of psychiatry, there is a field concerned with the nature of disordered behavior, how it emerges, and what can be done about it. Especially in practical approaches to the core disorders, areas of agreement are broad. Nevertheless, sectarianism persists. Psychiatry in different countries is dominated by characteristic supertheories that determine the overall orientation and interests of psychiatrists and color aspects of practice. In Germany, Holland, and Switzerland, for example, there is currently a strong interest in the schools of existentialist psychiatry. In most of the Communist countries, Pavlovian theory is pre-eminent and officially indorsed, although the strength of its practical impact cannot be assessed easily. Depending upon the affinity of a supertheory to a certain culture, the supertheory will be accepted or rejected, particularly if such a theoretical system is based on certain bold assumptions rather than hard facts.[36] In the United States, the strong interest in dynamic psychotherapy is explained, at least in part, by the typically optimistic American belief that man can be and should be helped to actualize himself and overcome weaknesses, by a characteristic sense of social justice which holds that wrongs committed during infancy and childhood for which the individual is not responsible should be undone, and finally, by the assumption that the rational should replace the irrational. One also finds various polarizations of opinion, informal "schools" where adherents flock around a leader whose observations and assumptions are highly revered. Failure to accept the total system leads to ostracism.

Robert J. Lifton has compared the indoctrination in such schools with various manifestations of political and religious totalism,[29] but to imply that these schools are indistinguishable from dogmatic religious sects and totalitarian parties would be erroneous. The subject matter, after all, is not an ethical or cosmological system, but a body of practices and theoretical propositions that can be proven or refuted or, at the least, pragmatically assessed over a period of time. This, in fact, is precisely what has happened, and such schools often rapidly disintegrate after the death of the creator and leader. What is of value usually survives in the general body of knowledge. For instance, the psychobiological school of Adolf Meyer today really no longer exists, but it has influenced and enriched American psychiatry. In any of the developed sciences where methods are different and the reliability of facts in dispute, one finds that polemic precedes consensus, and free empirical inquiry tends to be replaced by a technical authoritarianism. In a scientific atmosphere, such abuses tend not to survive, and this is true even for the young field of psychiatry.

John MacIver and Fredrick C. Redlich[31] pointed to a split in psychiatry in the United States into two large camps, which somewhat transcends any particular schools. One is an analytic-psychological group, referring to themselves at times as dynamic psychiatrists, who are usually practicing psychoanalysts or engaged in analytic psychotherapy. They see their patients for a fifty-minute hour several times a week. They express little interest in organic problems, rarely carry out physical examinations, and prefer not to make home calls or take care of emergencies. They tend to be related to a select coterie of admirers and to be somewhat alienated, or at least isolated, from the larger community, and certainly from accustomed modes of medical intervention. In contrast, the second group, the directive-organic practitioners, carry out directive and supportive psychotherapy, use a variety of organic therapeutic procedures and, perhaps, may respond more to the expectations of the patient and family for authoritative and mechanically efficacious treatment. They have the benign authoritarian orientation that is characteristic of the medical profession.

The student of psychiatry, it should be clear, is under no obligation to polarize his own practice along these lines. With the emergence of a more scientific psychiatry, this division should become less pronounced and be based more on areas of special interest and competence rather than ideological differences. In fact, the growing trend toward community psychiatric facilities and the efficacy of pharmacotherapies appears to be engaging both groups, and leading to interchanges and shifts of values.

Psychiatry and Medicine

Psychiatry is the child of medicine, and whereas some psychiatrists have little doubt about their filial allegiance, the problem of professional identity is in fact complex. Treatment of behavior disorders requires a more thorough knowledge of behavioral sciences than does any other medical specialty. The more interested the psychiatrist becomes in psychosocial and psychotherapeutic problems, the more he must master scientific areas that are not taught in the traditional medical curriculum. This is apt to produce in him a sense of estrangement from the medical profession. The fact that the primary data of psychiatry are derived from experiences with patient care and from treatment and observational procedures is, in turn, largely ignored by many biological as well as behavioral scientists who lack this practical experience. Practitioners of medicine too often treat psychiatrists as outsiders, on the fringe of the profession, yet most psychiatrists are happy to belong to the powerful medical brotherhood and enjoy the prestige and some of the ancient privileges that society accords the physician. Thoughtful psychiatrists, however, cannot deny the differences between themselves and the average physician. It is the peculiar position of psychiatry as a bridge institution—and the stress it places on psychosocial principles in the causation and treatment of disease—that has enabled psychiatrists to bring the behavioral sciences and psychoanalysis into the medical orbit. In general, this has had an integrating effect on the highly specialized healing arts and sciences.

Some psychiatric leaders have pondered the question not only of where psychiatry belongs at present, but what place psychiatry will enjoy in the future. Robert Felix has strongly reminded psychiatrists that they are physicians, and that their unique contribution to the mental health field lies in the fact that they are the only mental health specialists who have competence in medical and psychosocial techniques in diagnosing and treating behavior disorders.[11] Lawrence S. Kubie envisages a new practitioner of psychotherapy, who will have more training in psychoanalysis and the behavioral sciences, but less training in those basic medical and clinical disciplines that are tangential to the practice of psychotherapy.[25] Whatever develops, we are convinced that there will be a definite and continuing need for general psychiatrists, that such practitioners must be trained in both the medical and behavioral sciences, and should remain in the medical profession.

Psychiatry and the Public

Ernest Havemann called our time the "age of psychology." [21] In some countries, notably in the United States, throughout the vast spectrum of communications media, the interest in psychological and psychopathological problems is pandemic; experts and columnists tell the public how to have happy marriages, bring up children, learn efficiently, be successful, and make friends; psychiatric books are best sellers, particularly the how-to-be-normal-and-happy type of book and the sensational revelations of the gory unconscious. At a different level, the *Basic Writings of Sigmund Freud* in the Modern Library edition sold over 250,000 copies, and Benjamin Spock's book on child-rearing was a second all-time best seller after the Bible.

Gerald Gurin has shown that most people in this country are in fact quite ignorant about the nature, causes, and treatment of behavior disorders.[19] Seemingly they either feel unnecessarily pessimistic or else expect that psychiatrists can solve almost any problem—from personal difficulties to international crises. To some, the psychiatrist appears as an enemy of established values and is feared and hated. For others, he becomes the hope of humanism.[37] The field of psychiatry touches inevitably upon the unreasoning sources of human hope and despair; psychiatrists will always have to cope both with destructive pessimism and a belief in their "omniscience," all too often fostered by silent assent or readiness to advise on problems quite outside of psychiatric competence. Yet public interest in new expert knowledge has resulted in support that justifies an optimism that, for the first time in man's history, the problems of behavior disorders, of severe and excessive suffering, can be tackled by rational means.

NOTES

1. Walter E. Barton, *Administration in Psychiatry* (Springfield, Ill.: Charles C Thomas, 1962).
2. Virginia Bellsmith, "Social Work," in Silvano Arieti, ed., *The American Handbook of Psychiatry*, Vol. II, pp. 1857–1876 (New York: Basic Books, 1959).
3. Daniel Blain, "The Organization of Psychiatry in the United States," in Silvano Arieti, ed., *op. cit.*, Vol. II, pp. 1960–1982.
4. Wilfred Bloomberg, "A Proposal for a Community-Based Hospital as a Branch of a State Hospital," *American Journal of Psychiatry*, 116 (1960), 814.
5. G. Morris Carstairs, *The Twice Born* (Bloomingdale, Ind.: Indiana University Press, 1963).
6. Joseph W. Eaton and Robert J. Weil, *Culture and Mental Disorders* (Glencoe, Ill.: The Free Press, 1955).

7. Rudolf Ekstein and Robert S. Wallerstein, *The Teaching and Learning of Psychotherapy* (New York: Basic Books, 1958).
8. Erik Essen-Möller, "Untersuchungen über die Fruchtbarkeit gewisser Gruppen von Geisteskranken," *Acta Psychiatrica Scandinavica,* Suppl. VIII (1935).
9. Jack R. Ewalt, "Presidential Address," *American Journal of Psychiatry,* 121 (1964), 1.
10. Rashi Fein, *Economics of Mental Illness* (New York: Basic Books, 1958).
11. Robert R. Felix, "Psychiatrist, Medicinae Doctor," *American Journal of Psychiatry,* 118 (1961), 1.
12. Gail S. Fidler and Jay W. Fidler, *Introduction to Psychiatric Occupational Therapy* (New York: Macmillan, 1958).
13. Jerome D. Frank, *Persuasion and Healing* (Baltimore: The Johns Hopkins Press, 1961).
14. Sigmund Freud, "Psychoanalysis," *Encyclopaedia Brittanica* (Chicago: Encyclopaedia Brittanica, 1954).
15. Edward Glover, *The Technique of Psycho-Analysis* (New York: International Universities Press, 1958).
16. Erving Goffman, "Characteristics of Total Institutions," in *Symposium on Prevention and Social Psychiatry* (Washington, D.C.: U. S. Government Printing Office, 1958).
17. Mike Gorman, *Every Other Bed* (Cleveland: World Publishing Co., 1956).
18. Alan Gregg, "The Limitations of Psychiatry," *American Journal of Psychiatry,* 114 (1948), 513.
19. Gerald Gurin, *Americans View Their Mental Health* (New York: Basic Books, 1960).
20. Molly Harrower, *The Practice of Clinical Psychology* (Springfield, Ill.: Charles C Thomas, 1961).
21. Ernest Havemann, *The Age of Psychology* (New York: Simon & Schuster, 1957).
22. August B. Hollingshead and Fredrick C. Redlich, *Social Class and Mental Illness: A Community Study* (New York: John Wiley and Sons, 1958).
23. Robert R. Holt and Lester Luborsky, *Personality Patterns of Psychiatrists* (New York: Basic Books, 1958).
24. Maxwell Jones, *The Therapeutic Community* (New York: Basic Books, 1953).
25. Lawrence S. Kubie, "The Pros and Cons of a New Profession: A Doctorate in Medical Psychology," *Texas Reports on Biology and Medicine,* 12 (1954), No. 3, 692.
26. Alexander H. Leighton, *My Name Is Legion,* "Foundations for a Theory of Man in Relation to Culture" (New York: Basic Books, 1959).
27. Alexander H. Leighton, T. A. Lambo, C. C. Hughes, Dorothy C. Leighton, J. M. Murphy, and D. B. Macklin, *Psychiatric Disorders among the Yoruba* (Ithaca, N.Y.: Cornell University Press, 1963).

28. Bertram D. Lewin and Helen Ross, *Psychoanalytic Education in the United States* (New York: Norton, 1960).
29. Robert J. Lifton, *Thought Reform and the Psychology of Totalism* (New York: Norton, 1961).
30. Tsung Yi, Lin, "A Study of the Incidence of Mental Disorder in Chinese and Other Cultures," *Psychiatry*, 16 (1953), 313.
31. John MacIver and Fredrick C. Redlich, "Patterns of Psychiatric Practice," *American Journal of Psychiatry*, 115 (1959), 692.
32. Ørnulv Ødegård, "The Incidence of Mental Disease in Norway during World War II," *Acta Psychiatrica Scandinavica*, 29 (1954), 333.
33. Talcott Parsons, *The Social System* (Glencoe, Ill.: The Free Press, 1951).
34. Hildegard E. Peplau, "Principles of Psychiatric Nursing," in Silvano Arieti, ed., *op. cit.*, Vol. II, pp. 1840–1856.
35. Richard J. Plunkett and John E. Gordon, *Epidemiology and Mental Illness* (New York: Basic Books, 1960).
36. Fredrick C. Redlich, "Social Aspects of Psychotherapy," *American Journal of Psychiatry*, 114 (1958), 800.
37. Fredrick C. Redlich and June Bingham, *The Inside Story: Psychiatry and Everyday Life* (New York: Alfred A. Knopf, 1953).
38. Fredrick C. Redlich, John Dollard, and Richard Newman, "High Fidelity Recordings of Psychiatric Interviews," *American Journal of Psychiatry*, 107 (1950), 42.
39. Margaret J. Rioch, J. Elkes, A. Flint, B. Usdansky, R. Newman, and E. Silber, "N.I.M.H. Pilot Study in Training Mental Health Counsellors," *American Journal of Orthopsychiatry*, 23 (1963), 678.
40. Paul Sivadon, *Symposium on Preventive and Social Psychiatry* (Washington, D.C.: U. S. Government Printing Office, 1958).
41. Harry Solomon, "The American Psychiatric Association in Relation to American Psychiatry," *American Journal of Psychiatry*, 115 (1958), 1.
42. Leo Srole, T. S. Langer, S. T. Mitchell, Marvin K. Opler, and Thomas A. C. Rennie, *Mental Health in the Metropolis: The Midtown Manhattan Study* (New York: McGraw-Hill, 1962).
43. Erik Strömgren, "Beiträge zur psychiatrischen Erblehre auf Grund von Untersuchungen an einer Inselbevölkerung," *Acta Psychiatrica Scandinavica*, Suppl. XIX (Copenhagen, 1938).
44. Harry Stack Sullivan, *The Psychiatric Interview* (New York: Norton, 1954).
45. *Training the Psychiatrist to Meet Changing Needs* (Washington, D.C.: The American Psychiatric Association, 1963).
46. James S. Tyhurst, "The Role of Transition States—Including Disaster—in Mental Illness," in *Symposium on Preventive and Social Psychiatry* (Washington, D.C.: U. S. Government Printing Office, 1958).

CHAPTER TWO

The Evolution of Psychiatric Theory and Practice: I *The Beginnings*

◆ To grasp the problems with which current psychiatric theories and practice are concerned, it is useful to trace their development. It is never surprising but always sobering to discover that much of what we cherish as contemporary achievement existed before, and much of what we deride as obsolete and shameful still plagues us. The history of psychiatry, as Sir Aubrey Lewis remarked, is "checkered with reforms and separated by periods of recession." [10] Broadly, the development of psychiatry can be seen as taking place in three overlapping phases, the first of which is less a history of psychiatry than a history of madness from ancient times until the end of the eighteenth century. A coherent history of a recognizable psychiatry—the second phase—starts about 150 years ago with the consolidated beginnings of humanitarian practices and hospital reform. These beginnings developed from enlightened eighteenth-century philosophers and educators, movements on behalf of the "rights of man," as well as from the practice of a few influential physicians who felt that psychiatric patients properly belonged within the province of medicine. The third phase, that of scientific psychiatry, reaches back seventy-five years to a relatively small group of neurologists, psychiatrists, physiologists, and psychologists concerned with mental disorders. Working and teaching roughly between 1890 and 1945, Sigmund Freud, John Hughings Jackson, Emil Kraepelin, Pierre Janet, Eugen Bleuler, Ivan P. Pavlov, Julius Wagner von Jauregg, Adolf Meyer, Harry Stack Sullivan, and many others are quite literally the academic fathers and grandfathers of today's psychiatrists.

The Archaic Period

Antiquity

In prehistoric and ancient times, healing was in the hands of priests and sorcerers. Utilizing herbs, trance, and suggestion, such healers apparently exhorted the best in the patient—his soul—and exorcised the intruding demons. Through their authority, healers offered the patient an opportunity to relinquish the fear and overcompensatory behavior that can complicate disease processes. The likelihood, however, is that many of those afflicted were killed, a practice revived by National Socialism under the uplifting term of *Gnadentod,* or death of mercy. Madness was well recognized but hardly understood, either in antiquity or in the Middle Ages, and demonological concepts and practices have persisted in contemporary folk medicine and short-lived fads. Antiquity did not know hospitals in our sense; possibly the Saturnian temples in Alexandria might be considered the earliest medical as well as psychiatric treatment centers.

Reports of humane treatment date from the early recorded history of the Chinese, Indians, and Egyptians, but the father of medicine in Western culture was Hippocrates (460–377 B.C.). He was a keen clinician, describing epilepsy, postpartum psychosis, and toxic infectious disorders. He ascribed the pathophysiology of hysteria to the wandering of the uterus (Hystera), and his therapeutic recommendation of marriage is not very far from a "prescription" of a nineteenth-century gynecologist, cited by Freud, "*Penis normalis dosim, repetatur.*" [6] Hippocrates connected pathology of the brain rather than actions of gods and demons with persons who were mad, delirious, or possessed of apprehensions. He advanced a neurohumoral basis for temperament and madness from the purported effect of various forms of bile, a theory surviving in the term melancholia (derived from the Greek word for black bile). Perhaps of more contemporary relevance to our age of specialization is Socrates' advice to military surgeons, that the moral and spiritual well being of the patient—his soul—was as important as the treatment of a particular organ.

Ascelepiades (*ca.* 100 B.C.) distinguished between delirium and mental disorders, which he thought were caused by emotional disturbances, and for which he recommended music and well-lighted rooms. Aretaeus (*ca.* A.D. 150) described disorders of senescence and classified mental disorders from a prognostic standpoint as did Kraepelin almost two thousand years later. Soranus (A.D. 77–120) differentiated febrile delirium (an acute psychosis that occurs with fever and restlessness) from mania and melancholia, terms that embrace the schizophrenias of current terminology. According to Erwin H. Ackerknecht (whose little book on the history of psychiatry we highly recommend [1]) Soranus rejected the following popular methods of treatment: darkness, fasting, opium, alcohol, whipping, phlebotomy, music, and sexual love. Galen, the great medical eclectic (A.D. 130–200), considered the central nervous system the center of sensation, mobility, and psychic functions, and he thought of mental disorders as brain disorders; he held a multifactorial view of the cause of symptoms. Some of Galen's descriptive, and much of his speculative, writing survived as dogma for the Middle Ages; his experiments on the spinal cord and differentiation of motor and sensory nerves were not rediscovered until centuries later.

Early Views of Causation and the Mind-Body Problem

Theories of mind and body contain notions of the relationship of cause and action. Central to primitive or highly developed theories of the etiology and treatment of behavior disorders were basic ideas concerning the link of mental to bodily events. At question were various theories: about why matter moves (why it is "animated"); what agency "directs" or induces a mental or physical activity; the extent to which these activities are dependent upon the presence of life; and about the significance of the fact that we have a subjective sense of being moved (or motivated) to act. For the early Greek thinkers, animation was equivalent to behavior. It was observed in nature (in the "behavior" of the wind or in the moving of trees) as well as in man. The human's ability to act was equated with the activity of some homuncular "prime mover"—a spiritual or bodily substance, either external or located in the heart or viscera and endowed with the power to cause and direct. Vitality or power was equated with mental life and the major vital act was breathing (Greek, *pneuma*; Latin, *anima*). The Greek word *phren* means both mind and diaphragm: we are heir to such notions in the suffix, phrenic. The air contained the life principle that was processed within the body and activated it; psyche derives from a Greek word connoting pseudosubstantive air—"breath" or "odor." Inspiration refers both to respiratory and mental processes, and with death—with the departure of the life principle or soul—one has expired. Apparently the equation of mental life with warmth, breathing, and combustion was popular long before oxidative metabolism was found to define the limits for consciousness and coma.

The psychophysiology of the earlier Greeks evolved through various versions, and a remarkable variety of somatic locations or "seats" were found for the thinking, moving, and sensing powers. It took centuries—indeed, until our own—to move these mental "powers" securely into the head, and we still have to struggle to think in terms of processes and events rather than either simple mechanical links or mysterious executive powers. We still encounter "prime movers" in simplistic notions about the single-factor causation of disease, for example, the exclusive causative role of unconscious wishes or brain centers or bad mothers or chemical processes in psychosis.

It has not been easy to win the right to examine dispassionately the organization of events in nature, including psychological events. Man was seen as a part of nature by the animists, by Eastern philosophies and also by nineteenth- and twentieth-century biology, which, however, tended either to ignore lawful behavior or to exempt the symbolic and experiential—a good part of what is "psychological" about man—from scientific scrutiny. The special or transcendental nature of man and his self-consciousness was developed by Western philosophy, theology, and psychology. Yet at times certain mentalistic views of man threaten entirely to launch the mind both from the world of nature and from the body. The fact that psychological, social, and biological systems are operationally distinct frequently leads to a failure to perceive their organizational relatedness and the continuities and discontinuities of man and animal.

We encounter homuncular and animistic thinking about behavior because we are heirs not only to history but to our own more primitive childhood theories. Every child develops theories about why his body works in the way it does, and what causes the events in his head, his body, or in nature. The way one makes things happen, the way an urge seems to become an act, is taken to be a cause for events. This subjectivistic model obviously does not tell us how a behavioral event (thinking, moving, defecating, or breathing) is, in fact, organized or accomplished, nor how mental and physical events are related. Subjective and introspective data are a necessary but not a sufficient part of the required evidence. Therefore, it is only through growth and education (or occasionally psychotherapy) that each of us transcends this heritage of childhood, but we never entirely yield the subjectivistic model. Where cause, motive, drive, instinct, or stimulus, as well as volition and will are discussed, such problems of initial causes, of prime movers, recur. Indeed, wherever different operationally defined systems are to be related (mental and physical events or—at the synapse—electrophysiological and biochemical events), skill is constantly required to avoid unwarranted chicken-egg problems. Essentially, the history of psychiatric thought comprises the variety of ways in which systems relevant to the link of mental and bodily events are viewed. As with other styles of thinking, similar solutions tend to recur and fade, whatever the era.

The Middle Ages

After the fall of the Roman Empire there was a decline in the existing knowledge. What today we call psychiatry fell entirely into the hands of exorcising priests and persecutors of witches.[1] Although most historians maintain that the medieval socioeconomic system was stable, it certainly did not abound in comforts, and the restlessness of the time was reflected in reports of what might be considered mass psychoses, such as tarantism (a dancing mania), and flagellantism, in which hordes of people injured themselves and others. Another medieval form of insanity was lycanthropy, the delusion of being a wolf, for which amputation was attempted in order to convince the patient (with this therapeutic extremity) that he was not a wolf.

Theology and psychology were inextricably linked. Theologians were preoccupied with studies of the physiology and temperament of demons, dignified with such details as their possession of bodily form, lack of heat, and ability to vanish in smoke. This period also saw the canonization of psychiatry's patron saint, Ste Dympna of Gheel. According to legend, Dympna, the daughter of an Irish king, refused to marry her father after her mother died. Fleeing to Gheel in Belgium, she was there trapped and beheaded by the insane monarch. Witnesses of the crime built a chapel, people began to bring their insane to Gheel, and when they were not cured they stayed on as boarders and the colony, still extant, developed.

The rationale for medieval "therapies" is expressed in the infamous "The Witch's Hammer" (*Malleus Maleficarum*). In this book two monks, Sprenger and Kramer, put down not only their own sadistic and misogynous beliefs, but also the common beliefs of the time: that witches and sorcerers have of their own free will become heretics and have chosen the devil as their master; that they perform evil deeds and seduce others to their evilness; that they can be diagnosed by stigmata (in modern terms, signs and symptoms of hysterical reactions, sociopathies, depression, and schizophrenia); that these evil deeds range from peculiar practices, such as having intercourse on certain days, to monstrous crimes such as causing plagues, famine, and impotence; that they must be made to confess these deeds by any means including cruel torture and then be punished by death (the ultimate therapy). The great savants and physicians of the time concurred, and countless numbers of victims were tortured, notably at the beginning of the sixteenth century, precisely when the old order of the Middle Ages had begun to collapse. It is puzzling that an epoch producing a physician as humane and practical as Maimonides (who prescribed gentle environmental treatment for mania) or a theologian with the logic and grasp for which Thomas Aquinas is known, still bequeathed a vulgar and sadistic heritage to psychiatric practice and thought.

New and Old Concepts during the Renaissance

During the sixteenth century, at the time of the "collapse of the Middle Ages," some disagreement with these beliefs began to be expressed. Philippus Aureolus Theoprastus Bombastus von Hohenheim, called Paracelsus (1493–1541), an alchemist and mystic, wrote about mental disorder in *Von den Krankheiten die der Vernunft Entrauben* ("Of the Diseases Which Deprive of Reason"). He held that true insanity was caused by the stars or by the distillation of vapors from excreta which rose to the brain and turned into worms (a neurohumoral theory). His treatments, while not specific, were generally medical rather than theological and, with some exceptions, ameliorative in intent rather than sadistically reformistic. Johannes Weyer (1515–88) wrote a famous dissent in his "*De Praestigiis Daemonum*," in which he held that the devil was not a material being. This perforce meant such deeds as sexual intercourse between the devil and witches were fantasies. Weyer and a few contemporaries believed that many witches were mentally ill and should be treated by physicians and not by priests. While this period has been referred to by Gregory Zilboorg and George W. Henry[14] as the first psychiatric revolution, witches were still being sentenced to death in Poland, Mexico, and Switzerland until almost 1800.

With the Renaissance and its new explicit focus on man, there gradually emerged a less anthropomorphic and less demonic view of moving forces. With a secure place for man, there came to be room for nature. Johannes Kepler began with the notion that the planets are moved by souls but came to believe that they were controlled by natural forces. René Descartes, who at times believed he had clearly separated matter and spirit, applied mechanical explanations in terms of matter and motion, not only to the movement of planets but to inorganic matter and—more critically—even to the physiologic processes in organic bodies. The latter extension was consequential for future developments in psychophysiology. Purpose became less homuncular; bodily functions were now conceived to operate in the manner of "the movements of a clock or other self-acting machine or automaton [which] follow from the arrangement of its weights and wheels"—a model for what makes a person tick! Descartes was aware of sentience in animals which, however, lacking pure reason, lacked a soul.

Descartes spoke of "animal spirits" supported by a special combustion, but these spirits were particles which transmitted information and energy to the body. (We would call this the nerve impulse.) He shrank the location of the soul to the tiny pineal gland, very slight inclinations of which could direct the motion of animal spirits of the brain to motor nerves and thus execute actions willed by the soul. This has been termed a conception of "guidance without work done," [11] that is, a conception that in contemporary terms would be called communication, signaling, or information transfer between systems, rather than the passage of large quanta of energy from one system to another. Descartes's non-material soul was insignificant in terms of space but critical in terms of mental function. Operating through the rudder of the pineal, the soul was responsible for man's reason and thus was endowed with what we would term regulatory functions; in view of man's fine adjustments to a variety of situations it also had adaptive functions. The clear-cut dualism of Descartes and his highly speculative physiology are generally deplored; his models and terms of discourse can, however, be seen to have polarized the issues and to have opened up a challenging program for subsequent empirical research into the nature of man and his psychophysiological functions.

MEDICAL CONTRIBUTIONS In the seventeenth century, we encounter physicians more clearly recognizing behavior disorders as problems in the general practice of medicine. Leading physicians of the seventeenth and eighteenth centuries provided astute clinical descriptions, which, in fact, were of far more consequence than Robert Burton's *Anatomy of Melancholy,* which has received much literary acclaim. Thomas Sydenham (1624–89) recognized that hysterical and hypochondriacal reactions were the most widespread and complex of illnesses. The great anatomist and clinician,

Thomas Willis (1621–75), first described general paresis (much later identified as CNS syphilis); he also differentiated mental deficiency from the deteriorating illnesses. The Scottish physician George Cheyne (1671–1743) was probably the first to describe neurosis under the name "The English Malady," by which he meant disorders that later were called hypochondriasis, hysteria, and neurasthenia; according to him about one-third of all medical patients suffered from this malady. George Ernest Stahl (1660–1734) divided diseases into sympathetic (organic) and pathetic (functional) diseases, a distinction that, of course, still survives. Even with these clinical advances within general medical practice, a truly clinical psychiatry did not appear until the beginning of the nineteenth century. It began with the problem of hospital care for the incapacitated "core" population of behavior disorders.

Humanitarian Changes in Patient Care

The Age of Enlightenment

In Europe the first mental hospitals recognizable as such appeared in the twelfth century, and Bethlehem Hospital, the infamous "Bedlam," in London was founded in 1377. These hospitals in reality were little more than dungeons. Moslem countries had earlier enjoyed a flowering of the medical arts, and mental hospitals were there established as early as the eighth century. Arabic innovations were particularly evident in Spanish medicine; the first asylum in the New World in which mental patients were treated in a more or less humane fashion was founded by Bernardino Alvarez at San Hipolito, Mexico, in 1566.

By the beginning of the nineteenth century, a belief that man was a part of nature, that mental diseases could be treated, and the strong philanthropic interest of the time induced a number of men in different countries to press, in word and action, for reform of mental hospitals. The need was great. Patients, at the mercy of their keepers and of other patients, were brutally mistreated. Institutions were run by overseers who made certain that the able-bodied contributed to their upkeep by hard labor and severe punishment. Patients were often exhibited to the public for small fees; this was customary at the famous Narrenturm, the Fool's Tower, built in Vienna in 1784.

With the belief that organic disease and injury could affect the higher or "moral" faculties, medicine could be sanctioned to care for the core population of behavior disorders. It is customary to credit Philippe Pinel (1745–1826) with the freeing of mental patients from chains, although other physicians and reformers in several countries were also active. Pinel was Professor of Hygiene and Internal Medicine at the University of Paris and also Director of the Asylum of Bicêtre and the famous women's hospital of Paris, La Salpêtrière. While his colleagues appreciated his work in internal medicine,

Pinel's *Traité médico-philosophique sur l'aliénation mentale* (1801) became internationally influential.

Pinel classified mental diseases as mania, melancholy, dementia, and idiocy. Dementia (which he attributed to sex debaucheries) was characterized by incoherent thinking and probably consisted of cases of schizophrenia and general paresis lumped together. He thought heredity played a role but felt that irregularity in living and education had a more important etiological role than somatic factors. Pinel worked out rules for the running of mental institutions, replaced overseers with medical superintendents, and separated the mentally ill from idiots and thieves (now, once again, we are inclined to view all of them as "sick"). Dunking, strongly recommended by a famous eighteenth-century physician, Hermann Boerhaave, was replaced by the more agreeable hydrotherapy. Pinel used drugs sparingly, an advance over the earlier heavy-handed use of purgatives, phlebotomy, and herbals, and he strongly recommended good aides and attendants. It is perhaps inevitable that such a man would be a therapeutic optimist; he felt that over half of the manias and melancholias in this four-part classification could be cured after eighteen months of treatment.

William Tuke, a Quaker layman (1732–1822), pursued similar interests in England and influenced a coreligionist, Benjamin Rush (1745–1813), the father of American psychiatry. One of the signers of the Declaration of Independence, Rush was not only the first real teacher of psychiatry in the United States, but an exceptional man, opposing slavery and the death sentence, and working for humane reforms of institutions. His therapeutic beliefs, though, in contrast to those of his contemporaries, entailed bleeding and purging, and a rotating chair (referred to as "the tranquilizer"), which was as bad as its British counterpart (called Darwin's chair, after Charles Darwin's grandfather, Erasmus Darwin).

Nineteenth-Century Reforms and "Moral" Treatments

The Tuke and Pinel families sustained their friendship throughout the nineteenth century, and Daniel Hack Tuke (1827–95), the great-grandson of William, became a humane, learned, and judicious leader of British psychiatry. Reforms were carried on in many countries and had the character of a social movement. Who was to be reformed? In part, the general educated community—legislators, committee, and board members—whose beliefs would make one or another pattern of patient care more likely, and in part physicians and psychiatrists residing outside the few centers of progress. At that time, advances in metropolitan psychiatry were not reflected generally in the provinces. (Even today, there is a wide variation in the quality of patient care in the various hospitals of a single city; every medical student applying for specialty training knows this.) Throughout most of the century, the task of building mental hospitals, of improving the status of the mentally ill, and organizing their aftercare dominated British and American psychiatry; hospital administration was the all-consuming interest. Isaac Ray (1807–81), an American hospital superintendent, described the "good superintendent" in quite modern terms,[14] as the center of the patient's system "around which they all revolved, being held in their places by the attraction of respective confidence." He encouraged talking with patients so that one could get a "glimpse of their inner life," which he thought might be helpful in treatment. In 1844, thirteen superintendents in the United States formed the American Association of Medical Superintendents of Insane Asylums (later to become the American Psychiatric Association), and founded the Journal of Insanity (later the American Journal of Psychiatry).

A number of therapeutic experiments through the century were notably enlightened, but the all-too-familiar process by which reform becomes overweeningly evangelical was also encountered. Among therapeutic experiments were the so-called moral treatments of humanely administered small institutions, the "open door," and special training for nurses or supervising personnel. "No restraint" therapy became the hallmark of British psychiatry. At the turn of this century, English and American psychiatrists debated about the use of the wetpack (a cocoon of wet sheets wrapped in blankets, ensheathing the patient from neck to feet), the Americans (through the 1940's) generally considering the device tranquilizing, and the English condemning it as an imposition. Dorothea Dix (1802–77), a retired schoolteacher, bolstered the aims of a new humane psychiatry to treat behavior disorders; in a virtually single-handed crusade, she aroused public interest and organized the aftercare movement both in this country and in England.

It was largely neurologists, welfare workers, various philanthropic groups (and the usual peripheral complement of variously motivated social dyspeptics) who were active in an association imposingly entitled the National Association for the Protection of the Insane and the Prevention of Insanity (NAPIPI). Albert Deutsch, examining these movements, speaks of the "cult of curability"—the "totally unfounded idea" that in its earlier stages mental disease was not only curable but that therapeutic devices were already at hand.[4] Today, we are familiar with the difficult problems involved in establishing criteria for improvement, in controlling and matching populations and drawing accurate conclusions about incidence, prevalence, and therapeutic efficacy from statistics. But in 1840, asylum heads often claimed 90 per cent cures; Deutsch cites one claim of 100 per cent cures.

By exploiting this myth of curability, the reformers succeeded in bringing the mentally ill clearly into the province of medicine; explosion of the myth (shortly after the Civil War) and the expanding population which increased the numbers of patients to be cared for, then led to a period of apathy and to the notion of "once insane, always insane." This kind of sentiment and the practices derived from it had to be coped with by a successor of that formidably named NAPIPI, the influential National Committee for Mental Hygiene (1908), later the National Association for Mental Health. This committee was founded by Clifford Beers (1876–1943), a graduate of Yale University, who had written a stirring book, *A Mind That Found Itself*, about his unfortunate experiences in mental hospitals. The mental hygiene movement became world-wide and has become enormously influential in educating the population about mental health and illness and in promoting better practices.

Expansion of Psychiatric Services

Associated with this movement were two developments that led psychiatry into broader fields than the care of the adult psychotic. A clinic and school for children, established by the psychologist Lightner Witmer in Philadelphia in 1897, took cognizance of the new intelligence tests, and by 1908 psychiatrists, such as William Healy, began to work and later to lead in what came to be called the child guidance movement. Mental hygiene clinics were established in connection with juvenile courts, institutions for delinquents, prisons, mental hospitals, schools, and general hospitals. By 1905, social workers who had been active for some time in poorhouses and prisons began to work in mental hospitals and child guidance centers. Psychologists were sporadically occupied either in directing clinics or in testing, but the "team" was not established until the beginning of World War II.

Another development, the extension of therapy to non-psychotic adult patients, came largely under the impetus of European and American neurologists, who frequently encountered the neurotic patient. In the United States, the neurologist S. Weir Mitchell (1829–1914) invented a total rest treatment (punctuated by stimulants to "tone up" the nervous system) for the neurotic battle-casualties of the Civil War. This treatment was ultimately discarded (although a similar therapy, the Morita method, developed under Zen influence, is still in vogue in Japan). Mitchell, who had been active in NAPIPI, founded the outpatient department at the Pennsylvania Hospital in 1885, for the treatment of those suffering from "incipient mental diseases." Again, psychiatrists proved adaptable, as evidenced by the modern proliferation of psychiatric outpatient clinics and private practice.

Legal Reform

New legislation on the status of hospitalized mental patients evolved when adequate mental hospitals became available. In some states, at least, detention of lunatics in prisons, jails, or houses of correction was forbidden (New York, 1827). Commitment was informal until the nineteenth century (Benjamin Rush wrote on a scrap of paper: "J. Sproul is a proper patient for the Pennsylvania Hospital . . ."), a state of affairs modern psychiatrists, beset with paper work, would like to recapture. Isaac Ray and workers from reform movements helped to shape appropriate laws. In the 1860's, the famous case of Mrs. E. P. W. Packard, who claimed she had been "railroaded" into a mental hospital, aroused public interest and led to the first modern commitment laws in the United States. Our concern with the problem of crime, responsibility, and mental illness stems from reforms in the nineteenth century and is taken up in the chapter on Law and Psychiatry (Chapter 24). Until this century of reform, the mentally ill and the criminal, sane or insane, had no rights and no defense. Their property was confiscated by the state or municipality without recourse.

The Emergence of a Scientific Psychiatry

Psychiatry as a Medical Specialty

After the French Revolution, the civilized world became increasingly aware of severe mental disorders as a social problem requiring public concern, humane treatment, and medical attention. As the demons were put to rest in both the cosmic and the biological world, new sciences began to develop that were basic for the diagnosis and treatment of behavior disorders. Through the research of the nineteenth century, the earlier concept of animal spirits was replaced by notions of natural forces, subject to observational and experimental scrutiny. Gradually, by the twentieth century, it became clear that information in the world within and around us does not terminate in any "seat" of consciousness but rather in complex interneural functions, synapses, which could be studied in their anatomical electrical and physiochemical characteristics. Reports of introspection (which philosophers hitherto had treated as unquestioned "givens") were challenged at the beginning of the nineteenth century by the astronomers' discovery of the "personal equation" (or individual differences in measurements of reaction time). Later, the physiologists proved that, in spite of subjective impressions that a stimulus leads to instantaneous perception, neural processes do not proceed with the speed of light, but take more time. This led to the notion that it was feasible to measure and study psychophysical processes, perception, and the contents of consciousness. Last, and perhaps foremost, Darwin's discoveries about the evolution of man set the scene for a very different, essentially developmental approach to the study and treatment of behavior disorders[8]—an approach that is still evolving in the contemporary scene.

Brain and Behavior

The nineteenth century saw psychiatry grow with advances in biology and medicine and in the midst of widespread debates about the spiritual (psychic and moral) or somatic nature of mental disorder. In the phrenology of Franz Josef Gall (1748–1828), we bump into an unsuccessful attempt to relate configurations of the skull with brain anatomy, and both with specific psychological traits. Yet such a theory required that feelings and character traits as well as physiological functions have a localized seat in the brain, and further that experience must affect the size of portions of the brain. While this parlor pastime could not be taken too seriously by scientists, the idea of localization did stimulate neurobehavioral research and, on the psychological side, compelled careful description of complex behavior by psychiatrists such as Jean Etienne Dominique Esquirol.[5, 13] Further, the growing ability in medicine to discriminate diseases encouraged that clinical empiricism, which carefully observes and describes the course and symptoms of a disorder. Toward the end of the century, descriptions of aphasia and other higher symbolic dysfunctions began to appear, and detailed psychiatric observations of neurosis as well as psychosis were published. The right of scientists to be interested in any aspect of human behavior—including sexual, subjective, symbolic, and emotional aspects—was beginning to be asserted.

Emotions in Neurobehavioral Theory

Empedocles had emphasized the role of love and hate in behavior, and Plato had given Eros a special role, but medicine treated aspects of emotions somewhat as a stepchild. At the beginning of the last century, emotions were still given a "seat" in viscera apart from other mental operations; perhaps this was in part due to the apparently "autonomous" anatomic features of the paraspinal sympathetic chain and the scattered parasympathetic ganglia. Whatever the reasons, it is surprising but true that it required an evolution of thought in order to observe emotions as explicitly suitable for description and to ascribe to them some consequence, both in psychopathology and neurophysiology. Major advances such as studies of the hypothalamus and limbic system were not developed until our time.

The Relationship of Brain and Mind

The argument between proponents of the organic or psychic nature of mental functions was epitomized in the peculiar slogan of physiologists and philosophers, "no psychosis without neurosis," meaning that there could be no "higher psychic faculties" without neural activity. Later, in psychopathology, this meant that disorders of mentation were dependent on basic disturbances of nerve function. Ernst von Feuchstersleben (1806–49), bringing the terms "psychosis" and "psychosomatic" into psychiatry in 1845, argued the opposite, that is, any change of nerve activity was dependent upon psychic factors. And there was yet another view, which spoke for the "unconsciousness" of sequences of neural activity ("neurosis without psychosis"), as in a number of reflexes. Finally, some organicists, lacking insight into the integrative action of the nervous system, thought it incredible that there could be disturbance in nerve function without histological evidence. The fact that, unlike most diseases, "mental disease" could be diagnosed only in the living and not at autopsy, did not deter those overly keen neuropathologists who "discovered" a variety of microscopic lesions. These lesions generally turned out to be a nineteenth-century version of endowing spirits with material reality. Although contemporary philosophers tend to view psychic and physical phenomena as parallel or as two aspects of the same thing, there are still unsettled issues of fact, which await research with modern tools and methods.[2]

Somatic Theories of Behavior Disorder

Two theories were characteristic of the somatic orientation that dominated the theoretical scene in the late nineteenth century: the localization theory and the degeneration hypothesis. *Localization theories* concerning the specificity of brain areas for particular complex behavioral functions were advanced by experiments of nature as well as in the laboratory. Exciting speculation about the relationship of brain, consciousness, and willed action followed the demonstration in 1870 by G. Fritsch and E. Hitzig that electrical stimulation of discrete areas of the cortex produced discrete motor movements in both animals and man. Paul Pierre Broca (1824–80) had examined an old resident of a mental hospital who could vocalize but not talk (motor aphasia), although he communicated intelligently by signs. In 1861, discovering a lesion of the foot of the third frontal convolution of the left cerebral hemisphere at the patient's autopsy, Broca asserted that this convolution contained a center for language and that mental functions had a precise localization. Later, Carl Wernicke described a lesion of the left superior temporal gyrus which led to an inability to understand language (receptive aphasia) in the presence of an intact sensory system. The discovery of aphasia launched important basic and clinical research by John Hughlings Jackson, Sigmund Freud and, in the twentieth century, by Kurt Goldstein and Karl S. Lashley. These workers argued, in effect, that both localizing and general factors have to be considered, and that any specialized apparatus of the brain is profoundly affected by supporting and connecting parts—in brief, that an *organization* of neuronal operations and brain systems is involved in complex mental functions such as language. (See Chapter 16.) The notion of complex interactions and organizations of forces as partly accountable for complicated behavioral operations would prove to be important in future analyses of behavior disorder.

The *degeneration hypothesis* also had consequences in preparing the ground for a more highly developed clinical psychiatry. Benedict August Morel (1809–73) taught that the mentally ill were degenerative deviations from normal types. Transmitted by heredity, progressive deterioration or degeneration would appear in subsequent generations until the species became extinct. For mental illness the steps over several generations would be:

nervousness, neuroticism, psychosis, idiocy, and degeneration recognized by stigmata. Various misinterpretations both of Darwin's theory and the new science of genetics contributed to the vulgarization and unwarranted therapeutic pessimism associated with the degeneration hypothesis. Viewed as a model and given modern context, there may be merit in the notion of familial transmission of behavior disorder over generations, operating through an interaction of psychosocial and genetic mechanisms. It is clear, however, that this modern version does not prejudice therapeutic action nor imply neuropathological degeneration as did the earlier degeneration hypotheses. Richard von Krafft-Ebing (1840–1902) wrote extensively about the degenerative basis of sexual psychopathies but nevertheless thereby brought detailed clinical descriptions of sexual behavior into medical scrutiny.

Neuropsychiatry

Clinical observations and theories about the brain and its relevance for mental diseases involved a close union of neurology and psychiatry. Two of the most outstanding representatives of this development were Jean Etienne Dominique Esquirol (1722–1840), a student of Pinel, and Wilhelm Griesinger (1817–69). Esquirol has been called the founder of French psychiatry. He taught at the Medical Faculty of the Sorbonne, and his primary interest was the psychoses. Esquirol recognized sociocultural factors in mental illness and identified the etiological role of isolation. On the basis of careful observations, *syndromes* of psychiatric disorders, whatever their cause, were delineated. Pinel described "monomania" (the coexistence of intellectual gifts and disordered behavior), and Esquirol observed that there could be serious psychopathology without delirium or gross disorganization. This was a critical step in expanding the range of psychiatrically relevant disorders. To read Esquirol's lively clinical descriptions is still a pleasure today. He expressed his eclecticism and clinical wisdom in the sentence, "In practice one must never be absolute." On his deathbed, he said to his students, among them most of the future leaders of French psychiatry, "Keep peace!"—an impressive statement in a discipline still plagued by dogma and sectarianism.[1]

Wilhelm Griesinger (1817–69), Professor of Psychiatry and Medicine at the University of Berlin, developed very advanced ideas. In his *Mental Pathology and Therapeutics*[7] Griesinger described psychic diseases as brain diseases; he believed that irritations of the brain could produce abnormal emotions and ideas. He emphasized the importance of emotions rather than of intellect; he did not believe in a clear split of normal and abnormal and considered dreams, febrile deliriums, and the behavior of intoxicated persons as analogous to mental disease. He also observed and reported certain courses of mental disorders: they begin with anxiety, lead to apathy and withdrawal, and end with a cessation of human relations. Griesinger held that to understand mental disease one must understand the premorbid personality. He assumed multiple factors to be of etiological importance: heredity, nervous constitution, sex disturbances in childhood, shock, grief, and many organic disturbances. He felt that there was in fact only one psychosis, with a great variety of symptoms. Griesinger recommended early treatment and favored hospitalization of mental patients, prescribing vigorous treatment with many drugs, cathartics, and emetics. With Griesinger, we see the beginning of university psychiatry, which later became a powerful influence on the European continent, particularly in German-speaking countries.

The emphasis of the university neuropsychiatrists was on brain pathology; even today in many European university clinics—and in Japan and Latin America, where early development followed the German and French patterns—a visitor is first shown the brain pathology laboratory. Of course, the number of organic patients and particularly of general paretics was very high. The contributions of brain pathologists such as Franz Nissl (1860–1919) and Constantin von Economo (1876–1931), the discoverer of epidemic encephalitis, are of lasting value. In the second half of the nineteenth century, German psychiatrists described a number of syndromes that are still considered valid: catatonia and paraphrenia by Karl Kahlbaum (1828–99) and hebephrenia by Ewald Hecker (1843–1909). The spur for these distinctions came in part as a reaction to Griesinger's monopsychosis and resulted in some appallingly elaborate classifications, now forgotten.

Fathers of Modern Clinical Psychiatry

Emil Kraepelin (1856–1928) studied under the neuroanatomist Paul E. Flechsig and the psychologist Wilhelm Wundt, worked in several mental hospitals, and occupied the academic chairs of psychiatry at the universities of Dorpat, Heidelberg, and Munich. The founder of the first psychiatric research institute, Kraepelin became, through his classic textbook,[9] the most influential psychiatrist of his time; and his impact is still strong. Kraepelin was a clinician; he observed and described his patients' behavior in convincing detail and developed what became known as descriptive psychiatry. Kraepelin stressed the importance of heredity and constitution, feeling that psychological causes were of minor significance. His most incisive achievement was to base a system of classification of diseases on prognosis as well as on symptomatology. This enabled him to regroup various entities into the complex of dementia praecox, differentiating these from manic-depressive psychoses and setting both apart from psychoses caused by brain diseases and toxic states. Kraepelin's diagnostic system has been much criticized, yet—in the absence of a better one—it is still widely used. One criticism of Kraepelin cannot be refuted: he was, like so many of his contemporaries, a therapeutic nihilist.

Eugen Bleuler (1857–1939), a Swiss, was definitely interested in therapy.

Where Kraepelin had catalogued symptomatology of dementia praecox in the natural history of the disorder, Bleuler based his description on psychological processes.[3] The dysfunction of associative processes was thought to lead to the characteristic symptoms of what Bleuler called schizophrenia. Thus, Eugen Bleuler became the first important modern psychological psychiatrist—in contrast to Kraepelin and the other neuropsychiatrists. Bleuler coined the psychiatric household words *depth psychology, ambivalence*, and *autism*. His influence on European and, more indirectly, American psychiatry is enduring.

Swiss-born Adolf Meyer (1866–1950), professor of psychiatry at Johns Hopkins University, and one of America's famous psychiatrists, also took issue with Kraepelin's ideas and particularly with his nihilistic approach to the treatment of mental disorders. Meyer was, in the best Anglo-American medical tradition, a very pragmatic clinician, who studied patients from both the biological and psychosocial points of view. He established the so-called psychobiological school and developed a classification and terminology of his own, which have not survived him. The view of behavior disorders, not as diseases, but as reactions to multiple psychobiological stresses related to the life cycle and current life situation was Meyer's most important contribution.[12] Teaching at John Hopkins University, Meyer put American psychiatry on its feet. His personal impact on his students was great; Phyllis Greenacre (who, like many other students of Meyer, became a psychoanalyst) said that he was a Christlike person. For a while his students filled most of the important posts in American psychiatry. Meyer is usually described as an antagonist of the psychoanalytic system, and, like some other prominent academic teachers, he was clearly jealous of Freud. Meyer's ideas, however, were manifestly modern and not incompatible with psychoanalytic thought, and at various junctures his administrative decisions helped psychoanalysis to become established in the United States. Although some consider Adolf Meyer neither a dynamic nor an American psychiatrist, we regard him as the first dynamic American psychiatrist of great distinction. Others, such as Morton Prince (1854–1929) and William A. White (1870–1937), pioneered in effectively advancing psychodynamic principles and bringing them into psychiatry. We have come then to the modern phase of a more scientific and "dynamic" psychiatry. In the next chapter we will highlight the development of these modes of thought and practice.

NOTES

1. Erwin H. Ackerknecht, *Kurze Geschichte der Psychiatrie* (Stuttgart: Enke, 1957); *A Short History of Psychiatry*, translated by S. Wolff (New York: Hafner Publishing Co., 1959).
2. Ludwig von Bertalanffy, *Problems of Life* (New York: Harper Torchbooks, 1960).

3. Eugen Bleuler, *Dementia Praecox, or the Group of Schizophrenias* (New York: International Universities Press, 1950).
4. Albert Deutsch, "The History of Mental Hygiene," in *One Hundred Years of American Psychiatry* (Washington, D.C.: American Psychiatric Association, 1944); *The Mentally Ill in America* (2d ed.; New York: Columbia University Press, 1949).
5. Jean Etienne Dominique Esquirol, *Mental Maladies: A Treatise on Insanity,* translated by E. K. Hunt (Philadelphia: Lea and Blanchard, 1845).
6. Sigmund Freud, "On the History of the Psychoanalytic Movement (1914)," *Standard Edition,* Vol. 14 (London: Hogarth Press, 1959).
7. Wilhelm Griesinger, *Mental Pathology and Therapeutics,* translated from German 2d edition (New York: Wood's Library of Standard Medical Authors, 1882).
8. David A. Hamburg, "The Relevance of Recent Evolutionary Changes to Human Stress Biology," in S. Washburn, ed., *Social Life of Early Man* (Chicago: Aldine, 1962).
9. Emil, Kraepelin, *Psychiatrie: Ein Lehrbuch für Studierende und Ärzte* (Leipzig: Barth, 1909–15); *Clinical Psychiatry: A Text-book for Students and Physicians,* translated and adapted from the 7th German Edition by A. Ross Deifendorf (New York: Macmillan, 1921).
10. Aubrey J. Lewis, "Melancholia: A Clinical Survey of Depressive States," *Journal of Mental Science,* 180 (1934), 277.
11. William McDougall, *Mind and Body* (Boston: Beacon Press, 1961).
12. Adolf Meyer, *Collected Papers of Adolf Meyer,* E. E. Winters, ed., Vols. I–III (Baltimore: Johns Hopkins Press, 1951).
13. Pierre Pichot, "Die franzoesische Psychiatrie der Gegenwart," *Deutsche Medizinische Wochenschuft,* 84 (1959), 912.
14. Gregory Zilboorg and George W. Henry, *A History of Medical Psychology* (New York: Norton, 1941).

CHAPTER THREE

The Evolution of Psychiatric Theory and Practice: II *Modern Times*

The Development of a Dynamic Approach to Behavior

Observation and diagnosis advanced in neuropsychiatry, but the individual tended to be lost in a web of classificatory schemes based on what Otto Pötzl called "brain mythology." A more satisfactory explanation of symptoms awaited a new motivational psychology. Such a psychology is deterministic and may deal with a "prime mover" or with multiple acting mechanisms at various levels of integration. It takes account of need, states of deprivation, and associated goal-directed activities. From the medical physiology of the nineteenth century, epitomized in Claude Bernard's writings, notions of adaptation, of regulating factors maintaining constancy in the internal milieu, were in the air. The phylogenetic relationship of homologous structures, the notion of hierarchies of levels of organization and the adaptedness of structures to the environment were contained in Darwinian theories, although the overriding "model" for neuropsychology was usually derived from the senior science, physics. Thus the laws about the conservation of energy and the constancy principle were important to all scientifically trained men who believed in a physical basis for mental phenomena.

John Hughlings Jackson

The English neurologist, John Hughlings Jackson (1835–1911), creatively adapted the thinking of his day to the nervous system and became one of the most important dynamic thinkers in modern psychiatry. Interested in the "evolution" and dissolution of nervous functions, he saw the nervous system as organized in hierarchical fashion.[30] Under conditions of trauma, fatigue, or strain, there was "regression" of neural functions to lower levels. He clearly enunciated the doctrine of concomitance, "for every mental state there is a correlative physical state," a parallelism that permitted scrutiny of the organization of neural and psychological functions, each at its own level. The notion of a correlation of states meant that sets of (physical) events rather than each discrete physical event could be related to mental states. Jackson viewed mental disease as inherent in the organization of psychological functions and as emerging when lower levels were not "kept down" by the function of higher levels of integration. He thought of a symptom as the end result of a struggle among conflicting discharges—the survival-of-the-fittest state in terms of the internal circumstances of the individual. In analyzing the effects of brain damage, Jackson distinguished between negative symptoms or the loss of function (the loss of "government") and positive symptoms ("the anarchy of the now uncontrolled people"). More recently acquired functions were lost, and more primitive modes emerged as compensatory symptoms were formed. Symptom formation was thus the combined consequence of the negative symptoms with the effects of the positive symptoms, a notion, which as Erwin Stengel points out, Freud (quite aware of Jackson's views) used implicitly in his work.[65]

Jackson spoke of the "dynamics of the nervous system" to refer to the function of nervous matter that, for him, was to "store up and expend energy." These essential activities of the nervous system, the consequence of which we study either in physiological or psychological phenomena, are the primary dynamic forces. The activity of "lower levels" of organization, "although unattended by any sort of conscious state is essential for energizing of the highest mental states."

This model for viewing the relationship of neural and mental states and for studying the forces determining these states implicitly requires a view of prior development in order to understand regressive phenomena. It is also of obvious importance to the growth of a "dynamic psychiatry" and is related to the depth psychology that was emerging toward the end of the century. Depth psychology had to take account not only of phenomena that were conscious, but also to consider the activity and consequences of nonconscious—"lower level"—processes in determining the emergence of manifest behavior. How behavior develops—both over long periods of time and how it is "built up" or constructed from moment to moment—became questions of scientific interest. The forces that structured and determined clinically relevant mental and behavioral phenomena had thus come to be ready for study.

The Introspectionists

Jackson, among others, mentioned that insights both into the nervous system and psychological functions could be observed by study of dreams, jokes, and by use of experimental drugs. Deliriums and states of fatigue were recognized as conditions in which interesting mental phenomena occurred. The gifted English gentleman-scientist, Francis Galton (1822–1911), perhaps the father of statistical psychometrics (and an undisciplined advocate of applied eugenics and psychology), systematically studied the data of introspection, compiling a "statistics of mental imagery." He stressed unconscious processes that occur in "the antechamber of consciousness," and he produced the phenomena of psychosis simply by systematically assuming every animate and inanimate object was a spy. The English psychiatrist Henry Maudsley (1835–1919), interested in chemistry and mental function, published in 1867 that "mind" was *not* coextensive with consciousness; philosophers and physiologists argued that perceptions were "built up" and then noticed, and that ideas were kept below the limen of consciousness in a "state of tendency" pressing to rise above the threshold. E. von Hartmann synthesized some of these trends in his famous *Philosophy of the Unconscious* in 1869.

Hypnosis

It was, however, hypnosis rather than introspectionism, philosophy, and physiology that vividly presented problems for a depth psychology. In part, this may derive from its application as a therapeutic technique, which seems always to command attention even though it may lead scientific inquiry astray. Franz Anton Mesmer (1734–1815) claimed to cure all illnesses by the touch of a rod permitting equalization of a magnetic field that filled the universe, its distribution influencing health and illness. His pretensions were finally exposed, but his influence, indirectly at least, outlasted his charlatanry. Mary Baker Eddy (1821–1910), the founder of Christian Science, was a Mesmerian, as was the Marquis de Puysegur (1751–1825), who established modern hypnosis in France. It is probable that only the discovery of nitrous oxide, ether, and chloroform kept mesmerists from becoming anesthesiologists. James Braid (1795–1860), a British surgeon, called the phenomenon a "nervous sleep" (hence hypnosis), which he explained in a doctrine called "neurohypnology." Induction of hypnosis was first attributed to a specific physiological control of sensory fixation. There were, however, early observations that pointed to suggestion as crucial in both the induction and the subsequent trance. Ambroise August Liebeault (1823–1904), practicing hypnosis at Nancy with hysterical patients, was impressed by the role of suggestion and taught Hippolyte Berheim (1840–1919), who investigated post-hypnotic suggestion, or "latent memory." He "implanted" suggestions during the trance, which the patient later performed but with amnesia for the suggestion, its source, and circumstances. Bernheim believed that these amnesias were essentially normal phenomena; he found suggestion operating in many disorders and was among the first to speak of "psychoneurosis." His pre-eminent contemporary, Jean Martin Charcot (1825–93), maintained that hypnotic phenomena occurred only in hysterics and were therefore abnormal, since hysteria, to him, was a disease of the internal capsule.[12] Charcot's demonstrations in the Salpêtrière of the hypnotic dissolution of symptoms in excellently performing cases of "grande hysterie" attracted physicians, society, and the demimonde of Paris.

Pierre Janet

One of Charcot's students, Pierre Janet (1859–1947), a fine clinician and brilliant modern thinker, reported in 1889 that some neurotic patients recalled traumatic memories in their hypnosis and became well after such ideas were made conscious. Janet evolved his own therapeutic methods, essentially emotional re-education and teaching patients how to live, but his theoretical notions remained generally confined to French psychiatry. Janet defined the role of dissociation of mental processes but did not believe this to be triggered by repression, as Freud later argued. Rather, he thought of an integrating tension or energy that normally held the stream of consciousness together; constitutionally determined generalized lowering of this energy led to psychasthenia (roughly, phobic, compulsive, and anxiety symptoms) and specific lowering led to hysteria and fugue states.[31] Freud gave Janet credit for his part in the discoveries of the clinical significance of unconscious processes and of cathartic therapy.

Sigmund Freud

The greatest disciple of Charcot and Bernheim, although they did not know it, was Sigmund Freud (1856–1939). An authoritative biography of his life and most particularly of the evolution of his work was provided by Ernest Jones, Freud's colleague and student.[32] Freud's theories and approaches affected psychiatry in many of its perspectives and practices; we will outline these approaches in some detail in the following section.

Freud's father, a Jewish merchant, moved his family from Freiberg, a small Moravian town, to Vienna when Freud was a child. As a medical student, Freud became interested in biological sciences, but he opened a neurological practice in 1886 to earn a living. His earliest publications were in comparative neuroanatomy, neurological studies of diseases of children, and aphasia. In his experiments with the psychological effects of cocaine, he thought he had a chemical cure for human woes and came close to discovering its anesthetic function.

Neurological practice involved many neurotic patients. Freud noted he had little success with hydrotherapy, massage, Weir Mitchell's rest cure, and the then popular electrotherapies. Nor was he satisfied with the methods of direct hypnotic suggestion, which he had learned in fellowships with Charcot and Bernheim. Some years earlier (in 1883 and before the Janet publications), Dr. Joseph Breuer, an elder and established practitioner of medicine, had deeply impressed Freud with an informal account of a hysterical patient whose amnesia and symptoms had disappeared when whole areas of her forgotten experiences were spontaneously talked about and relived under hypnosis. Freud later spoke about this to Charcot, who was not especially interested. He finally, then, resumed discussions with Breuer, and began a collaboration that resulted in their publication (between 1893 and 1895) of the *Studies in Hysteria.*[9]

Freud's experiments with Breuer impressed him with several features that were to remain themes throughout the subsequent development of psychoanalysis. *First* of all, internal events, such as memories, were crucial. The organization of these memories and thoughts was governed by an associative process that could be disrupted by strong emotions leading to amnesias, experiences of confusion, disruptions of the personality, and symptoms. *Second,* the existence and lifting of amnesia revealed another consciousness or a split consciousness—a forgotten world that could "intrude upon" normal states disrupting orderly thinking and leading to a less unified personality. Accordingly, conscious and unconscious processes were important. *Third,* conflict was at the center of mental problems. Such conflict resulted either from traumatic sexual experience or from sexual drive opposed to moral standards (conflicts between the demands of reality and instincts). *Fourth,* conflict induced a protective forgetting or a repression of the sources that instigated it. There were usually multiple "dynamic" reasons for the dissociations in personality and for ensuing symptoms. *Fifth,* such forgotten conflicts still had a power that could be relieved by recall. *Sixth,* memories apparently had an emotional charge; when the charged memory was exposed, there was a discharge or abreaction of emotion, and the patient's symptoms disappeared. This treatment was called catharsis.

It is interesting that notions of the multiple mechanisms underlying symptom formation and relief were advanced; apparently emotional energy could shift about. If a conflict led to a situation where the charge of emotion had to be defended against or warded off, then the quantity of energy might be displaced to the body in the form of hysterical paralyses. Instead of consciously remembering and dealing with a situation—instead of absorbing the charge of the emotion or letting it wear away (by association with other mental acts)—the patient repressed both the charge and the unpleasant memory and developed symptoms. With the recovery of the memory and its associated, but hitherto "strangulated" charge of emotion, the nervous system could now achieve its "principle of constancy" by abreacting the emotion. The expressive channels were now unblocked, and the symptom and the force of the conflict could disappear. The charged memory could now take a proper place alongside other, more neutral, thoughts. Loosely bound energies led to fragmented thoughts; less mobile or "bound" energies corresponded to a more orderly mode of thought. This notion provided one basis for understanding the "economy" of the mental apparatus and demonstrates the extent to which observations of subjective experiences in the form of verbalization and associations were quite early linked to theories of how the mind fundamentally worked.

A major consequence of this early work lies in the method of free association, which Freud slowly evolved. At first using direct therapeutic suggestions that a symptom would disappear, he later used suggestion to persuade the patient to remember and finally abandoned hypnosis and simply asked the patient to concentrate (occasionally pressing his hand on the patient's forehead) in order to recall experiences. Finally, he simply allowed the patient to relax and talk. He told the patient to suspend censorship, to say anything that came to mind: the method of free association. Under these conditions, the patient's memories and ideas—his associations—would be organized by internal psychological forces. As associations emerged or were interrupted, they would directly or indirectly reveal conflict, which could then be interpreted. This would allow further forgotten wishes and memories to emerge.

Freud learned over the years that there were numerous obstacles to be overcome in this process: patients forgot rather than remembered. Even when they remembered, they showed "resistance"—confused or otherwise diverted the therapeutic process. If the patient was embarrassed or conflicted, he avoided, evaded, denied, or otherwise defended himself. Further, the patient displaced ("transferred") onto the physician the same patterns of striving for attention and gratification that had characterized earlier behavior and wishes toward parental figures. Without realizing it, patients made "false connections" between forgotten events and wishes and the present situation. Hence, they represented earlier memories in current behavior. Accordingly, one had to analyze not only impulses and wishes, but the motives for their currently covert and displaced expression. Freud continually developed and refined these concepts of resistance, transference, and defense as they operated during the treatment.

As Freud's work advanced, he increasingly focused on inferring underlying and intervening processes which lead to a wide range of behaviors: from dreams to memories to slips of the tongue and symptoms. Momentarily shaken by the finding that many reports of sexual seduction in childhood were simply fantasies, he then discovered the remarkable power of wishes and fantasies in organizing mental life. At bottom, he felt that such wishes and images were connected with basic drives (or instincts, as we customarily but inaccurately translate the German, *Trieb*). The energy of these drives was manifest not only in personal relations but in images, dreams, memories, thoughts, and actions and represented determining conditions for neurotic symptoms. Some of his earliest ideas are contained in letters to his friend, Wilhelm Fliess.[2] We find there a remarkable "model" for how the brain could produce these phenomena, which he called his "Project." His major published theoretical formulations first appeared in the famous Chapter 7 in the *Interpretation of Dreams* (1900). In this book, Freud took an every-night occurrence—a dream—seriously and attempted to see what could be learned about such a phenomenon. He tried to create a picture of a "mental apparatus" and the forces and counterforces that could conceivably produce a dream. Among many major notions, a theory of cognitive processes emerged: the "first thought" was a hallucination provoked by the absence of the mother, the need gratifying object; thinking at the outset was organized but primitive and linked with bodily needs. Dream images were disguised primitive thoughts provoked by wishes and revised by a "censorship." Symptoms also were instigated by instinctual wishes and shaped by at least some regard for reality. The meaning of both dreams and symptoms could be unraveled through the process of free association. In discovering the significance of this usually forgotten form of consciousness, Freud undertook self-analysis and came more clearly to appreciate the persistence of childhood theories about sexuality for which most adults normally have an amnesia. Only with the "regression" of sleep would dream thinking emerge and express wishes normally out of consciousness. Because this was a general theory of a common part of mental life—exempting no one—the book was not kindly received.

Some of Freud's most important books exposing the pervasive operations of unconscious wishes were: *The Psychopathology of Everyday Life* in 1904, and *Wit and Its Relation to the Unconscious* in 1905. In 1905, he also published *Three Essays on the Theory of Sexuality,* in which he stated his views and observations on the existence of infantile sexuality and its persistence in normal adult sexuality, a book that shocked the intellectual world. Roughly in a period between 1910 and 1930 he began a final formulation of his theory, which will be briefly described later. Some of the most important points are contained in *Inhibitions, Symptoms and Anxiety* (1923).

Freud did not simply treat patients and develop ideas. Rather, he created a movement, and by 1902 there were a number of disciples. As in all revolutionary movements, there were both extremely gifted and some rather disturbed people; some of the turbulence in the history of the psychoanalytic movement bears this out. Of his early close great colleagues, only Karl Abraham and Ernest Jones stayed with Freud; Alfred Adler (1870–1937), Carl Jung (1875–1961), Otto Rank (1884–1939), and Wilhelm Stekel (1868–1940) left to form movements of their own. Sandor Ferenczi (1873–1933) never seceded, but he developed ideas about "active" interventions to bypass (rather than "analyze") resistances, which Freud criticized severely.

Although Freud felt the theoretical superstructure of his observations could be eliminated or changed, he showed little tolerance for the deviations of his students. This dogmatic spirit has, unfortunately, remained characteristic of the orthodox psychoanalytic movement. Since 1909, when (at the invitation of G. Stanley Hall and the neuropathologist James Jackson Putnam) Freud and Jung delivered their famous lectures at Clark University, Worcester, Massachusetts, the psychoanalytic movement has become world-wide. Of all countries, the United States has been most receptive to psychoanalysis; this is ironical because Freud never liked the "New World," although he loved and admired England. Freud felt ambivalent about Vienna, but he preferred to live, practice, and teach there. He was past forty when he began his work with psychoanalysis and spent his last two score years, often in pain from a carcinoma of the jaw, constantly developing his science. Only the political events of 1938 forced him to emigrate and seek refuge in London, where he died in 1939.

Freud saw himself as a discoverer, not as a genius, but undoubtedly he had the self-mastery, perseverance, and courage to convert the gift of insight into an astonishingly detailed, extensive, and relevant body of knowledge. It may be added that Freud was not attracted to medicine and thought of himself primarily as a scientist. His dissatisfaction with the medical profession that, particularly in Vienna, showed so little understanding of his work is also expressed by his strong endorsement of "lay" or non-medical psychoanalysis.

Psychoanalytic Theory

In contrast to his clear methods and convincing observations, Freud's theoretical statements are complex and often bewildering. The basic aim of Freud's interpretations was to account for the inner and subjective life of man and to infer links between subjective experiences, their determining mechanisms, and overt behavior. He first limited the definition of psychoanalysis to a science of unconscious mental processes, but in his later writings and in his incessant reformulations he appears to have aimed at a comprehensive theory of all psychological life. We can see this as a major attempt to formulate one way of thinking about behavior and not, certainly, as the ultimate product of scientific inquiry into the organization of behavior. Freud had far less difficulty than many of his followers in explicitly distinguishing between observations, binding inferences, and speculative ones. In none of the twenty-three volumes of his work can one find a systematic and comprehensive "final" theoretical statement. Rather, Freud generally took up a set of observations (amnesias, dreams, fetishes, perversions, slips, and therapeutic failures) or an issue about psychological forces and carried it as far as he could in terms of theory, starting afresh if a different set of observations or ways of thinking seemed desirable. We think his "theory" can best be viewed as a set of orienting principles, which in certain areas quite closely follows observations and in other instances involves frank speculation.

Freud staked out several nuclear points of view in order to explain psychological life.[8] He divided his theory into (1) economic concepts, (2) dynamic concepts, and (3) topographic concepts (the "regions" of the mind) that were later largely superseded by his structure theory (the id, ego, superego). In other words, for Freud, a complete description of any behavior would involve statements describing the psychic energies involved: their mode and economy of discharge (economic concepts); the psychobiological forces and reactions determining or "driving" behavior (dynamic concepts); the relationship of these unconscious forces to the preconscious and conscious processes, which oppose the press of drive derivatives for discharge (topographic concepts); and the intrapsychic organizations, which function to shape behavior (structural concepts).

Dynamic concepts deal with the interaction of forces that lead to behavioral expression or to conflict. Freud postulated that drives were such forces and comprised the most important determinants of behavior. Originally, he divided instincts into the self-preservative drives and the sex drives and later combined these into Eros (instincts of love and life—the tendency to unity), and counterposed Eros to the aggressive instincts of Thanatos (the forces of death, destruction, and dissolution). For Freud, drives referred to basic tendencies that have a psychic force. The drives provide the ultimate impetus for behavior, and their mode of operation basically molds the operations of behavior. The drives are the "psychical correlates" of somatic pressures. They represent ". . . the demands made upon the mind for work in consequence of its connection with the body." The drives evoke activity to reduce their pressure and have the aim of discharge and satisfaction. Where drive and object are rigidly attached, there is "fixation."

Freud came to the critical conclusion that what was most variable about a drive was its object. He derived this (perhaps now obvious) conclusion from examining the wide variations of sexuality (homosexuality, fetishes, or the range of special preferences that everyone shows in sexual life). A variety of "accidental" (experiential or environmental) factors in development could come to link a drive, such as the sexual drive, and an object. A "complementary series" consisting of experience and endowment would codetermine and condition behavior. The instinctual forces could be in a conflict or at odds with forces serving self preservation and the demands of society. The bulk of these conflicts are unconscious. The instincts may also undergo "vicissitudes": fusions of love and hate or modifications, or "taming," making them socially acceptable and desirable, which Freud called sublimation.

Sexuality, for Freud, comprised a range of bodily activities that were integrated at maturity into genital sexuality. A child's "auto-erotic" strivings for pleasure with his own body and his search for pleasure from parents and peers would color his adult "object relationships." Each stage of this development would prepare for the next, and fixations of interests or fears at various developmental stages could leave their mark on adult behavior. Freud referred to this biography of the sexual and aggressive instincts as *psychosexual development;* he observed some of this development and inferred much of it from his analytic work with patients. The infant's first pleasure interests are centered around intraorganismic needs: interactions that provide food, bodily stability, and comfort. The chief organ of pleasure is the mouth, hence, the *oral period* of development. As the infant develops the capacity for discrimination, he begins to cope with objects about him as having first an existence dependent only upon his bodily satisfactions and frustrations, and later an existence independent of them. The first two years are dominated by incorporative activities (passive and aggressive oral strivings) and gradually an infant develops a capacity for delay and for controlling the anal and urethral sphincters. Interest in these functions becomes the center of pleasure, attack, conflict, and, eventually, of mastery, and these concerns and their derivatives color the total behavior of the period. Freud named this phase the *anal period,* after the instinctual investment in the dominant zone for pleasure and mastery. This is followed by an immature genital or phallic interest and excitement, with strong attachments of the child to the parent of the opposite sex. In the *phallic phase,* the child fantasies importance for himself and his wishes to possess the parent. He also exaggerates his fears of abandonment and punishment for his ambitions ("castration anxiety") and is mortified about failures to meet requirements he is not equipped to fulfill. As he gives up his attachment to his fantasies of domination of his parents, there is a resolution of the "Oedipus complex." The child learns to exercise internal controls. Play, work, and learning with peers become dominant. After this phase of relative drive "latency," the mature sexual instinct develops in puberty. The broad outline of some of these developments (which we shall review more extensively in later chapters) is gradually being revised by detailed and reliable observational data. That childish sexual theories and notions persist in adult life is inescapable from clinical observation. We doubt, however, that the dual instinct theory has much—apart from orientation—to contribute to the theory of the future.

Economic aspects of psychoanalytic theory are comprised of highly abstruse hunches concerning the fundamental modes of operation and distribution of psychic energies. The energy of the sex instinct is called libido; the energy of the aggressive instinct has been termed by some authors destrudo. Libido invested in the self and the body was called narcissistic libido. In assuming that psychic energy is constant and that organisms strive to keep excitation low (constancy principle), Freud not only sought an ultimate explanation of why behavior "behaves" but treated psychic energy according to principles similar to the first and second thermodynamic laws. The damming up of psychic energy causes pain and tension (and perhaps activates mental and behavioral events); the release of energy produces pleasure or gratification. Basically, human beings act according to this "*pleasure principle,*" by which Freud meant tension reduction, although sometimes he also referred to consciously felt pleasure. As they grow up, under the exigencies of their environment, human beings act increasingly according to the "*reality principle,*" which requires the postponement of satisfactions and the temporary tolerance of pain. Freud considered the tendency to repeat the same thing—the *repetition compulsion*—as an expression of the death instinct (fundamentally a notion related to entropy). He derived this from the observation of the remarkable persistence of neurotic and self-destructive behaviors, as well as the difficulty most adults have in establishing new behavior patterns.

In his lighter moods, Freud referred to various of these deductions as "our mythology." A number of analysts and behavioral scientists have discarded the libido theory and inferences about energy, some because the laws regulating psychic energy could not possibly conform to those of physical energy. There are others whose pragmatic bent did not require such broad explanatory assumptions and who see notions of instincts as prime movers, as prescientific and unnecessary. Finally, there are some who, perhaps uncomfortable with the emphasis on sexuality, hope to diminish the observationally derived significance of this component in behavior by dismissing its theoretical underpinnings.

Freud used the term primary process in part to characterize the energic processes in instinctual activity, their fluidity, and their press for immediate discharge, as in the kaleidoscopic images of dreams. Secondary processes (thought to be characterized by binding rather than ready displacement of highly mobile energies) became dominant in the course of development; they are reality-oriented and underlie what general psychology calls higher mental processes. In some of his writings, Freud speaks of primary and secondary process thinking. He described *primary process thinking* as impervious to the categories of time, causality, and logic. Hence it is highly plastic, sensory, and drive-dominated; essentially it is wishful and imaginal thinking "short-cutting" reality. *Secondary process thinking* corresponds to the reality-oriented and categorical thinking of mature adults. Dominance of primary process thinking is characteristic of dreams, many forms of abnormal behavior and also, to a certain extent, of humor, play, art, literature, and music. What Freud said about the laws that govern primary and secondary process cuts across the dynamic, economic, and structural divisions of his theory. Perhaps they should be conceived of as a continuum of modes of organization of thought.

TOPOGRAPHIC CONCEPTS Freud asserted that not everything that is mental is conscious. His reasoning reveals the breadth of factors—biological as well as perceptual—that for him constituted mental life. He noted that somatic activities, unlike conscious events, occur continuously, so that consciousness cannot be the whole story. Just as physiologists were coming to view nonconscious reflexes as consequential for integrated behavior, Freud viewed non-conscious somatic activities as having a psychic or mental consequence. The mental value of unconscious activities has to be discovered by inference and translated into the language of conscious life. For example, he noted the patient might say one thing but behave as if he meant something else; the "as if" component represented the force of unconscious drives. Both what is noted (or conscious) and what can become noticed (or preconscious) were influenced by the driving pattern of the unconscious forces.[4] Thoughts and memories could be organized according to a logical frame of reference but also according to a drive frame of reference. Forces of the unconscious, pressing for expression, and the counterforces of the preconscious, censoring what was coming to the surface, were said to determine the content of cognized mental events such as dreams and associations. This, then, is the topographic theory—the theory of "regions of the mind" operating as dynamic systems.

It should be noted that Freud, with his notion of drive derivatives, brought together aspects of behavior that the psychologists, with compartmentalized "faculties," had been unable to interrelate. Thus, for Freud, acts, wishes, fantasies, subjective perceptions, images, dreams, and symptoms—and their occurrence in childhood as well as adulthood—were parts of a whole scheme. Freud thereby contributed to a new view of mental functions by emphasizing the role of wishes and impulses—the role of drive organization—in perception, thought, motor action, and memory.[52]

STRUCTURAL CONCEPTS Freud had focused upon demonstrating unconscious drive organization in a wide range of behaviors. But existence of drives demands some structure to implement their press and aim. It also became clear that much of our highly organized ability to cope with conflicts occurs automatically, and without consciousness. Not only drives, but defenses are unconscious. Therefore, "the unconscious" cannot be the repository solely for drives. Structure theory was advanced—largely replacing the topographic theory—to deal with enduring functions and modes of organization of instincts (the id) and of the steering and controlling functions (the ego and superego). Consciousness was reserved as a quality pertaining to some but not all of the ego and superego functions. Robert Waelder has rightly emphasized Freud's observation that what the analyst calls id, ego, and superego can operationally be differentiated only when there is conflict.[68]

Id is thought of as the innate reservoir of instincts and totally unconscious; it blindly drives, and it is known by its effects, and not directly. *Ego* refers to that organization of psychological functions that structures the external and internal world for the individual. It mediates adaptive internal adjustments, overt response, and environmental demands. It provides psychological regulation of the senses and motor apparatus; through the ego, we are somewhat independent both of our sense organs and our wishes. Through its cognitive and "executive" and synthetic functions, it is involved in: integrations of perception, thought, feeling, drive, and action; facilitating or inhibiting gratification of appetitive needs; and in protecting the organism from unbearable affects and dangerous impulses through defense mechanisms. The ego should not be confused with the neurological sensorimotor system (although there must be some bridge that has yet to be conceptually built); rather it represents psychological sorting and controlling mechanisms, which—according to Heinz Hartmann—serve adaptation.[34] In human beings, adaptive aims often are in conflict with instinctual aims.

The third major organization of the psychic apparatus is the *superego*, which is the largely unconscious counterpart of conscience. This organization internalizes reward and punishment and thereby delays impulsiveness. This involves a process by which the child comes to possess, if not the parents (as he wished at the height of the Oedipal strivings) at least the attributes of the parents. He *identifies* with them or their expectations in order to control instincts and to win, instead of constant attention and gratification, at least approval; this develops into self-approval and self-esteem, or self-punishment and guilt. Freud called the superego the "heir" to the unreasonable demands of the Oedipus complex. Inner standards and goals are called the *ego ideal.* These internalized controls are at first black and white, harsh and, in any case, closely reflect the lack of modification and judgment and the intensity of the drives that evoke such controls. The logic of such punishment follows the talion principle (an eye for an eye) and the rule of magical thinking prevails (a bad thought is equivalent to the deed). The organization of the superego continues to develop throughout life, its strictures modified and goals enlarged in accordance with reality. But the earliest patterns of demand and control may persist without awareness, leading to overly strict, unbearable, and maladaptive controls. Superego lacunae, or the suspension of controls, may occur. A person then persists in asserting the rights of infancy—to have given to oneself what one wants exactly when and how one wants it.

Defenses describe various mental operations that cope with painful, dangerous, and conflicting experiences. Descriptively, that which cannot be coped with is repressed and kept out of consciousness; dynamically, this is an activity of the ego in response to the signal of anxiety. "Signal anxiety" evoking defenses was the ego's way of warding off dissolution and overwhelming helplessness. A number of ways of avoiding or detoxifying the meaning of unpleasant and dangerous wishes or events have been described. Freud observed that these defenses did not rob a conflict of its power to influence behavior, and "the return of the repressed" could be observed as a determinant of dreams or of symptoms—various compromises by which the ego rendered tolerable that which could not otherwise be integrated or handled; a fear of a wish to show off might be expressed as a phobia for crowds and travel. Such attempts to put a distance between forbidden impulses and their expression are neurotic symptoms, compromises that contain a reference to —are in touch with—both the impulse and the reaction against it. These mechanisms will be discussed in subsequent chapters.

Freud's loyal followers contributed to further systematization of the structure theory, bringing wider ranges of data into focus. Freud's daughter, Anna, documented the various mechanisms of defense that are generally accepted by students of abnormal psychology as descriptively apt.[20] From the biological and social sciences, Hartmann brought broad viewpoints into analysis to show that not all the products of psychological development derive from conflict or solely for the satisfaction of instincts.[28] He advanced the notion of conflict-free areas of the ego and rudimentary ego functions that have an autonomy and maturation of their own. This fundamental concept made it possible for analytic theory to consider a wide range of determining factors and operations other than drive. Yet psychoanalysis did not develop an explicit learning theory. Perhaps the closest to it (apart from the notion of identifications of the child with the parent) was Hartmann's notion of neutralization. By this, he implied that drives—particularly aggression—may be de-energized and "bound energy" can become readily available to the ego for its coping and synthetic functions. In other words, the ego has the equipment for acquiring information but is not entirely independent from the drives in so doing; nevertheless, the laws determining this acquisition are obscure.

Psychoanalytic theory thus first explored the patient's conflict with reality, then focused upon the drive component in the organization of behavior, and finally moved to account for the interaction of drive and the steering and coping functions of the ego, which was now viewed as the internal and dynamic representation of reality. This shifted therapeutic emphasis from an exclusive preoccupation with uncovering hidden meanings of behavior to equal attention to modes of coping and adapting. It also led to some confluence of interest between academic and psychoanalytic psychology, especially in the areas of thought, attention, learning, and memory. Erik H. Erikson acknowledged the role of specific social patterns and worked out a psychosocial scheme of development that interlocks with the psychosexual scheme delineated by Freud.[15] David Rapaport and Merton M. Gill noted that Freud's work contained genetic and adaptive points of view and added these to the dynamic, economic, and structural propositions in an attempt to complete the groundwork and provide the basic dimensions by which analysts can study and explain behavior.[53] Thus modern psychoanalysis is not satisfied to be a psychology of the unconscious, but attempts to provide a most general and comprehensive theory of psychological phenomena. This aim manifests itself not only in the emphasis on ego psychology by classical analysts and neoanalysts and in Erikson's attempt to bridge the intrapsychic and social aspects of behavior, but also in the stress on the concept of object relations by W. Ronald D. Fairbairn.[17]

It is possible that psychoanalysis would be better served by fitting its data into a more open behavioristic scheme, so avoiding premature theoretical systematization. There is doubt in the minds of many, including the authors, whether the structure theory, and especially its intricacies, constitutes real progress over Freud's earlier thoughts.[52] At best it seems to be a mixed blessing. Any theory of behavior requires the assumption of enduring structures and of mechanisms coordinating component parts; but whether the strict divisions into id, ego, and superego will further advance knowledge is doubtful. These concepts are easily highly reified—almost as if they were actors on the stage of psychic drama—and this can retard as well as simplify knowledge of how behavior is, in fact, put together and organized. The concept of id in particular—as a cauldron of unconscious, untamed innate drives—is almost untranslatable into a behavioristic system. Fundamental differences of drive behavior, discriminating and controlling behaviors, exist and must be accounted for, but their impetus and linkages are only roughly comprehended in animistic terms.

Some of Freud's followers feel that nothing he wrote should be omitted, revised, or questioned. Nevertheless, there is a continuous movement to sharpen the formulations and extend the observations of analysis. The violent attacks by those who thought Freud undermined morality appear absurd today. In our opinion, the methods and data of psychoanalysis, and the dimensions of behavior revealed by it, are of more lasting importance than its supertheories. While highly subjective (rendering predictive or postdictive verification difficult), these methods and the most important data of analysis have stood the test of time for about seventy years. A thorough grasp of psychoanalytic method and, consequently, of psychoanalytic data will often be found to be absent among both friend and foe of psychoanalysis. Critics attack, overly enthusiastic experimentalists' "test" straw men, and spurious issues are provided not only by easy misreadings of Freud and avoiding direct experience with the method, but by all too correctly reading theories advanced by some Freudian practitioners. The chief problem in communication has been to translate the theoretical jargon and shorthand into explicit behavioral data—something experienced analysts do automatically but rarely patiently and publicly. An appreciation of the contingent nature of Freud's theoretical formulations, and a greater exposure to the facts of psychoanalytic observation and the method by which they are determined, should lead to a more operational approach than that which characterizes what Arthur Koestler called the Freudian Infantry, in contradistinction to Freud and his serious students.

The "Dissident" Psychoanalytic Schools

Jung, Adler, Rank, and the so-called Neo-Freudians, had original ideas of their own and also reacted critically—and sometimes overcritically—to limitations of analytic theory or therapy. Wilhelm Stekel once wishfully remarked that a dwarf on the shoulders of a giant might see further than the giant. Certain neoanalytic concepts have touched on soft spots of the classical theory and extended our knowledge.[46] These concepts are of intrinsic interest; it should also be recognized that they serve to justify various departures from Freud's therapeutic methods.

Carl C. Jung's complex theory of personality, which we will mention briefly, seems closer to archaeology, history, literature, and mythology than to the concerns of clinical psychiatrists. Some of his observations, especially those on the extroverted and introverted personality types, are widely accepted today, and his description of "archetypes" has attracted a good deal of attention. Such archetypes are certain images of man, as the good and omnipotent father or God, the bad father or devil, the bad mother or witch, the wise man, the tragic hero, and the like. They are living heritages containing a record of basic strivings from the past of mankind. For Jung, the unconscious is not an individual, but a collective characteristic, determined by the experiences of countless past generations. Unfortunately, many of Jung's penetrating observations seem lost in lush and dark mysticism.[33] His therapy, in part, is aimed at helping the patient recognize his primitive wishes in the context of larger philosophic schemes.

Alfred Adler's "individual psychology," although not a systematic theory, stressed such concepts as organ inferiority and inferiority complex, which evokes striving for support, power and dominance, and in women, "masculine protest"—a wish to be like a man.[2] Individuals develop unique goals, styles of life, and coping methods. Psychotherapy is a re-education, and neurosis is based on faulty compensatory devices and is responsive to cultural factors. Adler's ideas found general acceptance in our culture, but in their detailed presentation they had limited appeal for scientists and therapists. *Otto Rank*'s contribution to theory was small; it is his active therapeutic approach rather than speculations about birth trauma which has been widely incorporated by many psychotherapists.[51] *Melanie Klein* will be remembered for her imaginative therapeutic approaches and for some of her assumptions about mental operations in infants and adults.[35] Her conceptions of the universal importance of the paranoid and depressive attitude of the infant and of good and bad introjects (fantasies and primitive perceptions of parents) are penetrating psychological models and, in this sense, of lasting value. *Karen Horney* took issue with the libido theory and was an early advocate of a characterological concept of neurosis, which considers basic anxiety and rage as learned traits that stand in the way of growth and self-realization.[29] She stressed cultural determinants and kept a keen clinical focus in her various writings. *Erich Fromm* emphasizes cultural conditions as responsible for neurotic development;[22] he elaborated on Karl Marx's concept of alienation. Fromm views alienation as a result of a capitalistic marketing orientation, creating goals and practices that estrange one from one's own needs. The assembly line, for example, removes the worker from his product and isolates him from other producers and consumers. Fromm's therapeutic orientation is strongly influenced by what he, as well as many great men throughout history, consider the basic needs of mankind: to free individuals from primitive bonds, to help individuals to discover freedom, reason, love, and productivity. A socialist and idealist, Fromm's works are marked by a missionary note.

Harry Stack Sullivan (1892–1949) based his "interpersonal" theories on clinical work.[66] Eluding summary, his writing is brilliant, complex, and evocative. His impact came through his students, for whom he broadened both concepts and approaches to therapy. Many of his ideas are strikingly similar to Freud's basic concepts: around critical bodily zones and activities there are interactions with significant objects, the experience of which sets up modes of communication both to the self and others. Sullivan sees the human infant as helpless. For the satisfaction of his basic drives, the infant interacts with other people, particularly the "mothering one." If satisfaction is absent, tension and anxiety, rather than security, result. The behavioral rather than instinctual aspect of internal states (for example, anxiety and security) are stressed: anxiety or related emotions in the mother, evoked by the infant's response, are empathically relayed back to the child. This results in a structuring of insecurity and anxiety into behaviors that are meaningful and mutually regulating or disruptive. Sullivan calls the earliest communication of such interpersonal relationships *prototaxic;* when gestures and linguistic symbols convey the messages, he speaks of *a syntactic mode.* Uncommunicative, misleading, and unintelligible messages are called *parataxic.* If the child's responses are met with anxiety, the child considers such reaction as a reflection of his own lack of worth and arrives at the concept of the "bad me." If such experiences are very strong and painful, the child reacts with dissociation and finally with elimination of his self-boundary, a state Sullivan called the "not me." "Bad me" and "not me" become the matrix for deviations that lead to neuroses and schizophrenia. Sullivan also paid considerable attention to the importance of authority figures (for example, parents, teachers) and culture (also represented by parents and teachers). If the demands of culture and authority are not too severe, hypocritical, and "degrading" normal development ensues. If they are excessive, the child learns to deceive authority and also himself, which leads to "malevolent transformation." When parents are too severe, too weak, or too inconsequential, their behavior is not responsive to the process of building meaning, and socialization is impaired. A child thus handicapped may not be prepared for the constructive experience of intimacy in homoerotic relationships of puberty. This, in turn, may prevent the adolescent and young adult from experiencing intimacy in heterosexual relationships. If difficulty in adult relationships arises, the individual will revert to earlier "dynamisms," or habitual modes of coping. Some of these dynamisms, such as obsessionalism, selective inattention, dissociative emotionality, and paranoid mechanisms, occur in all persons. In mentally ill persons these dynamisms become extreme, dominant, and lasting. Sullivan's focus on communication and feedback processes in interpersonal behavior, on the behavioral rather than instinctual meaning of subjective experience, provides a ready grip upon the determining role of subtle but objectifiable transactions in behavior—an approach toward which many developments in psychiatry (family therapy) in one way or another appear to be moving.

Developments in Psychology and Physiology and Their Impact on Psychiatry

As a dynamic depth psychology developed, where was general psychology? Until the last sixty years, it was almost exclusively preoccupied with the elementary data of introspection—sensation, perception, and their physiological underpinnings. In spite of the work of Charles Darwin, Herbert Spencer, and Jean Baptiste de Monet Lamarck, psychology tended to ignore the continuities and similarities between man and animal, as well as psychopathology and the autogenesis of human behavior. After 1860, experimental techniques were increasingly applied to such processes as memory and association. Kraepelin, more than others in psychiatry, paid attention to the contributions of the new experimental psychology. Around the time of Freud's early work, there began to emerge a school that studied mental "acts" as well as mental contents—the act of seeing the color as well as the particular color seen. Judging, accepting, rejecting, wishing, and the like, were recognized to be just as "mental" as perceptions were; stable expectancies or attitude or "sets" became objects of investigation. In brief, the factors that structure psychological reality for an individual were becoming important for academic psychology. After 1900, motivation was brought into psychology by William McDougall and others. Robert S. Woodworth, later a professor at Columbia University, dubbed this "dynamic psychology" around 1910. The notion that behavior is not the sum of isolated or irreducible elements, but rather consists of configurations of events in a context, developed out of various movements in both Gestalt psychology (introduced into psychiatry by Kurt Goldstein[24] and Paul Schilder[60]) and biology. These movements undoubtedly influenced psychiatry, but they did not have the momentum or impact of Freud's work, which, free of academic strictures, grew more directly out of clinical concerns. Until the beginning of this century, the reflex was left largely to neurologists until Ivan P. Pavlov in Russia and Edward L. Thorndike, Robert M. Yerkes (and, much later, J. B. Watson) in America, created a new approach to the study of behavior by discovering and exploring the conditionability of reflexes and of behavior in general. This development in physiology and experimental psychology has become of increasing importance in its influence upon psychiatry.

Pavlov's Contribution

More than anyone else, the genius of Ivan Petrovich Pavlov (1849–1936) extended the horizons of our knowledge of the brain and behavior.[49] Pavlov was born in Ryazan, Russia, the son of a village priest. He studied first in a theological seminary and later at the University of St. Petersburg. In his early career as a physiologist, he explored circulation and innervation of the heart. "The Work of the Digestive Glands" was awarded the Nobel Prize in 1904 when he had already shifted his attention to a new career announced in a lecture, "Experimental Psychology and Psychopathology in Animals." Pavlov was strongly influenced by the father of Russian physiology, I. M. Sechenov, who was one of the first to propagate the idea that all behavior is controlled by the brain and may be explained by physiological methods. A contemporary, the outstanding neuropsychiatrist, V. M. Bekhterev (1857–1927), and

Pavlov had violent quarrels, although their ideas show considerable similarity. In "teaching" the salivary gland to respond to a bell, Pavlov established the momentous concept of the conditioned reflex as the material (not spiritual!) link between the environment, the central nervous system, and behavior. Instead of inputs being linked solely by mentalistic phenomena (ideas, images), a property of protoplasm was responsible, and this could be objectified, even in lower animals. The animal's "perception" would no longer be inferred but be known by the objectifiable relationship of stimulus and response, which depended on intact cortical tissue. Pavlov "supplied a body to the mind." [54] For Pavlov, psychic phenomena were distinguished from the physiological only "in degree of complexity." Later, he extended his ingenious experiments to observations of conflicting reflexes and was able to produce experimental disintegration of behavior—"neuroses"—in dogs. In his theoretical expositions he used the concepts of nervous inhibition and excitation in a complex theory of behavior and nervous activity.

Pavlov became interested in language and symbolic processes. He thereby entered the field of human psychology and, at the age of eighty, asserted that his main concepts were directly applicable to human behavior disorders. Pavlov was a notably astute observer but—as Freud—he was at times carried away by his creative originality and enthusiasm. From some of his statements one gets the impression that he was less adamant about his theories than some of his clinical followers, especially after his system was adopted as the foundation of psychiatry in the Communist countries. Pavlov was acclaimed by the Bolshevik government which, with a Marxist-materialistic ideology, welcomed the stress on brain and environment. Initially he disclaimed Communism and only gradually changed his views.

The Pavlovian system is a comprehensive deterministic theory of the brain and behavior based largely on experimental rather than on clinical evidence. The concept of the reflex is basic. Reflex, as Pavlov understood it, is not the elementary reflex of the neurophysiologist, but rather a behavioral stimulus-response sequence with afferent, central, and efferent segments. The *unconditioned reflex*—for example, salivation as a response to the presence of food in the mouth, is innate; the *conditioned reflex* is based on a linkage of a *conditioning stimulus* (a bell) with the *unconditioned stimulus* (food), and the conditioned stimulus can evoke a similar bodily response as food. One basic assumption was that the presence of cortex is necessary for the establishment of conditioned reflexes. Isolation of cortical from other cerebral activity was considered an important element in the causation of behavior disorders. Pavlov expressed the idea that cortical excitation and inhibition are responsible for the occurrence of unconditioned and conditioned responses. He distinguished between various types of conditioned and unconditioned excitation and inhibitions. One type of inhibition is neuroparadoxical inhibition by overload or response to extreme stress, which he considered particularly important in human behavior disorders. He conceived of sleep and also of hypnosis as general states of inhibition of the central nervous system. In general, operational definitions of such postulated brain processes have not been forthcoming.

He succeeded in producing experimental neuroses in dogs by conditioning them first to different sets of stimuli that evoked either food-seeking behavior or pain-avoidance. In the second phase of the experiment, the stimuli for these incompatible responses were made more and more alike and finally indistinguishable. The behavior of these dogs then resembled some aspects of human neuroses. The animals no longer performed previously learned skills, were disturbed on entering the experimental room, showed appetite changes, and the like. After rest, retraining, and administration of sedatives and stimulants, these experimental neuroses could be "cured." Pavlovian psychiatrists claim that these experiments are a basic model for the etiology and treatment of human neuroses.

Pavlov also noted that different dogs reacted differently to the stress of conditioning. These observations led him to assume different constitutional types, which he extended to human beings, reviving the Hippocratic divisions of cholerics, sanguinics, phlegmatics, and melancholics, and adding an artistic and a meditative type. With each type, he associated characteristic psychopathological traits. To Western clinical psychiatrists, these classifications and certain generalizations about hysterical and paranoid types appear to be rather naïve and not particularly useful.

One of the cornerstones of Pavlovian theory is the differentiation of the first and second signal systems. The *first signal system* is the totality of all internal and environmental stimuli to which animals respond with unconditioned and conditioned reflexes. Man, however, has developed a *second signal system*, consisting of signs that stand for the stimuli of the first signal system. The second signal system is essentially a system processing symbols akin to Freud's secondary processes.

The Pavlovian system is an impressive attempt to bridge the areas of the psychosocial and the neurophysiological with both objective techniques and supertheory. To Western clinicians, the Pavlovian theoretical system is bold but is usually considered not sufficiently close either to the clinical or to the neurophysiological data it is supposed to explain. Actually, most stimulus-response schemes of behavior do not adequately account for the self-structuring, directive, and integrative aspects of behavior. American behavior theory and Western neurophysiology profited from Pavlov's observations, but developed along different lines. Recently, there has been an interesting approximation of Western physiological psychology and Eastern physiology of higher nervous activities as exemplified by the work of Jerzy Konorski.[36] Some of Pavlov's students have extended his principles to many facets of corticovisceral relationships (relevant to psychosomatic medicine), to an exploration of the growth and development of human beings and animals, and to conditioning of semantic and higher processes. It seems that even in the Communist countries the influence of Pavlovian theory on psychiatry has decreased. On the other hand, this fundamental experimental approach to the functions of the central nervous system and social learning has been heuristically valuable for our field and incalculably important to the behavioral sciences.

Neurophysiological Contributions

Neurophysiology, advanced through the work of Edgar D. Adrian,[2] Charles S. Sherrington,[61] and others had a definite impact on psychiatry. The broad impact of modern biological thinking of such men as Walter B. Cannon[11] and Ludwig von Bertalanffy[5] is exemplified in the liberal use of such concepts as adaptation and "open systems." The brain can now be pictured as having the complexity that careful observation of behavioral arrays and their interactions would predict. For example, the complexities of passiveness, excitement, fierceness, and orality in mating behavior have a neuroanatomical and neurophysiological interrelationship in the limbic system[39] mapped by Paul MacLean as the "visceral brain." Degrees of awareness may be explained by shifts in the activity of reticular activating systems with their activation of both peripheral motor and cortical cells.[40] Processes of learning and component sequences of emotional behavior have been studied with implanted electrodes. From the effect of tranquilizers, it is clear that behaviors previously thought to be inevitably linked are fractionable, for example, sedation without drowsiness. Neural systems that maintain either reward or aversive behavior are systems that affect the motivational but not the motoric aspect of behavior; the self-stimulation experiments by James Olds provide a demonstration of almost pure directional and regulatory activity within the brain.[47] In brief, the organization of known behaviors, inferred mechanisms, and overlooked behavioral and organismic states, for example, sleeping, waking, and dreaming, have begun to be revealed.

It has been clear throughout this chapter that everyone has his commonsense notion of "cause," of how the body and brain work to bring about events. "Pure" psychological theories attempt to circumvent the question by not speaking openly about such assumptions. Yet neurobehavioral facts as well as subjective experience provide essential information about the organization of behavior and are important to psychiatry, both for providing models and analogies ("conceptual nervous systems") and for demonstrating mechanisms that define limits. Although chided for "neurologizing behavior," some behaviorists nevertheless advance new "models" of brain as new facts emerge and, at least, make their thinking explicit. Freud's unpublished "project" was a construction of a nervous system that could perform important psychological activities, and it heralded his later work with analysis.[21]

The newer drugs and neurophysiological techniques have given impetus to study of the neurochemical organization of behavior, and psychiatrists should realize that there are limits beyond which a change in brain chemistry is consequential for behavior. For example, Sebastian P. Grossman could selectively initiate either eating or drinking behavior by injecting microquantities of specific autonomic agents in the lateral hypothalamus,[26] and various components of sexual behavior have been similarly elicited with hormones. Changes in the metabolism of endogenous brain substances are evoked with psychoactive drugs, and these studies indicate that small local changes in brain chemistry may have profound general effects.[19] The fact that psychiatric syndromes may be composed of numerous different pathophysiologic processes is widely accepted and often forgotten. There is a possibility that some disorders will be found attributable primarily to an altered neurochemistry.

Developmental Approaches

Developmental approaches derived from biology and psychology have become important; among them are Heinz Werner's interesting observations. Werner's developmental theories are not as widely known in psychiatry as in psychology.[69] Following the thinking of Darwin and Herbert Spencer, he characterized developmental levels, starting from the undifferentiated whole and proceeding to differentiation into parts and integration of interdependent parts. Differentiation, followed by integration, can occur in longitudinal development or with "microgenesis" in the contemporaneous development of a thought or perception. Regression is characterized by primitivization and "physiognomic" mentation, where perception of form is personalistic and has animistic qualities. The rules articulating the coordination of elements at various levels of organization in ontogenesis, psychopathology, or in primitive and advanced cultures, and the role of bodily adjustments in perception and cognition have been a focus for Werner's work, which psychiatry has yet to fully exploit.

Jean Piaget has provided remarkable and important documentation of the growth of the child's organization of reality and concepts of space, causality, and time.[50] He evolved ingenious clinical tests and a scheme to account for the assimilation of meaning from the environment and the growth of thought structures. Psychiatrists have recently been introduced to him through the writings of Elwyn J. Anthony[3] and Peter Wolff.[72] His investigations have stimulated workers in child development as well as serious students of cognitive processes in man.

Experimentalists have identified "critical periods" in the growth of animals during which deprivations (for example of "stimulation") have biological and behavioral consequences at later phases of life (often but not always maladaptive). Similarly, critical periods for the suppression or de-suppression of various enzymes important for function and metabolism have been noted, and both biochemical and conditioning studies of embryonic development show that behavior reactive to the milieu can begin *in utero*. Specification of the operative mechanisms in genetics should lead to clearer understanding of points in which the interaction between nature and nurture can be crucial. A number of mental deficiencies have been differentiated on the basis of enzymatic defects, many of which control amino acid metabolism. These have activated a search for biochemical determinants of other behavioral disorders. In general, however, psychiatrists are attracted to broad psychobiological schemes that seem to sanction current clinical theories rather than to detailed studies. While an experimental approach is increasingly applied to many problems arising from clinical experience, experimental psychology and biology are yet to be integrated into clinical psychiatry.

David A. Hamburg has forcefully stressed the importance for psychiatry of an evolutionary point of view and pointed to the significance of ethology, the science that studies the behavior of animals in their natural habitat.[27] Konrad Lorenz and others have traced the development of major drive behaviors in many species. The obvious and not so obvious similarities between ontogenesis and phylogenesis ought to remind us constantly in our clinical work that *we* are—as Lorenz put it—the "missing link." [38] Comparative studies permit an insight about the articulation of neurobehavioral components into the sequences of complex behavior we study at the human level.

Learning Theories and Psychiatry

John Dollard and Neal E. Miller made perhaps the most ambitious and thorough attempt to link learning theory with clinical phenomena.[14] For them, a stimulus or cue as well as capacity for response must exist to make learning possible. There must be drive and reward for response, and theoretically the primary reward is the reduction of drive. Rewards in the ordinary sense of the word—secondary rewards—will allow for complexities in behavior. Punishment is either the prevention of drive reduction or the administration of a painful stimulus. Another basic concept is generalization, seen clinically, for example, in transference. Extinction is the disappearance of a response when not customarily rewarded. Drives can be reinforced or inhibited. If a cue evokes fear, then fear rather than corrective stimuli mediates behaving. Symptoms are acquired to reduce tension; for example, a phobic response of avoidance will *relatively* diminish the anxiety provoked by confrontation with danger. The theory does not adequately explain important clinical phenomena such as self-destruction, and self-punitive and masochistic trends in man. Many symptoms are apparently learned and unlearned in single-trial learning, and this cannot easily be accounted for by classical theories, although Miller has advanced interesting approaches to these problems (including the role of competition of inputs of new information as well as timing and prior equilibriums in determining response).[45] The naming of constructs such as anxiety or drive is, of course, less consequential than defining conditions under which behavior is predictably changed, and this is better developed in animal than human studies. Hans J. Eysenck,[17] Joseph Wolpe,[73] and others have advocated simple therapeutic approaches of conditioning, which, although welcome, are so far not particularly impressive. The approach is restricted by problems similar to that of other psychotherapies—simply naming a process deconditioning or abreaction does not identify the operative factors.

The approach of B. F. Skinner's students in operant conditioning is interesting to clinical psychiatry because of their concern with the history of the individual organism in its response to environmental contingencies.[63] The organism tends to operate directly or indirectly upon the environment, which, in turn, tends to structure its behavior; learning is transactional. The laboratory rat strikes a lever on a predetermined schedule and "makes" the experimenter reward him. Because the organism operates upon the environment, the structure of the milieu can preferentially "shape" behaviors; it cannot "implant" them. It is the law of effect, the consequence of behavior upon the environment, the changing of it, which is reinforcing to the operating organism, not a stimulus "evoking" a response. The psychotherapist might be viewed according to this psychology, as a non-punishing audience providing occasional positive reinforcements when desirable responses occur; his general lack of activity ("acceptance") should lead to extinction of responses that represent undesirable behavior. Acquisition of new behavior depends on prior behavior and present contingencies; it proceeds best with rewards and if the introduction of new material is made when the organism calls for it. Such material is offered in small and explicit increments rather than great leaps, points that are quite relevant both to teaching and psychotherapy.

Like other important psychologies, operant conditioning has indicated that behavior is lawful and that both man and animal are subject to these laws. Further, the operational nature implicit in this antitheoretical psychology (which "programs" the conditions for reward by machinery) forces specification of factors that may be controlling response, and it tends to limit reification of intervening variables. Operant procedures have been applied to complex problems, including verbal behavior and perception[23] and, at the least, have clearly demonstrated (as have most experimental approaches) that theorists and often experimentalists tend to be unconscious of the operative factors leading to conclusions perilously called "results."

The psychoanalyst looks behind a symptom or sequence of thought for operations that are determinant; he searches for the covert consequences and goals of the patient's behavior. Over a period of tested observations he comes to be able to specify these; that is, he now "understands." In the same manner most experimentalists, with their procedural stress (control over stimuli), do not take the subject's word for it but rather manipulate variables to see what actually produced a change in behavior; they try to see in terms of contingency and response what the behavior is behaving for. The hard-core

Skinnerians tend to avoid physiological data, in part in a belief that behavior should be studied in its own right. They also avoid with almost phobic intensity those internal environments and organizations that we call motive and that selectively seek environmental reinforcement. How operant conditioning will deal with such complex behavior in man and with self-initiated, self-sustaining sequences of behavior remains to be seen.

The explanatory value of all these approaches varies, but it is clear that psychiatrists can expect that behavioral science methodologies will more and more become a part of their discipline. On the other hand, psychiatrists respond with amusement or annoyance when basic scientists become therapeutic enthusiasts; they may not only forget their basic science, but Socrates' advice to consider the person as well as the method.

The Influence of the Social Sciences

In the social sciences, a theory about the relationship of personality, social systems, and culture was most highly developed by Talcott Parsons;[48] John Spiegel and other psychiatrists brought Parsons' concepts of "role" to the study of families and their interaction, as well as to the therapeutic interaction.[64] The relationship between culture and personality was also explored by the anthropologist Ralph Linton[37] and the psychoanalyst Abram Kardiner,[34] who developed the concept of a basic personality dependent on the culture in which the person lives. Some offshoots of these approaches lead to "diaper-ology" (for example, the "personality of nations" can be described according to whether the infant is swaddled or left free), but the fact that social factors condition behavior and the explicit mechanisms by which this is achieved is of crucial importance to clinical work. Many contributions that are relevant for psychiatry were made by David Riesman.[55] The most important one is his division into inner directed, outer directed, and tradition directed characterological types and their relationships to culture.

The most comprehensive and psychiatrically relevant view of the social psychology of man will be encountered in Erik H. Erikson's work.[16] His are bridging concepts that describe how an individual born into a community internalizes the values of the group and matches his biological and personal needs with the structure of specific environments encountered throughout the crises inherent in development, from infancy to old age. Numerous cross-cultural epidemiological studies have involved sociologists and anthropologists together with psychiatrists in the empirical study of social factors that contribute to the etiology of behavior disorders. A new strong interest in group therapy, family therapy, and the therapeutic impact of the community has further contributed to the liaison between psychiatrist and social scientist. With the emphasis on "community psychiatry" the resources of a wide range of skills and agencies may be employed.

Communication Theories

The business of psychiatry is to attend to its own data and also to remain accessible to knowledge from other disciplines. Generally, psychiatry has accepted different models and methods for viewing behavior when these are absorbed and introduced by psychiatrists. Information and communication theory have had considerable impact on the biological and behavioral sciences. They provide a general language for a wide range of phenomena that deal with the regulated relationships between input and output. Machines capable of goal-directed (and goal-modifying) behavior, servomechanisms such as thermostats, guided missiles, and computers, act "according to purpose." Norbert Wiener has termed the science of international feedback cybernetics, derived from the Greek word for steersman.[71] Such machines receive and process information and control their actions by regulating input. The unit of information—a "bit"—is dimensionless and in a sense permits comparisons of inputs regardless of their material source. Information transfer involves exchange of highly coded patterns in which "significant information" can be defined as *that part of the pattern that is retained in the transfer.*[13] Such exchange of codes and patterns can occur whether we deal with a cog and wheel, a molecule serving as a template to replicate itself, or events at a synapse. It is conceivable that many messages critical to the internal operation and guidance of a behavioral system could occur without keen awareness, and there are a wide range of biological mechanisms from the molecular to the behavioral in which such information transfer could occur.

Some interesting applications of information theory to biological and psychosocial problems have already been undertaken. The neurophysiologist and psychiatrist, Warren McCulloch, brought symbolic logic and information theory to problems of the brain.[43] Herbert A. Simon applied concepts of information theory to behavior. Unfortunately, these mathematical essays are difficult to grasp for the average psychiatrist.[62] The popular presentations by Norbert Wiener,[71] and Karl Deutsch's application of information theory to political behavior[13] are more appropriate introductions. Such attempts—in our opinion, of great interest to psychiatry—promise to provide a different approach to formulating questions, which in turn can lead to better prediction and control of behavior. At least, the new metaphors may help us to view our data in a fresh light. Nonetheless, it will take some time for clinical disciplines to assimilate these developments.

Jurgen Ruesch and Gregory Bateson[57, 58] have applied communication theory to psychiatric problems and feel that this, along with linguistic theory, ego psychology, learning theory, and action theory are converging into a common approach. We concur with this belief. It may be possible to group our data in terms of the monitoring of incoming stimuli, of storing and scanning of signals and transmission of their messages, and the programming of these in the use of outgoing messages to drive and control other sequences. When codes are understood by the receiver, meaning is established. This is a far cry from subjectivistic and intuitional descriptions of behavior. Of course, if one is overly impressed with machines which "think," it should be remembered that the determination of their ultimate purpose depends on their creator—man—which may or may not be relevant to philosophy and theology.

Ruesch and Bateson, differentiating the messages conveyed by language, distinguish language and metalanguage. In metalanguage the use of language is qualified, for example, metalanguage expresses whether a statement is made in play or jest, whether it is to be taken literally or seriously, and the like. In certain behavior disorders, particularly schizophrenia, metalanguage is impaired. Ruesch stresses that in psychosis, nonverbal communication is particularly important, as it is in infancy and early childhood. An impressive number of psychiatrists, behavioral scientists, semanticists and linguists deserve credit for bringing the crucial importance of language to the attention of psychiatry, a development that stems from the impressive pioneer work of Edward Sapir and the investigations of Benjamin Lee Whorf.[70] The practical impact of all these developments has been to jar the clinician loose from hackneyed jargon and to force him to view the behavior of his patients afresh and consider the range of significant factors through which behavior is organized.

Some Attempts to Integrate Theories into a Unitary System

A number of thinkers in our field, dissatisfied with existing monolithic theories, have attempted to fuse several theoretical systems. Attempts to integrate learning theory and psychoanalytic propositions have already been mentioned. A similar broad attempt has been made by Jules H. Masserman, who created an integrative theory that embraces neurophysiological, behavioral, and psychoanalytic data derived from experimental and clinical approaches to man and animals.[41] He states four principles: (1) Behavior is motivated by physiological needs. (2) The organism does not react to absolute reality but to its own interpretation of the world (a principle previously stated by Jacob von Uexküll).[67] (3) When goal-directed behavior becomes blocked by external obstacles, the organism develops substitutive methods to reach its goals. (4) If two or more motivations come into conflict the organism experiences mounting tension, and ambiguous, maladaptive, or disorganized behavior may result.

Roy R. Grinker made an interesting attempt to arrive at a unitary theory of man; his theory applies John Dewey's thoughts on the transactional process and utilizes the role concepts of Parsons and Spiegel and the propositions of communications theory and field theory.[25] David McK. Rioch's model of behavior utilized concepts of modern neurophysiology, cybernetics, Sullivanian psychodynamics, and a social field theory.[56] Unfortunately, Rioch has not presented his theories in condensed form, and the student has to glean his thinking from his extensive writings.

Systems theory is based on elements of mathematical, biological, psychological, and socioeconomic theories, and data in support of this approach have been advanced by James G. Miller, Ralph Gerard, Anatol Rapoport, and other investigators at the Michigan Neuropsychiatric Institute.[44] This complex, ambitious theory aims to explain the data of any system—from cell to societies—with language borrowed from biologists, economists, and communications engineers. All systems have subsystems and boundaries or regions where energy or information exchanges take place. Information may be coded or uncoded at input or output. Analogies and mathematical models are widely used. In psychology, the system is the organism—the input, a stimulus; the output, a response. Inputs may be loads and lead to disequilibriums or strains, which, unless equilibrium is restored, produce mental and physical illness or ultimately death. Miller and his associates believe they have not merely invented a new terminology but a system that permits more precise formulations of propositions, laws, and predictions than others. Whether psychiatry will accept and be able to handle systems theory remains to be seen.

Existential Philosophy and Psychiatry

In recent years, psychiatrists have again turned to philosophy. The work of existentialist philosophers has been interpreted and modified by a number of psychiatrists and thus become accessible to the profession.[42] Their holistic and highly subjective theories (or deliberations) embrace a wide variety of rather different approaches. The earlier philosophical foundations were provided by Sören Kierkegaard's and Friedrich W. Nietzsche's rebellion against the reductionist theories of essence. The dilemmas man experiences; his very experience, rather than abstract formulations of it, are stressed. The values and goals men arrive at, the anxieties they cope with, are vividly grasped or suggested in some existential approaches. Contemporary philosophers primarily sparking existential psychiatry are Carl Jaspers, Martin Heidegger and Jean-Paul Sartre. Jaspers, who was influenced by Edmund Husserl, is essentially a phenomenologist; his book on psychopathology is a contribution of lasting importance. Erwin Straus and Eugene Minkowski also should properly be called phenomenologists rather than existentialists. They pursued and developed the detailed phenomenological analysis of Husserl and Jaspers, and they applied their reflections to the analysis of man's perception of time and space, body schema, and the relevance of these concepts for psychiatric disorders. Heidegger's extremely complex and, to the non-philosopher, obscure concepts of being in the world, nothingness, transcendence, and the like, have been introduced into psychiatry by Ludwig Binswanger[6] and

Medard Boss.[7] Binswanger, in a very original way, analyzed life experiences of schizophrenic and manic patients in terms of their existence or being in the world. (See Chapter 14.) Sartre, like Boss, has essayed a fusion of psychoanalysis and existentialism.[59] Among existential philosophers, Sartre seems to be the clearest to non-philosophers, and some of his concepts on freedom and responsibility seem quite relevant for psychiatry, although they hardly form the basis for a psychiatric system. Victor Frankl sees as one of the most important functions of psychiatry its aid to patients in their search for meaning.[18] In our opinion, this exceeds the task of modern psychiatry.

Existential psychiatry has grown into a sizable movement, which even has its own journals; yet few pragmatic psychiatrists can do much with these extremely subjective and introspective concepts, which do not lend themselves to operational analysis. Existential psychiatry admittedly deals with fundamental problems but casts aside the advantages of a scientific approach. It also ignores any biological and developmental consideration. Some consider it philosophic extravagance of psychiatrists who try to solve the very problems of mankind; others see in it a reaction to an alleged bankruptcy of the dominant psychiatric systems. Still others feel that the subjective and radically holistic approach of existential psychiatry is making a positive contribution by avoiding meaningless reductionism, by talking about the world as a man experiences it, and by facing such fundamental issues as the meaning of life and death. We believe, however, that a behavior theory (or non-theory!), to be useful to psychiatry, needs to be closer to the total range of data relevant to the development and structure of behavior than existentialist approaches are.

Recent Advances in Clinical Psychiatry

Between World Wars I and II, organized psychiatry, particularly in North America and the United Kingdom, had begun to change; not only through its academic development but through the expansion of therapeutic interest beyond provision of humane housing for the core psychotic population. By the end of World War II, it was apparent that a large number of casualties were "psychiatric" and that many psychiatrists were able to diagnose these with more acumen than was apparent in the "shell shock" cases of World War I. Psychiatrists in service were able to treat and manage many of the transient behavior disorders with effectiveness and an understanding of the meanings and determinants of symptoms. By 1946, these developments, particularly in the United States, had generated a widespread public interest in behavior disorder, its psychological causes, and its possible cures. This was manifest in the explosive growth of psychiatric residency training programs and the expansion of medical school teaching in psychiatry and its basic sciences. These developments and the public's concern for "readjustment" of returning veterans and their dislocated families, coupled with a new and unexpectedly less parochial leadership of organized psychiatry, led to the large government programs in the United States.

Psychiatry is a practical discipline; diagnostic and therapeutic discoveries by psychiatrists contributed as much to the growth in size, scope, and importance of the specialty as did the development of its basic theories and sciences. Of the new biological techniques, the discovery of the electroencephalogram (EEG), reported in 1929 by Hans Berger (1873–1941)—a neuropsychiatrist—was particularly fruitful. Some of the most useful psychodiagnostic tests were devised by physicians, such as Alfred Binet (1857–1911), who developed the first widely used intelligence test; Hermann Rorschach (1884–1922), the Ink Blot Test; and Henry Murray, the Thematic Apperception Test (TAT).

Among the important events in the first half of this century that changed the status of psychiatry were the advances in therapy. The most important organic therapies were malaria therapy of general paresis, for which Julius von Wagner-Jauregg (1857–1940) received the Nobel Prize in 1927; treatment of pellagra with Vitamin B by Joseph Goldberger in 1915; the insulin coma therapy developed by Manfred Sakel (1900–1957); the chemical convulsive therapies, by L. von Meduna (1896–1964) in 1933; electroconvulsive therapies by U. Bini and U. Cerletti that were proposed in 1937; and the lobotomies introduced by Egaz Moniz, who was also honored with a Nobel award after he published his classical monograph in 1936. The enormous development of pharmacological therapies is still too recent to be viewed historically, but chemicals that produce behavioral sedation without impairment of complex thought processes have significantly influenced the nature of somatic therapies. Independently of the growth of the somatic therapies, depth psychological techniques were increasingly applied, not only in the offices of psychoanalysts but in mental health clinics, experimental schools, and, by a few bold persons, even with psychotics. The psychosocial therapies (milieu therapy in the hospital and in the community, family, and group therapy) are developing in an unprecedented fashion, with ambitious goals, new problems and new jargons. The new observations and methods have had an enormous influence, not only in psychiatry proper but in other fields as well. The broader applications reached the arts and humanities and contributed to the emergence of a new and more realistic image of man and his destiny.[10]

The humanitarian and scientific approaches of the past two hundred years have eventuated in the recognition of a range of factors that determine the organization of belief and conduct, both normal and abnormal. These have become a proper subject for rational study and intervention. For psychiatry, with rare exceptions, the broad-scale training of specialized scientific and research personnel has less than a ten-year history, but such workers have, finally, a broad foundation on which to build.

NOTES

1. Alfred Adler, *The Practice and Theory of Individual Psychology* (New York: Harcourt, Brace, 1929).
2. Edgar D. Adrian, *Research on the Central Nervous System* (London: Frome, 1936).
3. Elwyn J. Anthony, "Significance of Jean Piaget for Child Psychiatry," *British Journal of Medical Psychology*, 29 (1956), 20.
4. Jacob A. Arlow and Charles Brenner, *Psychoanalytic Concepts and the Structural Theory* (New York: International Universities Press, 1964).
5. Ludwig von Bertalanffy, *Problems of Life* (New York: Harper Torchbooks, 1960).
6. Leon Binswanger, *Grundformen und Erkenntnis der Menschlichen Daseins* (Zürich: Niehaus, 1942).
7. Medard Boss, *Psychoanalysis and Daseinsanalysis* (New York: Basic Books, 1963).
8. Charles Brenner, *An Elementary Textbook of Psychoanalysis* (New York: International Universities Press, 1955).
9. Josef Breuer and Sigmund Freud, *Studies on Hysteria* (1893–95), (New York: Basic Books, 1957).
10. Norman Brown, *Life against Death, the Psycho-analytical Meaning of History* (Middletown, Conn.: Wesleyan University Press, 1959).
11. Walter B. Cannon, *The Wisdom of the Body* (rev. ed.; New York: Norton, 1939).
12. Jean Martin Charcot and Paul Richer, *Contribution à l'étude de l'hypnotisme chez les Hystériques* (Paris: A. Delahaye et Lecrosnier, 1881).
13. Karl W. Deutsch, *The Nerves of Government* (New York: Macmillan, 1963).
14. John Dollard and Neal E. Miller, *Personality and Psychotherapy* (New York: McGraw-Hill, 1950).
15. Erik H. Erikson, "Identity and the Life Cycle; Selected Papers," *Psychological Issues*, Vol. 1, No. 1 (New York: International Universities Press, 1959).
16. Hans J. Eysenck, *The Structure of Human Personality* (London: Methuen, 1953).
17. W. Ronald D. Fairbairn, *An Objects-Relations Theory of the Personality* (New York: Basic Books, 1954).
18. Victor E. Frankl, *The Doctor and the Soul* (New York: Alfred Knopf, 1955).
19. Daniel X. Freedman and Nicholas J. Giarman, "Brain Amines, Electrical Activity and Behavior," in Gilbert H. Glaser, ed., *EEG and Behavior* (New York: Basic Books, 1963).
20. Anna Freud, *The Ego and the Mechanisms of Defence* (London: Hogarth Press, 1937).

21. Sigmund Freud, *Origins of Psycho-Analysis,* Marie Bonaparte, Anna Freud, and Ernst Kris, eds. (New York: Basic Books, 1954).
22. Erich Fromm, *Escape from Freedom* (New York: Rinehart, 1941).
23. Israel Goldiamond, "Perception," in Arthur J. Bachrach, ed., *Experimental Foundations of Clinical Psychology* (New York: Basic Books, 1962).
24. Kurt Goldstein, *The Organism* (New York: American Book Company, 1939).
25. Roy R. Grinker, "Introductory Chapter," in *Psychiatric Social Work* (New York: Basic Books, 1961).
26. Sebastian P. Grossman, "Eating or Drinking Elicited by Direct Adrenergic or Cholinergic Stimulation of Hypothalamus," *Science,* 132 (1960), 301.
27. David A. Hamburg, "The Relevance of Recent Evolutionary Changes to Human Stress Biology," in Sherwood Washburn, ed., *Social Life of Early Man* (Chicago: Aldine, 1962).
28. Heinz Hartmann, *Ego Psychology and the Problem of Adaptation* (New York: International Universities Press, 1958).
29. Karen Horney, *Neurosis and Human Growth* (New York: Norton, 1950).
30. John Hughlings Jackson, "Croonian Lectures on the Evolution and Dissolution of the Nervous System," *Lancet,* 1 (1884), 555.
31. Pierre Janet and Fulgence Raymond, *Les Obsessions et la psychosthénie* (Paris: Alcan, 1903), 2 vols.
32. Ernest Jones, *The Life and Work of Sigmund Freud* (New York: Basic Books, 1953).
33. Carl G. Jung, *Contributions to Analytic Psychology* (New York: Harcourt, Brace, 1928).
34. Abram Kardiner, *The Psychological Frontiers of Society* (New York: Columbia University Press, 1945).
35. Melanie Klein, *Contributions to Psycho-Analysis, 1921–1945* (London: Hogarth Press, 1948).
36. Jerzy Konorski, "Trends in the Development of the Physiology of the Brain," *Journal of Mental Science,* 104 (1958), 1100.
37. Ralph Linton, *Culture and Mental Disorders* (Springfield, Ill.: Charles C Thomas, 1956).
38. Konrad Lorenz, *Über das Sogenannte Böse* (Wien: Borota Verlag, 1963).
39. Paul D. MacLean, "Psychosomatics," in *Handbook of Physiology,* Section I, *Neurophysiology,* Vol. III (Washington, D. C.: American Physiological Society, 1960).
40. Horace W. Magoun, *The Waking Brain* (Springfield, Ill.: Charles C Thomas, 1958).
41. Jules H. Masserman, *Principles of Dynamic Psychiatry* (Philadelphia: Saunders, 1946).
42. Rollo May, Ernest Angel, and Henri F. Ellenberger, eds., *Existence* (New York: Basic Books, 1958).
43. Warren S. McCulloch, *Finality and Form* (Springfield, Ill.: Charles C Thomas, 1958).

44. James G. Miller, "Mental Health Implications of a General Behavior Theory," *American Journal of Psychiatry*, 113 (1957), 776.
45. Neal E. Miller, "Some Implications of Modern Behavior Theory for Personality Change and Psychotherapy," in D. Byrne and P. Worchel, *Personality Change* (New York: John Wiley, Inc., 1964).
46. Ruth Munroe, *Schools of Psychoanalytic Thought* (New York: Dryden Press, 1955).
47. James Olds and P. Milner, "Positive Reinforcement Produced by Electrical Stimulation of Septal Area and Other Regions of Rat Brain," *Journal of Comparative Physiology and Psychology*, 47 (1954), 419.
48. Talcott Parsons, *The Social System* (Glencoe, Ill.: The Free Press, 1951).
49. Ivan P. Pavlov, *Lectures on Conditioned Reflexes*, translated and edited by W. H. Gantt (New York: International Publishing, 1941), 2 vols.
50. Jean Paiget, *The Construction of Reality in the Child* (New York: Basic Books, 1954).
51. Otto Rank, *The Trauma of Birth* (New York: Basic Books, 1952).
52. David Rapaport, "The Structure of Psychoanalytic Theory, a Systematizing Attempt," *Psychological Issues*, Vol. 2, No. 2, Monograph 6 (New York: International Universities Press, 1960).
53. David Rapaport and Merton M. Gill, "The Points of View and Assumptions of Metapsychology," *International Journal of Psycho-Analysis*, 40 (1959), 153.
54. Gregory Razran, "The Place of the Conditioned Reflex in Psychology and Psychiatry," *Symposium #9, Group for the Advancement of Psychiatry* (March 1964).
55. David Riesman, *The Lonely Crowd* (New Haven: Yale University Press, 1950).
56. David McK. Rioch, "Psychiatry as a Biological Science," *Psychiatry*, 18 (1955), 313.
57. Jurgen Ruesch, *Disturbed Communication* (New York: Norton, 1957).
58. Jurgen Ruesch and Gregory Bateson, *Communication: The Social Matrix of Psychiatry* (New York: Norton, 1957).
59. Jean-Paul Sartre, *Existentialism and Human Emotions* (New York: Philosophical Library, 1957).
60. Paul Schilder, *Medical Psychology* (New York: International Universities Press, 1953).
61. Charles S. Sherrington, *The Integrative Action of the Nervous System* (New Haven: Yale University Press, 1906).
62. Herbert A. Simon, *Models of Man* (New York: John Wiley, 1957).
63. Burrhus F. Skinner, *Science and Human Behavior* (New York: Macmillan, 1953).
64. John Spiegel, "The Social Roles of Doctor and Patient in Psychoanalysis and Psychotherapy," *Psychiatry*, 17 (1954), 369.
65. Erwin Stengel, "Hughlings Jackson's Influence in Psychiatry," *British Journal of Psychiatry*, 109 (1963), 348.

66. Harry Stack Sullivan, *The Interpersonal Theory of Psychiatry* (New York: Norton, 1953).
67. Jacob von Uexküll, *Umwelt und Innenwelt der Tiere* (Berlin: Springer, 1929).
68. Robert Waelder, *Basic Theory of Psychoanalysis* (New York: International Universities Press, 1960).
69. Heinz Werner, *Comparative Psychology of Mental Development* (Chicago: Follett Pub., 1957).
70. Benjamin Lee Whorf, *Language, Thought, and Reality, Selected Writings of Benjamin Lee Whorf,* John B. Carroll, ed. (New York, M.I.T. and John Wiley, 1956).
71. Norbert Wiener, *The Human Use of Human Beings: Cybernetics and Society* (2d rev. ed.; Garden City: Doubleday Anchor, 1954).
72. Peter H. Wolff, "The Developmental Psychologies of Jean Piaget and Psychoanalysis," *Psychological Issues,* Vol. II, No. 1, Monograph 5 (New York: International Universities Press, 1960).
73. Joseph Wolpe, *Psychotherapy by Reciprocal Inhibition* (Stanford, Calif.: Stanford University Press, 1958).

CHAPTER FOUR

Normal and Abnormal Behavior

A Pragmatic Approach

In this chapter we will present some principles underlying normal and abnormal behavior that are pertinent for psychiatry. A few clinicians and behavioral scientists have advanced elaborate schemes of what the "beast," behavior, is like—of how it is put together and of how its functions are regulated. Yet, in spite of serious efforts, a completely acceptable supertheory on which psychiatry can generally rest its work does not exist. For the psychiatrist who wishes to construct simply an adequate working scheme, certain salient units must be selected out of the wealth of behavioral, biological, and environmental events for special scrutiny. Such a selection must currently be based on observations and assumptions that, through practice, tradition, and experimentation, have been found practical and useful. Today, a student of behavior must have the zest and discipline to approach the various avenues for the study of behavior openmindedly and with curiosity, since with increasing research and experience, dominant theories and terminologies will change. It is certainly not easy to find order and design in phenomena that are as variable and complex as behavior and behavior disorder. Yet in a relatively short time our field has increasingly become able to appreciate at least the nature of the problems to be attacked.

Behavior Is Lawful

As a technology based on the behavioral and biological sciences, psychiatry takes a deterministic point of view. This does not mean that all phenomena in our field can be explained, or that there is no uncertainty. It merely commits us to a scientific search for reliable and significant relationships. We assume causation—by which we mean that a *range* of similar antecedents in *both* the organism and environment produces a similar *set* of consequences. In general, we follow the procedures of basic sciences and attempt to determine the limits within which a range of antecedents has a high probability of producing similar results. Where an input produces an unexpected output, we search for unsuspected differences in the organism or environment. Human beings, like all biological systems, are goal-seeking and goal-modifying organisms. We not only look for antecedents as causes but try to discern purposes in the system. We examine the factors that determine goals and the means by which behavior is structured toward them. The apparent difference between causal and teleological explanations has been reconciled by cybernetics with the fundamental concept of feedback. This notion permits us to view purposive or goal-directed responses in guided missiles, amoebae, or in humans as guided by determinable antecedents—internal or external signals that activate, stop, modify, or correct sequences of psychobiological events.

The principles and basic methods of studying normal and abnormal behavior in individuals and in populations, in clinical practice, as well as under experimental conditions, are the same as in other naturalistic sciences. The methods must be reliable and enable us to repeat the same operation. Our findings should not be the result of chance, and we can assess this through the use of *appropriate* design, controls, and analysis of data. Findings must be valid or relevant and referable to empirical observations. Indeed, our concepts—as Percy W. Bridgman emphasized [8]—are determined by our operations, by what we do or omit doing in order to acquire information. Operationalism forces us to put our cards on the table. Although quantitative data gained from carefully controlled studies are gradually beginning to guide the practitioner, most of our clinical activities are still based on qualitative and incomplete information. Thus as practicing clinicians, psychiatrists must show wisdom, which has been defined as the courage to proceed with half-knowledge.

Multiple Determinants

In both medicine and psychiatry, single factor explanations have long ago been found inadequate. Even in those diseases in which an essential and necessary cause has been found, such as in many infections, we still need to understand the interaction of microbe and host in the environmental context in which it occurs. This approach leads not only to more adequate explanations but also points to quite specific sets of variables (such as factors of resistance) that require separate study. All etiological considerations must include the biological properties of the patient, his physical and social environment, and particularly the transactions involving other human beings in the present and in the past. The subjective representation of these transactions in thoughts, memories, and feelings—psychological variables—also critically govern human behavior.

Multiple causes may converge toward a major effect; in behavior, *any response* serves a number of different functions and has multiple consequences.[64] This usually leaves much room for interpretive speculations. Our task is to establish how antecedents and consequences are correlated and to specify the conditions under which a behavioral event is most likely to occur.

In practice, we assess the dominance or interaction of the various determinants and in each new case attempt to formulate a hypothesis about their probable role and outcome—which in medical parlance is diagnosis and prognosis.

A Simplified "Model" of the Behavioral System

We view biological organisms, including the human, as information-processing and physical energy-transforming systems. A biological or behavioral system—indeed, any feedback system—is comprised of arrangements for goal assessments and the capacity for internal rearrangements to initiate activities that meet or modify the goal. Any and all of the components of a behavioral system, whatever their nature, are articulated and connected through coded patterns. The highly regulated physical energy exchanges of the body may—conceivably—provide signals that lead eventually to behavioral activity, but these processes primarily maintain cellular function. Important behavioral problems related to "power failure" (for instance, fatigue) are encountered, but we are equally concerned with the processing of information, the transfer of coded patterns.

The organism receives such information through stimuli or input from the physical and social environment, from the body, and from its own stored data, and reacts with responses or output. The output consists of motor, visceral, chemical, electric, and acoustic responses carrying information, and such information may be received either by the transmitting organism itself or may be communicated to others. Within the organism, input and output are linked by a variety of intricate systems. Two fundamental phenomena of these systems are the capacity to store and recall processed input (memory) and feedback, or the return to the input of a part of the output.

We distinguish information that triggers innate patterns of active behavior—often with irresistible force—or drive behavior; information that has affective value (and hence signals and modulates various innate and learned "programs" of response); and information that controls, modifies, and inhibits or delays drive and affect-initiated behaviors. Finally, there is information that leads to cognitive functions ranging from simple discrimination to complicated logical and problem-solving activity. Encoded messages may be briefly stored to be sampled, shunted, matched, selected, or rejected by previous programs of information, which can function as filters, comparators, probabilistic computers, and so forth. Matching of the input to internal programs, partial matching or mismatching can generate the search for new input or retrieval of other programs; this leads to corrections, repetitions, or to complex and novel combinations. These arrangements thus permit both error and guidance through memory as well as learning and novelty through new combinations and selections of input.

Physical and Psychological Language

The internal rearrangements and channels for communication prior to and concomitant with overt behavior are important in a behavioral system. Similar inputs may have quite different effects (and different inputs may lead to similar effects) depending upon the internal arrangements, history, and current environment of the organism. Thus a part of the meaning or consequence of a simple input or a simple act is determined by the internal state and history of the organism, and in psychiatry we inquire into "what this act or event means for this person." A part of our objective data includes the report of subjective experiences (for example, the sensation, red) as well as events occurring in the realities of time and space, which we report in physical language (for example, wave length and frequency of light). There are usually reasons that make it more practical to report in one or the other language. Some of our most intricate, subtle, and indispensable data are reported in psychological language, the language of consciousness and of meaning.

Conscious and Unconscious Processes

If we are to conceive of a goal-modifying and goal-achieving organization that can move itself flexibly or automatically toward its own ends, some information about what it is doing or seeing—about its own state (either momentary or reflective)—must occur. In higher organisms these functions seem to be equivalent to consciousness. Consciousness, as James Grier Miller and others have noted,[52] refers to widely differing phenomena. It denotes *awareness* of the environment, the body, and the self. It also denotes the stages of *alertness* in contrast to coma, stupor, and sleep. The term may also refer to deliberate conscious *control* in contrast to regulation through habitual and automatic behavior.

What is this mysterious human quality of consciousness? Obviously much information flows through the organism without consciousness. As Karl Deutsch puts it, only some information produces secondary messages—messages about messages—which characterizes consciousness.[14] It seems that an optimal degree of awareness, alertness, and control is necessary for the proper functioning of higher mental processes in human beings, but what is optimal depends on the task. The optimal degree of consciousness differs for artistic and scientific activities, for mere action or for explanation. The psychotomimetic drugs illustrate that there are various components of consciousness that can be altered. They induce a vivid heightening of awareness but a diminished control over the events that reach awareness; with hypnogogic reverie or with opium, on the other hand, there may be rich dream imagery but obtunded awareness of stimuli. In other states, consciousness is intent but highly focused as in concentration for work. No current theory adequately accounts for the fact that both primitive and highly organized thoughts can vary so much in focus, control, and intensity.

When the contents of consciousness are organized in a loose, plastic way we speak of primary processes; where logic abounds we speak of the operation of secondary processes. Intrusion into consciousness of unwanted primary processes, of normally suppressed modes of experience, may occur in highly coded disguise in neurosis and less disguised in upsetting dreams and in many psychoses. Where the filtering of unwanted input fail, there is, in psychoanalytic terms, a lack of autonomy of the ego, a weakness of its attentional function that regulates the access of messages to consciousness.

The meanings most psychiatrists connect with the concept of unconscious behavior derive from Freud's observations and concepts.[23] Those experiences of infancy and early childhood that never reach the level of clear consciousness comprise the *archaic unconscious.* We infer the archaic unconscious from direct behavioral observations of infants or psychotics, from interpretations of derivative experiences (as in fantasies), and from metaphors that palely reflect infantile urges (for example, to "chew somebody out" in all likelihood is related to unconscious archaic cannibalistic urges). *Primal repression* was said to keep the origin of such derivatives from distinct awareness. This type of unconsciousness was distinguished from experiences and wishes that were once explicitly conscious and then, for certain reasons, eliminated by repression proper. The latter is called the "*repressed unconscious,*" because repression is the most important mode of rendering psychological processes unconscious. We infer its existence by the analysis of neurotic behavior, dreams, slips of everyday life, and by the phenomena of posthypnotic suggestion, of which the subject is unaware. The repressed unconscious is probably the most important single concept of dynamic psychiatry.

We know a third major type of unconsciousness that is related to the automatic aspects of behavior and to many controlling operations, such as defenses and certain processes of learning. Innumerable useful skills are also unconscious and appear to be automatic; for example, the movements involved in expertly playing an instrument, driving a car, sailing a boat, and so forth. These various behavioral operations (which include aspects of many cognitive processes such as attention and memory) are, of course, vulnerable to disruption by conflict.

We find the terms conscious and unconscious operationally valid and descriptively useful in simply denoting degrees of awareness in clinical and therapeutic phenomena. A neat line of demarcation between conscious and unconscious probably applies only to symptoms such as hysterical conversion and amnesia. In most cases the boundaries are nebulous, justifying Paul Schilder's comparison of consciousness to a planetary system with the greatest degree of consciousness in the center and decreasing consciousness in the outer spheres.[61] Clinically, we notice not only reductions of consciousness but also a heightened illusory sense of awareness in certain states of ecstasy, intoxication, and schizophrenia; in obsessives there is a heightened sense of consciously controlling events. Too much self-consciousness obviously leads to inefficiency.

We use the term preconscious for psychic processes that are not fully conscious but that can be rendered so without great difficulty. Freud used the term not only as a descriptive label but also as a "region of the mind"—the gateway through which derivatives of archaic processes were permitted to reach consciousness; the preconscious was seen as lurking in the background of focused consciousness. Wishes and affects intertwined with loosely organized thoughts and fantasies are preconscious. Such psychic processes abound in children and primitives. They are also characteristic for artistic expression and occur in humor, daydreams, and in nocturnal dreams. The content and organization of preconscious processes (coupled with our observations over time of behavioral patterns and tendencies) permit us to make inferences about the organization and function of unconscious processes.

These processes of consciousness are indispensable attributes of our notion of man. But how are we able to differentiate a memory trace (which is conscious) and a "real" perception? It does seem that to determine and locate what comes from the internal world and what comes from the external world requires more than consciousness. Certain additional operations—discriminative functions—must be acquired, and these clinically are described as reality- and value-testing.

Meaning

Much of psychiatric inquiry begins with the search for meaning. Without this, our work would become an irrelevant cataloguing procedure. Meaning refers to the connectedness of a known with an unknown item, which makes the latter meaningful. A word in a foreign language has meaning if we can translate it by a word of our own language. A concept gains meaning if we can define it by known concepts or available data. An affect, a wish, or a complex experience also gain meaning if we are capable at least hypothetically of re-experiencing or testing it. Meaning may be shared or remain private; when such private meanings are inaccessible to awareness we speak of unconscious meaning. Much of the world of a psychotic and to a lesser degree of the neurotic remains entirely private, infantile, and idiosyncratic. They are unable to communicate their world and hence are often desperately alone. Psychiatrists are expected to have a remarkable capacity to experience or translate the wide range of strange thoughts, affects, wishes, and overt acts of their patients. Sometimes this is achieved by an intuitive grasp or understanding of the patient and his problems; in other cases, this is achieved only by a slow and painstaking process of progressive interpretation and cross-validating investigations. In practice we may *infer* an underlying state: a patient's bravado is a reaction to his "basic" fear and loneliness; in which case the inference becomes a prediction to be tested. We may actually *observe* loneliness followed by bravado or, as an archaeologist, we *reconstruct* events from the details of history and clinical evidence gathered in treatment. Such relationships can be not only intuitively grasped but often objectively demonstrated.

Psychoanalytic psychiatry has made enormous progress in decoding and explaining the hidden unrealistic and confused meanings of many psychopathological experiences and behavioral acts. While phenomenological psychiatrists believe that only empathic understanding is possible, general psychiatrists attempt explanations (establishing the determinants of a given event[32]) and are interested in an ever increasing system of explanations that permit predictions and identifications of the variables controlling behavior. To do this we depend heavily upon history and biography for understanding how variables operate in the single or unique case—an approach that epistemologists referred to as the *ideographic*. Contrasted with this is the *nomothetic* approach, which arrives at general laws by observing similarities and differences in many cases.[1] To treat behavioral data in a manageable and useful way requires the best "objective" judgment, whether the source of information is derived from empathy or the collection and testing of a number of observations. In such continued search we generate new concepts, new observations and applications and enlarge our scientific comprehension of the meaning of behavior and its disorders.

Self-Systems

The Self-System and Self-Representation

Normal adults experience themselves as distinct entities. Even if such consecrated platitudes as "the human being as a whole" or fancy existentialist terms like "being in the world" may not be very useful, we recognize the individual or person as a meaningful and distinct unit that persists through changes of time and circumstance. Man always must represent his own actions and feelings to himself in *some* way, and much of our work and skill derives from detailed knowledge of the ways in which humans represent their needs to themselves and to their therapists. The self is the totality of one's own psychological processes introspectively viewed. The self-system (or more properly, the self-systems) recognized by the experience of unity and distinctness is predicated on the distinctness of the body, but self-representations comprise far more than this. The ability to reflect or to take oneself as an object of attention is distinctly human. A person may take himself as an object or a subject (as the source that acts or is acted upon). So there are various representations that comprise an "internal referent system" recognized in the pronouns "I," "me," and "myself." Some psychological schools do not include a self-system; self-understanding is not relevant to many aspects of conditioning. Yet no comprehensive theory and no theory aiming at personal growth can leave the self-system out of account. Of course, the language of subjective motivation—your notion of why you behave in a certain way—is not a sufficient explanation of how behavior is determined, although it does represent a part of the necessary evidence. The lawful links of the rich variety of subjective events to wishes and acts are a key focus of psychoanalytic psychology.

Insight

Self-awareness, or insight through introspection, often "unlocks" the hidden meaning of otherwise puzzling and apparently incomprehensible behaviors. The term *insight* is used to designate various degrees of understanding of one's behavior and one's difficulties. Insight is not exactly equivalent to knowledge. We must ask what function insight serves. Is it geared to action or "appreciation," to the acquisition and application of new skills? If so, it can lead to significant restructuring of behavior. Or is it a part of morbid self-awareness, a substitute for action? It would be an oversimplification to say that the sicker the patient the less insightful he is; some schizophrenics have an extraordinary capacity to discern unconscious processes in themselves and in others, but they are quite incapable of using such insights adaptively.

The Self and Reality

Throughout development, the self-system differentiates with both bodily and social experience. Psychiatrists are interested in the relationship of the self and others, of the inner and outer worlds, and in the correspondence between publicly and privately structured information. Information about the outer world can never be complete, never wholly accurate. In spite of this, human beings have an exceptional capacity to investigate and test reality and to communicate about it. E. Bibring pointed out that there is an inherent gradient in all humans toward approximating the requirements of reality and toward valuing what is expedient, and therapists, indeed, always count on this trend.[3] On the other hand, in virtually all behavior disorders the slope of this gradient is shifted. In the course of development the child's notion of self and reality are differentiated; learning about the response of others can enhance learning about oneself and vice versa. Psychiatric patients show selective or general arrest in this process. They suffer from distorted views about themselves or about the environment (or both); their capacity for reality- and value-testing is, therefore, to some extent impaired.

Body Image and the Psychological Self

The range of attitudes toward and perceptions of the body as a whole and its parts have been loosely lumped into the concept of body image as the ever changing sum of information about the body.[19, 87] Representations of the body are based on perceptions of surface and internal sensations; these differ in health and disease, during wakefulness and sleep, and organismic states such as hunger and fatigue. The body image is influenced by what we have learned about our body from infancy through interactions with others. Brain diseases can produce far-reaching changes in the body image and such symptoms as denial of a hemiplegia (anosognosia) and denial of blindness. The body image may be altered in severe neuroses and psychoses.

The boundary of the body is the skin; the boundary of the psychological self—the boundary between what is me and what is not me—is often called the ego boundary. The rational adult has a very sure if not explicit sense of what is psychologically "me and not me." In such normal emotional states as being in love, being a part of a crowd or group, or during the periods of falling asleep or waking, the ego boundary becomes much less distinct and more diffuse and extended. Different cultures preferentially reinforce self-definitions along a continuum from a narrow, highly focused "I-ness" to an extended "we-ness," but the preferred boundaries will be marked by stability. In many psychoses, in intoxications, and in acute and chronic brain diseases, the experience of "what is me and what is not me" is profoundly altered, and the boundaries of the self-system are loose. Usually such changes of ego boundary are concomitant with many other misinterpretations. For example, such patients readily confuse the intentions of other persons and personalize the significance of gestures and communications. A broad category of pathological experiences that are characterized by a subjective feeling of strangeness of the self is referred to as *depersonalization;* if the world is the focus of the feeling of strangeness, we refer to *derealization.* If such experience is not too rapidly masked by compensatory symptoms, the patient observes these changes as someone apart and complains of *estrangement.* Symptoms and traits that are not accepted as part of the self are called *ego-alien* or *ego-dystonic;* for instance, the hand-washing symptom in a compulsive neurotic may be felt by the patient to be unwanted and strange. This is in contrast to ego-syntonic symptoms and traits; the patient with excessive irritability may deem this simply a "natural trait." A strong feeling of psychological disunity is seen in neurotic double personalities, in some schizophrenics, and in the identity crises of adolescents.

Self-Esteem and Self-Love

Man not only encounters and perceives himself, but he takes himself as an object of love (so-called narcissistic love) and evaluates himself (with the result of a certain level of self-esteem). The latter is acquired as the child learns to evaluate himself through the evaluation of others, especially his parents. One's self-esteem may be realistic or unrealistic. The child's and the megalomaniac's feelings of omnipotence are utterly unrealistic. Self-esteem depends on one's conscious and unconscious levels of aspiration (corresponding to the psychoanalytic concept of ego ideal). It also depends on experienced reward and punishment and particularly on one's conscious and unconscious needs and criteria for self-reward and self-punishment. Consciously experienced self-esteem may be at odds with the preconscious and unconscious criteria. We may then notice in an overtly self-assured person subtle signs of self-derogation and attempts to invite criticism and abuse. The patient who privately interprets his possibly reasonable wishes as bad or excessively ambitious may commit a reprehensible act that leads to a decrease both of guilt and self-esteem. It is as if he sought both punishment and forgiveness in this awkward way. Many pathological acts, on the other hand, represent desperate attempts to restore self-esteem. The impact of one's "internal judges" on self-esteem is clearly considerable.

Conceptually we try to differentiate a feeling of worth and self-esteem from self-love, although they are related. Freud contrasted narcissistic self-love with the capacity to love others and also with normal egotism or the trait of having a healthy regard for one's interests. Undesirable egotism springs from chronically unsatisfied self-regard and a compensatory need for self-love. A need for continual and excessive self-love impairs the ability to appreciate others as persons of interest or importance in their own right. Narcissistic persons tend to see others purely as extensions of themselves and in their relationships with them satisfy their excessive needs: for example, the researcher who can perceive no other work than that which reflects his own glory. Such people are usually irritating to others and are isolated from the comfort and adaptive corrections that come with accessibility to others. A normal part of romantic or parental love includes the enhancement of the self through another person who completes a part of one's self-image; but a capacity for relative distance and a perception of the real qualities of others are also generally present. In severe psychoses, pathological narcissism is evident in the tenuous relationship with others and the extreme personalization of all stimuli and interactions.

Ego Identity

We are indebted to Erik H. Erikson for the concept of ego identity. Erikson did not offer simple definitions;[17] although the concept has been stimulating, it is far from clear. Erikson referred to ego identity as a continuity of personal characteristics, the silent doings of ego synthesis—an internal structuring that integrates coherence out of the individual's past. It may be evident in a style or mode of operating that permeates much of a person's activities and approach; thus identity comprises more than self-image. Since it involves an active process of building a recognizable self it is not quite equivalent to the more static concept of personality or character. There are clinically demonstrable differences in how identity is maintained and shaped.

Obsessive-compulsive persons may retain their identities with rigidity. Hysterical persons (who seem compelled seductively to invite and attract expectations rather than fulfill them) maintain an identity, paradoxically, by readily shifting roles and apparent goals; they substitute excitement for fulfilment, which because of their still lively early attachments is interpreted as taboo. In schizophrenic and schizoid persons, serious splits and incongruities of identity are noted; these people may react with oversensitivity and disorganization to the slightest indication of imperception on the part of others of their self-image, which, in any event, is highly unstable. Identity diffusion entails either a temporary moratorium for "trying it out" (as in adolescence) or an arrest of further development, with persisting difficulty in sexual and occupational identity. Malignant identity diffusion may entail defiant stances. A delinquent may be proud of what he is *not*, and this negative identity covers the underlying confusion and discomfort. He may become trapped with this identity, since being a delinquent is all, in a coherent way, that he can be.

Drive Behavior

The concept of drive behavior is complicated and far from satisfactory. The various notions about behavior and its impetus—about what makes behavior "go"—are subsumed under the label of instincts, drives, needs, or presses. A number of fundamental behavioral patterns appear to rest on internal arrangements and to unfold—often with inexorable persistence—upon internal as well as external cues. These fundamental states of disequilibrium can be subjectively experienced as frustration, urgency, tension, or want, and the tension is often discharged by certain instrumental responses leading to a state of subjective gratification and relative restfulness. Objectively, we observe the activation and diminution of behavior which appears to restore a state of balance; for example, the termination of hunger by behavior which leads to the ingestion of food.

What are man's basic drives? We are most certain about physiological drives regulating intake of air, food, elimination of excreta, sexuality, sleep activity, rest, and the avoidance of pain. Such activities have intrinsic somatic correlates, neurochemical sequences of feedbacks that start and stop the activation of bodily and behavioral responses that serve the need. Freud finally assumed two basic drives in man: sexuality and aggression. Other biological theorists still point to activities of the organism as centered around self-preservation and species preservation. Lorenz spoke of five basic instincts or directions in behavior—sex, hunger, fear, aggression, and social or group instinct.[44] It might simply be convenient to assume that states of disequilibrium within the organism produce information that results in behavioral and physiologic activity patterned along these dominant lines.

Such patterns quite early acquire a personal and interpersonal history and significance; hence, for the psychiatrist, drive behaviors are not only important in adult conduct, but their roots in early development are considered crucial. As complicated behavior unfolds, there are innumerable internal and external signals or stimuli that guide, correct, warn, change rates, or start and stop the unfolding process. Automatisms appear to unfold without sufficient external stimulus control; but generally drive behaviors are modifiable or conditionable, influenced by neuroendocrine as well as experiential factors, and it is the task of modern neurobiological research to sort these controlling systems into some comprehensible order.

In any case, we are inclined to assume that an array of basic directions in behavior, which we call drives, are of fundamental importance for clinical considerations. Of course, many forms of clinically significant drive behaviors, such as the need for status and esteem, support, or friendship, may be derived from one or several basic drives. Abraham H. Maslow described a hierarchy of drives[49]—safety, love, esteem, and self-actualization—which appears to be clinically useful. Essentially, then, it is a conceptual convenience to epitomize certain fairly universal trends in behavior as drives, and at this juncture in our knowledge it is most practical to be clear about our clinical definitions while we await clarifications of basic issues.

Clinical Aspects of Drive Behavior

The two drives that have the greatest clinical significance are sex and aggression. They are characterized by great plasticity and the capacity for modification by learning. The clinician has several reasons for learning to diagnose drive behaviors. For one, sexual and aggressive impulses get people into trouble. Secondly, we find that early drive conflicts acutely recur in the adult, particularly in situations involving a current threat or temptation and satisfaction. The majority of the child's strivings center around bodily needs; derivatives of early conflicts and unresolved early confusions influence future goals and relationships and permeate self-representations in both normal and abnormal behavior. Thirdly, an infantile drive component may chronically permeate and infiltrate the most highly developed behavior and at times functions to derail or divert mature goal-directed performance. Highly developed adult skills are often harnessed to childish needs; the *effective* program of reward and punishment is hidden behind acceptable current incentives and goals. These drive goals, and the guilt about them may, then, underlie other aims unbeknown either to the patient or his cohorts. An example is the capable man who seems to defeat himself recurrently. If his underlying achievement in work and love-making is primarily to be bigger and better than his father, a guilty fear can lead to impotence, to fear of success or to compulsive, competitive sexuality, or to depression and unhappiness in the presence of real or impending achievement. Such a man behaves as if he were still a child, trying to test his father rather than accepting his adulthood and realizing its frustrations and pleasures.

The clinical hallmark of drive problems is urgency, "drivenness" and an irresistible press for expression and discharge; a compelled search for immediate, usually sensory satisfaction or defense against it is characteristic for drive-dominated behaviors. These drive components are manifest not only in clear-cut symptoms but in dreams, in images and self-representations, and in motor and affective expression; they often are surprisingly hidden in character traits.

We recognize as sexual behavior not only sexual behavior in the narrow sense but a range of erotic, sensual, and social strivings. The sex drive develops, as does any complex behavior, through differentiation and then integration of component subdrives into the social behavior that is aimed toward genital gratification and mutuality. In normal adult sexuality, the heterosexual genital drive has integrated the partial or pregenital drives—the narcissistic, oral, tactile, visual, anal, phallic, and homosexual drives. The sexual drive has the greatest plasticity of all drives, both in its direct expression and "on loan" as a vehicle for expressing other conflicts. It also seems often to run counter to what we call self-preservation, adaptation, and reality sense, thus causing conflicting and inefficient behavior. In psychopathology, sexual, passive, and aggressive needs fuse into complex sadistic and masochistic drive behavior. A more detailed discussion of the psychopathology of the sex drive will follow in the chapter on neuroses (Chapter 12).

"Aggression" refers to attack behavior, but it can refer also to the intensity and style of approach to persons and tasks and to assertiveness. Destructiveness and hostility are specific aspects of aggression and, together with such other derivatives as dominance and rivalry, these play an important role in normal and abnormal behavior. *Passivity* refers both to avoidance reactions and to a range of behaviors where the aim is not to do but to be done unto. At times it refers to a marked need to receive and to be dependent; at other times to a lack of responsiveness and apathy. A quiet and alert receptivity is important both in maternal behavior and in the conduct of any good participant observer. Aggressive and passive behavior often occur together in complex syndromes, for example, provocative behavior that masks passive yearnings for care and attention. In a general way, passivity and aggressiveness are sex-linked, a linkage biologically based and culturally reinforced from infancy through adulthood. Yet biological determinants alone scarcely account for highly differentiated cultural patterns where the male may or may not be characterized by a higher degree of aggression in his various social roles and tasks than the female. In our culture the sex-linkage of sex and aggression gives rise to characteristic problems: envious striving for power and denial of passive yearnings. Freud felt that the fear of passive latent homosexual strivings in men and penis envy in women are characteristic expressions.[21]

We are inclined to consider the human need to interact in groups as both basic and clinically significant. The primitive horde, the family, the small and large groups based on the care and protection of infants, the sharing of tools and beliefs, are deeply ingrained human needs. Without the consideration of these traits, the needs to become a member of a group, to defend or conquer territory, neither human history nor human behavior could be understood. Much of psychopathology is concerned with the description, understanding, and treatment of deficits in the motivation and capacity to interact in groups, and also with the inability to retain one's individuality in such interaction.

We are also inclined to view fear or flight behavior as a basic drive and not just a secondary response to sex and aggression; again, as long as a physiological energizing substrate has not been established this is an academic question. Even in this regard, it should be recalled that all drive behaviors are conditionable and may appear as primary or secondary depending on circumstances. Certainly flight or fear behavior is of the greatest clinical significance; recognizing this, we will deal with the affects of fear and anxiety in some detail in the following section.

Drive behavior may be manifest not only in clear-cut "instincts" but may be hidden in character traits. For example, if a person's pleasure in argument primarily is the sensory quality of hearing his own voice, or the excitement of "arousing" others and causing them to lose control, or the fantasy of "killing" with words, we would suspect that these drive satisfactions rather than the cogency of the debated arguments were dominant and directing behavior. As a lawyer, such an impassioned advocate could lose the case for lack of caution, although he would have achieved some hidden pleasure in his argumentative display. Early drive experiences may condition adult fantasies so that a woman who thinks of intercourse as brutal and dirty may unknowingly tease and provoke her husband to violence; many marital tragedies are based on the maladaptive persistence of childish fantasies and theories. Character traits such as ambition or style of approach and avoidance have an inevitable drive history. A particularly harsh sibling rivalry in childhood, reinforced in peer relationships, may condition the tempo and pattern of conduct in the prime of life; in itself this is neither good nor bad but becomes a problem only when, for example, competitive needs become so conflictful or dominant as seriously to interfere with current adjustments and satisfactions. Sometimes we find that thwarted drives of curiosity, the need to look and peek, may evolve into a drive-dominated career choice. Think of the well-known confiscator of pornography who, instead of destroying his dubious booty, protected society by sitting in an office surrounded by filing cases bulging with notable examples of what repulsed him. Many such "reaction formations" underlie the behavior of the extreme reformer. Indeed, it is the "extra" energy, the zeal, frenzy, and push that may indicate a drive problem to the clinician. Where behavior is less compelled and compelling, where choice and alternatives seem more available, behavior is deemed less drive-dominated, less motivated by idiosyncratic and immediate sensual concerns and—in Freud's terms—less libidinized. It is, of course, possible for a mature champion of a cause to pursue it with selectivity, judgment, and relative freedom from the restrictions imposed by dominance of persisting infantile drive problems.

Affects

Emotions, affects, or feelings are essential components of behavior. These psychological states are usually concomitant with drive behavior. The most basic affects, such as pleasure and displeasure, are seen in human infants and also in higher animals. In the adult human, affects can be highly organized and differentiated. Since affects are both felt and expressed, some investigators refer to the subjective component as affects or feelings and to the patterned behavioral expressions as emotion. Affects act as signals alerting a person to attend to his current concerns. They carry basic orienting information as to value (good or bad, safe or dangerous) and degree of value (more or less dangerous). Affects carry information, not only about the internal state of readiness to respond (referred to as level of activation or arousal), but about the direction and implication of the latent state of readiness: a gesture, posture, a tone of voice, are "telling" in their impact. One of the social functions of affects lies in their capacity to evoke crude predictions of immediately forthcoming behavior. From Darwin to modern ethology and "kinesics" [5] there has been interest in documenting the phenomenology of affects, gestures, and language (inflection, tone) and their role as communications regulating our social interactions.

While the viscera express affects, evisceration does not abolish them since affects develop from centrally organized behavioral arrays (related to the basic self-preserving reflex systems). The neural equipment for laughing and crying, for eating, grooming, lip-smacking, smiling, grimacing, or baring of teeth is demonstrable by electrical stimulation of contiguous limbic and brain stem structures; peripheral input functions as a part of the feedback system to activate, to guide and to pattern the sequential behaviors. It is only with differentiation in behavior that a particular affective display becomes a meaningful "tag" reliably indicating a structured internal state with social implications; an infant can smile reflexly before it begins to smile in response to significant persons. The phylogenetic history of these basic and indispensable arrays of dispositions and their integration into differentiated behaviors should provide an important perspective on the meaning of man's affective displays. In this respect, the detailed observations of ethologists coupled with comparative neurophysiological studies are important.

Thus, affects are not identical with their neural substrates and they also require appropriate signals and objects to be released.[65] Affects, for example, may be felt when autonomic responses are pharmacologically blocked;[28] they may be repressed when the body is responding. There has been much work in the conditioning of visceral correlates of affects (which often persist when associated motor learning has been forgotten) and this is an important area for understanding man's affective and psychosomatic disorders.[24] Other approaches to the psychophysiology of affects show that individuality is both biological and psychological. Studies both of infants[46] and adults indicate that there are individualized and preferential autonomic responses (blood pressure in one, skin temperature and heart rate in another) that most readily respond to the arousal of affects.[40] Finally, with the observation that drugs and hormones influence mood and affect, the chemical organization of affect states comprises an important area for investigation.

Affects: Clinical Considerations

We infer the existence of affects from behavioral observations, from motor and visceral phenomena, from subjective reports, and from our own empathic ability to predict the consequences of affective states. While we can listen to and track the spoken message, we customarily "hear" the affective message by responding to it. Indeed, early affects constituting the first maternal-child communications involve action and the interplay of response states and bodily dispositions. The psychotherapist learns to not act but to pause and to sort affective messages by monitoring his initial responses as well as specific cues from the patient. The patient, on the other hand, can also learn to pay attention to his sensations and feelings, and these will lead him frequently to recall the situation that evoked the feeling. In other words, there is information value in affects. The therapist must thus determine when an affect is simply a discharge and when it is a true interpersonal communication or a reaction to an underlying painful and secret affect. Fortunately, people, no matter how masked, tortured, and complex their adult expression of affects, were presumably once children. Thus, the decoding of intricate defenses and feelings in behavior disorder may be complex, but the basic troublesome affects—anger, envy, injured pride, anxiety, dejection, loneliness, and the like—are universal and, in this sense, simple.

Often the identification of a single affect such as anxiety or rage is difficult because affects are often blurred and fused, and, unless carefully monitored, their onset and termination are difficult to track. We recognize a polarity of affects called *ambivalence*. This probably consists basically of a coexistence of opposing feelings such as love and hate; it is a paralyzing inability simply to focus on one of a set of feelings in those states where there is general impairment of directed attention. In more organized states, rather than a coexistence of multiple feelings, we find alternating love and hatred, and such ambivalence will influence decisiveness. In adults, enduring affect or *mood* generally is in the background of consciousness and becomes subjectively or objectively evident only on appropriate occasions or with special attention. Affects, as other behavioral operations, thus occur and differ at various levels of organization. This again indicates the importance of the first two or three years of development when relatively undifferentiated intense experiences (infantile rage or anxiety over helplessness) precede the child's capacity to make distinctions. It is thought that some persons may require years before they can cope with and adapt to consequences of these early experiences, which for them were somehow not integrated into the later steps of development. A two-year-old is helpless enough, and continued helplessness, inadequacy, and inferiority is an injury to self-love and integrity and can impair development of initiative and of autonomy.

Emotions and the Motor System

The word "e-motion" implies a close relationship of emotions to *motor systems*. Motor systems are integrated in the total response repertory of the organism—in exploring and changing the outside world as well as in expressing feelings. A child—and some adults (and not only psychotics)—practices and rehearses thinking through doing (moving parts of the vocal apparatus and possibly his hands with a thought). Gestures and "acting it out" externalize what is internal. Often a person will gesture or signal (sometimes to the therapist) before he can "catch a thought" and verbalize it. Specific motility patterns are highly characteristic for individuals and groups with common value systems. We recognize people by their posture and their facial and bodily movements. The motor link between "inside" and "outside" (between affect, and expressive or instrumental behavior) is changed not only in the developing child achieving mastery and control, but in altered states of consciousness—in sleep, in dreaming, and in various behavior disorders. Hypermotility or hypomotility occurs in anxiety,[45, 48] rage, and depression. In catatonic schizophrenics, very characteristic abnormalities of movements are noted ranging from stuporous immobility to extreme psychomotor agitation: posturing, grimacing, occasionally accompanied by waxy flexibility of the muscles, and various automatisms. Patients mimic actions (echopraxia) or speech (echolalia). Automatisms and related primitive reflexive mechanisms (such as sucking and grasping reflexes) also occur in behavior disorders associated with brain syndromes and in certain epilepsies. The inability to stop and to change an ongoing motor activity or speech (perseveration) and certain release mechanisms like compulsive laughing and crying, are characteristic motor syndromes in organic behavior disorders. These symptoms are not *only* expressions of cerebral pathology, but also have psychological meaning. Compulsive crying and laughing is not completely devoid of emotional content, and perseveration may acquire a mocking quality.

Specific Affects

Strong affects may occur sporadically or as perennial and enduring states. Such chronic pathological affects are of great clinical significance.

Anxiety has been called the alpha and omega of psychiatry. Anxiety is an affect accompanying a set of responses to threats to the internal equilibrium. When an appropriate stimulus can be linked with the affect we speak of *fear*. When the fear occurs suddenly and is startling, we speak of *fright*. If the anxiety is intense and disorganizing, it is called *panic* or terror. When the threat is based on an inability to assess the realistic alternatives, or on the personalized and immature evaluation of wishes, conflicts, or demands, we speak of neurotic or unrealistic anxiety. Unrealistic, anticipatory fears with displacement of the fear to relatively innocuous objects are referred to as phobias; a child's fear of bodily harm from the parent in retaliation for bad thoughts may be masked and displaced as a phobia for animals that bite. If a person—or an experimental animal—learns to respond to a cue with fear and tension in anticipation of punishment that has not yet occurred, many inappropriate behaviors can ensue. Unrealistic anticipatory fears that are learned (even "copied" from parents) are important in psychopathology. Even unrealistic fear may be a requisite precursor to adaptive action; tension is not equivalent to conflict and may be mobilizing rather than disorganizing. Obviously, we must make fine distinctions along the continuum of activation and its behavioral and affective correlates, and we should avoid lumping everything into one catchall category such as anxiety. As everywhere in behavior, level of organization is critical and differentiating.

Anxiety may be conscious, preconscious, or unconscious. It may be subjectively perceived as well as characterized by motor and visceral responses: dryness of the mouth, anorexia, constipation, vomiting, diarrhea, gastric hypersecretion, changes in heart rate and blood pressure. Some persons become agitated, overactive, or show motor tension and tremor; others become unresponsive and immobile, frozen. In early stages of infancy and childhood strong unconscious, unfocused, unverbalized anxieties occur. Freud clearly linked such affect with the incapacity to cope; he called the earliest anxiety "automatic" anxiety. This occurs when an overwhelming need or input can neither be mastered nor gratified; there is excessive excitation, flooding of the "stimulus barrier." In our opinion, this pervasive state of pain, displeasure, and frustration is a forerunner to more structured forms of anxiety. Freud first viewed anxiety as the *result* of repressed sexuality and dammed-up libido; for certain anxiety states, he persisted with this "neuroendocrine" theory. His major emphasis, however, shifted, and he later thought of anxiety as a part of the defensive equipment of the organism and spoke of "signal anxiety." This is evoked by perception of potential inner and outer danger. Signal anxiety then occurs first and, with varying degrees of success, either initiates repression or action; any "return of the repressed" wishes or thoughts again evokes anxiety. The inner cues are bodily signals, dangerous fantasies and wishes, as well as memory traces of outer stimuli that once provoked distress; the most important outer stimuli are aggressive threats.

In human psychopathology, the conscious and unconscious fear of injury to sex organs and the fear of death play a particularly important role. In view of the intense pleasure of stimulation and relief, the occasional pain and recurrent demand that the mysterious ingestive and excretory functions represent, bodily organs should have an intrinsically high value and interest for the child. His capacities for assessing reality are limited, and he quite early equates himself and the world with his body. The interest is enhanced not only by parental attention but by the child's equating the parents' body and organ size with parental power. Anxieties concerning the function and intactness of genitals thus seem to be inherently highly probable; they in turn probably rest on a more nebulous fear of annihilation or obliteration of the self. This nebulous though basic fear requires a concrete bodily or social "scapegoat" for direct expression. Thus it may be the child's propensity for translating fear and pleasure into concrete bodily terms rather than any direct threats to his person that accounts for the universal equation of genital threat ("castration anxiety") with a great variety of fears.

Anger or *rage* is the affect which is concomitant with aggression. In the helplessness of early infancy, when neither attack nor escape is possible, rage can hardly be differentiated from anxiety; but even later in life rage occurs just as often mixed with anxiety as in a pure form. Just as anxiety can be maximized when escape is impossible, rage may be enhanced by frustration. An acute outburst of anger—certainly in its proper context a "normal" response—is of less interest than irritability, or chronic rage and hatred, which are clearly pathological affects. One of the ugliest forms of hatred—cruelty—is probably a mixture of sexual and angry affects. There are many varieties of chronic anger. Some are accompanied by destructive behavior; some are more silent and manifest in psychosomatic or neurotic symptoms. Clinically, we are particularly interested in the covert, suppressed, and unconscious forms of hatred and self-hatred. Manifest behavior, then, may not be ostensibly "angry," but the *consequences* of overly passive behavior may be thoroughly destructive. This is what we might call the "critical equation" in psychiatry: whatever his expressed intentions, the consequences of the patient's behavior are such that it is *as if* he were angry, guilty, ashamed, and so forth.

An important basic affect is sadness or *dejection*, which is linked with losses of persons and possessions as well as a loss of pride and self-esteem. Ultimately this affect refers to a need to depend on persons and situations for internal stability. In early infancy these responses are akin to anxiety; beyond eight or nine months we can see pure sadness or *grief*. The complex behavioral manifestations of dejection may range from stuporous unresponsiveness to general retardation or to extreme psychomotor agitation. Between the ages of two and five, shame and guilt emerge.[56] These may undergo complex fusion with anxiety, rage, and grief. *Shame* is an emotion closely related to fear, dejection, and inferiority. It is often evoked by being discovered in sexual, exhibitionistic, or aggressive activities (or even wishes, which are often confirmed by the blush). The reaction is to hide, if not to cower; one feels momentarily too inferior to participate in a current community, be it a child in his family or an adult in his society. "Dirty" deeds may be reacted to by the allied emotion of *disgust*, usually associated with unpleasant gastrointestinal sensations.

Guilt is a complex emotion; it is closely related to anxiety, disgust, and shame. It is the response of the child or adult who fears punishment, disapproval, and loss of love; in part it is painful because it involves anticipation and dread of unnameable forthcoming consequences. Tension may arise in anticipation, before a rule is broken; guilt may be felt following the infraction. It is important in clinical work to recognize that guilt may be fully or vaguely conscious or unconscious. When unconscious, guilt is often betrayed by self-punitive or self-destructive acts; the patient is "answering to" some internal referent system (superego) which punishes, goads, rewards, and must be bribed, bypassed and, in any event, attended to. Some persons seem to search for a situation that externalizes and expresses their internal tension, conflict, and guilt; they commit antisocial acts and subsequently feel guilty but remain unaware of the underlying motive. Socially valuable guilt leads to tactful and appropriate reparation and concern. This is quite different from the excessive, self-centered suffering of the depressive, or acts of atonement based on unrealistic estimates of the fault and involving no appreciation for realistic means of repair. Some individuals stay glued to their "bad" or unacceptable impulses, bribing their punishing and critical self by repetitively atoning. Others resort to bribery of objects in order to gain approval and direction when they cannot develop an authentic and responsible self-control.

Other enduring affects or moods play an important role in psychopathology. *Apathy*, or general emotional underactivity, is not easily differentiated from passivity, depression, or from dullness and anergy that occurs in deficit states. It may be a genuine lack of responsiveness or a protective and defensive reaction to extreme hurt. As a defense, it could be translated into the logic or illogic of words: "If I cannot feel, I cannot be hurt." It may represent a malignant and general giving-up of all adaptive effort, and we are aware of physiologically unexplained states of simply wasting away, especially in elderly people. *Oversensitivity* is often coupled with anxiety. Paired with anger or inability to resolve conflicts and mobilize choice, it is encountered as irritability. A heightened awareness can mean a diminished capacity to select and control.

The least understood of all emotions is *euphoria*, especially in the enduring states of exaggerated well-being encountered in the syndrome of mania and, in less extreme forms, in hypomania. It is often found abruptly changing into anger and irritability. It may be a dominant affect in organic deteriorations or a temporary concomitant of the loss of habitual structure occasioned by a sudden change of state. While euphoria carries with it an escape or transcendence of constraints and concerns, neither existentialists nor psychoanalysts have really elucidated this affect. One of the psychoanalytic hypotheses assumes that euphoria is essentially a reaction designed to counter a deep dejection.[43]

Behavioral Controls

Controls and organization permeate all of behavior and to some extent even the most fragmented behaviors. It is interesting that in explaining controls we tend to "justify" their need and presence as if apologizing for constraints upon our infantile omnipotence. Thus: since neither our physical environment, our culture, nor our own efforts lead reliably to complete gratification and since frustration is unavoidable, controls are said to be "required." Whereas it is true that most of our controls of instinctual behavior are in fact acquired, this acquisition occurs only to some extent by imposition. Fundamentally, many controls are built-in "brakes" and acquisition of controls appears to be based on an inherent need for order and a capacity for delay, timing, and pacing of behavior, as well as a pleasure in mastery and problem-solving. The two large classes of control behavior are inhibitory and delaying activities and problem-solving or cognitive activities. We refer to the internalized conscious system of rules, which specifies what is permitted and what is forbidden as conscience. This agency corresponds in part, at least, to the external values, the mores and folkways of a society. We have already mentioned the valuable assumption of an unconscious system of aspirations—the ego ideal—and an agency (the superego) that unconsciously rewards or punishes and plays a critical role in a vast number of motivational conflicts. There are patients—the so-called sociopaths—who seem neither to respond to extreme punishment nor to have an inherent tendency to control themselves.

Controls of drive behavior may be voluntary or involuntary. Unconscious controls by definition are involuntary, but they are often integrated into a larger system, which is under conscious controls. For example, some controls over physiological functions, such as the elimination of bodily wastes, are so deeply ingrained that under ordinary circumstances they operate automatically, but they can be conscious and are, within certain limits, subject to volition. Defense mechanisms, a very important group of drive and affect-controlling mechanisms (which we discuss in the next chapter), usually cannot be readily discerned by the patient because they are preconscious or unconscious. Although possibly conditionable, they are not usually subject to direct and volitional control. The psychiatrist infers them by examining the patient's behavior and may (or may not) make his inference available to the patient through interpretation.

In the last half-century, relatively little has been written about will or volition, yet psychiatrists can hardly avoid the problem. Psychiatrists are constantly asked whether persons who have committed certain asocial acts are responsible and, indeed, our concept of behavior disorder implies a degree of irresponsibility. In general we observe, apart from any legal considerations, that man is always limited in modifying unconsciously organized drive behavior and is often helpless when truly unconscious forces are dominant. The authentic subjective experience of freedom and autonomy of choice requires that drives and controls be in a state of flexible balance. If and when a prevailing motivation is strengthened by new information, the person experiences a feeling of freedom in the capacity to make a volitional decision. A research worker cannot decide whether to go on a vacation or continue to work on a project full of headaches. A friend proposes a trip, and he accepts the invitation, because the prospect of traveling in company seems attractive —that is, this additional information, arriving in a receiver prepared to hear it (and able to act), turned out to be motivational and broke the former deadlock. The decision itself was experienced as a conscious and voluntary act. If therapy can facilitate the disposition to hear new information, then we can and do enlarge the area of the patient's voluntary activity. There are many occasions when it is appropriate and timely to remind the prepared patient that he can exercise choice and restraint. The unconscious cannot be argued or willed away, but it can be (at least partially) understood and influenced with effort and work.

Cognitive Processes

Perceived stimuli may have drive value, affective value, and discriminatory or cue value; many stimuli combine several values. Perception of simple sensations and more complex cues has been explored more by academic psychologists than by psychiatrists (with notable exceptions, for example, Emil Kraepelin, Otto Pötzl); only very recently have such investigations begun to arouse wider interest in psychiatric circles.[35] The exploration of the mediating processes that we call thinking has been of considerable concern to psychiatrists. *Thinking* or *cognitive* processes are uniquely characteristic for human behavior. They provide steering and control. Cognitive processes involve the use of signs and symbols or man-made signs. Susan Langer spoke of symbolic thinking as essentially human;[41] at the mention of his master's name (a sign) the dog wags his tail and looks for his master, whereas the adult human can picture and relate to an object in its absence and evoke images independent of external cues. Linguistic symbols enable man to cope with his complex internal structures and to imagine and objectify a picture about the world, himself, the past, and the future. The capacity to link the internal and external through symbols and to re-represent signals underlies our highest achievements; it also renders us vulnerable to error and distortion. Obviously, emotional expressions as well as words can be similarly processed, symbolically represented, and distorted. Thought may or may not precede action. Some psychologists consider thinking processes a rehearsing for action. Thoughts that function as "blueprints" for action are plans. The ability to plan realistically and carry out such plans is called *judgment*. It involves not only cognitive processes but the capacity to select or channel and to initiate action or make decisions. Psychiatrists have been, for practical reasons, quite interested in man's ability to plan and to make unambiguous and unimpulsive decisions that are based on realistic and not on wishful thinking. The capacity to do this is referred to in psychodynamic parlance as ego strength, a vague but useful term.

Different psychological schools distinguish between primitive and elaborate cognitive functions, generally with the notion that children, primitives, and very disturbed people operate at lower levels. Of course, children and primitives differ from psychotics, if only in the use to which non-logical thought is put. As Norman Cameron remarked, children do not, as they grow up, recover from schizophrenia nor does the regressed adult become a child.[12] In primitive thought, the tendency is for emotional needs to shape and distort symbolic functions (both symbolic representations and their linkage) resulting in highly subjective, unrealistic, and wishful thinking. A readiness to condense or displace the meaning of symbols, their fluid use, and an imperviousness to reality, time, and logic are characteristic of primary process thinking.

Whether a thought is pathological depends not only on formal characteristics but on the *use* to which it is put. Normal persons endow objects with personal attributes and speak of the raging sea, or the caressing wind. They are not confused by metaphor and poetic language. When a patient sees swinging doors as truly chomping jaws instead of as metaphorically chomping jaws, when thoughts are associated only by rhymes and not by relevant relationships, we are clearly dealing with pathological thought. Thus, whereas abnormal thinking may be recognizable by a lack of adherence to the rules of logic and syntax, usually we spot pathology of thought by its inappropriateness—a lack of integration with total behavior. Highly logical thought isolated from a relevant emotional context may be just as abnormal as palpably disorganized thought. What makes some behavior pathological is not the thought itself but the consequence of such a thought.

Symbolic Distortions

All communication is subject to distortion, and symbolic communication creates special problems. Such distortions may be conscious and deliberate, as in political propaganda, or in parental rules and explanations that have the effect of denying, masking, and disallowing relevant experience. Charles W. Morris divides the rules that govern the use of signs and also of symbols (or signs of signs) into syntactic, semantic, and pragmatic rules.[54] Symbolic distortion at the syntactic level occurs when symbols are not used according to the ordinary rules of language. This is the case in schizophrenia and in the cognitive dysfunctions associated with brain diseases—aphasias, agnosias, and apraxias. At the semantic level, distortion occurs when the sign or symbol does not denote the facts that it is supposed to represent; an inaccurate or false map misguiding its user would be an example. The inappropriate use of words, false generalizations, and stereotypes occurring in all behavior disorders fall into this category. For example, a young man has an unfortunate love affair and afterward labels all women as treacherous. The third type of distortion occurs at the pragmatic level: sender and receiver of a message attach different meanings to it. A wife tells her husband that he must love her, by which she means he has to endure and satisfy her excessive neurotic demands; to the husband, the word love means something else. Even more important than the above-mentioned classes of distortions is the fact that many symbolic distortions are built into group life and occur unnoticed by either sender or receiver.

Lawrence S. Kubie noted three levels of meaning in any symbol:[39] snake, for example, at the conscious level refers to reptiles; at the preconscious, it evokes metaphoric meanings of temptation or danger: snake-in-the-grass, the Garden of Eden; its bodily and unconscious root would be penis or feces. Aside from its specific adult references, "woman" might mean an object that gives or withholds care and pleasure and at even earlier levels tactile and oral comfort, or simply the equivalent of desired or dreaded engulfing or engulfment: the experience of internal satiation or a frightening or contented self-obliteration. While three levels of meaning can coexist, the choice of symbols would be multiply determined and dependent upon the dominant process (primary or secondary) organizing the ongoing cognitive activities.

The inherent plasticity and capacity of symbols to represent a number of events in one package can, if logically organized, facilitate abstracting. But their plasticity and the fact that they need not be logically organized probably accounts for the subtle distortions that are present in dreams and reveries and in all forms of artistic and religious activities as well as in neurotic acts. We can roughly gauge the severity of behavior disorder by an informal appraisal of the patient's ability to realize and correct distortions.

Dreams

Dreams are primitive cognitive but emotionally charged processes that occur largely during "fast sleep," the stage of sleep which is characterized by fast brain waves. While being dreamt, dreams are unshared. They consist mostly of visual imagery but also of acoustic, kinetic visceral, and, rarely, of olfactory and gustatory sensations. These sensations are accompanied by affects but generally are marked by the notable absence of actual motor responses. This lack of organized motor response could be viewed as the concrete correlate of the lack of reality-testing in the dream state. For Freud, the psychobiological motive in dreams was sleep protection. The psychological means by which this was achieved was through an attempt partially to fulfill instinctual wishes that might otherwise disturb sleep. Increases in excitation during sleep represent an upsurge of wishes and are coped with by dreaming, thereby allowing a discharge through other than motor routes. These wishes are usually connected with some unfinished or frustrating experience from the day preceding the dream and also with much older and more basic and enduring instinctual needs.

These strivings are prepared to "find" a current input that is appropriate as a vehicle for expression and are easily triggered by the residual thoughts and experiences of the day, which often were given only the briefest attention. Pötzl proved in ingenious experiments,[58] which were verified and elaborated by later investigators,[18, 36, 62] that tachistoscopically exposed pictures (upon which the patient concentrated but about which he could verbally report only a small portion) were represented in the dream imagery of the subjects. The clusters of infantile sexual and aggressive wishes are not compatible with the dreamer's conscious personality and will occur to him only when his vigilance is reduced in the regression of sleep, and even then in a disguised form. Freud called *dream work* the job of transforming latent drives and affects into "dream thoughts" and these into imagery that can suitably express and discharge the drives and affects without waking the dreamer. The "censor" acts to revise dream imagery until the manifest content is within tolerable limits. Freud saw these processes of distortion, self-expression, and compromise as occurring in dreams as well as in symptoms, forgetting, parapraxias (slips), and jokes. The coded disguise reduces the affective impact of dreams and protects the dreamer from awakening, just as symptoms prevent "waking up" to the unpleasant facts or confrontation with what—from the patient's special view—is intolerable danger.

The so-called dream symbols appear to have a relatively fixed meaning in dreams, and "universal symbols" are of great interest; perhaps they are based on common bodily experiences in infant development. Nevertheless, not all oblongated objects are phallic nor all cavities female genitalia.[2] If properly interpreted, dreams convey something about the dreamer's unconscious conflicts—the "latent dream thoughts" lying behind the manifest dream constructions (which in themselves reveal strivings and a style of coping).[7, 17] The interpretation of dreams, however, is usually difficult, although Freud believed that it was far easier than decoding covert strivings as they occur in the ongoing therapeutic interaction—in the transference. Dream interpretation requires the cooperation of the analysand, who "free associates" to the elements of the dream and thereby provides specific items to aid in translating the text of the dream. Typically, the analysand learns to analyze his productions. Despite Freud's penetrating work,[20] the decoding of dreams remains more an intuitive art than a science. Many complex and lengthy dreams of adults cannot be understood, even by skilful psychoanalysts. Children's dreams and also the "actual" dreams reported by subjects wakened during periods of EEG fast sleep and rapid eye movements are simpler.

Fantasies

Hypnagogic reveries of drowsing states and fantasies or daydreams are similar in content and structure to true dreams. As the latter, they are a way of thinking and representing the self to the self, but the distortion of reality is less marked. Fantasies range in structure and purpose from childlike theorizing (that is, linking of cause and effect with relatively primitive fantasies), to wish fulfilment and to rather realistic daydreams. The mental mechanisms that work to disguise or "detoxify" what is forbidden and sacrilegious are similar in night- and daydreams, in humor, folklore, art, and children's play. The play of children provides an arena for pleasure and experimentation that prepares the young for the exigencies (as well as leisure) of adult reality; the child's fantasied friends and playing are often "transitional modes" of dealing with current family relationships. As real dreams, fantasies are also adaptive, preparing the dreamer for a task (for example, communicating a problem to the therapist) or serving as a retreat from reality. Imagination, or the capacity to have fantasies, endows thought with rich connections; it may be constricted in some neuroses and impoverished as in depression or organic deficit. In some schizophrenias, manic symptoms, or toxic psychoses, imagination is uncontrolled. Fantasy in some situations can provide a path of retreat to autistic adjustment. Excessive imagination and playing is considered abnormal in our rationalistic culture, yet we usually cannot classify dreams and fantasies according to their content as normal or abnormal.

Hallucination and Illusion

Hallucinations are usually described as experiences of perception without any (known) objective stimulation to evoke them. Illusions are distortions or misinterpretations of perception; both hallucinations and illusions occur in a wide variety of regressed states and also in states of keen anticipation. Both illusions and hallucinations may be motivated—although not necessarily caused—by the need to reduce anxiety, and both may help the patient to adjust to frightening reality. Like dreams, hallucinations may be interpreted as attempts at wish fulfilment or as projections—ways of representing unacceptable experiences. Freud conceived of hallucinations as primitive representations or thoughts; the hungry infant "hallucinates" the absent mother's breast, and the use of sensory images in thought persists in adult life. Today most psychiatrists focus on the meaning of hallucinations, their dynamic value and their social function rather than minute descriptions of form and content (which might yet be useful in differentiating mental states). An emphasis on meaning and dynamics should not, however, lead us to confuse cause and effect; hallucinations may be a consequence of neural and chemical conditions that are the occasion for their occurrence. Fatigue, isolation, toxic conditions, as well as intense desire or fear provide conditions in which discrimination is impaired and in which a range of misinterpretations may occur: everyday slips, mishearings and misreadings, dreamlike absorption in memories, fantasies, delusions, and hallucinatory projection of internal ruminations and debates. The power of psychological "set" is evident in "anticipatory" hallucinations, illusions, and slips; the misinterpretation of examination questions by a tense student, or the distortion of overheard fragments of conversation if one is self-conscious, or of shadows as a trespasser, are common examples. Obviously, the psychological setting or levels in which these distortions occur, the overall organization and balance of reality and wish, are the differentiating factors determining the nature and function of misinterpretive phenomena. Cultures that strongly reward categorical rather than perceptual thinking, inhibit hallucinatory experiences, which may, in some settings, be a normal way of thinking certain thoughts and adapting.

Auditory hallucinations in the major psychoses are more frequent than hallucinations involving other sensory organs. They often appear to reflect internal conflict, the voices chastising or approving. The fact that self-esteem, reward, censure, and punishment are subjects of the internal debate reveals not only the current needs but the structure and source of these internalized experiences. In learning to regulate oneself, there has been an "incorporation" of the parental voices that were directive; the patient has proceeded to improve when he can identify these vividly heard voices (or, at another level, thoughts) as his own, something for which he has responsibility. Occasionally compelling hallucinations not only warn and scold and defend the patient, but direct him to act, and the innocent may be victims of these commands. Many patients attend to hallucinatory activity episodically, apparently shifting their interest from ongoing events to internal preoccupations; we do not know what environmental or internal factor determines these shifts. In some toxic and organic states, in contrast to chronic schizophrenia, the content of hallucinations appears strikingly amenable to suggestion and to concurrent environmental changes.

Encountered in many severe disorders with regressive features, hallucinations are signs of a shift in level of functioning but are not diagnostic of the particular underlying disorder. In view of what has been learned about the psychobiological determinants of dreaming (Chapter 6) we have much to learn about the interneural and intracerebral conditions that may facilitate, induce, or compel hallucinatory experience. Visual, auditory, visceral, tactile, and olfactory hallucinations are experienced as part of epileptic seizures and can be induced in man by electrical stimulation of temporal lobe structures. Even here, however, the detailed content can be determined by psychological factors, including the situation at the time of the seizure. There clearly are a number of different pathways by which hallucinatory behavior may become manifest in behavior.[47] Sensory and sleep deprivation and psychotomimetic drugs induce states in which hallucinations may be experienced.

These experimental conditions induce an alteration in the capacity to organize and implement an ongoing experience, a regression in which logical and illogical thinking coexist and in which habitual modes of response come into play less readily. Customary experiences become novel and portentous; processing of input requires more work and the usual filtering and suppressing mechanisms seem impaired.[63]

Hallucinations frequently occur when corrective and adaptive procedures and regard for reality are reduced especially by severe deprivations and intense anxiety; experimentally induced thirst, for example, does not produce perceptual distortion similar to that of a man genuinely stranded, overactivated, and deprived who then experiences a mirage.[35] Since hallucinatory phenomena are indeed experienced and "visualized" in the "mind's eye," they compel belief, and their occurrence may be real enough. What the patient requires to overcome them is the motivation and capacity to identify their source—to discriminate the internal and the external. If the patient hears or sees things that are in fact not there, we can view this as a distinct way of thinking at a particular level of organization such as that of a dream or a psychosis. At a higher level, such hallucinations may be replaced simply by images—or by something to be thought about.[57] As the patient who hears loud voices shouting instructions improves, the voices either recede or he does not notice them. The patient may then merely know what he is doing without the help of hallucinated instructions: awareness, judgment, and discrimination have "replaced" hallucinations.

Delusions

Delusions are incorrigible false beliefs that are not shared or sanctioned by a group. As we ordinarily encounter them in psychiatry, delusions are unshared experiences, although we recognize delusions of groups. It is startling to find that both the content of the patient's delusion and his primitive mode of thinking can be traced in part to familial experience. The difference between a deluded patient and his somewhat prejudiced family lies in part in the capacity of those not ill to cope; they seem to utilize family myths and rationalizations in a manner that does not dangerously impair reality functioning. The formal aspects of the delusion need not differentiate the patient and his family. The same distinctions also apply to group delusions and group beliefs. As with perceptual experiences, the context in which such thinking occurs and the way it is handled and integrated into the totality of behaving is critical.

Both delusions and hallucinations are primitive experiences in which strong drives and wishes operate. Freud showed conclusively that such drives, affects, and related thoughts are projected into social molds in the form of constructions or explanations that can guide the patient and still satisfy internal requirements. Delusions have a defensive, expressive, and regulatory function, and the patient's identity and contact with the world often appears to hinge, for a time, solely on his delusions.[55] This strategic function of the delusion in the presence of defective reality-testing makes such belief systems rigid and inaccessible to reason; even slight modification of the "dogma" seems impossible. Persons who doubt, who advocate correction, are seen as enemies and are incorporated into the system.

Delusions may be coupled with hallucinations and illusions (particularly in regressed and disorganized patients). Among the more common types are: paranoid delusions or delusions of persecution; delusions of influence and reference, in which patients feel themselves observed or subjected to strange forces inducing them to act in an antisocial or immoral manner; hypochondriacal delusions in depressions, schizophrenias, and organic reactions; and rigid denial of illness. The loss of control and autonomy over what is transpiring and compensatory efforts in the face of such loss are apparent in these phenomena. In the group of delusional denials of illness are interesting cerebral syndromes, which were previously mentioned, such as denial of hemiplegias, which occur with lesions in the non-dominant hemispheres, denial of blindness, and the syndrome of a phantom limb (which occurs after amputations).

Intelligence and Problem-Solving

There is no completely satisfactory definition of a total capacity for problem-solving behavior, which we call intelligence. The prevalent, simple, and operational definition—intelligence is what is tested in intelligence tests—begs the question. Many view intelligence as a general factor, characteristic of most mental operations, and unique skills are then usually considered separately. From a clinical point of view, we are concerned with such abilities as (1) capacity to learn and perform logical operations and solve abstract problems; (2) judgment, or the capacity to discriminate, perform correctly and relevantly in practical and especially social situations, as well as the capacity to plan and to make realistic choices in which thinking precedes or underlies action; (3) fund of knowledge; (4) memory, attention, concentration, and the primitive capacity for orientation. In any case, intelligence is essential for the assessment of reality although such assessment does not solely depend on intelligence per se, but on the proper use of intelligence without undue interference from drives and affects. The routine tests in clinical psychiatry are generally conducted in the context of a clinical interview during which the psychiatrist can directly or indirectly explore the patient's intellectual capacity, his fund of knowledge, and make a quick, practical assessment of orientation, memory, and attention. Our interest in special abilities and skills is stimulated by a concern with occupational rehabilitation. Little is known about the range of these and particularly of creative abilities, although some are accessible to special testing by psychological techniques. The evaluation of biographies of creative men do not show a close association of high creativity and mental health. Biologists have speculated that a negative correlation could represent the costliness of special gifts—another instance of the link of desirable and undesirable traits that frequently occurs in selection.

If we are to have stability, each event in the world cannot possibly be perceived as novel; rather, input must be linked with some stable internal framework. Such internal referent systems (known as "sets" or attitudes) appear to "anticipate" input and to coordinate ongoing behavior. A simple and unpleasant example would be a prejudice in which minimal information is required for elaborate ideas and often important decisions. These internal referent systems are also called hypotheses, cognitive structures or maps, schemata, or conceptual tools.[25] Experts in cognition believe that human intelligence does not vary in what can be taken in; rather, it depends on salient "keys"—strategies—which simplify the steps in problem-solving. Some of these operations have been built into machines. It is speculated that such devices may be involved in human problem-solving: coding of the input (such as in mnemonic devices) can speed performance, and such steps as "successive approximations" are devices for testing and eliminating irrelevant categories and narrowing down to a probable choice (as in the game of twenty questions). In order to solve problems there must be occasional checks on the applicability of ongoing strategies or "stocktaking"; this involves the ability to shift sets, and this capacity is found to be impaired in organic deficit states and schizophrenias.

Intellectual Deficit Reactions

The pathological inability to solve problems is called intellectual deficit. As with normal problem-solving, deficit reactions cannot be viewed in isolation. As a matter of fact, in all deficit reactions the emergence of otherwise controlled drives is quite important and often responsible for the excessive disorganization and "desocialization" of such behavior. Desocialization refers to diminished social contact and appreciation of social values, meanings, and relationships.

Deficit reactions, whether innate or acquired during infancy and early childhood, are referred to as *mental subnormality*. The mentally subnormal individual lacks the equipment, motivation, or opportunity to learn—or at least to acquire knowledge—at the usual pace. We distinguish between the *mentally deficient* with cerebral impairment and the *mentally retarded* without impairment. Many problems of the retarded are not created by the primary deficiency but by the attendant psychological and social stresses, which will be discussed in some detail in Chapter 19. The deficit reactions acquired in later life are divided into *organic deficit reactions* associated with demonstrable brain diseases and those that are not. The organic deficit reactions are usually, though not accurately, divided into *acute deficit reactions* occurring in relatively active brain diseases, and *chronic deficit reactions* in persons with relatively permanent cerebral deficits. Chronic and acute deficit reactions may occur simultaneously or alternatingly in the same patient.

The *acute deficit reactions* are seen in active cerebral diseases, in injuries and intoxications with rapidly changing cerebral pathology (often manifested by seizures), and in certain states of sensory deprivation—and possibly also in severe panic states. The hallmark of acute organic deficit states is disturbance of awareness, attention, memory, and orientation. The patient, unable to process the input, loses his reference points about reality and himself. He is bewildered and frightened. His anxiety and inability to solve his problems are usually enhanced by some dim preconscious perception of his acute illness.

The *chronic organic deficit reactions* occur in diffuse, slowly changing, or permanent cerebral lesions resulting from brain diseases and injuries. The severe deficits observed in old age usually fall into the category of chronic organic deficit reactions. The organic deteriorations are characterized by disturbances in abstract and complex thinking, memory defects, and the inability to learn new skills. In patients with organic deficits, a tendency to adhere to accustomed practices and an avoidance of exposing themselves to new situations is marked. In extreme cases this inability to shift, change, assume new roles, and perform creative tasks takes on the form of perseveration of thought, language, and behavior. The clinical syndromes of acute and chronic organic deficit states are taken up in Chapter 16. The most puzzling deficit reactions are the *schizophrenic deficit reactions,* which we will describe in detail in Chapter 14. In such reactions, thought and language are strangely irrelevant and incoherent. Affective responses and drive behavior seem inadequate and also inappropriate. Reality and self are grossly misjudged and responded to in highly unconventional ways. The essence of this disturbance is at present not well understood or explained.

Thinking may become accelerated in hypomanic and manic states, called "flight or pressure of ideas," or slowed down, referred to as "retardation" (not to be confused with retardation in mental deficiency) in depressive states. Depressive retardation is at times not too easily differentiated from "blocking" of thought in schizophrenia. In this particular thought disorder, thinking moment only becomes arrested, "withdrawn" or "emptied." Impairment of task efficiency occurs not only in psychotic but in many neurotic reactions which involve a milder degree of misjudgment of reality and the patient's needs and usually is produced by a motivational disturbance rather than a lowered capacity. In obsessive disorders, thinking becomes rigid; sophistry tends to replace a more plastic and flexible use of words and concepts. In hysterical patients, playful and dramatic, symbolic, and allegoric thinking is manifest, which is also more easily subject to correction than the thinking disturbances of the psychoses. What is common to all these disturbances of thinking is the intrusion of drive-dominated behavior that permeates the "cue-oriented" behavior of cognitive processes. In neuroses it is less marked and more easily reparable. According to Norman Cameron, all deficit states are characterized by disorganization, desocialization, and regression.[13] We submit that these phenomena exist in varying degrees in all behavior disorders.

Attention and Orientation

We refer to the capacity to focus and concentrate on tasks as attention. In a wide variety of psychiatric syndromes, this ability is disturbed. Such patients are easily distractible or preoccupied, and sometimes their orientation or ability to identify themselves as to time, place, and the spatial and temporal coordinates of this situation is disturbed. We observe this in anxiety states, in many schizophrenic reactions, and most pronouncedly in the delirious syndromes, where basic disorientation and confusion are the most striking symptoms. Patients seem unable to decide whether to attend certain stimuli; their vigilance for certain classes of stimuli is impaired, though at times they seem under the pressure of drives and affect, or hypervigilant to irrelevant stimuli, or subject to overanticipation and false alarms. We also speak of a disturbance of "orienting" functions—the work of getting ready or set for what may come. There is much to learn about the various levels of control that influence focusing and attention, but it is clear that a crucial sign of impaired organization is whether attention is felt to be compelled or is under self-control. Relative autonomy of the organism with respect to control over attention and concentration appears to be a prime sign of optimal functioning. Experimental studies are beginning to map out the basic capacities of the operations involved in the intake of information,[51] its retention, and processing in normal and abnormal states.[9,10]

Edwin A. Weinstein and Robert L. Kahn drew attention to complex psychosocial factors contributing to disorientation and disturbances of attention.[66] In many instances, patients with a delirious syndrome (already restricted in function) are so alarmed by their illness that they have to deny it. They also find their surroundings uninteresting or so unacceptable that they reject them. Under such conditions it is of little import to the patient where he is or how and when he got to the hospital. Nor does he wish to know what happened to him; he only feels desperately in need of support and care by familiar persons. Conditions of sensory deprivation or a reduction of (meaningful) sensory input occur in persons isolated in unstimulating environments, such as in wards for chronic mental patients. For such patients, one day is like the next, existence is completely routine; it hardly pays to know the doctor or nurse in charge. Clearly, there are reasons to deny that one is incarcerated, and the wish to be free, at home or with friends, is also obvious, especially when one can be with them in wish rather than in a less perfect actuality. All of these determinants could produce some disturbances of attention, orientation, and memory—and subsequently confabulation in normal persons—and would particularly do so in severely regressed persons. If we turn the problem around and ask what *can* a regressed person attend to, we recognize his very real limitations of the moment and a feature of all attentional dysfunction—the lack of flexible control and autonomy over attention. In organic states, the *major* reason for attentional dysfunction and for error and misconception is not motivational but biological. As Jackson saw it, the patient is now in a more automatic state and, besides his "not knowings" due to organic deficit, his "wrong knowings"—his misperceptions—are due not solely to compensatory moves, but to the level of organization biologically available.

Memory

Memory is the capacity to retain, recall, and recognize psychological data; it underlies conditioning, learning, and higher mental functions. *Retention* and *recall* occur with awareness or without it, as in a retained behavioral pattern occurring on cue. Continuity and stability in a changing environment are guaranteed by our capacity to reproduce and recognize familiar elements in the milieu. The enormously developed memory capacities of man link past and present in a unique fashion and also enable him to plan for the future by making choices based on past experience. They make of man a creative being, conscious of time and bound by it. Clinically, we usually examine memory by testing recall, or the task of reproducing or recognizing previously learned stimuli. In experimental work in man and animals, behavioral scientists test memory by comparison of repeated trials of learning and conditioning.

The capacity to retain and recall structured and coded data is much greater than the capacity to retain relatively amorphous data. It is easier to retain organized material than less meaningful material learned by rote. One of the causes for the so-called amnesia of childhood is the fact that material that is not structured by linguistic symbols is difficult to remember; another is, as Freud discovered,[21] the power of repression. The same explanation also applies to the recall of more primitive perceptual and ideational data such as dreams and reveries.

Loss of memory may be brought on by factors ranging from neural to psychological events. It may be general or specific; it may involve the most important identifying data (such as name, age, and address in so-called total amnesia), which may also be regarded as a form of disorientation. In acute brain injuries, the amnesia for events extends only over a limited period of time before or after the injury (retrograde or antegrade amnesia, respectively). In diffuse brain damage, for example, in advanced senile disorders and in organic deficit states, memory is generally impaired. Motivational factors also play a role in such memory defects as can be demonstrated in patients with an organic dymnesic syndrome who relearn material in which they are interested, and which is not conflict-laden, faster than other material.

The selective intake of information, its consolidation, its storage and retrieval, can be studied at many levels; lesions of the hippocampus, for example, are thought to interfere with the consolidation of input so that current events are only fleetingly recallable.[53] Memory disturbances with experimentally altered brain chemistry, for example, procedures changing the rate of catabolism of brain acetylcholine, are under study, and the role of nucleic acids such as ribosenucleic acid, important in the "memory" of immunity and genetics, as well as the role of small molecules, is currently of interest.[11,15,29,30,59] Hypermnesia is seen in certain, usually early, psychotic states, often with trance and drug states, and in a sense in traumatic neuroses.

A major advance in our understanding of dymnesic behavior came from Freud's discovery of what he called the psychopathology of everyday life:[22] forgetting names, slips of the tongue, and other banal errors. Freud pointed out that such behavior is caused by emotional conflict; a name or event that is associated with unpleasant, unethical, or dangerous needs is repressed if it clashes with protective or controlling needs. The analytic method enhances the conditions for remembering and may help the patient to recover the forgotten word, event, or object, and also to identify the rather complex motivation for the repression and the loss of memory. Memory, it should be noted, is often contained in actions as well as images; it is surprising how often a minor ritual or a major "acting out" is a "choreographed" memory of conflict, which cannot otherwise be expressed.

Under the impact of a psychodynamic orientation, we are apt to overlook the fact that there is something like simple forgetting due to disuse. Psychologists have pointed to the phenomenon of retroactive inhibition: the learning of newer responses has an inhibiting influence on the old response; the learning of a new language will tend to inhibit the recall of the symbols of the older language. Experimental and clinical study of forgetting and pathways for retrieval or recall has much yet to discover and teach.

Normal and Abnormal Behavior

After reviewing some of the principal categories and relevant operations underlying behavior, we are in a better position to discuss the concepts of normal and abnormal behavior.[6,60] The concepts of normality and abnormality are more complex in psychiatry than in general medicine, and some people have suggested abandoning the concepts of normal and abnormal behavior entirely because simple concepts of health and disease do not apply. Marie Jahoda[31] and other social psychologists are using the concept of positive mental health, which is supposed to designate more than an absence of mental illness. Three traditional approaches to the concept of health in psychiatry can be distinguished: (1) the statistical approach, (2) the clinical approach, and (3) the normative approach. The statistical approach focuses on average behavior and determines what deviates from the statistical average. Few exact data, however, are available on the frequency and distribution of behavior traits. Such an approach presupposes that behavior is quantifiable and measurable, but obviously many forms of behavior are not. Good examples of this approach are the data supplied by Alfred C. Kinsey *et al.* on sexual behavior,[33, 34] socioeconomic data—income, consumption, and production of goods—as well as the broad investigations of intelligence. Few data, however, exist on the prevalence and the incidence of psychiatric symptoms, such as anxiety, hallucinations, phobias, and so forth. Statistical data are, of course, not helpful in determining whether a given individual is sick or well, which may have something to do with the fact that clinicians have, without justification, a deprecating attitude toward morbidity statistics.

The clinical approach defines as abnormal anything that does not function according to its design. This approach is useful in somatic illness, including brain disease, but it is less helpful in behavior disorders, because all too often we do not know what design or function a certain behavior pattern serves. Heinz Hartmann[27] and also George L. Engel [16] view adaptation as a crucial criterion for normality. We find this concept, which is supposed to explain just about everything, only of very limited use in differentiating normal and abnormal behavior. Hartmann's concept of the "average expectable environment," however, is useful for an assessment of normality because it stresses that normality of behavior is judged not under extreme conditions of stress but under average conditions. In general terms, clinical normality is not ideal performance but minimal performance, just above the level of pathological performance for a given individual.

Another practical attempt to define normality in terms of maturity has been suggested by John G. Whitehorn;[67] adult and mature behavior are normal; infantile and immature behavior are abnormal. Much of what clinicians consider abnormal is immature behavior. Carl Binger pointed out that a two-year-old with temper tantrums, endowed with the physical and intellectual abilities of the adult, would be a veritable monster.[4]

An important clinical and theoretical approach is Kubie's assumption that predominance of conscious and preconscious motivations over unconscious motivation of behavioral acts determines normality.[38] Normal behavior is flexible and characterized by the capacity to learn. Unconscious behavior is rigid, repetitive, and insatiable. In criticism of Kubie's proposals, one may point to the fact that in many types of normal and socially desirable behavior, unconscious and preconscious motivations occur: in passionate love or in ecstatic religious experience, or in projections and identifications that are instrumental for the appreciation of art or empathy with our fellow human beings. In an effort to meet these objections, Kubie differentiated more rigorously between preconscious and unconscious motivations; the unconscious acts, according to him, are tantamount to bad, irrational, non-adaptive behavior, a psychosocial orientation that he wanted to avoid. Kubie's theory also fails to apply to phenomena like mental deficiency and many forms of abnormal behavior determined by brain disease.

In the authors' opinion, most propositions on normality and abnormality depend on value judgments. Take Karl Menninger's statement: "Let us define mental health as the adjustment of human beings to the world and to each other with a maximum of effectiveness and happiness. Not just efficiency, or just contentment, or the grace of obeying the rules of the game cheerfully. It is all of these together. It is the ability to maintain an even temper, an alert intelligence, socially considerate behavior, and a happy disposition. This, I think is a healthy mind." [50] There is nothing wrong with such a statement, as long as it is recognized as a value proposition; abnormality depends on the cultural values of defining persons. What is normal drinking? In many Irish, French, Italian, German, and Scandinavian families, moderate drinking is normal; to Protestant fundamentalists and Moslem believers, any imbibing of alcohol is abnormal. Prostitution is accepted in some cultures but not in others. There are remarkable differences in aggression, sexuality, and dependency needs in the different social classes of a single culture, and there are notable differences in the acceptance of mental illness in different cultures. The Indian sage, Ramakrishna, was considered a prophet and a saintly man by many of his companions, but he would have been judged as mentally disturbed by Western psychiatrists (and in all likelihood he also would have behaved differently had he lived in a Western cultural setting). Although some social scientists do not accept a relativistic point of view, it would seem that only extreme forms of behavior, such as indiscriminate murder, cannibalism, or absolute disregard for property are almost universally rejected. The more severe a behavior disorder, the more likely is it considered abnormal, regardless of the cultural context. In actual practice, psychiatrists use a composite approach; they diagnose behavior as clearly abnormal when it is seriously disabling, frustrating, deviates from established cultural norms, hence occurs relatively rarely; however, in borderline cases such an approach does not work well.

One of the revealing pieces of empirical research on normality is by Roy R. Grinker, Sr., *et al.*, who studied homoclites, or persons who follow the common rule.[26] Their subjects were male students of a college that specializes in teaching group work, recreation, and physical education. Grinker found these students amazingly free of disabling symptoms. The subjects were of average intelligence, worked well, but were not ambitious or creative; they had adequate stable adjustment to reality. They were middle-of-the-roaders and had warm human relationships with parents, teachers, friends, and girls; they had a firm sense of identity, with relatively few areas of conflict. Grinker noted the following contributing factors: good health, parental cooperation in child-rearing, strong identification with parents, sound early religious training, reasonable and consistent punishment and also definite limitations set on behavior, early work history and eagerness to tackle problems in a common-sense fashion, a disinclination to introspection, and an emphasis on good fellowship. For these people money was only a means and not a goal.

In summary, the concept of health and normality is still quite muddled, with empirical research mostly lacking.[6] Only gross deviations are clearly recognized and agreed upon in all civilized societies; borderlines of normal and abnormal behavior are fuzzy and overlapping. Cultural relativism with respect to milder disorders is the rule. The judgments of psychiatrists cannot in reality be far removed from those of the common man of the societies and cultures in which psychiatrists and patients live. At present, we cannot make precise statements about normal and abnormal; we can, however, define to a certain extent the psychiatric sick role.

The Psychiatric Sick Role

Diseases and injuries put the patient into the sick role, legitimately excusing him from work and social obligations and granting him the right of special attention, while requiring him to do his best to recover. Psychosocial losses are balanced by certain advantages that are quite similar to those offered by neuroses (the secondary gains). Patients may exploit their somatic illnesses to evoke support and avoid obligations. Illness may become a style through which comfort can be achieved. Symptoms of somatic illness may become a part of one's identity, inducing the patient to stay entrenched in incapacity rather than to adapt more creatively to his limitations. Such factors are contributory but remarkably potent in sustaining behavior disorders related to physical illness.

The "psychatric sick role"—a term that may be questioned by purists—is considerably more complex than the medical sick role. The bulk of psychiatric patients are not sick in the ordinary sense; if the term were less awkward we might speak of a "disordered behavior role." We suggest two basic types: (1) the sick role of the patient with severe behavior disorders; (2) the sick role of the patient with mild to moderate disorders. The first group corresponds to the psychotic and severely neurotic groups. In all technologically advanced societies, such patients require attention and psychiatrists and other mental health workers are charged with this task. Patients need not be cooperative; if necessary, society enforces treatment and confinement to psychiatric institutions. Such patients, like medical patients, are excused from work and other social obligations; they are not considered accountable for antisocial acts. If the patients with obvious and unequivocally severe behavior disorders commit crimes they are treated—or at least restrained—in psychiatric rather than in penal institutions, although Western society is far from certain what it should do with the less obvious behavior disorders associated with criminal acts. In patients with severe disorders, the goal of therapy is to free the patient from his most severe, undesirable, and crippling symptoms. In treating these patients, therapists employ a wide variety of therapeutic means, ranging from the biological to the psychosocial; moreover, generally speaking, they maintain a medical therapeutic role. In the light of new empirical knowledge the sick role of patients in mental hospitals is quite complex. Daniel L. Levinson and Eugene B. Gallagher examined patienthood or the human conditions in a mental hospital.[42] They view the mental hospital as a quasi-bureaucratic institution—somewhere between a prison, a boarding school, and a general hospital—with a therapeutic-educative-corrective task. In such a system, patients assume complex patient-student-inmate roles. The patient role in the second group is quite different. Patients in this category, roughly corresponding to the moderate to moderate-mild group (which cannot be readily differentiated from the "normal" general population), request therapy or are advised to seek therapy, not because they are helpless or severely troubled in most spheres of living; rather, they hope for the realization of their capabilities. These patients are accountable for their acts; they do not receive, generally speaking, the benefits of the medical sick role, such as being relieved from work and other social obligations. Their relationship with the therapist is, at least in adult patients, a voluntary one, and the goal of therapy is the patient's self-actualization. The therapy of this group is entirely psychosocial. The extent to which the sick role is granted to neurotics and sociopaths is far from settled, both in the minds of experts and the general public.

These two types surely do not encompass all possible variants of the psychiatric sick role. Indeed, many people come to psychiatrists neither in total despair nor for self-actualization; they come for temporary relief of a troublesome state. Yet the distinction between the two basic roles can be helpful in answering: "Who becomes a psychiatric patient?" Psychological status and behavioral signs alone do not establish what a case is; the process of becoming not only disturbed but a case depends on those social and cultural factors that determine the sick role. Beyond any doubt, the psychiatric sick role depends on socioeconomic status and ethnic factors, as well as on the availability and general orientation of therapeutic facilities.

NOTES

1. Gordon W. Allport, *Pattern and Growth in Personality* (New York: Holt, Rinehart and Winston, 1961).
2. Gustav Bally, *Einführung in die Psychoanalyse* (Munich: Rowohlt, 1961).
3. Edward Bibring, "Symposium on the Theory of Therapeutic Results of Psychoanalysis," *International Journal of Psycho-Analysis*, 18 (1937), 170.
4. Carl Binger, "What Is Maturity?" *Harper's*, 202 (1951), 70.
5. Ray L. Birdwhistell, "Contribution of Linguistic-Kinesic Studies to the Understanding of Schizophrenia," in A. Auerback, ed., *Schizophrenia* (New York: Ronald Press, 1959).

6. Sidney J. Blatt, "An Attempt to Define Mental Health," *Journal of Consulting Psychology*, 28 (1964), 146.
7. Walter Bonime, *The Clinical Use of Dreams* (New York: Basic Books, 1962).
8. Percy W. Bridgman, *The Way Things Are* (Cambridge: Harvard University Press, 1959).
9. Donald E. Broadbent, *Perception and Communication* (London: Pergamon Press, 1958).
10. Enoch Callaway, III, R. T. Jones and R. S. Layne, "Evoked Responses and Segmental Set of Schizophrenia," *Archives of General Psychiatry*, 12 (1965), 83.
11. D. Ewen Cameron, "The Process of Remembering," British *Journal of Psychiatry*, 109 (1963), 325.
12. Norman Cameron, *Personality Development and Psychopathology* (Boston: Houghton Mifflin, 1963).
13. Norman Cameron and Ann Magaret, *Behavior Pathology* (Boston: Houghton Mifflin, 1951).
14. Karl Deutsch, *The Nerves of Government* (New York: The Free Press of Glencoe, 1963).
15. Joel Elkes, "Subjective and Objective Observation in Psychiatry," in *The Harvey Lectures, Series 57* (New York: Academic Press, 1962).
16. George L. Engel, "Homeostasis, Behavioral Adjustment and the Concept of Health and Disease," in Roy Grinker, ed., *Mid-Century Psychiatry* (Springfield, Ill.: Charles C Thomas, 1953).
17. Erik H. Erikson, "Identity and the Life Cycle," *Psychological Issues: Selected Papers*, Vol. 1, No. 1 (New York: International Universities Press, 1959).
18. Charles Fisher, "Dreams and Perception," *Journal of the American Psychoanalytic Association*, 2 (1954), 389.
19. Seymour Fischer and S. Cleveland, "An Approach to Physiological Reactivity in Terms of a Body Image Schema," *Psychological Review*, 64 (1957), 26.
20. Sigmund Freud, *The Interpretation of Dreams* (1900) (New York: Basic Books, Inc., 1955).
21. Sigmund Freud, "New Introductory Lectures on Psycho-Analysis (1933)," *Standard Edition*, Vol. 22 (London: Hogarth Press, 1964).
22. Sigmund Freud, "The Psychopathology of Everyday Life (1901)," *Standard Edition*, Vol. 6 (London: Hogarth Press, 1960).
23. Sigmund Freud, "The Unconscious (1915)," *Standard Edition*, Vol. 14 (London: Hogarth Press, 1955).
24. W. Horsley Gantt, "Principles of Nervous Breakdown—Schizokinesis and Autokinesis," *Annals of the New York Academy of Science*, 56 (1953), 143.
25. Riley Gardner, Philip S. Holzman, George S. Klein, Harriet B. Linton, and Donald P. Spence, "Cognitive Control: A Study of Individual Consistencies

in Cognitive Behavior," *Psychological Issues,* Vol. I, No. 4 (New York: International Universities Press, 1959).

26. Roy R. Grinker, Sr., Roy R. Grinker, Jr., and J. Timberlake, " 'Mentally Healthy' Young Males (Homoclites)," *Archives of General Psychiatry,* 16 (1962), 405.
27. Heinz Hartmann, "Psychoanalysis and the Concept of Health," *International Journal of Psycho-Analysis,* 20 (1939), 308.
28. David R. Hawkins, John T. Monroe, Myron G. Sandifer, and Charles R. Vernon, "Psychological and Physiological Responses to Continuous Epinephrine Infusion—an Approach to the Study of the Affect, Anxiety," in Louis J. West and Milton Greenblatt, eds., *Explorations in the Physiology of Emotions* (Washington, D.C.: Psychiatric Research Reports of the American Psychiatric Association No. 12, 1960).
29. Oscar Hechter and I. O. K. Halkerston, "On the Nature of Macromolecular Coding in Neuronal Memory," in *Perspectives in Biology and Medicine,* 7 (1964), 183.
30. Holger Hyden, "A Molecular Basis of Neuron-Glia Interaction," in Francis O. Schmitt, ed., *Macromolecular Specificity and Biological Memory* (Cambridge: Massachusetts Institute of Technology Press, 1962).
31. Marie Jahoda, "Toward a Social Psychology of Mental Health," in Arnold M. Rose, ed., *Mental Health and Mental Disorder* (London: Routledge and Kegan Paul, 1956).
32. Karl Jaspers, *General Psychopathology,* translated by J. Hoenig and Marian W. Hamilton (Chicago: University of Chicago Press, 1963).
33. Alfred C. Kinsey, W. B. Pomeroy, and C. E. Martin, *Sexual Behavior in the Human Male* (Philadelphia: Saunders, 1948).
34. Alfred C. Kinsey, Wardell B. Pomeroy, Clyde E. Martin, and Paul H. Gebhard, *Sexual Behavior in the Human Female* (Philadelphia: Saunders, 1953).
35. George S. Klein, "Need and Regulation," in Marshall R. Jones, ed., *Nebraska Symposium on Motivation* (Lincoln: University of Nebraska Press, 1954).
36. George S. Klein, D. P. Spence, Robert R. Holt, and S. Gourevitch, "Cognition without Awareness: Subliminal Influences upon Conscious Thought," *Journal of Abnormal Social Psychology,* 57 (1958), 255.
37. Lawrence C. Kolb, "Disturbances of the Body Image," in Silvano Arieti, ed., *American Handbook of Psychiatry,* Vol. II, pp. 749–769 (New York: Basic Books, Inc., 1959).
38. Lawrence S. Kubie, "The Fundamental Nature of the Distinction Between Normality and Neurosis," *Psychoanalytic Quarterly,* 23 (1954), 167.
39. Lawrence S. Kubie, "Influence of Symbolic Processes on the Role of Instincts in Human Behavior," *Psychosomatic Medicine,* 18 (1956), 189.
40. John I. Lacey, in "Timberline Conference on Psychophysiologic Aspects of Cardiovascular Disease," *Psychosomatic Medicine,* 26 (1964), 445.
41. Susan K. Langer, *Philosophy in a New Key* (Cambridge: Harvard University Press, 1957).

42. Daniel J. Levinson and Eugene B. Gallagher, *Patienthood in the Mental Hospital* (Boston: Houghton Mifflin, 1964).
43. Bertram D. Lewin, *The Psychoanalysis of Elation* (New York: Norton, 1950).
44. Konrad Lorenz, *Über das Sogenaunte Böse* (*Zur Naturgeschichte der Aggression*) (Wien: Barota Schoeler, 1963).
45. Alexander R. Luria, *A Nature of Human Conflicts: or Emotion, Conflict and Will, An Objective Study of Disorganization and Control of Human Behavior* (New York: Liveright, 1932).
46. Seymour L. Lustman, "Rudiments of the Ego," in *The Psychoanalytic Study of the Child* (New York: International Universities Press, 1956), Vol. II.
47. George F. Mahl, Albert Rothenberg, Jose M. R. Delgado, and H. Hamlin, "Psychological Responses in the Human to Intracerebral Electrical Stimulation," *Psychosomatic Medicine*, 26 (1964), 337.
48. Robert B. Malmo and C. Shagass, "Electromyographic Studies of Muscular Tension in Psychiatric Patients under Stress," *Journal of Clinical Experimental Psychopathology*, 12 (1951), 45.
49. Abraham H. Maslow, *Motivation and Personality* (New York: Harper, 1954).
50. Karl Menninger, *The Human Mind* (3d ed.; New York: Alfred A. Knopf, 1946).
51. George A. Miller, Eugene Galanter and Karl Pribram, *Plans and the Structure of Behavior* (New York: Holt, 1960).
52. James Grier Miller, *Unconsciousness* (New York: John Wiley and Sons, Inc., 1942).
53. Brenda Milner, "The Memory Defect in Bilateral Hippocampal Lesions," *Psychiatric Research Reports*, 11 (1959), 43.
54. Charles W. Morris, *Signs, Language and Behavior* (Englewood Cliffs, N.J.: Prentice-Hall, 1946).
55. Rafael Moses and Daniel X. Freedman, " 'Trademark' Function of Symptoms in a Mental Hospital," *Journal of Nervous and Mental Disease*, 127 (1958), 448.
56. Gerhart Piers and M. B. Singer, *Shame and Guilt* (Springfield, Ill.: Charles C Thomas, 1953).
57. William L. Pious, "A Hypothesis about the Nature of Schizophrenic Behavior," in Arthur Burton, ed., *Psychotherapy of the Psychoses* (New York: Basic Books, 1961).
58. Otto Pötzl, "Experimentell Erregte Traumbilder in Ihren Beziehungen zum Indirekte Sehen," *Z. ges. Neurol. Psychiat.*, 37 (1917), 278.
59. Karl H. Pribram, "The New Neurology: Memory, Novelty, Thought and Choice," in Gilbert H. Glaser, ed., *EEG and Behavior* (New York: Basic Books, 1963).
60. Fredrick C. Redlich, "The Concept of Normality," *American Journal of Psychotherapy*, 6 (1952), 551.

61. Paul Schilder, *Medical Psychology*, translated by David Rapaport (New York: International Universities Press, 1953).
62. Howard Shevrin and Lester B. Luborsky, "The Measurement of Preconscious Perception in Dreams and Images: An Investigation of the Pötzl Phenomenon," *Journal of Abnormal Social Psychology*, 56 (1958), 285.
63. Sanford M. Unger, "Mescaline, LSD, Psilocybin, and Personality Change," *Psychiatry*, 26 (1963), 111.
64. Robert Waelder, *Basic Theory of Psychoanalysis* (New York: International Universities Press, 1960).
65. Marvin Wasman and J. P. Flynn, "Directed Attack Elicited from Hypothalam Stimulation," *Archives of Neurology*, 6 (1962), 220.
66. Edwin A. Weinstein and Robert L. Kahn, *Denial of Illness* (Springfield, Ill.: Charles C Thomas, 1955).
67. John C. Whitehorn, "Guide to Interviewing and Clinical Personality Study," *Archives of Neurology and Psychiatry*, 52 (1944), 197.

CHAPTER FIVE

Etiology I: Psychodynamic Models and Development

Clinical Relevance

Scientifically based clinical practice differs from quackery because the therapist tries rationally to account for behavior disorder and to learn about it from his activities with patients. In this chapter, we will review some general models and key concepts related to the etiology of behavior disorders. We will consider the operation of psychological factors, the role of personality dynamics—of conflicts and defense—and developmental sequences as they are related to symptom formation and behavior pathology. In Chapter 6, we will review the etiologically important physical and social variables. From our previous discussion, it is clear that it is unlikely that we can establish a single definitive cause of a behavior disorder or assign an invariant course for most dysfunction. Rather, we must test hypotheses about the probable outcomes of the interactions of many variables.

We retain the traditional medical etiological categories more for purposes of exposition than for their intrinsic value as scientific guideposts in the study of behavioral processes. Thus, we customarily distinguish between necessary and sufficient factors; between predisposing factors, which create a fertile ground for pathogenesis, and precipitating factors—the proverbial straw that breaks the camel's back. Other traditional divisions that are conceptually misleading though operationally convenient are: the psychological and the physiological, the organismic and the environmental, and the physical and the social environment.

We usually encounter considerable difficulty when we try to specify what is fundamental or primary and what is secondary. Fatigue, for instance, with its altered capacity for processing information, may be viewed as a primary state, and irritability, as a *concomitant symptom* or perhaps as a consequence, or *secondary symptom*. If fatigue occurs as a resistance to a task (such as the housewife who is always tired when her husband wants to have intercourse), frigidity becomes primary and fatigue secondary. This is more than a game with words; in therapeutic work, we would very much like to differentiate such important secondary characteristics as compensatory and reparative symptoms from primary symptoms. It would undoubtedly be useful if it were always possible clearly to distinguish onset of disorder from incipient disorder and both from premorbid factors, if only from the standpoints of prevention and prognostication.

Yet, however much we desire clear-cut answers to these issues, the general rule for proceeding in our therapeutic work is relevance to the practical clinical problems. The psychiatrist must gather relevant data about the specific behavior of the individual patient and learn *when* to ignore interesting data which might or might not lead to an academically comprehensive explanation of the patient's behavior. The therapist happily making sense out of the dreams and other personal struggles of the patient who never mentions his addiction to alcohol has missed a key item in that patient's behavior. He has been more entranced by the inherent connectedness of things than by searching for and selecting what is relevant to the therapeutic task at hand. This requires a sense of timing that specialized training seeks to foster. It also requires experience to learn how usefully to employ and ignore textbook abstractions about the flux of living events. The psychiatrist soon finds that talking or thinking *about* behavior and behaving *with* another person are mutually complementary skills which he must learn to integrate if he wishes to be effective. Appreciating what behavior is like, the psychiatrist should proceed to leaf through a number of possibilities, to consider alternative interpretations and interventions in order to cope with a specific problem.

Etiological Models

In a broad sense, two models dominate psychiatric thinking about etiology: a *motivational model* derived largely from Freud's study of neurotic behavior (which emphasizes competing wishes—their drive or press for expression—and compromise solutions) and a *neurobiological model.* The latter is based mainly on the clinical study of brain pathology (which stresses deficits and impaired capacities, "release" or loss of controlled behavior, and lowering of the level of organization) and was stated most clearly by Hughlings Jackson.[19] If we ignore the details of these models and instead extract the emphases of each, it will be clear that both are relevant to our thinking about the etiology of *any* behavior disorder. The critical variables that are recurrently encountered are: (1) the function or purpose of the symptoms; (2) motivation; (3) factors relating to capacity, to limits and intrinsic strengths of drives and controls; (4) regression and level of organization—its causes and consequences; and (5) the role of reinforcement and learning, about which we perhaps know the least. These variables may be viewed independently, but they are, in fact, interacting. The capacity to integrate and cope and the relative strength of impulses have organic as well as psychosocial and developmental roots, as do the laws of learning and reinforcement.

Symptoms serve a *function* in the over-all economy of the organism; symptoms occur in order to maintain a relatively stable state. Freud expressed this adaptive view of the symptom's purpose (which differs somewhat from a motive or intention) as the primary gain to the over-all economy; Jackson spoke of the symptom as the "survival of the fittest state" in terms of the internal circumstances and prevailing resources. Both Jackson and Freud emphasized the importance in symptomatic behavior of *regression,* or the emergence of more primitive levels of function in the presence of trauma or stress. Freud eventually thought of internal conflicts and forces (coupled with the capacity of the ego) as largely responsible for the occasion and character of the regression; both the vicissitudes of development and constitutional endowment influenced the strengths and weaknesses as well as the direction of the operative forces. Given a *current* stress, the ensuing behavior represents what the organism can muster and acquire with the equipment, reinforcement, and motivation available.

The term *motive* is not to be equated with all possible causes or determinants of behavior. Motives constitute subjective wishes, their conscious and unconscious press for expression. They may be positively or negatively *reinforced* by the environment (which offers "incentives") and by internal factors. To a greater or lesser extent, there is a motivational component in all behavior—in the brain-damaged patient, in the regressed schizophrenic, as well as in the neurotic. It is also true that we are always making judgments about the consequences of developmental arrests (whatever their origin) in which drives and controls may be enhanced or inhibited. We always try to assess the level at which the patient is able to function, his *capacity* to function, or his "ego strength."

In establishing etiology, we encounter problems in evaluating how much weight to give to the motivational component or to components related to capacity. The most common error of dynamic psychiatrists is confusion of antecedent motivations; the secondary is mistaken for the primary, the visible effect for the covert cause. Description of motivations is mistaken for an adequate assessment of pertinent variables; too often, both are substituted for objective description of overt behavior.

Having a clear description of how the patient behaves—of his everyday "tactics"—we can then discern underlying strategies. In doing this, we must distinguish between *psychodynamics* and *psychogenetics* and between both of these and those physical and psychosocial interactions that both reinforce and limit the range of possible responses. Clinically, we describe the dynamics or forces operating in a disorder first by inferring and then by identifying the patient's characteristic basic wishes, fears, and defenses as they are evident in his various behavior patterns. We extend our view by describing his social setting and its reinforcements. When we do this, we can more clearly demonstrate what the patient contrives to do in the everyday drama of his life; the patient aggressively provokes but fears punishment for competing and seems always to be a loser in school, in love, at work. When we discern *how* a dynamic pattern was established in childhood (psychogenetics), we can predict what personal factors, wishes, and situations are apt to be "loaded" and meaningful for the patient. The patient acquired this pattern in the context of being punished for competing with his younger brother, who was habitually rewarded with comfort and attention for which the patient yearned; he now tends to see his boss as a parent and is disappointed when his awkward and brash bids for attention are not rewarded, and at home he reacts to his young son with inexplicable hostility. Both approaches describe how the patient functions, and neither approach fully explains why the behavior persists or changes. The patient's behavior becomes understandable and coherent, but the reasons for its entrenchment, the conditions required for a change in pattern require some contributions from an as yet inadequate clinical learning theory.

The error of the organicist may be to view limitations as nonrestorable even though—with motivation and skill in techniques of retraining—paths to new learning can often be found. In all rehabilitative or therapeutic work, defects, whatever their origin, are best faced and dealt with by fostering realistic compensations and helping the patient to avoid unnecessary struggles. To do this, the therapist must be able to make realistic assessments of what factors, from moment to moment, are impeding the patient.

The result of both cerebral and psychological trauma is to a greater or lesser degree impaired capacity or efficiency, impaired ability to learn or to employ cognitive, social, and emotional skills. There is regression, loss of control, desocialization, and disorganization. Just how efficiency is impaired and repaired depends on the nature of the trauma and the prevailing resources and level of organization. In the subsequent adjustments, the organism must cope as best it can with the facilities available to it. Depending on the initiating traumatic circumstances (behavioral or cerebral), the *reparative* pathways do, of course, differ. In hysterical reactions, for example, the motivational factor seems primary, and analysis of the defense and motivating wish may be sufficient to restore efficient activity. In brain-damaged patients, the dysfunction may be viewed as being primarily but not completely the result of damage to the equipment, and the symptoms represent the way in which information can be organized in the presence of such damage. At times helplessly, at other times deliberately, we shift from one mode of explanation to another.

Fortunately, our practical dilemma is easier than our theoretical conflicts. We know how to restore function in a transient situational crisis by providing new information or changing the social situation. In the brain-damaged patient and in some manic-depressive, schizophrenic, and delirious patients, we find it difficult or impossible to change behavior solely by such informational input and resort to methods (such as drugs) that are designed to modify the equipment. Of course, we could say that such severely disturbed persons do not "want" to organize themselves, that they or their families are poorly motivated; but it seems more tenable to believe that, if they could change, they would—or at least might if they have the chance to do so. Thus, as we work on the "equipment," we must not forget that reinforcement or motivation is always of *some* importance and that, on the other side, without any consideration of equipment or the laws of learning, a motivational therapy becomes unrealistic. In making these distinctions, in assessing both limitations and capacity for change in the treatment of all types of behavior disorder, the psychiatrist employs his highest clinical skills.

Psychological Stress

Stress is produced by an overload that the organism cannot handle; the equipment may be inadequate, the environmental input may be extreme, or both. In general, every organism has its breaking point. Organisms not only differ in "how" they will break but also in their innate, acquired, and learned attributes to forestall stress, cope with it, and the resilience to recover from it. One general immediate result of man's exposure to severe psychological stress is an experience of psychological trauma or, in psychoanalytic terminology, of narcissistic mortification;[7] one feels helpless, frustrated, "hurt."

An apparently small overload may produce stress and precipitate disordered behavior. We are forced to resort to two explanations: (1) the overt stress may appear innocuous to us because the subject did not experience it consciously and fails to report it fully; (2) the present stress is interpreted in terms of past or *predisposing* stresses, and the small overload may be experienced as a severe stress. What is taxing for one person is surtaxing for another. Subsequent behavior will vary depending on whether the person finds a realistic solution or fights stress by defensive maneuvers at the expense of a general or selective diminished awareness and coping ability. The range of symptoms and behavioral deficits that can flare up as a response to overload is impressive, but so is the fact that many persons do adjust to chronic and recurrent excessive loads. Some individuals acknowledge their deficits and institute ways around them rather than constantly and blindly fighting the inevitable with symptoms.

We attempt to differentiate between the direct impact of the traumatic load, the measures that defend the organism against overwhelming affect, and mechanisms that repair the damage or establish new equilibria. Actual "restoration" may not in fact be "biological" or possible in nature, but there clearly is a tendency continually to re-establish limits for relatively stable states. There are many specific as well as general homeostatic mechanisms. These can compete with one another, become over- or underactive, or respond to wrong cues. Thus symptomatology arises that is secondary to the initial overload. Dickinson W. Richards criticized an overly benign notion of "the wisdom of the body," which too often is presented as a victorious St.

George of homeostasis defeating the dragon of stress and damage.[36] In shock, cardiac failure, and asthma, for example, the attempts at reparative processes generally lead to more difficulty than the primary lesion. A component of a system may adapt to its overload to the detriment of the total system. Integration and coordination of the various specific adaptive and regulatory mechanisms is achieved, but frequently not without cost to some components of the system.

Hans Selye viewed stress as a comprehensive pathophysiological adaptation, which he called "the adaptation syndrome." [38] His theory, with its emphasis on the pituitary adrenal-cortical system and certain biochemical interactions, does not attempt to account for responses to complex psychosocial stresses and has only limited utility for psychiatry. In general, the neural, biochemical, and behavioral components of a variety of stressful states have yet to be disentangled and are poorly comprehended by measurement techniques currently available. Psychiatrists must also more adequately define the nature, occasion, and consequence of the stress that they study in a variety of forms in the clinic. We will discuss the chemistry of stress in Chapter 6. The role of peripheral vascular change (for example, carotid sinus pressure) in activating or inhibiting cortical-reticular-limbic mechanisms and the various levels of activation under various types of stress has been a focus of psychophysiological investigation.[24, 28] The methodology for linking altered states of consciousness induced by stress with peripheral and EEG measures has been advanced, in part, by psychiatrists and psychologists concerned with the technological advances required in space biology.[4]

Daniel H. Funkenstein and his co-workers[16] explored stress in normal subjects and distinguished among acute stress or emergency reactions, prolonged stress reactions, and chronic stress reactions. They found that their subjects could be divided into three basic types, characterized by anger-out, anger-in, and anxiety response. Anger-out and anger-in responses occurred in subjects whose fathers were dominant in the family, whereas anxiety responses occurred in subjects whose mothers were the dominant parent. Anger-out reactions were to be correlated with the secretion of a norepinephrine-like substance, and anxiety reactions correlated with epinephrine secretion. Mastery of stress—adaptation—after several stress experiments depended on quite different developmental variables. Whether such correlations in fact prove to be generally valid, future psychobiological studies will require some such consideration of various sets of genetic, developmental, and personality factors determining vulnerability, reaction, and resistance to various categories of stress. Obviously, psychiatrists are particularly interested in psychophysiological responses—not to laboratory-contrived horrors, but to psychological trauma as it occurs in real life: deprivation; separation; loss; failure; overstimulation and temptation; overprotection; harsh and inconsistent punishment; and a variety of threats including those of disease, injury, pain, and dysfunction.

Conflict

It is rare that a simple overload or stress is critical in the etiology of neurotic and related behavior disorders; rather, an individual is exposed to many stresses that conflict with one another. Much of behavior pathology consists of descriptions of the often unconscious clashes of drive and control behavior and the resultant impairments in social, emotional, and cognitive function. The simplest type of drive control is avoidance of instinctual gratification—and even of temptation. A normal young man who is tempted to have sexual intercourse with an attractive prostitute will simply avoid such contact if there is reasonable expectation of acquiring a venereal disease or if the act offends his values. The drive is still present and recognized, but checked. Another solution is inhibition, which results in diminished drive behavior; under the threat of infection or disapproval, the young man has lost his desire or is impotent, and his behavior is thereby checked. A third possibility is vacillating and indecisive behavior, which, as the result of the interaction of drive and control behavior, may become ingrained as a character trait. In the face of real or imaginary threats or temptations, a person may permanently renounce his sexual or aggressive and dependent desires. He may be fully or dimly aware of the temptation and what he is doing about it, or he may be utterly unaware of it (repressing or denying his needs) and justify his misery by various rationalizations and reaction formations. Both the *perception* of temptation and *response* to it may be influenced by conflict. Symptoms and pathological character traits may be the visible remnants of such struggles between drive and control.

Apart from neurotic symptoms and traits, it is difficult to try to explain all those conditions that eventuate in severe disorder on the basis of such conflict alone. Indeed, beyond the fact that conflict is part of life, it is not always clear that conflict is necessarily predisposing. Conflict may produce resistance, strength, and ability to cope. In some disorders, conflict may be a consequence of faulty personality structure and engendered by inherent weakness in the capacity to integrate personality resources toward realizable goals. Given this level of organization, the continuing or additional stresses may secondarily provoke more conflict. The matter is one for study. Whatever the basic personality structure, any stress that weakens current ability to cope may induce disorganization and release or activate demands for imperative "here and now" satisfactions. Some people eat or smoke under mild stress; others become irritable and demanding or become aware of primitive, angry or sexual thoughts and impulses that frighten them or annoy others. An increase of conflictful aggressive or sexual behavior may then be a consequence of frustration and not the primary cause. This can create cycles of conflict. The pure motivational model would hold that conflicting wishes were the major determinants in predisposition as well as precipitation of the regression and subsequent symptom formation. In its modified form the model would assert that conflicting wishes as well as diminished capacity to cope lead to repetitively inadequate "solutions." This view would guide clinicians to ferret out what was motivational and what was a function of the availability of internal and external resources. He then—with understanding and perspective—may demonstrate to the patient the occasion for his "solutions" to major early conflicts and the consequence to him of such persistent and inadequate behavior, when in fact alternative solutions are available.

Defense Mechanisms

When faced with stresses and conflicts and the unpleasant affects produced by them, an individual, whenever possible, will attempt to extricate himself by flight, fight, or problem-solving behavior. But often this is not possible because the situation, particularly for infants and children, severely limits these alternatives. Psychological processes that defend against anxiety and provide temporary security were called defense mechanisms by Freud [14, 15] and security operations by Harry Stack Sullivan.[40] Usually, they are inefficient. Generally speaking, an individual is unconscious or dimly conscious of the defense and of what he defends against. The basic defense maneuver is *repression.* It is implicitly present in all defenses. Freud once termed it the precursor of judgment; perception of offending reality is "automatically" ejected from consciousness, leaving no opportunity for selective judgment about the danger. Repression is a mental device evoked especially with internal danger (which is inherently difficult to perceive, grasp, and identify), and it is closely related to primitive flight mechanisms; unpleasantness is thereby avoided, not perceived or forgotten.

What represses? Freud ascribed this function to the ego. Yet we hardly know the mechanisms through which awareness is dimmed, nor why an experience—although relatively inaccessible—yet retains its motivating power and produces derivative experiences and various disguises. We do know that elimination from consciousness may involve simple or complex perceptions, thoughts, memories, affects, and motivations. Repression may be complete, but far more frequently it is incomplete and accompanied by a symbolic distortion (changes of meaning) of the past or concurrent stimuli; a person may be aware of feelings but ignorant of their source and motivation. A partial blotting out of offending stimuli, "the blind spot," is called *scotomization.* The raw impulse may be relatively untouched (such as in schizophrenias, depressions, and some sociopathies) or the warded off impulse may return to consciousness in a disguised form, or be expressed behaviorally in inhibitions and restrictions of coping functions. Often the defense seems more troublesome than the dangerous impulse; the cure can be worse than the illness. In general, however, one makes the other necessary, especially in terms of the patient's personal interpretations of safety and danger.

Repression differs from *suppression,* or deliberate inattention to needs, affects, and thoughts. Conscious restrictions of the self, or of dangerous drives (curiosity, for example), are common modes of coping with feared wishes. The affect or the meaning of unpleasant, overstimulating, or dangerous situations may be repressed while the content remains conscious. Both an unpleasant idea or wish and the affect may be "conscious," but the individual makes no connection between them; in effect, one is aware of an event without knowledge of its meaning or significance. Such *isolation* of content and meaning occurs frequently as one of the chief *intellectualizing* defenses of obsessional neurotics. "It's true I have homosexual thoughts, doctor, but that is ridiculous since they don't mean anything," one such patient remarked. *Rationalization,* or intellectualizing about one's behavior, is ubiquitous. It is perhaps the main "perversion" to which we put our intellectual endowment; we obfuscate our fears, needs, and obligations by elaborately or deceptively justifying an avoidance, conflict, injury, or temptation.

An important type of reality distortion is referred to as *unconscious denial,* the negation of threatening realities about the self and others, such as the existence of defect and dangers, and especially of illness. According to R. Waelder,[41] it is the foremost defense in the psychoses; the denial of reality can marshal a large part of the personality to strengthen the defense, and hence such consequences are major. To a greater or lesser extent, many defenses isolate or "split" parts of the personality, and such *dissociations* impair flexible adaptation or realistic assessment of the range of changing demands and needs that life normally entails. Analysts refer to this segregation of major portions of the personality as "*ego splitting.*"

In the important defense of *projection,* one's own unacceptable wishes and fantasies are placed outside the self. One psychological explanation of hallucination, illusion, and delusion assumes that these are manifestations of such projections. Where inside and outside cannot be easily distinguished, the tendency is to disown unpleasant states (or forbidden pleasant wishes) and to locate their cause as alien to the self. This may be the basis for defensive projection. It is a fundamental mechanism closely related to locating, orienting, and object-seeking and as such is seen in both normal people and patients. As a mental mechanism rather than a defense, the projection of one's feelings onto others is thought to characterize early emotional learning and the later capacity to anticipate the feelings of others and to identify with them. A milder form of defense related to projection is *displacement,* such as kicking the garage door rather than one's wife, or being grouchy with one's wife rather than kicking the boss. Displacement also characterizes a fundamental capacity for representational plasticity in mental life, as in symbols, where one sign stands for another.

Studies of primitive cultures and of children reveal elaborate magical rituals employed to ward off anxiety. Some of these formulas are institutionalized in many cultures as ceremonial and superstitious practices. At another level, we encounter a similar mechanism in the study of obsessive and psychotic patients, referred to as *undoing;* every spoken bad thought must be magically warded off or atoned for by a ritual, a process often consuming all the patient's time and energy. *Reaction formation* consists of overly strong and inflexible traits that express the opposite of what is feared; excessive cleanliness rather than a tolerable range of messiness; exaggerated pity and concern motivated by fear of sadistic and envious feelings.

Defenses as well as anxieties (and the related emotions against which we defend) become complex parts of our character structure. But defenses per se are not necessarily pathological. They may undergo a change of function in development and, as many higher functions, be less influenced by immediate needs and become "adaptive." It is the degree of inflexibility of the defenses and drive-derivative behaviors—their relevance to the total context of behaving—that measures the excessive or neurotic component in the behavior.

Humor and the related techniques of wit and comic devices are examples of normal defenses; they can reduce anxiety, turn grim reality into something more acceptable, and gratify forbidden impulses. Humor and teasing may provide sadistic-masochistic gratification. In caricatures, anger turned either on others or on the self is seen frequently. Turning about or "*reversal*" of the instinctual wish is a basic mode for many defensive operations; exhibitionism versus peeking, hurting or being hurt, loving or hating, ridiculing or inviting ridicule, are common examples. Benign uses of defenses are seen in repression and denial in the face of approaching death in malignant illness. Another commonly useful defense is the use of fantasy and daydreaming under certain conditions, permitting instinctual gratification without anxiety; excessive daydreaming, of course, may interfere with the normal reality perception. One might say that without the controlled use of projection we could not understand another person or a work of art. Since we cannot conceive of a healthy person without an array of these defenses, we define defenses as mental mechanisms—their use in different contexts defines their "defensiveness." Two important mental mechanisms that often have a defensive function, *identification* and *regression,* will be discussed later.

Fixation, Regression, and Repetition Compulsion

We have already mentioned that conflicts may be prepared for in advance; they are—when properly studied—often discernible early in the course of behavior pathology. Whether or not there is a causal link, current conflict can usually be "traced" to earlier conflicts in the patient's life. Just as success breeds success, the present lack of success seems often to be modeled on earlier experiences of failure or maladaptation. Modes of behavior are astonishingly persistent.

Thus, early stresses and conflicts provide guideposts, either determining the specificity of later frustrations or creating "fissures," along which trouble, once started, can spread. Freud called these developmental road blocks fixation points. He developed a complicated theory of fixation but essentially believed that fixations divert the subsequent courses of development. After experiencing severe stress or conflict that cannot be mastered, man and also animals fall back on earlier, infantile modes of behavior.

Looking at such a sequence from the adult viewpoint, we denote the use of infantile modes of behavior as regression. Regression describes employment of earlier modes of behavior that were at one time appropriate in problem-solving. It may be partial and select; massive; fleeting; or persistent. It may variably involve perception; aspects of cognition; affects; adaptive and defensive mechanisms; or all of these. It may be psychologically or organically induced and may represent flexibility, or fixation and impairment. It may be defensively or more rarely adaptively employed. As an unconscious defensive response, regression can have, in some instances, a stabilizing and anxiety-reducing function. Regression also seems to express the sentiment: "I am only a frightened child who is not responsible and needs help and protection." Liability and resistance to regression presumably have both experiential and constitutional determinants. Regression, as the retreat of an army, can be orderly or chaotic; Ernst Kris referred to the former as "regression in the service of the ego," [22] a mechanism employed in creative work, play, and humor. The end result of any such retreat depends not only on the magnitude of the retreat and the developmental level at which it comes to a halt, but also on what controls or compels the regressive movement and the resources for progressive thrusts.

Analysts speak of regression to phallic and the "pregenital" anal, oral, and narcissistic phases of development. In more neutral behavioral terms, one could speak of regression of adults to adolescent, puerile, and infantile modes of behavior. Theoretically, an astute observer, watching the course of development, might be able to note and predict the conflict or trauma fated to become the focus for trouble for a particular future stress and even how these earlier, reactivated conflicts become "pathogenic" in the current conflict, determining the choice of symptoms. It seems that a current problem picks its most suitable ancestor. Much remains unclear: why do we fall back on earlier conflict instead of regressing to problems that were mastered? Possibly we can merely state that man endlessly repeats his unconscious mistakes. Freud referred to this tendency as the repetition compulsion. There seems to be an inertia and "stickiness" of unconscious drives, affects, thoughts, and conflicts; no corrective learning takes place, and infantile patterns of wish and problem-solving are rigidly maintained.[23]

Symptom Formation

Most psychiatric symptoms become manifest in disorganized interpersonal reactions. In severe behavior disorders, we can clearly discern a "loss" of coping facility—negative symptoms in Jackson's model. Positive symptoms would represent psychological operations that can be carried out with the available "equipment" and includes those symptoms resulting from a release of more archaic mechanisms. For example, the delusions of schizophrenia represent inefficient and primitive methods of explaining and coping with reality, and the capacity to cope is clearly impaired. The factors of motivation and reinforcement, as being etiologically (rather than descriptively) important, come into sharper focus in those conditions in which there is less profound regression and impairment of coping facilities. Here, the basic psychoanalytic model—the view of symptoms and abnormal characterological traits as a compromise between impulse and defense—has wide application. Some symptoms betray their instinctual origin clearly; the pelvic thrusts of an hysterical seizure are strongly reminiscent of the motivating sexual urge. If the strong repressed conflicts surface again with certain symbolic distortions, they become manifest in abnormal behavior that attempts to disguise the original conflict; the over-control of drives by the obsessive refers to a constant rebellion and urge to make a mess. The symptoms and psychopathological traits are compromise formations, heirs to the original conflict. Symptom formation permits token gratification of such forbidden wishes and provides punishment for this through suffering; it also impairs coping abilities and limits realistic solutions while reducing the original psychological distress. Once symptoms occur, they may be maintained or reinforced by the sociocultural advantages that symptoms provide through the sanction of the sick role. Freud distinguished between the *primary gain* through symptoms, by which he meant establishment of an equilibrium through partial gratification of the forbidden drive. By *secondary gains,* he meant the psychosocial advantages the patient derives from his neurotic symptoms: sympathy, care, and excuse from responsibility. Jay Katz reviewed the complicated writing on the subject[20] and stated that the strict differentiation into primary and secondary gains is tenuous and that it is better just to simply speak of gains through illness.

In practice, the precise sequence in which a symptom was formed is not only difficult to reconstruct but is not easy to conceptualize. Our explanations leave many questions unanswered: why the unpleasant emotion is successfully reduced in some cases and not in others; why inefficient behavior and inhibitions to new learning become so persistent; and why some solutions through symptom formation are harmless and others are crippling and dangerous. The fact that we can make *ad hoc* explanations when we encounter a specific case should only serve to warn that we know little about the general principles of learning, the laws of reinforcement and extinction, applied to clinically relevant behavior.

In most instances, we are unable to predict the "choice" of a specific symptom and can only discern the meaning of symptoms once they have appeared. That a symptom is probable, that it has biographical roots, that the ground has been prepared for it, is often evident; but why we find a paralysis rather than an amnesia, or a paranoid rather than a depressive syndrome, all too often is unclear. Freud resorted to an answer that most workers employ, namely: the interlocking of constitutional factors and acquired behavior appears to set up the possibilities for various fixation points to be critical. For example, I. Arthur Mirsky demonstrated that a constitutional factor[30] (high pepsinogen level) plus certain stressful experiences predispose toward ulcers as a symptom. Thus, symptom "choice" must be due to convergence of factors about which, at present, we know far too little. We have already mentioned that symptoms have many "causes." They also have multiple purposes and consequences. A simple example is the fact that most patients hurt not only others but also themselves.

Normal and Abnormal Development

By now it must be obvious to the reader that the growth and development of a person throughout the phases of life is the context in which our investigations and therapeutic activities are conducted. Qualitative and quantitative factors depending on genetic patterns, constitution, environmental loads, and learning can be consequential for pathological or normal outcomes. We usually call what is programmed in the chromosomes hereditary or genetic. The sum of what is biologically given (whether determined by genetics or intrauterine environment) is referred to as constitutional. We will discuss the importance of genetic and constitutional parameters in more detail in Chapter 6. The unfolding of biologically given factors and their manifestation at critical periods in the life history are referred to as maturation, a somatically programmed schedule. The opposite of maturation is involution. The maturing organism, interacting with the impact of physicochemical events and the infinitely more varied psychosocial input from the environment, produces changes in the organism. When these changes consist of organic growth, of differentiation and diversification, or of physiological and behavioral activities, we speak of development. The issue is never nature versus nurture, but rather the role of each, in each and any item under investigation. The role of constitution and environment should seriously be considered in assessing *each* predisposing and precipitating factor in a behavior disorder. The social environment that meets the growing human being is of decisive importance for shaping the detailed events of development.[9] Our review of development tends to be clinically biased and emphasizes an outline of psychosocial and psychosexual development, which appears to be most relevant. The psychobiological mechanisms and controls regulating the development of sensorimotor, perceptual, cognitive, as well as psychosocial and psychosexual processes, are beginning to be investigated in detail. Our understanding of clinically relevant development will undoubtedly change as our field incorporates the results of such investigations.

The Learning of Disordered Behavior

In general, we postulate that neurotic behavior disorders, including sociopathies and addictions, are in a major sense learned forms of disordered behavior. We are less sure of the extent to which such learning is pertinent for the specific etiology of schizophrenia, manic–depressive behavior disorders, and psychosomatic diseases, although learning undoubtedly plays its part.

We distinguish three basic patterns in human learning: (1) classical conditioning or linking of responses to conditioned stimuli; (2) instrumental learning or performance, and selective response acquired through rewards or punishment inherent in the environment; (3) one-trial learning, in which the higher mental processes are involved. Much of human learning, apparently casually acquired in one trial, occurs in very complex social situations. Such learning includes creative learning, but also the learning of disordered behavior. What are the factors that interfere with phase-specific learning as new abilities come into play; what causes the entrenchment and reinforcement of particular patterns, the transfer of others, and the readiness to shift to new patterns? The development of a clinical learning theory is one of the great challenges of modern psychiatry and the behavorial sciences; this is more than a pious hope, since discernible beginnings have been made in spite of the distance that remains before clinical facts and problems can be reached.[6, 32] The role of consciousness in the acquisition of skills and behavior that appear to be automatic has yet to be worked out; and a learning theory that takes into account unconscious processes is required.[35]

The order of learning that is psychiatrically significant has to do with the ability to identify emotionally and socially meaningful stimuli and respond with the psychologically appropriate relationships. If, for emotional reasons, a patient is unable to tell whether a person is friendly or hostile, he is unable to respond appropriately. The basis for impaired emotional regulation may be faulty learning, faulty equipment, or both. If the child is taught that it is bad to have angry thoughts, he can disown and deny them and in so doing distort his development and capacity to function. If he has inherent or acquired defects in his capacity to grasp what is relevant in what he is told, this can affect his ability for role-taking, for internalizing standards, and for seeing what others see; and hence his object relations and social relations may be impaired. Disturbance of brain-mediated capacities to process input can inhibit early and sustained learning. Although proof for such interactions as etiological in most major disorders is absent or scarce, it is suspected in some cases of autism,[11] and it operates in many cases of mental deficiency and in convulsive disorders where, however, the emphasis has been on tool skills rather than deficient role-learning. In the learning situation the individual must be motivated to make the correct response and be rewarded for it. Many learning problems depend on faulty or inhibited motivation or drive, which, in turn, may be related to the individual's history of psychosocial reinforcements. This is true over a wide spectrum from underachievement in school to the mislearning of social and sexual responses.

Identification

The learning of social roles within the framework of the family and peers depends in part on models for imitation and identification. The concept of imitation connotes a conscious deliberate copying of models. By contrast, identification is an unconscious process of internalizing parental behavior, attitudes, and expectancies. Of course, whenever we speak of learning and teaching, we refer to a host of poorly appreciated processes whereby response-patterns and dispositions are reinforced and acquired. The processes involved range from explicit tutoring to the various mechanisms by which environmental response is internalized and integrated into the structures controlling an individual's behavior. The child retains and internalizes parental values and he shapes internal standards and images of what he wishes to be or achieve. Through these internal or self-initiated regulations (which at first are crude copies of parental attitudes), the child can retain an internal attachment to his parents by allegiance to their rules and wishes and at the same time further his independence from their moment-to-moment regulation of him. Having "internal" parents, he is somewhat freer to make wider attachments and additional relationships. According to Freud, this internal structure tends to crystallize at the time the child gives up his close Oedipal attachments and turns his attention to other matters. Once the child's incorporation of values has taken place, expectation of strong reward and punishment becomes somewhat less important. We commonly call the conscious and preconscious part of this incorporated value-system conscience. These internal structures can be a source of great difficulty because they are frequently primitive and sporadic. We know from clinical experience that the proper values may be rejected, or have never been taught; the capacity for learning may be impaired, or the "wrong" values may be learned. All children are literal. Until they develop in judgment and self mastery, punishment may be interpreted far more extensively than the parent intended. The child may be harsher with himself, and less discriminating (and less consistent) in dispensing punishment toward himself or (in fantasy) toward others than the adult realizes. Needing structure, the child may provide it by self-imposed restrictions, where the environment lacks structure; needing love, he may resort to overt inhibition or provocation to win attention, to express defeat and unworthiness (which he believes accounts for the deficit of love), or to gain forgiveness for imagined or real wrongs. When such patterns persist in adulthood, we deal with neurotic and sociopathic problems.

Identification provides the child with human ingredients out of which he can fashion what he and others will recognize as most characteristically his "self." Building and guiding himself through identifications, the child not only complies with instructions, but extracts attitudes, modes of coping, and values, which he then makes his own. The building blocks for an identity derive from relations with others, which is not surprising, since we require some concrete way to realize our potential for becoming social and "human" beings. This capacity proceeds in tandem with psychosexual and cognitive maturation and skill acquisition. One can identify with desirable or undesirable models, with one or many, and with selected attributes of such models.[43] If different role expectations cannot be reconciled, conflict and role diffusion are apt to emerge.

Identification is genetically related to the more primitive need to fuse with the loved and revered objects by incorporating them and also to destroy dangerous and hated objects by such incorporation. The infant wants to incorporate or take as part of himself what he needs. What is good and pleasant becomes part of one's self—such as the good mother—and it is only later that she is differentiated into the object that makes one feel good. What is bad, such as the frustrating bad mother, is also introjected, felt to be within one and is separated from the good, forming the nucleus of alienated feelings, which we often see in devisive internal wars between the good and the bad, especially in psychotics. These introjects (representations of internalized projections and guiding images) are deemed important for further development, especially by Melanie Klein, and also by Harry Stack Sullivan. Klein believes that the "bad mother" introject is the principal determinant for what she calls the basic paranoid and depressive dispositions that underlie all behavior disorders.[21] To the young child, such an introject evokes a basic attitude: I am deprived of love (the paranoid position); I am undeserving of love (the depressed position). These attitudes and attachments continue through further development, in her view.

Both incorporation (with its bodily meanings) and identification (with its more behavioral and interpersonal referents) operate in the fantasies of young children and in psychotic individuals, in ritualistic cannibalism in primitive cultures, and in the oral and gastric metaphors of neurotics and "normals." An obese patient, in a moment of emotion, patted his paunch and announced, "Doctor, when you're with me, you're *in* me." In some of our most significant religious ceremonies, bodily incorporation plays a significant part. Identification, then, is a primitive mode of relating to significant persons and provides a bridge to emotionally satisfying relationships, through which the child acquires authenticity and reliability in employing and expending his skills. It is a step to achieving a stable identity, mature relationships with persons, and the general quality of self-possession.

Identification may serve a defensive function, too. Anxiety may be warded off by "identification with the aggressor," as Anna Freud pointed out.[12] She tells of a little boy who, just after seeing the dentist, spent his time with her in exceptionally aggressive play, thus mastering his previous pain and fear by being the aggressive one. By "being" another person, rather than realistically and maturely relating to him, one can borrow strength. The insecure child can do what others do before he is confident of his own choice and skill. In identifying with another person, one can avoid the painful or forbidden aspects of a relationship; in this sense, identification takes the place of object relationships. Negative identification is the result of an unconscious wish not to be like the model. Hostile identification is manifest in punishing the self, as one was unjustly punished, and of treating others as one did not want to be treated. At times, it appears that psychiatric patients are grasping for some leverage in order to differentiate themselves from these primitive identifications with another person; a repetitive "acting out" of the seductive or punitive patterns, which a parent employed toward oneself, may dominate a person's life; but such behavior also "spells out," through action, the problem that could not be solved. Our job is to "read" and hopefully to translate the message in a way that effectively helps the patient to stop the cycle. Such patients often complain that they find themselves with an unpleasant habit, which they had always condemned in their parents. And, this undesired loyalty to traits of others, this archaic way of being close, represents the failure of identification processes to continue into self-differentiation, into a self that empathizes with others but has a "place of its own" from which to relate to them.

Faulty Child-Rearing and Behavior Disorders

Psychiatrists have become aware of certain patterns of child-rearing that are found with high regularity in the anamnesis of psychiatric patients. The most important of them is maternal deprivation. Although gross neglect is not uncommon, such behavior patterns as maternal overcontrol, masking of feelings, and various forms of imperception bordering on indifference can profoundly influence development. The mother who is infantile, or frightened of or envious of infants, or who sees the child as a doll or a toy to be artificially manipulated, can effectively deprive the infant of needed experiences. Sally Provence and Rose C. Lipton[34] demonstrated the role of human objects and their importance for subsequent regulations. They found that infants quite impersonally reared in a large orphanage tended (perhaps surprisingly) to be compliant and pleasant but to become upset and disruptive (not psychotic) when they were offered opportunities for strong ties to specific persons; and it is just such ties that we believe are important if the adult is to function adequately in marriage, work, and as a parent. René Spitz and Katherine Wolf [39] found that during the early oral stage, abandonment or ostensible severe neglect of the infant by the mothering person *could* cause severe depression and physical wasting of the *infant*. Although these findings were challenged,[33] other investigators lent additional weight to these deprivation theories, which have remained quite powerful in developmental psychiatry.[8] These notions have been bolstered by the experiments of H. Harlow, who showed that rhesus monkeys also showed significant disturbances in development when they were not reared by their natural mothers, but by artificial contraptions.[17] The infants of "wire mothers" showed striking defects in adulthood in their mating and mothering behavior. Lest we assume that this demonstrates what stuff "schizophrenigenic mothers" are made of, such misbehavior is not refractory to learning, since it may dissipate after several pregnancies. Persistent research is required to evaluate the detailed sequence of conditions through which infantile experience influences later development, to identify "critical periods," and to discover for what specific processes they are critical. The observation that rats that were petted and fondled in infancy grew to be sturdier adults than neglected rats might speak for the importance of mothering and bodily contact in early development; on the other hand, painful electric shocks in infancy gave similar results.[26] In both instances, the operative factor was the stimulation and activation of stress mechanisms. Fondled mice, on the other hand, developed less adequate stress responses. In general, interactional and feedback systems, properly phased and timed, are required for adequate performance in later epochs of development; but the crucially important details and mechanisms differ among the species and, probably, among persons. From clinical evidence, separation and maternal deprivation have been held responsible for a wide variety of psychosomatic, depressive, and schizophrenic reactions in adult life. These assumptions derive mostly from retrospective inference and could be on somewhat shaky ground. All humans have to endure, at least temporarily, intense pain, hunger, and separation during their earlier phases of life, when they are most dependent and helpless; only some, however, become permanently crippled. Early rejections, and psychological loss and separation that are maladaptively compensated in all likelihood provide necessary predisposing—though not sufficient causes—for later severe behavior disorders.

Parental overprotection also has been blamed for a wide range of behavior disorders.[27] Overprotection interferes with the ability to learn to master anxieties, fosters a propensity for the growing individual not to free himself from parental bonds, and leaves one confusedly bereft of an inner confidence and firm identity; a patient concluded, "My mother lets me have everything—so long as it's not mine." Another factor equally disruptive to the learning process in all phases of development is an unpredictable inconsistency in reward and punishment.

Some sources of unresolved conflict and possible behavior disorder are located in the inconsistencies of child-rearing. Again, this view of the role of confusing input derives support not only from clinical observations but from a very large body of evidence gained in conditioning experiments, and studies of experimental neuroses. There remains the problem of explaining why not all children exposed to a very inconsistent environment become impaired. All parents are human and inconsistent; a purely logically consistent parent would be "inhuman." What we look for is not consistency as much as some degree of relevant coherence. Successful child-rearing obviously is a matter of mutual regulation between the particular child's needs and the optimum range of inconsistency for him, and this cannot be programmed in the form of specific rules for parents. Nor are determinants of parental misbehavior easy to specify. Parents are vulnerable to the specific temperament of their child and the child's fittedness for the parents' current phase of life and adjustment. Ongoing changes in the child activate and touch on forgotten conflicts from the parents' childhood; instead of focusing on the child's real difficulties, or ways of keeping him out of trouble, the parent is unknowingly distracted by his own blind spots and unsolved problems.

Another general category of stress and conflict is sexual temptation and seduction in childhood. In his early work, Freud was impressed that most of his patients had severe sexual traumatic experiences in their childhoods. He later recognized that he mistook common though vivid fantasies for actual trauma and revised his theories. Yet the fact that many psychiatric patients have been exposed to unmanageable excitement, handling, and stimulation, and to unusual temptation, seduction, and severe conflict over sexual behavior, cannot be disputed; only our interpretation of such data has changed. The noxious factor is not the traumatic sexual experience per se; it is, rather, the fact that such seduction and persistent temptation are expressions of very faulty child-rearing practices in general, which do not permit the child to make proper identifications and develop the integrity and autonomy necessary for development. We observe mother–son incest usually only in the history of some schizophrenias or severe character dysfunctions, in which the parent–child relationship is generally extremely disturbed; but exceptions have been documented in which incest was not followed by behavior disorder. Today, neither psychoanalysts nor anyone else adheres to a "pansexual" etiological theory of behavior disorder. There is no "prime mover" or single causative factor in the etiology of behavior disorders; rather, many factors interact in the most complex way in the system we call behavior.

The last general pattern of faulty child-rearing, which we mention briefly, is unreasonable, cruel punishment, which either produces overt, aggressive, rebellious, or very passive attitudes, both interfering with adult adjustment. As the punished child not only fears and fights the punitive parents, but also identifies with them, the net result of such mistreatment is exceedingly complex. We can trace overt personality traits of aggression, defiance, and passivity, as well as the stern self-punitive attitudes as deriving from unconscious identification with a harsh, unloving parent. Sociopathic patients often have such cruel but also overindulgent parents.

Strict legalistic controls, as many tyrants—and many parents—have experienced, are quite precarious and inefficient. Of course, there are many adaptive responses of compliance that permit the desired performance without internal assent. Generally, it is much easier if rules are understood, accepted as appropriate (because they are advanced appropriately), and become part of one's own value system, thereby being regulated by internal authority and control. The child needs someone who knows better than he; who knows how and when to advance rules, and to expect and reward compliance, as well as self-expression and autonomy; he needs someone who, in doing this, finds overall pleasure in the job. A child must be taught to respond to a degree of pain or frustration by tolerating it; he can learn this if others are trustworthy and assured, rather than anxious, guilty, or overbearing. Parents who police not only behavior but feelings can only impose confusion and provoke rebellion. A child can be told what to do without questioning his basic worth; his feelings may be recognized, but they need not be so catered to that he misjudges the importance of his impulses. Authoritarian parents may wish to lay down firm principles to control inappropriate behavior once and for all; instead of simply stopping an instance of misbehavior, the parent may question the child's basic dignity. For example, having made a mess, the child may be led to feel he has spoiled not the floor but a better part of the universe. Having made an error, he is not wrong but ruined. A cartoon shows a child as a debased derelict slumped against a lamppost on Skid Row, and the caption echoes the parents': "I don't know what's to become of you."

Developmental Phases and Crises

The concept of developmental phases and crises assumes that each so-called period of development carries with it characteristic tasks, the mastery or failure of which influences the future course of development. It is also assumed that during a given "critical" period of life, certain categories of events are selectively meaningful. Anna Freud was able to demonstrate that wartime evacuation and separation from parents was not particularly meaningful and traumatic for two-year-olds, but highly traumatic when children reached the Oedipal phase.[13] Sigmund Freud's "psychosexual" scheme (Chapter 3) sketched the links of early drive characteristics and object attachments, especially as revealed in the study of adult neuroses and dreams. The language with which Freud traced psychosexual development, although rich in psychological meaning, hardly represents the actual complexities. The satisfaction of bodily zones (oral, anal, genital) is basic in patterning conduct, fantasies, and wishes, but it is not a peripheral bodily zone that directs, powers, and steers development, since cognitive, emotional, social, motor, and linguistic elements are similarly evolving. The body orifices and sensitive zones are a "referent" for experiences of pleasure and pain but are coordinated with many patterns and mechanisms, through which the infant grows and develops. A child requires more than sucking experience to develop "oral behaviors" and more than the trauma of toilet training to display the patterns of thought, rebellion, and autonomy associated with Freud's anal phase of development. No child in the late phallic phase has been arrested for incest or exhibitionism; rather, it is the normal development or pathological fixation of his vivid attachments and concrete experiences that—as precursors—are consequential at later developmental levels, when new object and social attachments and satisfactions are capable of being sought. A child would be grossly defective if he did not elaborate primitive theories and experience impressive pleasure and concern around the satisfaction of his bodily functions. It is the power of these experiences, interpreted with the concreteness of childhood, and organized into covertly directive attitudes about the self and others that, if insufficiently integrated and contained by development (or repression), are striking in psychopathology. It should be remembered that the level and context in which behavior occurs affects all the components in it, and that, for example, achievement, intellectual level and capacity are as determining as disturbing emotions and confusions in the events that comprise development. It should also be kept in mind that the following discussion pertains primarily, though not exclusively, to development in the upper and middle classes of Western culture.

Early Infancy

The infant is a true nestling,[31] a helpless receiver, regulated largely from within; hence, we speak of the "narcissistic" or pre-object phase of development. The mothering person is experienced—probably—as a global equivalent to internal pleasure and relief of pain and through months of interactions emerges less as an extension of internal states and gradually as an object. The main instrument of contact is the mouth; hence, we also tend to speak of the oral phase of development; and a good part of the mother infant transactions are organized around this phase-specific zone. Behavior evolves from global and undifferentiated expression to discrete expression, and it becomes patterned through basic precognitive operations: orientation and search (to the feeding apparatus); discrimination (of what goes in); delay (in swallowing and getting fed); and generalization (to other objects to be mouthed).[5] The infant must regulate his receptive activities in order to "get hold of" the various styles by which he will be given attention, food, and so forth. His readiness for response, for "shaping" his component activities into identifiable behavior is met differently by different persons and cultures. The modalities of the culture—the ways by which giving, getting, and getting-to-be-given-to (demanding) are generally organized—regulate far more behaviors than feeding and represent the pattern by which sequentially developing social behaviors will be integrated.

With the appearance of more active motor behavior (at the oral, biting phase), oral, visual, and manual grasping, letting go and holding on to objects—later, taking hold of anything in sight—is characteristic. In the infant's getting hold of his world (getting "a bite" on his problems), we see the beginnings of self-stability and continuity; we also see the beginnings of the equivalents of attention, focus, concentration, and the discrimination of objects in depth and dimension. The child now moves in space, having been prepared by innumerable rehearsals (experiments in head lifting, sitting, creeping, and, by the age of two, in toddling). The mother's response (and her smiling encouragement when he falls and wonders whether to cry) becomes his courage;[37] he is guided by the affective cues he "takes in." Trusting what he sees and hears, he develops self-trust. Confidence and faith have begun to develop out of the early receptivity, which, behaviorally, is an expectancy that he will receive, or can get done, what is needed. But as he can achieve, he is weaned; he loses as he gains. Erikson views this "age-specific" crisis as the origin of optimism or pessimism ("being left empty").[10] Impulsive greed, clinging, and demanding behavior; or deep feelings of internal division, distrust (giving up), and reactive rage; and needs to bite, fight, and take rather than receive, are "oral behaviors." In various derivative forms, they are evident in some severe behavior disorders of adults. The social psychology of faith, reunion, and communion is also based on these early "oral" attitudes, which permeate many metaphors and rituals of adult life; there is a continuity from feeding of infants to alumni feasts at the alma mater. We already mentioned the effects of early oral deprivation and separation and their possible consequences. All adults inherit primitive responses even to slight separation and change; they may anticipate anger and catastrophe or experience deprivation and loss of esteem, even when the change is clearly "reasonable." Psychotherapists are rightfully alert for such automatic unconscious responses.

Late Infancy

Ability to think, conceptualize the world, and communicate meaningfully continue to evolve. Infantile babbling and imitation first express feelings, then acquire directive qualities before words are used for objects and activities. Early inferences are built according to concrete, perceptual, and personalized principles rather than generic categories: all men are "daddy." The child is puzzled if someone else has his name and only gradually assumes play roles.

With the developing musculature and discrimination, the child at two is still very dependent, but by no means helpless. Aggressive, he struggles now with his growing autonomy, ready to stand and walk on his own, and to risk falling. There is also the perception that the enlarging world may be fearful and hostile, which is coped with in part by insuring protection and love through his affection for his mother. Encouraged to control his anal and urethral sphincters, he can please and torment by retaining or eliminating. As he has notions of omnipotence as well as doubts, he can experiment with the power of holding back, and of letting go. He can both fear and enjoy defecation or urination and associated fantasies (and the social consequences with his mother). A frank, more mature reporter of five years remarked: "It feels good when I let it go."

As the child experiments with autonomy and overestimates his thoughts (which are more powerful than his ability to implement them) he may develop rituals to try to assert control. The self-will and negativism; the childish experiments with decisions; his yesses and noes; and the compliance and dawdling, which occur with the struggle for mastery of internal physiological forces, all partake in the prevailing zonal mode, retention–elimination. The phase-specific crisis of the two- to three-year-old is shame and doubt about control and loss of autonomy. Instead of experimenting and developing initiative, he may be absorbed in defiance, stubborn rebellion, and attention to the presumed autonomy of others (siblings). These various concerns are carried into later phases and generalized into the "anal" characteristics of putting things into their place, time, order; and of meticulousness, compliance, or rebellion; and if shame and doubt are paramount, stubbornness and overcompensatory control (instead of autonomy), and zealous reform or compulsive cleanliness, are characteristic. An adult, feeling impotent, abandons autonomy, initiative, and industry; he is absorbed instead in doubts; he is preoccupied with envy of what others are doing; and he shows a retentive, stubbornly meticulous greediness about his rights and a magical overestimation of his thoughts. Earlier and later modalities ("oral" greed and "anal" retentiveness) may thus combine and underlie such regressive traits. Excessive reactions (becoming a "good boy") designed to placate the mother and bring a truce to prevailing warfare may later become permanent character traits.

Whether the symptoms of severe obsessive-compulsive neurosis are simply a consequence of toilet training is doubtful. We also feel quite uncertain whether the assumption that the symptoms of many psychosomatic diseases can be traced to vaguely specified trauma during the oral and anal phase is correct. We believe, however, that important beginnings of later character traits, such as cleanliness and dirtiness, orderliness and sloppiness, punctuality and disregard for time, rebellion or defeat and avoidance, clearly are found at this stage of development.

Early Childhood

With a growing cognitive ability and a growing capacity to internalize and conceptualize relationships, the child of four to five can grieve, worry, anticipate, and brood. As he tries to locate himself in his family, he is egocentric, and he personalizes conversational fragments that must refer specifically to him. He frightens himself with his ability to imagine and wish. He believes his thoughts should be known without words, or he dreads that they are apparent (since others appear to know what he wants, when he has "to go," and so forth). He falls down and projects the blame to his mother for not watching, and he is insulted if she intrudes. It is a concrete world of magical rules, literal controls, charming compliance, and new skills—as well as undisciplined wishes—reflecting the child's zest but general inexperience and dependency, and shifting only with the growing capacity to discriminate relationships, categories, and time. With developing cognitive and motor skills, and sphincter control, he shows a growing initiative; he begins to make things out and, as Erikson notes, "is on the make." [10] Able to talk well and to locomote his body skillfully, he can now pause to fashion things with his hands and with growing interest to regard his body parts. Much earlier, his genitals, purposefully or aimlessly manipulated, provided pleasant sensations; and a variety of masturbatory activities can be observed. The little boy begins to find himself and to wonder what he is, to poke into things, to ask and intrude comments, to see and be seen, to show off and to peek, and to measure himself and his body against the differences of others. Little girls show these "phallic" assertive and exhibitionistic interests, as well as a developing dominance of receptive behaviors; for example, in doll play and in relationships to the father. But their "penis envy" is literally evident in their wishes and attempts to show off like a boy, to urinate standing and make the stream a boy can make.

In locating themselves in the scheme of things, children look now to both parents. They believe that when they grow up they will take the exclusive and proper place of a grownup, of mother or father. It requires a step in development for the literal child to recognize that, as a grownup, he need not possess his (ageless) parents in order to possess something like what father or mother possesses. Wishful fantasy intermittently abrogates the difference between a boy and a man; a girl and a woman; or a girl and a boy; and these fantasies can guide later sexual identification. The male child, blithely assuming his own importance, frequently wants to be united with his mother and to eliminate the father (except when he needs him); this is the love affair Freud called the Oedipus complex, after Sophocles' drama. The daughter, entranced with her father, considers the mother at times as a deadly rival; she likes to think she can do better in taking care of father; and she is sensitive about the attention that father shows her and any knowing disapproval that her mother might indicate: the Electra complex. These domestic politics are quite complicated, as Freud recognized by speaking not only of a "positive" but of a "negative" Oedipus complex: the attractions between parent and child of the same sex, which coexist with the heterosexual attachments. For his wishes, the male child characteristically expects punishment in the form of castration; fear of death can, after all, only be translated into a meaningful frame of reference—fear of loss of body parts, status, and love. The phase-specific crisis is between initiative (or misplaced ambition) and guilt. The solution of this stormy romantic experiment results in the boy gradually renouncing his wishes and identifying with his father, thus beginning the groundwork of growing into a man through acquiring skills and pleasures actually within his reach. The little girl, interpreting her penisless existence as castration and deprivation (imposed by both or either parent), is inclined to master her disappointment and go in the footsteps of the mother, thus finding a way to be a woman who can win a man and have babies. The father is an "object choice" to be related to with affection rather than sensual excitement. If the father continues to like her she "has" him to relate to, until she can have a man of her own. If she cannot temper her possessive and erotic fantasies, or if he withdraws, she "has" him by "being him" or being like him; she identifies with him. If this is dominant, if her sexual organ and role are too disappointing, disorders in adult roles and sexuality may be expected.

Freud noted that identification with a parent of the same sex after the dissolution of the Oedipus conflict involves internalization of values and sanctions in the form of conscience, superego, and ego ideal. These identifications represent an internal commitment to a future goal, an intention to come to possess attributes that will bring future pleasures while winning contemporary support and security. Both parents provide a picture of what is sought and how to seek it, and the child selects and rejects aspects of both. This era in development clearly represents a crisis in role-taking for the child and heralds the industrious building of a real present. From infancy forward, the parents' preformed expectancies condition the child's roles and values. Individual or cultural differences in the parents' attributes can change the script, but, up to this point, not the number of acts in the play. It should be kept in mind, as Alexander Mitscherlich pointed out in a thoughtful book,[31] that the father's significance in modern society has decreased and that some of the evils of our time, such as alienation, may be related to the fatherless society.

When the conflict is not resolved through the appropriate identifications, certain culturally accepted qualities of the parent of the opposite sex (a certain aggressiveness of the male and a certain receptivity of the female) may appear as abnormal characteristics (excessive and eroticized passivity in males, aggressiveness in females); intense anxiety or guilt are also apt to occur. Indeed, volumes could be written documenting the variable adjustments individuals arrive at in this period. Hysterical behavior, in particular, has been related by psychoanalysts to an unsuccessful solution of the Oedipal conflict. Biographically, these attachments (whether fantasied or openly expressed) may be recalled as devotion, adoration, or a fearful awed admiration of the child for the parent. On closer inspection, such persisting bonds are often found to impair adult sexual ties and to lead to frustrating expectations and disappointments in adult partners. The universal stresses of unconscious castration anxiety, penis envy, and bisexual wishes—to be a man, a woman, or both—are mainsprings of behavior. In the history of antisocial personalities, inflexible attachment to hated and dreaded parental figures that never matures into tempered filial regard and affection is often found. Yet whether all these behavior patterns can be explained by exclusive emphasis on the traumatic impact of the Oedipus conflict has become doubtful.

Late Childhood

Erikson coined the sequence: "I am what I am given" (oral phase); "I am what I will" (anal phase); "I am what I can imagine" (phallic phase); and, for late childhood, which Erikson calls the phase of industry, "I am what I learn." Now in a period marked by problems of inferiority or successful industry, the child comes to be employed with the employment society anticipates for him: the acquisition of special skills; social values and patterns; and competition and interaction with peers and authoritarian figures in a grown-up world. In late prepuberty, his future vistas begin to gel: "I can see what I am to be." The child of eleven knows where his parents fit in society and locates himself accordingly.

The sex drive in this period is felt by psychoanalysts to be relatively dormant, except in overstimulated children. Hence, this phase is called the *latency* period. In fact, a shift in focus rather than a proven diminution of drives is observed. There may be a decline and social inhibition of early masturbatory activity; but a background of erotic interests persists and, to a varying degree, may permeate the highly competitive and intellectual activities of this phase. This is the first time the child looks beyond the family and engages in interactions with teachers and peers, and major feelings of social inferiority can emerge. School represents a new reality and new responsibility; of course, the relative importance of effort and of initiative differs profoundly according to culture and class. Neurotic, deprived, or abused children—long before they go to school—do not learn to listen or to use modes of communication on which teachers depend for their work with the child. Lack of preparation for the task to learn, or lack of pleasure in learning, aggravated by passivity and defiance, may lead to underachievement, which in turn leads to a lowering of self-esteem and to inferiority. Learning and failure are equated by the child with being morally good or bad and hence involve emotional and interpersonal factors. If learning from peers will not compensate for such handicaps, and all too often it does not, the ground for future troubles is laid.

The probability is that learning difficulties *precede* the latency period. By his third year, the child is in a limited way able to designate relationships, and it is probable that the maturation of cognitive abilities may aid the child to transcend his Oedipal struggle and to locate himself as one person among many. With the "thrust" of age-specific, problem-solving capacities, it is important that the environment meet the child's new needs. Any child will explore, but not all build or represent with crayons or even learn to listen to words with any attention (because it is not valuable to do so). If at this time a child is merely cared for physically, not expected to discriminate boundaries and objects (things to name, keep, and retrieve) or to put things together, he will be ill-equipped for future learning in a complex society. Recent objective studies show that a more primitive and magical—a less prepared—child arrives at school from a deprived home. The parents' failure to use language (they point, call different objects "this" or "that") is demonstrably critical. These studies show a marked effect of social factors on intelligence quotient; and it is sobering to find that as much "intelligence" develops in the first four years of life as in the next thirteen years—and 80 per cent of it before the child is eight. Environmentally contingent change in intelligence quotient occurred mostly before school age.[3] Thus, it appears that the basic framework for intellectual as well as for emotional development is markedly shaped by the age of six. A good part of the consequential remaining story is of the development and integration, the arrest, enhancement, and modification of what has been so stably formed in the way of implements, strategies, and attitudes.

Puberty and Adolescence

With pubescence, the hormonal shifts and secondary sex characteristics emerge after a period of relative consolidation of emotional and cognitive development. A restless "waiting" of the late latency period gives way to a phase that involves intense movements and rapid shifts, if only in "catching up" with physical growth and an altered body. In primitive societies, after appropriate initiating rites, the young are now accepted as full members of society, ready to step into what the past has programmed. In advanced civilizations, the license for mature sexual function is denied, and development is held open. The extended period of adolescence reactivates old conflicts and guilts, as old dreams become potentially realizable, and as sexual activity becomes consequential rather than simply fanciful. Attitudes and reactions toward the menarche in girls and toward a capacity to ejaculate in boys (often repressed) are consequential turning points. It is harder for a girl to be a tomboy, and it is more tension-arousing for a boy to be in physical contact with his mother and the women in his family. The sexual outlets are still restricted to crushes and infatuations with partners of the same or other sex, social dating, exploratory petting, and practices falling short of mature fusion of sexual and erotic needs. The most important outlet, masturbation, creates opportunities not only for genital gratification but for the fulfillment of archaic fantasies. These old forbidden wishes produce conscious and unconscious guilt, shame, and fear; and these can make masturbation, which is harmless in itself, a source of stress and concern. Tensions between parent and child mount and may be expressed in an intrusive prurient interest in the adolescent's behavior, or overconcern with his industry. All such concerns are heavy with the portent of consequences, of secret "perversions" and masturbation, forbidden intercourse, changed sexual roles, pregnancy, total failure, and the like. Both parent and child participate in these concerns. The young person may brood, retreat, or compulsively assert his new interests. He may provoke parental intrusion or cling to a vanishing childhood. He certainly requires timely parental guidance. Frequently, under favorable conditions, he turns his attention to philosophy and the advanced contributions of his culture, and to the sublimations of sex and aggression with activity in the social, athletic, and competitive modalities.

This is the time when the young shape what Erikson called "ego identity." In adolescence and young adulthood, the individual develops means (through what he does and the way he does it) for authenticating who and what he is and is to be; society has a range of ways both to ask this question of the individual and to recognize him. Too often, this mutuality fails. Ego identity implies both similarity and uniqueness; in continuity with those with whom he has identified (various males) a boy comes to be a man, but recognizable and unique—a man in his own right; *mutatis mutandis*, this happens in woman too.

Puberty and adolescence constitute one of the major crises in man's life. In these important times, irreversible role patterns and commitments for life are set up; a twelve-year-old may already be motivated not to trust "the power structure" and systematically to become what deprivation and inertia have outlined for him by example. The adolescent often asks implicitly for a postponement of any decision to assume adult sexual and social roles (Erikson's *psychosocial moratorium*). The adolescent is expected to learn many, and possibly too many, new roles; role diffusion at this time may easily become malignant. Psychiatric disturbances, ranging from transient "adolescent turmoil" to sociopathy and schizophrenic psychoses, are related to this period of precipitating stress and conflict. The danger of faulty sexual and social identity formation, which exists in all adolescents, is particularly great. Rather than healthy rebellion, malignant and diffuse identity may occur, which depends purely on protest rather than mastery of skills necessary for independent growth; this may lead to juvenile delinquency and adult criminality. In early adult life, estrangement from oneself, inability for intimacy with others, and particularly the other sex, and for productive work—alienation and isolation—may be striking symptoms of an arrest in development.

Adulthood and Decline

With the consolidation of identity, a reconciliation of the past, present, and future, the young adult assumes innumerable duties, rights, and frustrations. This is the time of the greatest freedom and the heaviest obligations. True involvement in the sexual, social, and occupational sphere, dreamed of in childhood, becomes possible in young adulthood. At this time, under circumstances that permit it, the most important commitments are made: a family is formed and a job is chosen or obtained. The crises of young adulthood are likely to be marital, social, and occupational conflict and failure. Many behavior disorders express themselves in the patient's incapacity to function in these spheres.

Whether adult males or females are more predisposed to behavior disorders has often been discussed. Apart from obligatory biological associations, it is impossible to point to any sex-linked predisposition of specific disorders, although epidemiological trends, to be discussed under specific disorders, are noted. In our society, competition and striving for superiority, and shame concerning passive yearnings generally are more meaningful to the male. However, at a time when the sex role of the female is changing rapidly, similar conflicts and problems in females are increasingly encountered.[29] Justice is not commonly encountered in nature, but it does seem in this case that both sexes have, or find, their crosses to bear.

For a mature adult, the incapacity to love encompasses more than a failure in copulation. In general, psychiatrists have ceased to act as judges of acme and standards in mature sexual performances. Mature couples achieve a range of genital satisfactions through a variety of techniques. It is the attitudes, conflicts, and aims in sexual life, and the integration of sexual activity into the total picture of behavior that are of psychiatric concern. Many psychiatric patients do not present themselves with sexual symptoms or notice them, but the fine details of their sexual lives usually contain and reflect the story of their psychosocial troubles.

Many of the difficulties of adult life express themselves in self-absorption and the inability to work happily and efficiently with others. Western society is an extremely competitive society; and the striving to attain love, power, territory, and possessions may manifest itself in early rivalry, persisting through life, with siblings and peers. Underachievement, not only during the school years, but in adult life, has serious secondary consequences. It not only lowers self-esteem, but an individual's chance to attain a status of respect and power, which, according to Alfred Adler[1] and later Harold Lasswell,[25] are such important motivations. Invariably, in our patients conflicts over such needs exist. In some of them, however, we are not impressed with the drive for power, but with the need to be submissive and passive, and the secondary consequences of such behavior. It is also crucial to diagnose "pregenital" needs for love, security, and childish affection, which so often are masked by seductiveness in the female, overcompensatory masculinity in the male, and denial of dependency needs by both sexes, through a gamut of behavioral and bodily symptoms. In many patients, a curious irrationality in handling money is matched only by Western man's irrationality in sexual matters. Money is the main instrument of many social manipulations; it is equated with power, independence, retaining, giving, and getting.

In the third decade, decline, or at least a shift in functioning, begins, as productiveness still increases. Evident only in certain tests (especially in the acquisition of new learning), there is also a decrement in muscular endurance and some physiological functions. From the fourth to the sixth decades, the involutional process becomes grossly manifest, particularly in the female, who loses her reproductive capacity in the menopause and undergoes marked physical changes. Changes in occupational and social effectiveness aggravate existing conflicts. Mild depressive and paranoid reactions are frequent responses to the stresses of not feeling useful and adequate and in being unable to deny the discrepancy between what has in fact been lived and the illusions that had made frustration bearable. There may be a "last fling," an upsurge in drive behavior. There also may be an increase in productiveness and creativity, or a generous concern with guiding the growth of other generations; with children, social organizations, or other fields of activity—what Erikson termed generativity. This does not entail surrender of personal interests, envy, or ambition but is a deployment of all these forces in the direction of building and care-taking.

Increase of experience, purpose, and organization may outweigh the decline of abilities for rapid learning; only in senescence do the catalytic processes predominate. Even then, the impairment of biological and social functions varies tremendously between different persons and in the same individual. Intellectual decline, regression to infantile need patterns, and a propensity to catastrophic anxiety, when new or unexpected situations (illness, retirement) are encountered, make old age a stressful period, taxing self-respect, not only for the psychiatrically ill but for many normal persons. General illness, in addition to cerebral malfunction during this period, seems the most serious stress that can precipitate major behavior disorders. Yet it is not completely hopeless. There is danger of despair or disgust for the elderly in society, and the rejection of life to which he clings; but there may also be a sense of integrity and tolerance for the solutions others achieve.

Some Consequences of the Developmental Point of View in Psychiatry

The principles that apply generally to biological development also characterize the movements in these epigenetic sequences in man; perhaps they apply also to behavior change and to learning. Integrated biological systems, as complex behaviors, are prepared for in advance.[42] In man, separate zonal interests coalesce into general excitement and then differentiate into the repertory of erotic genital and affectionate relationships of adult sexuality. We have noted several "weanings" in human development (in infancy, the Oedipal period, adolescence) that prepare both for adult individuality and mutuality. Environmental factors can influence events in these phases, and arrests and lags occur, visible to us as "pathology." Similarly, in embryonic development, component parts of a reflex appear first but show only a random responsiveness to stimulation; later, stimulation produces a mass body reflex, finally to be followed by specific sequential and circumscribed response of muscles.[18] J. Barcroft[2] compared this preparation to the tuning of individual instruments, but the moment comes when the orchestra as such breaks forth; individualized themes and solos can then develop against an orchestrated background.

When biologists conceive of growth, they do not see a little man in the embryo to which is added the accretions of adulthood; nor is the child an adult with certain features subtracted; nor does regression mean subtraction; rather, it is the earlier level *intermixed* with newer features. When sheep embryos were "regressed" with partial anoxia, the earlier mass reflexes returned but now intermixed with sporadic respiratory movements that, in integrated fashion, had characterized the preregressive stage.[2] The same principles apply to the adult who regresses; there is an admixture of adult and childish responses. These admixtures may be seen also in the "progressive" course of development and even in the "ups and downs" of therapeutically induced behavior change. When behavior changes, we deal with the consequences of rearrangements of familiar elements and the altered conditions governing them. The reproductions and new combinations, however, do not require the appearance of new "basic" laws or novel elements. The processes we call judging, thinking, perceiving, defending, and feeling operate at different levels of development, with different effects; we may view their "disorder" in behavior pathology not as a novelty but as a *consequence* of the prevailing level of organization. The operations we call conscience in the normal adult may, at a psychotic level of functioning, appear as hallucinated voices offering judgment (or thinking may appear as visual images). Since we grow through various levels of organization, it is not surprising to find past modes of operating coexisting with the present, whether in dreams, in symptoms, in new achievements, or in the surprisingly retained skills of the regressed schizophrenic.

How closely can we track behavior change: is it a progressive (or regressive) step-by-step linear process? This is doubtful. The emergence of a reflex, a thought (or an intuition), or of a new behavior seems to happen suddenly. As with crystal formation, a new structure emerges, and this would seem to oppose the "sensible" notion of continuity in development. Yet, in the world of physics, we have learned to live with quantum states that involve "jumps" and discontinuity between levels. In behavioral states, continuity must be integrated (as in the formation of personal identity); every day we bridge the quite disparate states of sleep and wakefulness; and the failure to integrate disparate states and levels of organization, the too vivid "waking dream" appears as behavior pathology. To achieve behavior change, neither the therapist nor the patient puts pieces of behavior together, as a string of beads; behavior change occurs through rearrangements within the patient; and he and we can perceive only the products of changed conditions and levels of organization—the altered behaviors, feelings, or perceptions.

The many levels of development through which the adult has emerged are mirrored clinically in many levels of meaning. When an adult speaks of "trust," we do not know whether he means infantile trust (that others will perform exactly what he needs without his participation), or the trust of confident self-reliance and mutual regard. The patient may speak of independence but mean he must, with distrust, excessively strive for tyrannical infantile autonomy. The "dependency" of a contemporary graduate student need not be played out at the infantile level; hopefully, he may show the strength to tolerate dependency and interruption and delay of his autonomy without the doubts, shame, and rebellion of a three-year-old. The more the psychiatrist grasps the meaning of the various levels of organization and their potentialities for behavior, and the more he appreciates the vicissitudes of growth and development, the readier he is to bring a cogent response to the suffering he studies as behavior disorder. For this continuing education in life, much more than textbooks are required; but we believe that a receptivity to the developmental point of view about behavior is a useful beginning.

NOTES

1. Alfred Adler, *Study of Organ Inferiority and Its Psychical Compensation; A Contribution to Clinical Medicine* ("Nervous and Mental Disease Monograph Series," No. 24 [New York: Nervous and Mental Disease Publishing Company, 1917]).
2. Joseph Barcroft, *The Brain and Its Environment* (New Haven: Yale University Press, 1938).
3. Benjamin S. Bloom, *Stability and Change in Human Characteristics* (New York: John Wiley, 1964).
4. Neil R. Burch and H. E. Childers, "Physiological Data Acquisition," in Bernard E. Flaherty, ed., *Psychophysiological Aspects of Space Flights* (New York: Columbia University Press, 1961).
5. Norman Cameron, *Personality and Psychopathology* (Boston: Houghton-Mifflin, 1963).
6. John Dollard and Neal E. Miller, *Personality and Psychotherapy* (New York: McGraw-Hill, 1950).
7. Ludwig Eidelberg, "An Introduction to the Study of Narcissistic Mortification," *Psychiatric Quarterly*, 31 (1957), 657.
8. George L. Engel and Franz Reichsmann, "Spontaneous and Experimentally Induced Depression in an Infant with a Gastric Fistula," *Journal of the American Psychoanalytic Association*, 4 (1956), 428.
9. Erik H. Erikson, *Childhood and Society* (New York: Norton, 1963).
10. Erik H. Erikson, "Identity and the Life Cycle; Selected Papers," *Psychological Issues*, Vol. 1, No. 1 (New York: International Universities Press, 1959).
11. Barbara Fish, "The Study of Motor Development in Infancy and Its Relationship to Psychological Functioning," *American Journal of Psychiatry*, 117 (1961), 1113.

12. Anna Freud, *The Ego and the Mechanisms of Defence* (New York: International Universities Press, 1946).
13. Anna Freud and Dorothy Burlingham, *Infants without Families: The Case for and against Residential Nurseries* (New York: International Universities Press, 1944).
14. Sigmund Freud, "Inhibitions, Symptoms and Anxiety" [1926], *Standard Edition* (London: Hogarth Press, 1959), 20.
15. Sigmund Freud, "Introductory Lectures on Psychoanalysis, I and II" (1916–1917), *Standard Edition* (London: Hogarth Press, 1961), 15–16.
16. Daniel H. Funkenstein, S. H. King, and M. E. Drolette, *Mastery of Stress* (Cambridge: Harvard University Press, 1957).
17. Harry F. Harlow, "The Nature of Love," *American Psychologist*, 13 (1958), 673.
18. Davenport Hooker, "Reflex Activities in the Human Fetus," in R. G. Barker, S. J. Kounin, and H. F. Wright, eds., *Child Behavior and Development* (New York: McGraw-Hill, 1943).
19. J. H. Jackson, "Croonian Lectures on the Evolution and Dissolution of the Nervous System," *Lancet*, 1 (1884), 555.
20. Jay Katz, "On Primary Gain and Secondary Gain," *The Psychoanalytic Study of the Child*, 18 (1963), 9.
21. Melanie Klein, *The Psycho-analysis of Children* (London: Hogarth, 1950).
22. Ernst Kris, "Ego Development and the Comic," *International Journal of Psycho-Analysis*, 19 (1938), 77.
23. Lawrence S. Kubie, "The Repetitive Core of Neurosis," *Psychoanalytic Quarterly*, 10 (1941), 23.
24. John I. Lacey, in "Timberlane Conference on Psychophysiologic Aspects of Cardiovascular Disease," *Psychosomatic Medicine*, 26 (1964), 445.
25. Harold Lasswell, *Power and Personality* (New York: Viking, 1962).
26. Seymour Levine, "Psychophysiological Effects of Infantile Stimulation," in E. L. Bliss, ed., *Roots of Behavior* (New York: Harper, 1962).
27. David M. Levy, *Maternal Overprotection* (New York: Columbia University Press, 1943).
28. Robert Malmo, "Activation: A Neuropsychological Dimension," *Psychological Review*, 66 (1959), 367.
29. Margaret Mead, *Male and Female: A Study of the Sexes in a Changing World* (New York: W. Morrow, 1949).
30. I. Arthur Mirsky, "Physiologic, Psychologic and Social Determinants in the Etiology of Duodenal Ulcer," *American Journal of Digestive Disease*, 3 (1958), 285.
31. Alexander Mitscherlich, *Auf dem Weg zur Vaterlosen Gesellschaft* (Munich: Piper, 1963).
32. John I. Nurnberger, C. B. Ferster, and John P. Brady, *An Introduction to the Science of Human Behavior* (New York: Appleton, 1963).
33. S. R. Pinneau, "The Infantile Disorders of Hospitalism and Anaclitic Depression," *Psychological Bulletin*, 52 (1955), 429.

34. Sally Provence and Rose C. Lipton, *Infants in Institutions* (New York: International Universities Press, 1962).

35. David Rapaport, "The Structure of Psychoanalytic Theory," in *Psychological Issues*, Vol. 2, No. 6 (New York: International Universities Press, 1960).

36. Dickenson W. Richards, "Homeostasis versus Hyperexis: Or Saint George and the Dragon," *Scientific Monthly*, 77 (1953), 289.

37. Daniel P. Schwartz, "The Integrative Effect of Participation," *Psychiatry: Journal for the Study of Interpersonal Processes*, 22 (1959), 81.

38. Hans Selye, *The Stress of Life* (New York: McGraw-Hill, 1956).

39. René Spitz and Katherine Wolf, "Anaclitic Depression. An Inquiry into the Genesis of Psychiatric Conditions in Early Childhood, II," *The Psychoanalytic Study of the Child*, II (1947).

40. Harry Stack Sullivan, *The Interpersonal Theory of Psychiatry* (New York: Norton, 1953).

41. Robert Waelder, *Basic Theory of Psychoanalysis* (New York: International Universities Press, 1960).

42. Heinz Werner, *Comparative Psychology of Mental Development* (Chicago: Follett Publishing Company, 1957).

43. Allen Wheelis, *The Quest for Identity* (New York: Norton, 1958).

CHAPTER SIX

Etiology II: Biological and Psychosocial Variables

Brain and Behavior Disorders

The roles of the brain, of neuroendocrine and biochemical control systems, and of heredity and constitution as etiologically significant variables in behavior disorders are usually not as clearly in the forefront of our immediate clinical concerns as psychological, psychodynamic, developmental, and environmental variables. They are, nevertheless, of basic importance. For the organic behavior disorders, the study of cerebral functions is obviously indispensable, but it has also been thought quite possible that a key to some riddles of at least a group of schizophrenias and affective psychoses will eventually be found by elucidation of pathophysiological processes involving the central nervous system. Essentially, we require an appreciation of the nature of the limits and organizations that underlie behavioral systems for an intelligent and basic understanding of the way in which behavior is organized. Our clinical data and theory will thereby gain, if not in validity, at least in focus and perspective. Through his medical training, the psychiatrist will be familiar with the fundamentals of neuroanatomy, neurophysiology, neurochemistry, and neuropathology. He should know the principal facts of scalp and depth electroencephalography, and the results from new micromethods of stimulating, destroying, or chemically altering cerebral tissue, which were developed by J. M. R. Delgado[27] and others. Our growing knowledge depends on more than acute experiments with stimulation or ablation of brain components. Experimentalists have begun to reconstruct how the brain is related to developing behaviors; and they have begun to identify the bits and sequences, the components by which an animal who needs to eat can organize itself to find the source of food and implement its intake; or recognize, orient to, and locate its prey; or acquire discriminatory skills. These neurobehavioral studies employ techniques for evoking and inhibiting behavioral sequences, for making phylogenetic comparisons in developing animals, and for studies of the learning and forgetting of cue and drive-organized performance in animals and man. In what follows, we can present only an overview, directed more to conveying some sense of how the nervous system might be related to normal and abnormal behavior, than to any specific systems and mechanisms. These will be discussed where relevant in the various chapters on clinical disorders. Of necessity, biological principles and mechanisms derived from animal experiment will be stressed, and data about the human brain will be cited where relevant (see Chapter 16).

Structure, Ultrastructure, and Information Transfer

The relationship between different subsystems or levels of brain organization (electrophysiological, neurochemical, vascular, behavioral) may be conceived as involving the exchange of information at critical junctures through a variety of transfer mechanisms. From a physical-chemical standpoint, the energies involved for the operations, as distinct from the maintenance, of this consequential organ are minimal. The brain is quite sensitive to a supply of oxygen for its integrity. Nevertheless, as Seymour Kety pointed out,[72] it takes no more energy to think a crazy thought than a sane one in terms of over-all oxygen consumption of the brain; rather, this gross measure defines the limits for coma or consciousness. With techniques developed by Oliver H. Lowry for measurement of metabolism in even single cells,[87] the role of energy changes as signals for neural events may be clearer.

From the peripheral receptor to the cortex, there are numerous points where direct or feedback mechanisms can filter and reduce the flood of input and thereby organize it. Even at the level of reflex, the prior state of neural activity, as well as the output, determines to some degree what the *next* stimulus is going to be. The fate of an ascending message in the neuraxis is determined at synaptic connections, where mixing and scanning (selection) of inputs can occur, and is influenced, in part, by interneural systems distal as well as proximal to the synapse and by graded states of subthreshold electrical activity, as well as molecular changes at critical membranes. An ascending message can also be dampened at the peripheral receptor by feedback loops (such as gamma efferents).

In a sense, the synapse, transforming input from one state to another, is where the physiologist first encounters the body–mind problem. There are approximately 10^{10} neurons (many with quite specialized architecture) and vastly more synaptic connections, which alone should indicate that simple switchboard models of neural operations are not adequate. There are ranges of interneural, chemical, and electrical sequences that determine what occurs at the synapse.[14] Some of these sequences occur in ultrastructures. Within the cell are vast stretches of coiled and configured membranes, structures, and channels comprised of double-layered arrays of stereospecific protein and phospholipid, which, in addition to maintaining structural integrity, provide (within the mitochondria) the sites for energy-trapping and energy transfer. Within the universe of the cell, there is a "traffic" of synthesized, stored, and released bioactive substances such as amines;[42] the binding and release of these substances at synaptic membranes may alter their polarization and the subsequent transfer of electrical messages. In addition, chemical, ionic, osmotic, and metabolic states may be consequential for thresholds at the electrical level. The brain is somewhat buffered from rapidly changing chemical events in the body by the "blood–brain barrier," which is comprised functionally of any number of enzymatically-controlled processes and which anatomically may be represented by a capillary-glial-neuronal assembly. The interposed glia appear to have some function in the transport of substances between vessels (which systematically differ in ultrastructure) [133] and neurons (which may differ in permeability).

Thus, the structure and ultrastructure of cells condition chemical traffic that can influence membrane excitability and, at another level, graded electrical events at the synapse. It should be noted that the brain is not only composed of highly differentiated cellular arrangements, but is also chemically inhomogeneous; its chemical structure varies regionally, providing a system for the "chemical coding" of behavior. These various junctures and membranes may be critical sites for both drug action and neurochemical dysfunctions of behavioral significance.

Sensory Filtering, Perception, and Integration

The processing of simple inputs in man can be tracked; for example, the cortical potential evoked by stimulation of the ulnar nerve or visual stimulation can be traced out of the complicated scalp EEG by computers.[116] Such studies have shown differences between some groups of psychotic patients and normals.[121] Similarly, parameters of the eight-to-fourteen-per-second alpha frequencies shift with graded states of consciousness and are said to differentiate some patient groups and drug states.[39, 53, 104]

The processing of input requires "filters," or gates, selectively admitting information as well as systems for recoding and saving various channels from overload. Integrations of sensory input (especially in man, who elaborates rich meaning from input) are relatively unstudied, but the role of sensory systems in organizing perception is clearly considerable. The cells of the retina, for example, structure input at the very outset.[63,108] Apparently, a light-stimulated receptor cell of the retina inhibits a neighboring unilluminated cell, allowing a boundary; and the stimulated cell, free from inhibition by its neighbor, fires more rapidly, sharpening the contour. This "packaging" of input, begun at the periphery, continues from the first synapse to the visual cortex. There, certain of a columnar "bank" of cells react, not to a retinal point, but to a particular, say, horizontal line of brightness on the retina. Another cell in the bank can monitor these specific stations for individual horizontal lines. This cell responds only to *any* horizontal line whatever its retinal location; other "monitors" respond only to any such moving line; and so forth. What is of general import is that perception, prior to symbolic alterations, involves an abstraction, or organization, of input. These arrangements allow for speed of response and comprise one of several mechanisms by which a world, rapidly changing in minute details, can be kept relatively constant. On the other hand, the ready adaptation of retinal cells to a constant input (subjectively, the input "fades" away) provides a built-in preparedness for the detection of change and novelty.[111]

Whereas the cellular, topographical, and hierarchical organization of specific inputs is important, we can barely perceive how all this complex activity gets put together, that is, how it provides integration and information, rather than noise.[14] Perhaps mathematics' topological principles may be required to explain complex neural function: simultaneous events at various scattered points throughout the brain may actually comprise a common "domain." It is likely that the future will bring to light integrating operations that we cannot even conceive of at present.

Centers, Steering Functions, and Consciousness

A search for the seat of consciousness and steering functions in behavior in the nineteenth century was literally a search for a common anatomical "integrative" point in the human brain. A confluence of input and output was sought in such median structures as the pineal, septum pellucidum, corpus callosum, or the third ventricle. In our day, functional systems have been offered as seats of consciousness acting as governing mechanisms: the rostral brain stem, the ascending reticular formation, or Wilder Penfield's centrencephalic system. Apart from the fact that both cortex and subcortex are necessary for the *experience* of consciousness, we do not know how the experience comes about nor how behavior is "directed." It is clear, however, that the simple instigation of behavior by stimulating a point in the brain does not describe the organization of that action nor the various pathways and neural interactions involved; one cannot equate the prime mover with a stimulating electrode. A center may be conceived as a timing or programming device, a group of neurons, which, among their other functions, sequentially fire to a number of different systems. Such a programming system could be stimulated by a variety of central and peripheral sources and conditions. Perhaps the "start-and-stop" systems (where animals work for or avoid electrical stimulation to brain areas) partially regulate input to centers.

Memory and Learning

What are the neural correlates of behavioral memory—the electrophysiological and chemical processes underlying the storage of information patterns (often called engrams)? With the connection fibers between the hemispheres severed, experiments in man have shown that both hemispheres can record memory, that motor feedback is decisive as to which hemisphere records and builds up simple sensorimotor memories (that is, for repeated action patterns), and that language and verbal memory are usually recorded only in the dominant hemisphere, whereas lesser functions are recorded in the nondominant one and transferred when required. We know little concerning the neural correlates of learning or conditioning, although an electrical event can apparently act as a conditioned stimulus,[28] and patterns of electrical rhythm (when a flashing light of specific frequency is the conditioned stimulus)[68] can be tracked in various subcortical and cortical areas during phases of learning. It appears likely that primitive subcortical systems play an essential role in the "reinforcement" or drive-reduction aspect of learning. With new input, new connections may be formed among the myriad synaptic knobs that rest upon a cell body; experience may cause increases in brain size.[115] Reverberating electrical circuits have been advanced as a model for memory (and isolated cortical slabs will sustain an excitation for a long time), but no empirical link to memory has been found. The role of the temporal lobe and its deep structures in recording memory is discussed in Chapter 16. Another engaging model conceives of memory as changes in the orientation of constituents of cellular membranes, similar to the polarization of a magnetic tape; and the effect of fields of electrical forces on learning and neuronal function has been studied.[118] Transmission of genetic information or of immune memory through molecular replications (involving the nucleic acid, RNA) provides yet another proposed model for behavioral memory.[31] Models for the retrieval of registered information run the gamut: electronic scanners, matching the input to a recorded sample followed by retrieval. These are models, however, not buttressed with data.

Development and the Brain

The ground plan of the brain essentially comprises parallel lateral systems of motor and sensory tracts and interposed systems that modulate sensorimotor function. Many neuronal assemblies are apparently organized in agonist–antagonist subsystems, the balance and prior state of which are important for response. Stimulation of an inhibitory system or inhibition of a facilitatory component could lead to apparently identical response. This is one intrinsic reason for exercising great care in inferring or diagnosing a brain mechanism solely from gross behavioral observation. These various systems presumably come under more complex control and coordination with experience and maturation.

The formation of the human cerebral nervous system begins in the second month of intrauterine existence, and there has been a growing body of work on the development of reflex activity and the EEG in the fetus.[62] Although the early chemical conditioning of behavior during critical periods requires further study, developmental periods are critical for the appearance, suppression or stimulation of certain brain enzyme systems,[112] some of which adapt to their environment. Approximately in the third year of life, the anatomical and physiological development of the brain is complete. Between the first and third years, functional cerebral hierarchies develop, which correspond generally to hierarchies of behavior. The role of experience or age is clinically important, since a number of lesions, for example, viral encephalitides, produce different consequences and rates of recovery in children and preadolescents than in adults. Dominance in cerebral function develops as do preferential behaviors; the plasticity of brain areas is thus a function both of age and experience. Neurohumoral events are critical for shifts from prepuberty to puberty and, finally, repeated experience (dependent in part on critical developmental periods) changes the organization and involvement of cells in various brain areas.[141]

Higher Functions

A great number of functional differentiations occur, at first primarily in the subcortical systems regulating bodily functions. Participating at the highest level of Jackson's hierarchy are the frontal and posterior cortical association areas, which, in concert with other systems, are required for the highest and uniquely human functions: the ability to use symbols, to control both impulses and input, to plan, to have foresight, and to learn. Higher functions require integration of complex and plastic neural organizations and are more vulnerable to disruption than more automatic and overorganized operations. Of course, we are still able to deal with only the simplest building blocks out of which perceptions and images may be achieved. How further abstractions such as thought, or experiences such as consciousness occur can be approached only through models and analogies and fragmentary objective data. Most of our knowledge concerning higher functions comes from clinical rather than experimental studies, but the studies of performance and learning by Hal E. Rosvold,[117] Karl H. Pribram, [107] and others are of basic interest. At the next level in the pre- and postrolandic areas are the cerebral stations for sensory input and motor output, connected through projection fibers. Vocalizations and speech, sensorimotor as well as behaviorally significant functions are integrated through cortical mechanisms; these complexities are discussed in Chapter 16.

Drives, Affects, and "Splits"

The primitive part of the endbrain, the limbic system with its phylogenetically older cortex and nuclei, is related to the expression of instinctual drives and emotions, for example, hunger and sex drives. Violent emotional outbursts, hypersexuality, orality, and bizarre placid states were observed with experimental lesions (now referable to the amygdala) several decades ago.

John Flynn has shown that emotions displayed after hypothalamic stimulation are psychologically valid outbursts of rage (for example, they are linked to objects), and not simply pseudoemotions.[89] The significance of the primitive endbrain for feelings of pleasure and displeasure is attested to by the subjective reports of patients with implanted electrodes, and has been demonstrated in self-stimulation experiments where animals will perseverate a behavioral response to achieve or avoid electrical input to these areas.[101] The very important investigations of Paul MacLean,[90] based on early work by Heinrich Klüver and Paul Bucy, James W. Papez, and others, have demonstrated that the limbic system is responsible for a range of functions that deal with bodily and behavioral activity, which subserves the preservation of the self and the race. The appropriate recognition of input as well as the organization of output related to a number of basic behavioral arrays—sex, attack, food—are affected by lesions of the deep temporal lobe structures. Later, we will discuss this system (and its hypothalamic and midbrain components important for visceral, autonomic, and metabolic regulations) with respect to its importance for psychosomatic medicine.

In a broad sense, it is clear that the old and new cortex provide an electrophysiological demonstration of dissociation: while integrally connected through the midbrain with sensorimotor and neocortical systems, the hippocampus can become a stage for "violent" electrical seizures without any evidence of change in motor or neocortical activity. This "split" in functions is of interest to clinicians speculating about the integrations and splits in affective and intellectual and motor behavior. R. W. Sperry's studies of split brain (disconnection of the hemispheres) in man and animal are also relevant. They indicate that there can be a doubling of attention, but more usually a competition between the hemispheres for attention, one being dominant.[127] Without the connecting fibers one side can only know indirectly what the other is doing; each has its own memory and can carry out complex behavior.

Activation and Subcortical Integration

Associated with the neocortical mantle and frontal lobes are functions related to the distance receptors: the location of distant sensory cues and the spatial structuring of them. This seems analogous to psychological functions dependent on the neocortex: the alignment of the past with future anticipations, or the appreciation of psychological distance—which functionally is delay. These operations appear to be "prepared" by "first-order" mechanisms. These cope with bodily and postural immediacy and orient the animal with respect to preparation for danger or pleasure; for such operations subcortical systems appear dominant. The brain stem reticular formation and its associated limbic system connections (and the thalamo-cortical projections) appear to be prepotent in bringing the physiology of the organism into immediate contact with the environment: through basic visceral, metabolic, and hormonal integrations; through postural, motor, and equilibratory mechanisms of the medulla, midbrain, and basal ganglia; through inhibiting or facilitatory influences on spinal input in preparation for motor outflow; and through its activating ("alerting") functions on rostral and neocortical neurons.

The activating functions of a brain stem system that is both motor and sensory, projects rostrally (through the thalamic projections) to the cortex and caudally to the cord, and provides a background against which highly specific sensory or motor functions are augmented and diminished. These functions are crucial for linking the *bodily* and vegetative components of behavior to such *behavioral* components as set, readiness to respond, intensity, attention, and alertness. Cortical and peripheral dampening and activation of these reticular systems may be critical in functions such as attention; if perceptual input could be dampened before it reaches cortical levels, an efficient gating and attention mechanism would be provided. Clinical findings such as those by Fredrick Redlich[110] and experimental findings by Horace Magoun[91] and Robert Livingston[84] established that the reticular systems in diencephalic and mesencephalic regions are crucial for a primitive consciousness and vigilance. These neural nets also reveal an intrinsic activity; they can dampen a "large" input but magnify a "small" one and this flux of activities, partially independent of specific inputs, permits variable and flexible function.

Activation and Intensity

One of Jackson's basic assumptions was that lesions disrupting a higher hierarchical level will produce deficit reactions and also will release the lower neural hierarchies and their behavioral concomitants, a view that, in France, has been revived by Henri Ey and applied to many significant psychiatric problems.[36] It should be clear, however, that intensity in behavior need not be a matter solely of release or disinhibition and lack of feedback control.[34] It may involve distinct organizations of neural activity; for example, activation systems, which, in some instances, are under higher control. In any event, the ascription of intensity to behavior can be more than an empathic or value judgment; it is an operationally specifiable dimension of behavior. What specific behavior or behavioral process is intense, depressed, or inhibited? This must first be defined, and we should be careful to distinguish between these labels and the actual mechanisms at the neural level.

In summary, the picture of the brain today is less exclusively "corticocentric," less geared to mechanical models, and more responsive to the coordinated facts of microanatomy, electrophysiology, neurochemistry, and behavior. These various approaches, coupled with information theory, have begun to break the mold imposed by older and looser metaphors and models and to lead to the picture of material systems that can operate to produce the complexities and subtleties we encounter in behavior and behavior pathology. We would strictly caution the student not to mistake analogies derived from such an extensive range of discrete studies as established, unalterable facts. The fact is, that whereas basic designs are becoming clear to us, the links between the brain, the peripheral receptors, and behavior must be spelled out in ever-increasing detail.

Neuroendrocrine Change and Behavior

R. W. Gerard once quipped that no twisted thought occurs without a twisted molecule.[48] We are, of course, a long way from understanding how it is that biochemical changes can become behaviorally manifest; in a rigorous sense there is an appalling distance between biochemical mechanisms and the particular substrata for perception and behavior. The problem inherently entails a detailed study of intrinsic control systems at a number of different levels from the enzymatic to the psychosocial. Yet in this age of drugs, it has become abundantly clear that chemical changes do influence neurobehavioral function, that periods of chemical change are consequential to the way in which behavior can be coordinated, and that there are a variety of chemically dependent linkages (such as phenothiazine-induced sedation without drowsiness) of which the nervous system is capable. We have begun to learn about the effects of electrical impulses of the brain on central and peripheral feedback mechanisms involving the hypothalamus. Stimulation of the hypothalamus evokes neurosecretory activity—the release of a variety of polypeptides that activate pituitary hormones regulating target glands (such as the adrenal and thyroid glands, and gonads) as well as chemical reactions.[56] In turn, the level of circulating hormone may affect neural function. The basic strategy underlying measures of hormones and chemicals rests on the fact that the limbic system and the hypothalamus as well as the caudal brain stem participate in the regulation of metabolic and chemical systems and are, in turn, affected by them; changes in body chemistry could, therefore, reflect changes in the activity (the integration and regulation) of small or large components of the central nervous system. The intent is to deduce the functional status of these consequential central systems through a variety of behavioral, psychophysical, perceptual, physiological, and chemical measures.

In general, we know more about a few of these sequences (for example, chemical control of thyroid activity) than about the effects of sensory input and neural activity upon the control of chemical systems which are localized in the brain and are important in synaptic function. There are, however, a growing number of studies that are laying the groundwork for our understanding of when and how environmental input to the brain can directly alter its chemistry—enzyme activity, concentrations of substrate, and changes in the blood–brain barrier.[40, 58, 126] In animals, the stress simply of intense exertion can change local brain metabolism of amines and not generally disrupt body physiology.[3,40] It is, therefore, not unlikely that we shall continue to find instances of how environmental events rather directly alter local brain chemistry. The capacity of but a few molecules of indole or catechol amines to produce profoundly altered mental states is impressive, and there is mounting evidence that the body contains the enzymatic machinery for synthesizing such psychotoxins.[50] The changes in brain produced by these substances occur at the level of ultrastructures and the order of magnitude of chemical change is in millimicrograms or less. The importance of such findings is not their immediate clinical relevance but rather the demonstration of the kind of biological mechanisms that must be investigated at the clinical level.

In the past decade we have learned something of the detailed biochemistry of those amines that have been thought to underlie "fight-and-flight" behaviors. A number of exotic and endogenous amines have been identified so that the "base vocabulary" is now available, and current research is directed at establishing the syntax, the rules regulating the activity of amines under normal and abnormal conditions, and their relationships to energy and fatty acid metabolism and to endocrine as well as neural function. Studies of the urinary metabolites of amines in depression and in schizophrenia indicate that these disorders can involve a shift in amine metabolism, at least as a consequence of the stress of the behavior disorder. Similarly, the role of abnormal electrolyte and water metabolism has been studied in a number of states, and in depression a decrease of CSF sodium has been noted.[51] Hormonal responses to various subjectively defined stresses in normal and depressed persons were explored by D. A. Hamburg and his co-workers,[10] who noted that protein bound iodine and 17-hydroxycorticosteroids were significantly elevated in depressed patients after the stressful experience of hospital admission. While it is clear that severe behavior disorder may be a stress, evoking steroid response, these effects appear to be relatively non-specific and not diagnostic.[16,17,18,76,98,106]

Current measures of endocrines in behavior disorders show values that, while correlating with stress, are still within the medically normal range, so that endocrine changes related to shifts in functional status require precise and fine measurement both of endocrine and behavioral variables. The appropriate use of rating scales and a variety of objective methods for assessing behavior has been a crucial development for this psychiatric research.[23,54] It has been recognized that measurement of endocrine response may prove to be most valuable in longitudinal studies focusing on fluctuations of behavioral and physiological status during the course of a behavior disorder.[18] This approach permits scrutiny of the sequence of mental and bodily changes in the individual patient. It is also apparent that the complex psychobiological and neurochemical events in different periods of stress require methodologically sophisticated investigation at both the basic and clinical levels. For example, the relevant measures of stress are not simply the levels of hormone or even various free and bound fractions, but also the changes in underlying microchemical and enzymatic mechanisms that affect many bodily processes and control rates of biochemical reactions. Stress, for example, can activate enzymes (histamine decarboxylase, tryptophan pyrrolase) that regulate substances active in autonomic and brain function. Thus measurements of catecholamines, and their metabolites,[93, 95, 119] lipid,[11] and liver metabolism (for example, hippuric acid), and hormones are employed in searches for simple correlates of anxiety and stress;[55] but little attention has yet been given to the neurochemical regulation of such substances in experimentally controlled pathophysiological or developmental sequences.

While we have much yet to learn about endocrine effects in local brain areas, gonadal hormones, acting upon the hypothalamus in early stages of maturation are known to organize neural tissues that later mediate the periodicity of hormonal patterns, mating behavior[5] and possibly sex-linked social behavior.[57, 144] Apparently the rodent brain is sexually dimorphic; it is the nature of the endocrine secretion at critical periods that patterns the characteristic male and female mating behaviors. By experimentally changing the endocrine stimulation—giving estradiol at the right time to the castrate infant male—female behavior patterns and hormonal rhythms ensue at puberty. This is an interesting demonstration of the role of interlocking feedbacks of developmental, genetic, neural, and chemical variables in determining behavioral patterns. The significance of hormonal disturbances for man is unclear. Man's behavior after castration, in contrast to animals, appears to be somewhat independent of the intact or disturbed function of his glands and relatively independent of endocrine-induced "triggering" of specific behaviors. Glandular dysfunction may tax this independence, but such factors are difficult to sort out. Some severe endocrine disorders ultimately affect the neurochemical organization of the brain and are correlated with behavior disorders, ranging from delirium and organic deficit states to mood and impulse disorders. In view of the toxic psychoses variably produced by therapeutic administration of hormones, their effects on mood, the unsolved role of hormonal shifts (especially in the psychological adjustments of women), and the fact that their neurochemical and biochemical effects are incompletely known, we should anticipate even more specific definitions of their role and consequence for behavior. In summary, brain dysfunction, perhaps of ultrastructural chemistry and the control of hormonal and metabolic function, remains a plausible but generally unproven causal and contributory factor in most psychiatric disorders.

Minimal Brain Damage

In the absence of gross neurological signs and in the presence of disordered behavior one should not rule out organic dysfunction. If we are serious about the biological roots both for the various "programs" of drive behaviors and the developmental and maturational schedules, we will be more alert to the possibility that clinical problems may be referable to equipmental variables. Some of these problems will be discussed when we review constitution and genetics. Minimal brain damage at critical developmental periods may produce a wide variety of developmental difficulties, which, possibly, in turn predispose to neurotic and sociopathic disorders.[102] Clinically, we are familiar with the various covert or subclinical seizure states such as psychomotor epilepsy. Due to temporal lobe dysfunction, this disorder sometimes leaves no histopathological trace. We often require special EEG techniques for detecting the dysfunction and it is important that we do so since the patient may respond to medication. If these disorders occur in early childhood they may episodically alter the child's perception and impulse control and hence give rise to a skewed development of compensatory traits, which in adulthood appear as rigidity, eccentricities, and mild paranoid reactions. We are, of course, far more familiar with a large number of developmental diseases and anomalies, infections and toxic reactions, metabolic diseases and trauma, which produce clear-cut cerebral damage and severe behavior disorder. These may be characterized not only by an inability to solve problems and by intellectual and sensory motor deficits, but also by disorders in drive control and in emotional regulation.

Modifiability of Brain Function

Students should be clear about the irreparable sensorimotor defects contingent on brain injury, but should not predict unalterable defects based solely on obsolete allocations of specific functions to specific brain areas. We know, of course, that psychosocial factors, motivations, and premorbid personality traits are important in the psychological adjustment of the patient with brain disease and injury, and we have noted the unconscious motivations of the brain-injured person to ignore his environment. It is clear both through animal and clinical observations that heredity and maturation, personality and prior experience influence the effects of small or large brain lesions. We also know that the acquisition of behavioral skills and their consolidation require different patterns of local and general involvement of the brain. For example, the retention of a skill requires less tissue than its acquisition. Following a lesion, the retention of certain skills depends both on the extent to which neuronal elements are specialized and also on the extent of prior practice and overlearning, and the period during which learning occurs. If a kitten is deprived of visual input, there are histological changes in the visual system and loss of cells, which does not occur in the blinded adult cat.[141]

The activating and steering functions of emotion can shape, power, sustain, or disrupt sequences of performance; without "evaluative" recognition and appreciation of input and modulation and coordination of output, human behavior appears inappropriate, "unfeeling," awkward, irresponsible, and asocial, if not impulsive. There are lesions (such as frontal lobe lesions) that affect the conditions for arousal and emotional involvement rather than impairing highly developed skills. Luria noted effects of cortical lesions related to arousal.[88] With frontal lesions, spoken words and instructions ("pay attention to this signal") had a diminished power to control performance, but a central stimulant such as caffeine temporarily improved performance. J. M. Fuster showed that stimulation of the reticular activating system in animals could lower thresholds for the recognition of tachistoscopically presented objects.[47] The effect of brain lesions on such perceptual thresholds could be critical in the integration of intellectual performance. Although it is not probable, neither is it inconceivable that ways will be found to influence these mechanisms in disease states.

Clinically, we are interested in the capacity of the brain to substitute and compensate for certain losses. Hans Lucas Teuber,[130] in extensive studies, noted improvements in function over a ten-year period in veterans with large penetrating brain injuries; they showed minimal defects and an overall intactness of general intelligence. Hemispherectomy, or excision of the cerebellum, in infants does not markedly impair function, but in general the marked plasticity of the infant brain is lost after two or three years. Nature provides a wide range of "surplus mechanisms," alternative paths and multiple foci for the recording of input and these are of value especially to the damaged developing organism. In the adult, the nature of the behavioral impairment and restitution depends in part upon differential specialization of contralateral areas. For example, handedness and cerebral dominance are correlated with the restitution of cortical functions; the left hemisphere in sinistrals and dextrals is normally dominant for speech and praxis, but for those individuals fortunate to have mixed dominance, restitution is more likely. Thus, whereas brain lesions are without doubt limiting and incapacitating, there are modifying restitutional as well as motivational factors to be considered.

Sleep and the Etiology of Behavior Disorders

Sleep and fatigue are organismic states that have intrigued physiologists, psychologists, and psychiatrists for a long time. In recent investigations much has been learned about sleep, a state of (apparent) inactivity, which not only punctuates but is integrated with our daily periods of mental and physical activity. As a state, sleep can be behaviorally and electrically differentiated from wakefulness, coma, stupor, or anesthesia. It not only represents a physiological need, but seems at *some* point to be crucial for adequate psychological integrations and functions. It is valued as a pleasure but frequently becomes the focus for disturbances in psychobiological function; it may have a

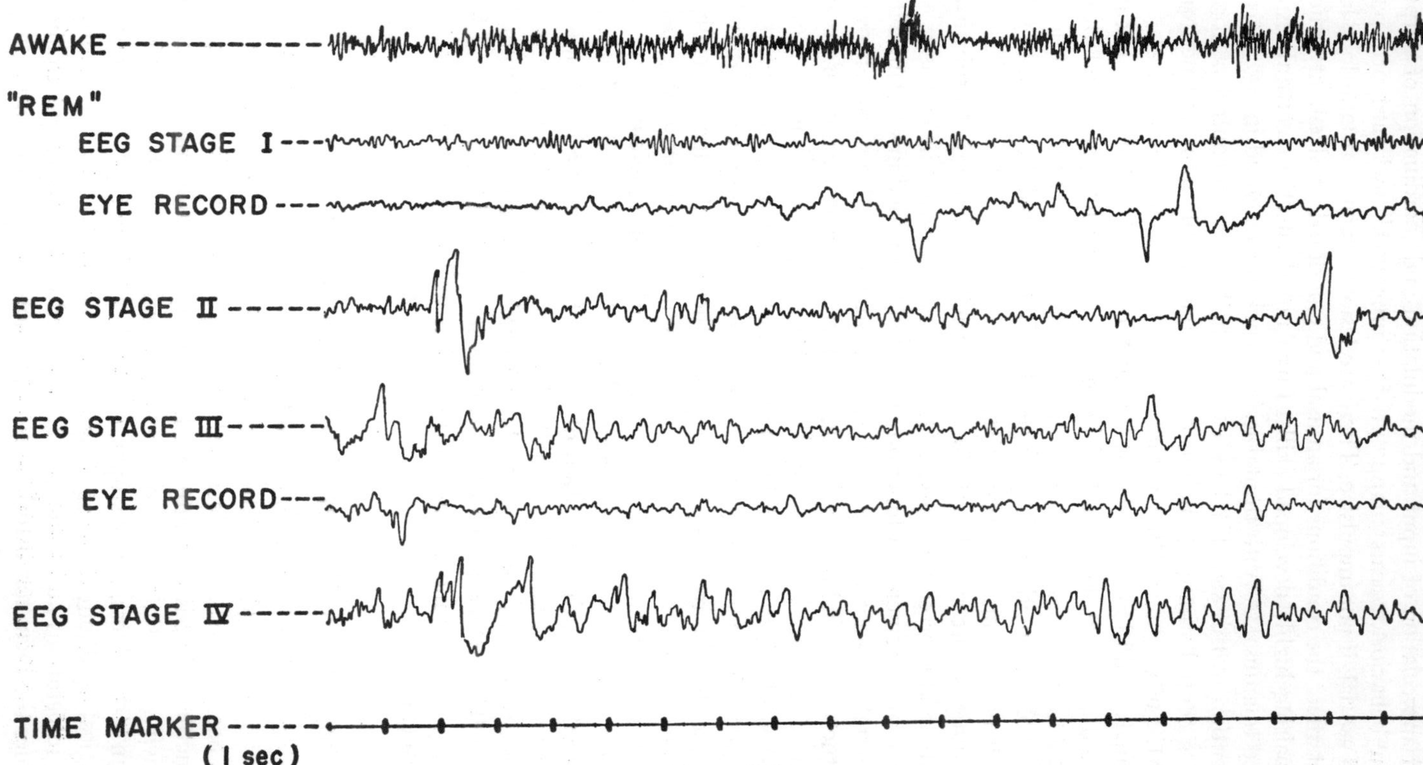
EEG SLEEP STAGES
AWAKE
"REM"
EEG STAGE I
EYE RECORD
EEG STAGE II
EEG STAGE III
EYE RECORD
EEG STAGE IV
TIME MARKER
(1 sec)

Figure 6–1.

defensive function (avoidance of reality) as well as represent danger (equation with death, or loss of control). How we are able to bridge the "lapse" in conscious activities represented by sleep and preserve continuity of mental functions, and how the state is related to physiological and psychological "rest" and restoration is still unknown. Nor is it easy to estimate the extent to which the psychobiological functions of sleep and sleep deprivation are related to the gamut of behavior disorders. Sleep dysfunctions can probably be causal and are certainly contributory; they can be concomitant or secondary symptoms in both the mild and severe behavior disorders. The increasing momentum of research has been reviewed by Nathaniel Kleitman.[74]

"Fast Sleep" and Dreaming

High-voltage slow waves interspersed with spindles and spikes recorded from the cortex were once considered characteristic EEG concomitants of sleep; a general muscular relaxation was thought to accompany the state. Sleep was differentiated by being light or deep. Recently, however, there has been a convergence of evidence, both from animals and man, which defines what Frederick Snyder called a special "organismic state" occurring during sleep.[125] Physiological activation uncoupled from motor response is characteristic. This special state is called activated or fast sleep (Figure 6–1). It is manifest by low-voltage fast activity, which, except for the relative lack of alpha rhythms, might be confused with waking EEG records. Fast sleep represents an activation of the cortex. This activation is thought to occur only indirectly through the midbrain activating system so important for wakefulness; rather, the more caudal pontine reticular nuclei may "trigger" fast sleep, and lesions of these nucleis produce striking changes including hallucinatory-like episodes. Certain thresholds for arousal are higher in this state (as if sleep were deeper) and particular muscle groups (for example, in the neck) show hypotonicity; yet respiration, palmar conductance, and heart rate indicate activation or arousal. This "paradoxical" phase of sleep occurs with varying durations in all ages in all mammalian species studied. It periodically

---

Figure 6–1. A composite of electroencephalogram (EEG) records from each sleep stage. When the patient is awake, increased muscle tone is present in all scalp (cortical) and eye electrode leads. When asleep, as demonstrated in all other cortical records, muscle tone is absent. As the patient begins to sleep, his EEG changes consecutively from Stage I to Stage IV. Stage I is characterized by low-amplitude fast (8–13 cps) activity; only in Stage I does the eye record reveal the large peaked waves (REM's or rapid eye movements) characteristic of dreaming. In Stage II the fast activity of Stage I disappears and large "K" complexes appear. Stage III is defined by several high-amplitude delta (2–3 cps) waves, and Stage IV is represented by an entire record of delta or "slow" wave sleep. Each stage tends to appear six times during a typical night's sleep. These EEG records are run at half the speed of the more conventional clinical records and hence the over-all pattern appears more compressed (see Chapter 18).

punctuates the other phases of sleep, which are characterized as drowsiness, light sleep, and a deeper, or "slow" sleep. Kleitman, William Dement,[30] and others discovered that the periods of fast sleep were characterized by rapid eye movements (REM's) and that the periodicity of sleep stages was characteristic for the individual. Ingenious experiments established that in man the REM's become associated with dream imagery; they represent not only activation but also the dreamer orienting to and scanning the dream scene. Comparison of these dreams with those recalled during the day is of potential clinical interest.[100,140]

During the night, and more frequently in the latter half of a night's sleep, there are four or five periods (of five to sixty minutes) of fast sleep. W. C. Dement, on the basis of considerable data, has postulated that fast sleep is a necessity, since deprivation of all sleep or interruption of fast sleep is followed by increased periods, or lengths of periods, of fast sleep.[29] Speculation about the "meaning" of this state of fast sleep (for example, preparing the organism for wakefulness by reordering the day's input—or a discharge, which, occurring in sleep rather than wakefulness, is a protection against psychosis) has far outpaced the research findings. With development, there is a gradual decrease in amount of sleep occurring in a twenty-four-hour period, and Kleitman believes that this is a function of maturation of the brain. The young infant has to "pay" with two hours of sleep for each hour of wakefulness, and the adult only with a half-hour.

Regulation of Periodicity

Intrinsic factors regulating sleep have been hard to define. With drugs such as atropine, and with certain neurological and mental conditions, the slow waves of EEG sleep may persist in the presence of behavioral wakefulness; alcohol, amphetamine,[109] and barbiturates alter the regulation of the various sleep stages. Chemical correlations of sleep are few; in animals brain acetylcholine levels are elevated during sleep, a change of unknown significance. The periaqueductal region of the midbrain is important for sleep regulation and is disturbed in such diseases as epidemic encephalitis. But neurophysiologists cannot agree whether there is a center that physiologically and actively induces slow sleep (perhaps in the medial forebrain bundle), or whether the normal wakefulness systems (the ascending reticular activating system—ARAS—and its interlocking limbic and cortical feedback systems) are simply diminished in their activity. Kleitman puts great emphasis on the role of muscular fatigue, with its associated diminution of input into, and output from, the ARAS—as the physiological motive for sleep.

The physiological basis for periodicity of sleep and wakefulness is even less clear; a theory that there is regular accumulation of toxic metabolites requires contemporary testing, and possible chemical regulators are under study. Social and psychological factors also influence the periodicity of sleep and wakefulness. A volunteer who stayed in a mock space capsule for a number of weeks reportedly showed marked shifts in periodicity only after his last contact with the structure of events in the social world was removed, that is, a clock. Individuals are aware of fluctuations in alertness even during a normal waking period, and cycles of wakefulness occur periodically throughout a long sleep deprivation. Our interest in the psychobiological determinants of periodicity is thus not confined solely to an alteration of sleep and wakefulness and the different stages of sleep, but also to periodicity of various stages of wakefulness.

Behavior during Sleep

The state in which thinking in the form of dream imagery predominantly occurs, the REM periods, obviously involves a crude consciousness with attendant defensive and cognitive operation. Fast sleep and shifts of muscle tone and heart rate occur in the congenitally blind, whose sightless dreams emphasize that thinking in some form, visual or not, is a correlate of this state. In animals and infants, we cannot, of course, firmly deduce mental content from the physiological indices, but some degree of activation of sensorimotor memories seems possible. Although levels of consciousness and the physiological measures of sleep generally appear to coincide, consequential mental activity can occur during slow sleep and probably in all stages. Problems are solved; discriminatory functions such as the measurement of elapsed time do occur;[41] some individuals habitually awaken themselves from slow sleep after a given period of time and others can do so on instruction in experimental situations. Certain automatic acts during sleep, for example, pressing a button on schedule to avoid pain, occur without full arousal. Somnambulistic phenomena have not been studied with physiological recordings, but sleep-talking and enuresis can occur during periods of large amplitude slow waves, associated with the moderately deep slow sleep.

In general, then, it seems there may be a coexistence of a number of psychological organizations during these different stages of sleep. Neurophysiologically, sleep should not be considered a matter of more or less over-all activity. Rather, it appears to be a different organization of activity. Edward V. Evarts has shown that the grouping of single cell discharges may shift,[35] and in the visual cortex increases are observed; thus, there is no direct evidence of a generalized Pavlovian inhibition or decrease of neural activity in sleep.

Sleep Deprivation and Fatigue

The psychological effects of sleep deprivation are irritability, illusions, and hallucinations as well as lapses or blocks in consciousness. Jolyon West described quite serious psychopathology following extended periods of sleeplessness.[138] The role of sleep deprivation in psychopathology is probably more crucial, at least as a precipitating factor, than is generally appreciated, but the sleep and dreams of psychotic patients have only begun to be definitively studied. It appears likely that deprivation, either of slow sleep (a stage that apparently is correlated with a sense of restfulness) or fast sleep, could lead to residual difficulties during the day and that different disease entities may be characterized by different patterns of sleep. With sleep deprivation, various physiologic measures show an increasing activation with increasing deprivation;[92] since this is also seen with certain psychotomimetic drugs, the neurophysiological organization of these states is of interest in investigating possible parallels in clinical disorders.

Relatively little is known about psychological and physiological fatigue. It is interesting that the bases for such common symptoms as malaise, weakness, and fatigue, in a great many general illnesses, are not well understood. These are ordinary sequelae of trauma, illness, and lack of sleep. In addition to anxiety, subtle neural and metabolic changes, perhaps ultimately mediated by pathophysiological processes in the brain (for example, the pyrogen-sensitive hypothalamus), may account for the almost imperceptible degree of intellectual and emotional malfunction that accompanies many such illnesses. In many respects, fatigue itself resembles depression. We will discuss clinical aspects of insomnia and fatigue in the chapter on psychosomatic diseases (Chapter 13).

Sensory Deprivation

As a primary etiological factor, sensory deprivation is probably not of crucial clinical importance. As a contributory factor, it may be of major importance in a few disorders. It is demonstrably so in delirium and senile disturbances, where the patient requires familiarity and stability of his surroundings and is sensitive to reduction of stimulation that can lead to panic and confusion. In general, all workers are impressed with the inhibitory effect of reality upon fantasy. Experimental studies of sensory deprivation were pioneered in Donald Hebb's laboratory at McGill University;[8] with translucent goggles, a uniform auditory field, and padded extremities subjects showed hallucinations, defects in psychological tests, and EEG changes. With many different isolating procedures, it is now clear that some but not all subjects show fantasies, illusions, and hallucinations, effects John Lilly and others characterize as regression and the need—related to a kind of "stimulus hunger"—to replace lost reality with fantasy.[82] The mechanisms are surely more complex. Some subjects are anxious, others relaxed; minimal input can be more disorienting (because there is some input present that must be interpreted) than no input. John Marcell Davis *et al.* showed that many "sensory" deprivation effects could occur in the presence of considerable meaningless "sensation" such as light patterns.[25] Thus, deprivation of meaning and structure is important, as is the level of anxiety. For some individuals, a dark room is terrifying and for others a relief. For many subjects, repetition of the experiment diminishes its "deprivation effects"—a case of familiarity breeding sanity. Not only symbolic and sensory deprivation, but motor restraint is also accountable for some of the phenomena, possibly in those for whom action is imperative for contact. Indeed, Jack Mendelson *et al.*[96] made acute observations of the effects of poliomyelitis respirators in inducing altered mental states and hallucinations.

The built-in capacity of the nervous system both to bring constancy to a variable environment and to be "prepared for" or disposed to new stimuli or novelty has been noted.[111] These needs may be critical in certain developmental periods. The effects of stimulus deprivation in early development have been extensively studied. For example, the Jackson Laboratory Group reported that puppies reared in isolation and then exposed to a normal milieu showed persisting motor and social deficits. However, rather than stimulus deprivation per se being accountable, it appeared that it was the sudden confrontation with a complex environment that elicited overarousal and interference with adjustment. This overreaction in the unprepared animal could be dampened by a few days of chlorpromazine during exposure to the novel environment; temperament influenced response, since some excitable terriers responded differently than placid beagles. Thus, when the organism is not equipped to handle novelty, or when isolation is coupled with high anxiety, overarousal and confusion may be the result. These components—as well as sensorimotor deprivation—may be clinically important in exacerbating disorders in various minor or major cerebral deficit states, if not certain schizophrenics. Sensorimotor deprivation per se is apparently less important than more complicated deprivations; a history of so-called "psychosocial isolation" (with deprivation of love, esteem, tutoring in skills, and stimulating relationships involving recognition, challenge, and satisfactions through personal and social feedbacks) is frequently encountered in our case material. It is obviously of great psychological importance to the already isolated patient that he be in contact with a community that can relieve him of his loneliness. The bulk of evidence shows that deprivation of meaningful and familiar structure, monotony, and social isolation are critically important psychological stresses for normals and for those with a wide range of disorders. The more elementary factors of sensory isolation or motor restraint play a variable role; their relationships to a variety of neurobehavioral operations are discussed in Chapter 16.

Heredity

We distinguish between population genetics, the study of hereditary traits and the distribution of genes in normal and abnormal populations; biogenetics, the study of the biochemical and biophysical aspects of the hereditary process; and behavioral genetics, or the study of genetically determined behavioral patterns. Strong emotional biases have worked against an advance in knowledge of genetics. Genetic propositions have often been linked with political and cultural beliefs. Psychiatry in National-Socialist Germany presented a blatantly horrible example: attempts to test the assumption that mass sterilization and genocide would improve mankind. On the other hand, there are irrational cultural biases, which decree that all genetic propositions about behavior ought to be disregarded, because they supposedly negate the role of the environment or "learning." In fact, geneticists assume that what is transmited, the genotype, is a "potential," which certainly does not rule out (and indeed requires) modifying influences resulting in the phenotype. In any event, prejudice is a poor substitute for critical thought and research.

The precise concepts of biogenetics obtained from the study of lower organisms have provided us with Mendelian rules, concepts of mutation, dominance, recessivity, penetrance, and expressivity; homozygous and heterozygous characteristics; and multifactorial inheritance. Human beings, with their long lives, limited offspring, complex environments, and their wealth of learned characteristics, do not behave as red and white peas or sea urchins; nor do they lend themselves to genetic experimentation. Yet recently, genetic research, coupled with biochemistry, has yielded extraordinary results in understanding hematological and metabolic diseases. The very important research in the chemistry of deoxyribose nucleic acid (DNA) has demonstrated biochemical mechanisms for genetic information transfer, and a new impetus has also come from microscopic studies of chromosomes; for example, the discovery of the extra chromosome in Mongolism, and from the study of the impact of nuclear radiation, not only on genes but on behavior.[46] These advanced methodologies have established that certain metabolic deficiencies, transmitted in a complex fashion according to Mendelian rules, are the essential causes of certain forms of mental deficiency. The best known are disorders of amino acid metabolism such as phenylpyruvic oligophrenia (phenylketonuria), in which a deficient enzyme, phenylalanine hydroxylase, leads to the disturbances of phenylalanine metabolism, excessive urinary secretion of phenylpyruvic acid, and the accumulation of a number of possible psychotoxic products; brain serotonin is reduced in experimental phenylketonuria. The ability to produce "model" mental deficiencies with various enzyme inhibitors or dietary manipulations has brought the biological and experimental psychology laboratory into the area, and it is hoped that the central neural and chemical effects and their linkage with behavior can be more clearly studied (see Chapter 21). An interesting example of a genetically determined psychosis is a recessive form of porphyria, which is triggered by the ingestion of barbiturates.[26] We are also interested in the role of genetics in the pathophysiological course of a disorder as well as in establishing links with simple etiological variables. In general, the notion of "one gene, one enzymatic defect" has given way to the observation of multiple defects.

Syndromes such as the recessive metabolic diseases are of great significance to psychiatrists, because they suggest the possibility of preventive measures. In general, these recessive diseases are very rare. So far, no major genetically controlled chemical defects have been found in the schizophrenias or in the manic-depressive psychoses. This is not ascribable to lack of effort. For example, Herbert Scheinberg's discovery of a disordered ceruloplasm metabolism in Wilson's Disease (involving the lenticular nucleus) suggested that it might be profitable to explore similar disturbances in schizophrenia. For a time, ceruloplasm in schizophrenics was linked to abnormalities in adrenalin metabolism; but, with adequate control of diet, neither adrenalin nor copper metabolism was found to be specifically disturbed.[94] Indole compounds, synthesized by the body, have had a long and doleful history of essentially unproductive research, but current studies show that changes in the metabolism of endogenous indoles can influence behavior. Disturbances of indole and catecholamine metabolism occur in some mental deficiencies and could conceivably be a factor in some of the schizophrenias. However, biochemical investigation has not as yet produced any differentiating chemical findings in this group of disorders and clearly none linked to genetic control. Isozymes, genetically determined variants of normally occurring enzymes, differ slightly in their protein linkage from the parent enzyme and, while catalyzing similar processes, differ in their optimal conditions for function; a change in the kinetics of normal processes might provide a genetic and biochemical link in schizophrenia. Some of these approaches are reviewed in Chapter 14.

Our knowledge about genetic factors in the major disorders rests, for the most part, not on biological findings but on studies establishing expectations of genetically determined traits in certain populations. To arrive at such estimates requires careful clinical observations, elaborate statistical methods, and ingenious scrutiny of environmental and genetic factors. The practical complexities of the task and our inability to define precise traits and symptoms in a manner appropriate for genetic explorations are responsible for the scarcity of reliable findings. The salient approaches are: (1) the family-history (or pedigree) method, (2) the census method, and (3) twin studies. Franz J. Kallmann[70] is of the opinion that pedigree studies, such as studies of diseases in certain families over long periods of time, are not particularly helpful. Observations of families as the Kallikaks, who exhibited mental deficiency and sociopathy over many generations, or the family of the royal house of Wittelbach of Bavaria, in which schizophrenias have occurred in many generations and in many of its members, are of intrinsic interest; they suggest a genetic problem but do not advance an answer. A simple polygenic theory of inheritance makes it difficult to disentangle the complicated genetic and environmental factors that obviously play a role in the etiology of these disorders. The census approach depends basically on knowledge of true incidence in populations, and so far this information is not available. In fact, a genetic statistician, W. Weinberg, showed conclusively that most of the early studies have been grossly faulty.[136]

The major assertions about hereditary factors in behavior disorders have been based on studies of twins. In a sense, these are experiments of nature. Ideally, twin studies would involve the comparison of homozygotic twins, preferably with a dichoroideal circulation, who were reared apart in significantly different environments. Such twins are rarely available; in lieu of this, intensive study of identical twins discordant for schizophrenia offers an opportunity to tease apart differentiating constitutional, physical, and psychosocial variables. Most twin studies have relied on the comparison of identical and fraternal twins. Usually, these studies were feasible only with hospital statistics and records (with their inherent unreliability) or with questionnaire, and somewhat cursory, interview techniques. The well-known major studies by Kallmann,[69] E. Slater,[124] and others reported high concordance rates for identical twins with schizophrenia, manic-depressive psychosis, and also in homosexuality. These have been challenged by Don Jackson,[64] who pointed to the importance of psychodynamic factors of mutual identification and other unique elements in twin relationships, explored by Dorothy T. Burlingham,[19] Theodore Lidz,[81] and others. Jackson also noted that only two pairs of identical twins, who were reared apart and unquestionably developed schizophrenia, were reported. Yet some ardent proponents of a psychogenic etiology of schizophrenia present such ghastly pictures of the psychological consequences for identity formation of twinship per se that one would expect a necessarily high incidence of psychogenic schizophrenia in twins. In fact, twins have rates of schizophrenia similar to non-twins. The area and the methodological problems have been dispassionately reviewed by David Rosenthal[114] in a painstaking, multidisciplinary study of schizophrenic quadruplets. Martin L. Pilot[105] has recently carried on studies of psychosomatic disorders in twins; he drew attention to such critical factors as different birth weights, different life stresses, and the somewhat nebulous concept of different ego struggles. He cautions against easy conclusions and generalizations in this complex field.

The importance of inherited characteristics in neuroses and sociopathies is no longer asserted except by Hans J. Eysenck and D. B. Prell.[37] Yet Sigmund Freud [44] also felt that hereditary and constitutional factors do play an important causative role in neuroses, although he pointed to acquired factors as most decisive in explaining the mechanisms and content of any specific neurosis. The extent to which neurotic mechanisms are repetitive and fixed, and their intensity, has never been satisfactorily answered on psychodynamic grounds alone. "More or less" aspects in neurosis, "thresholds" for conflict, and the like, may well have important biological if not genetic components.

Constitution

Constitutional factors have been emphasized from antiquity to the present. The anatomist, Julius Tandler, in his lectures, referred to constitution as somatic fate. In general, those factors that can be biologically transmitted across the placental membrane must be distinguished from genetic transmission and from physical-chemical influences on chromosomes in the process of division. The problem has been to specify discrete mechanisms and their consequences; but to isolate such mechanisms and to correlate them with human behavior is beyond our present research abilities. While the role of constitution is elusive (and is evoked often where precise data are lacking), constitutional factors are nevertheless "wanted" for explanations. Thus, the concept of constitution remains uncomfortably vague. Do we mean by constitution such important human characteristics as a highly developed brain, stereoscopic vision, erect posture, skilled hands (which enable man to use tools), possibly his social nature, his aggression, and the plasticity of his sex drive? Or should we limit it to reactivity or to discrete physiological mechanisms; or to body-build? How do these factors affect "temperament" and basic "dispositions" to perceive and respond differently (for example with placidity or irritability) to the world—factors about which we are far more familiar than knowledgeable. Temperament in animals can be genetically controlled, and this significantly influences behavior as any dog breeder knows. Psychiatry has not sufficiently explored man's basic dispositions to respond and the consequences of these to personality development and disorder, although some European psychiatrists concentrate on typologies, and an emphasis on various "styles" of cognition and perceptual defense has emerged in the United States.[24] For example, some persons tend to "sharpen" or take in perceptual differences, others to "level" or fail to observe them, and so forth. To objectify and select salient typical differences in psychological functions is, however, not an easy task.

In ordinary psychiatric parlance, constitution is often equated with body-build. In the nineteenth century, French constitutionalists spoke of the *type respiratoire* and the *type digestif*; these are similar to certain types of modern constitutional pathologies. Ernst Kretschmer[75] described four body types, the athletic, the leptosomic, the pyknic, and the dysplastic, which he matched with certain normal and abnormal personality types and with the predisposition to mental diseases. In spite of notably serious effort, Kretschmer was not able to demonstrate quantitative correlations between body type and mental illness or normal personality types. Nor did he account sufficiently for mixtures of types as William H. Sheldon, in more recent work, has done.[122] Sheldon's three basic somatotypes, the *endomorphic, mesomorphic,* and *ectomorphic* types, correspond rather closely to the pyknic, leptosomic, and athletic types of Kretschmer. The endomorph has large body cavities, round face, fragile extremities, weak muscles, and an inclination to obesity. The mesomorph is rawboned and muscular. The ectomorph is thin and asthenic and has angular features. Sheldon accounted for the mixtures of types by assigning each of the three a rating from one to seven in any one person. Sheldon correlates the body-build with a cluster of psychological traits—or temperaments. He calls the endomorph *viscerotonic* (corresponding very roughly to Kretschmer's cyclothymic and Jung's extrovert); the viscerotonic is a relatively uninhibited, emotionally expressive and hedonistic dionysian personality, one who lives through his gut.[123] The mesomorph is called *somatotonic:* an individual with vigor, powerful drive and resistance to fatigue—a muscleman. The ectomorph is a *cerebrotonic* (Kretschmer's schizothymic and Jung's introvert), a more inhibited though highly sensitive person, inclined to cogitate and speculate. Although Sheldon distinguishes and characterizes his types from a physical standpoint fairly well (somewhat better for men than for women), the psychological divisions do not express the clinical data well, and seem to strait jacket the wealth of phenomena actually encountered in life. Mathematicians have pointed out that the operation of a constitutional factor in clinical disorder ought to be revealed in at least bimodal distributions of traits (distinguishing distinct mechanisms or populations) rather than in normal distributions; and this criterion has not been met by the typologies investigated to date.

There have been other such attempts in psychiatry, for example, the division based on the dominance of sympathicotonic (adrenergic) and vagotonic (cholinergic) functions. This has never been conclusively correlated to a disposition to certain temperaments or types of neuroses. In child development, Arnold Gesell and his co-workers[49] stressed constitutional factors, and psychoanalytically oriented scientists such as Katherine Wolf[142] and others found marked constitutional differences in the behavior of very young infants.

Benjamin Pasamanick[102] and his co-workers[113] have made the important observation that subtle brain damage of the fetus may lead to varying degrees of behavior abnormality, ranging from cerebral palsy, epilepsy, or mental deficiency, to milder disturbances such as reading or speech disabilities, and to various behavior disorders of childhood. The causes of such disturbances may be prenatal toxemia in the mother, bleeding during pregnancy, and various infectious diseases; it is well known that German measles during early pregnancy may produce serious physical and mental maldevelopment. Pasamanick speaks of possible minimal damage being manifest, for instance, in clumsiness that eludes the ordinary neurological examination and is detectable only by special tests. Careful comparisons of large numbers of premature and full-term infants indicate that the chance of neurological damage increases as birth weight decreases, and we may expect more careful attention to these factors in future research on the major psychoses. Pasamanick found that neurological damage was much more frequent in lower socioeconomic groups, a finding that may possibly be ascribed, among other factors, to deficient prenatal diet. He also concluded, from trends in his data, that some of the damage in infant populations, which he studied in Baltimore, may be related to excessive summer heat at the time of conception and during early pregnancy.

The acute observations of ethologists such as Konrad Lorenz,[86] Nikolaas Tinbergen,[132] W. H. Thorpe,[131] and others are of definite interest for considerations of etiology since they indicate the possibility for a similar study of innate response dispositions in the human infant and adult. The fundamental observation concerns imprinting or the very rapid acquisition of habits apparently without learning.[59] Lorenz's original observation involved goslings who "adopted" and followed a human being as a "parent," after they were exposed to him instead of a goose. Imprinting not only demonstrates the "plasticity of instincts" but indicates that the infant comes prepared for select categories of "reinforcers." A duckling will rapidly learn a variety of behaviors (either to peck or not to peck a key, for example) other than following the mother, apparently in order to see the mother or mother surrogate on which it is imprinted.[103] Over a period of time this reward becomes less important as new capacities for reinforcement come into play. We must investigate what can go wrong in maternal infant interactions and influence a variety of adaptations because of improper timing and phasing of the environmental response. Ethologists have demonstrated that instinctual behavior (which Lorenz defines as "innate release mechanisms") can become maladaptive. Competition among a variety of instinctual behaviors is observed; a rooster paralyzed between fear and rage displays weak feeding movements. Such careful behavioral observations should lead to identification of underlying mechanisms and refine our notions of the inherent limitations and possibilities for the production of normal and abnormal behavioral patterns.

Individual, Social System, and Culture

Throughout this book we look at the behavior of an individual as a series of transactions occurring not only in a physical environment but in a social system. The rules for the conduct of the actors in such a social system are contained in the wide range of overt and implicit value systems—the cultures and subcultures. Alan Wheelis, following John Dewey, divides the value systems into ideological or institutional values concerning belief systems and into instrumental rules concerning tools and implements.[139] The fact that these value systems are communicated from one generation to the next through memory, learning, and traditional practices, rather than through inherited release mechanisms, is unique to man. Subcultures in particular, such as the value systems of religious, familial, or occupational groups, determine behavioral boundaries and expectations; these are reflected not only in clearly identifiable "social behaviors" and interactions but in each and every act we call behavioral (as distinct, say, from the purely reflexive). Newer views of behavior pathology locate a social unit as the focus of investigations; the psychotic behavior of an individual is comprehensible only as a disturbance in a small or large social system. Indeed, it is precisely for this reason that the psychiatrist usually first receives the patient. Thus, at times we look at man's total behavior in a social system; at other times we need to consider the individual as a correlative focus and in so doing isolate special aspects or components of an individual's behavior that are relevant for our work.

Social Groups

Man lives in groups, and it is important for students of normal and abnormal behavior to appreciate the consequences of this fact. Groups are aggregates of persons who interact, and whose behavior is, in part at least, determined by such interactions. Grazing animals, or people milling on Times Square, are aggregates or crowds; but a football team, a medical staff, or patients on the ward of a mental hospital, are groups. Results of such interactions are shared skills, rules, beliefs, and communication, which guide behavior. Specific assignments over a period of time are called roles. Role behavior and attitudes that are anticipated in a group are patterns called role expectancies. Patients in some psychiatric hospitals are expected not simply to suffer from disorganization or difficulties in coping but to act "crazy." Many role assignments, such as the role of therapist and patient, require a certain mutuality. Most of the signals that structure role behavior are hidden in the complex rapid feedbacks we call social behavior. A skill acquired by contemporary psychiatrists is the capacity to identify these signals either in the reported case material or in direct observation of transactions of patients and families.

The most important general role differentiation in a group is the one between leader and members of the group. The leader, regardless of whether he is a political, religious, educational, or therapeutic leader must, in order to be effective, express and carry out to a certain extent the common interests of the group. Members interact according to the intrinsic, innate, and acquired rules of conduct of the society to which the group belongs. In man, such interactions are extraordinarily varied. In general, human interaction is characterized by a high degree of aggressiveness and competition and also by the capacity for great sharing and mutual support.

We distinguish between intragroup behavior and intergroup behavior. The importance of understanding of the former is obvious; there is irrefutable clinical evidence that spontaneous and experimental groups can support and sustain their members or confuse and upset them. Groups can be psychonoxious or psychotherapeutic. William Caudill demonstrated this by studying the interactions of patients on a hospital ward.[21] The patients created a value system emphasizing acceptance of the hospital, cooperation with the therapist, as well as tolerance of the handicaps of fellow patients. The understanding of intergroup behavior is significant in hospital psychiatry where staff groups, such as psychiatrists, professional psychologists, nurses, social workers, clerical workers, and so forth, interact with each other and with the group of patients. Such interaction often generates false beliefs and assumptions about each other, which can reduce the task efficiency of the groups. Obviously, irrational interaction with massive distortion of communication between hostile groups is one of the major problems of national and international politics. Within the group, we note differences in the behavior of small or face-to-face groups and of large groups. The latter are in general more primitive, less capable of concerted effort, and more likely to be destructive.

Psychiatrists, in their search for etiological variables and methods of treatment, have been particularly interested in behavior of the small group. For fundamental work on such group behavior, we are indebted to Sigmund Freud,[43] Kurt Lewin,[80] Robert F. Bales,[2] and W. R. Bion.[9] Bales devised objective criteria for monitoring small-group behavior. According to Bion, any member of a group is threatened by losing his individuality in a group, and also by being rejected by the group. Such anxieties impair the task of efficiency of the group member and of the group. Group members defend themselves against such anxieties by making unconsciously what Bion calls basic assumptions. One of these primitive assumptions is the dependency assumption, which asserts that the group needs an omniscient leader to sustain its security. Such a leader is treated as if he were a godlike creature, and he is also ambivalently faced with covert hostility. The members of such a group see themselves as worthless, miserable, sick, and inefficient. Another basic assumption is the flight-fight assumption. The group wants action at all cost, is disinclined to think, and leans on clichés to justify such action. Individuals are unimportant and can be sacrificed. There is a sharp division between the ruling clique and the ruled. The third basic assumption is of pairing, usually of two or several members who feel they have common bonds, share secrets, and may produce an unborn leader; when no messiah emerges, they become disappointed and resort to distortions, rationalizations, and myth formation.

The Family and Behavior Disorders

The most important human group is the family. Again it was Freud who drew our attention to the relevance of studying the relationships of patients within their families. A rapidly increasing number of investigators has been exploring the families of neurotic and psychotic patients.[1, 65, 73] In general, psychiatrists are less impressed with the etiological significance of such gross sociological criteria as the "broken home" than with subtle disturbances of communication and psychodynamic relationships.[81] The consensus among most clinicians is that the effects of severe family discord (whether or not the home is a broken one) are important for the genesis of neurotic and probably of psychotic behavior disorders.[13, 143]

The basic concept of these recent family researches is that a person with behavior disorder comes from a "sick" family, or more precisely, a family with disturbed relationships; disorders of individuals derive from faulty complementary roles.[128] The cardinal point is that preferred or specific patterns of behavior, out of the range of behaviors possible to a person, are reinforced through a variety of communications. Currently, psychiatrists are learning to note generally overlooked modes by which people structure each other's behavioral roles and self-images; for example: a husband can politely tell his apparently helpless wife the time of day, and also communicate that she is helpless to find it out without him. The intricate regulations by which order and mutual positions—even territories—are maintained in a family group are perhaps "too close to home" to be seriously considered, much as our dreams were once too commonplace for investigation. A family, Warren M. Brodey remarked, spans the generations as a living organism, has its own "skin" and boundaries, as any daughter-in-law (or therapist) knows.[15] If roles are complementary, the family functions smoothly; if roles are incompatible, constant decision-making becomes necessary, or decisions cannot be made; and the aversion of crises will become unsuccessful. Perhaps the most crucial aspect of role structure in families (and actually in all groups) is its rigidity; once a preferential role is ascribed, it is difficult to shift roles and even to perceive the needs for such a change. The distribution of roles is a stabilizing and regulatory mechanism for the group and relatively impervious to corrective feedback for role change; however, looseness of the role structure may be troublesome too.

With an incompatible pattern, if not for marriage then for child-rearing, the establishment of desirable identifications may be inhibited, and infantile sexual patterns may be prolonged. John P. Spiegel points to manipulative techniques such as coercing, coaxing, and masking, as relatively ineffective.[128] Techniques characterized by insight and mutuality are more effective in the remedying and preventing of difficulties. Such techniques do not take place only between husband and wife and parent and child, but also among siblings in the family, and an even larger number of dominant actors in the extended family. For example, a too-helpful grandmother can retard her own daughter's growth as a competent mother and fulfilled woman. The illnesses or behavior disorders of one key member (grandparent, spouse, uncle, or child) can produce a major shift in the emotional give and take of the whole family group.

The troubles of the person who gets labeled as the patient often can be related to the mutual doings of these key members. This does not mean that the cure lies in changing the family after the damage to growth and development has been done; rather, the condition of the patient and his capacity for new learning and unlearning becomes the focus of therapy; and the family may or may not be useful as direct participants.

There is strong clinical evidence that the group can preferentially reinforce the pathologic behavior of one of its members; the group may "scapegoat" through him, or aid him; and this may or not lead to a change which offers the individual increased immunity from disorder. If groups do behave in this fashion, the factors that determine the population of "winners and losers" in these transactions remain to be identified. In brief, behavior is demonstrably responsive to the structure of groups and their values; but factors that reinforce behavioral patterns do not provide a complete explanation of the formation, persistence, character, and selectivity of behavior disorder.

The psychological mechanisms relevant to development and linked to social interactions are identification and internalization of values, including the unconscious values of one or several models. These communications do not occur magically, but through cues occurring in highly charged situations. We emphasize the importance of unconscious factors in identification that support both pathology and therapy, but we should not underrate the importance of conscious, cognizable communications that lead to information and to mastery of behavior modes essential for family as well as community life. Properly phased reinforcement of behavior patterns, or the absence of reinforcements (for example, adequate educational facilities), play a critical role both in psychological development and community life.

The Community and Behavior Disorders

The growing individual progresses from interaction with family members and peers to participation in the economic, social, and cultural organizations—the integrated sum of which we call the community. The functional effectiveness of the community is relevant for the mental health of individuals; and, to turn the coin, the mental health, particularly of leaders, determines to a certain degree the community's effectiveness. Alexander H. Leighton[78] presents a lively and thoughtful picture of such forces based on years of psychiatric studies of communities in the Maritime Provinces of Canada. He distinguishes two extremes, the model or ideal community with a high degree of effectiveness, and the maximally disintegrated and deficient community. In the ideal community, psychiatric symptom formation is markedly inhibited. According to Leighton, the indices of disintegration are: (1) high frequency of broken homes; (2) few and weak associations and poor communication between members of the community; (3) poor and weak leaders; (4) few and inadequate patterns of recreation; (5) rampant hostility, delinquency, crime, and reliance on alcohol and drugs to alleviate suffering. It will be important for future investigators to determine whether mental health or community variables are primary, and to what extent they constitute a vicious circle.

Poverty, starvation, and lack of opportunity for sexual and other need gratifications contribute significantly to poor mental health. Lasting unemployment as a source of apathy was demonstrated in the classical study by Paul F. Lazarsfeld and Hans Zeisel.[77] The decisive factors seem to be strongly related to low morale and also to effective and realistic counteraggression under such circumstances. Apart from economic and political causes, Leighton points to certain events that may produce disintegration in communities, for example:

a recent history of disaster, widespread ill health, cultural confusion, extensive migration, and rapid social change. The complex relationship of such events, called culture stress, to behavior disorders was also reviewed by Caudill.[20]

Social psychiatrists have begun to pay some attention to the hardships caused by malfunctioning of transportation, poor housing, or the breakdown of modern machinery used in everyday living. No matter how distressing such breakdowns may be, we do not track neuroses and psychoses to, say, a malfunctioning washing machine or abominable commuting facilities. There are several investigations about the extreme stresses individuals endured in disasters,[67, 134] in prisons, and concentration camps.[4, 7, 83] One effect commonly found in concentration camps is a tendency to apathy and lethargy, particularly in the older and sick inmates.[22] Another is the threat of corrosion of the ethical values of both inmates and jailers unless very effective countermeasures are taken. Yet, we cannot say with confidence whether the incidence of behavior disorders increases, even under the most harrowing conditions. In some cases, the very conditions that cause psychological breakdowns can mobilize powerful social countermeasures such as high morale, resistance movements, and also call out in the individual unconscious defenses and effectual action that prevent breakdown.

Social Class and Behavior Disorders

The impact of social class on behavior disorder and its treatment has been quite systematically explored. Sociologists define *social class* as a large segment of a population with certain common socioeconomic characteristics. Basic work on this concept was done by W. Lloyd Warner, John Dollard and August B. Hollingshead. Jurgen Ruesch was among the first to apply social class concepts in medicine and psychiatry. Classes can be delineated by objective criteria, for example: occupation, education, the area of residence, and the type of dwelling. There are many other distinguishing characteristics, such as source of income, recreational patterns, consumption of various goods, and the like. In studying the class structure in different communities, sociologists have found from three to six distinct classes or social positions and have designated them by descriptive terms such as upper-upper, lower-upper, upper-middle, lower-middle, upper-lower, and lower-lower classes.[135] (Hollingshead uses numbers to designate the different social classes.) Hollingshead and Redlich studied the relationship of social class to the prevalence of treated mental disorders.[61] They found a significantly larger proportion of mental disorders in the lower classes; and they found more psychotics and fewer neurotics in the lower classes than in the upper classes. To avoid misunderstanding, it should be stressed that these investigators studied only patients under treatment by psychiatrists, and not true incidence or prevalence rates. Leo Srole and his co-workers found similar differences in true prevalence studies of persons of different socioeconomic status.[129]

Psychiatrists are particularly interested in the differences in ethical values and in the use and meaning of aggressive, sexual, dependent, and possessive behaviors of patients in different social classes. It is likely that conscious and unconscious conflicts in the members of these classes differ, and these differences should have an impact on the type of disorders observed. Hollingshead and Lawrence Z. Freedman[60] noted that symptom neuroses and character neuroses occur mostly in the upper and middle classes, and that sociopathic disturbances are more frequent in the lower classes. Much of the earlier work on social class and behavior disorders has recently been confirmed by a number of investigators.

Robert L. Faris and H. W. Dunham studied the influence of upward and downward social mobility on mental disorders.[38] Contrary to some expectations, they found that downward mobility does not account for the accumulation of mental disorders in the lower classes. A simple downward-drift hypothesis in the case of schizophrenics was refuted. It is likely, however, that the grim living conditions of the lower classes, their loneliness, and their lack of therapeutic facilities contribute to a greater accumulation of schizophrenic patients at the lowest socioeconomic level. Many schizophrenic and neurotic and psychosomatic patients are characterized by strong upward mobility. On the other hand, we find some of the most difficult and therapeutically refractory psychiatric patients to be downward mobile—patients with extreme forms of self-destructive behavior, manifested by delinquency and drug addiction.

Cross-cultural Psychiatry

It seems that the main categories of behavior disorders are ubiquitous. Influences of ethnicity on abnormal behavior are subtle, complex, usually modifying rather than causing behavior disorders. There is no doubt that the sick role, and hence diagnosis, is to some degree determined by the culture. Some psychotic and neurotic reactions, such as Imu of the Ainus in northern Japan, Latah in Indonesia, or Arctic hysteria in Asiatic Russia, have been thought of as special diseases. Yet these reactions are rather unspecific and do not really constitute distinct and new disease entities. In all likelihood, the culture of Ainus, Malayans, or Chukchees modifies the symptomatology of neuroses and psychoses that occur anywhere, and give them a specific stamp and coloring.

Once a behavior disorder becomes "traditional" it is likely to be perpetuated in a group for some time. A number of investigators have made relevant observations about culture differences in behavior disorders, but most of the differences appear to be superficial.[6, 12, 33, 85] Whereas interesting statements are made, for instance, about different rates of suicide in different countries and social classes,[137] it has not been unequivocally established whether these differences are valid or, in part, artifactitious, and due to differences in reporting. Only with thorough study of the distribution, nature, and range of determining factors will we be able to tell just what the impact of culture is, and when and where in the course of a behavior disorder such impact is the difference that makes a crucial difference. Paul V. Lemkau critically reviewed current epidemiological studies in this country and abroad.[79] None of the epidemiological investigations permits a reliable assessment and comparison of existing cultural and social stresses and their impact on mental disorders. So far, we know only that severe behavior disorders occur in all known cultures and that social, economic, and ethnic factors alone cannot explain them.

Contemporary Living and Behavior Disorder

The question of whether contemporary living has increased behavior disorders is often asked. No satisfactory answer, based on definitive research findings, can be offered. Frequently the work of Herbert Goldhamer and Andrew W. Marshall is cited to prove that the incidence of mental disorders has not changed within the last hundred years.[52] These authors explored the admission of psychiatric patients to mental hospitals in the Commonwealth of Massachusetts. Although the number of admissions (relative to the present population) was fairly stable over a hundred years, the type and pattern of admissions did change. Currently, patients admitted are older and do not show the disease severity that was reported in the 1860's. Admission to hospitals, however, is not a good index of mental disease in any society; such data do not reflect the total incidence and prevalence of patients in the population as a whole, and make meaningful comparisons of different cultures impossible.

Undoubtedly, such social factors as racial discrimination and intolerance, both in their gross and subtle forms, are clearly demoralizing and stressful for individuals if not the society; such intolerance has always existed. Cultural stress is introduced in modern living by the malfunctioning of impersonal and alienated bureaucracies in industry, business, or government. Impressionistically, it would seem that none of the large ideological or religious systems is more apt to produce mental health or behavior disorder than any other. In the psychiatric literature of the communist countries, the claim is often made that capitalism, unlike communism, breeds mental disease. The opposite is claimed at times in the writings of Western countries, but substantial data are not cited by either side. In any case, such reflections do not loom large in our clinical considerations. The only generalization that one may venture is that consistently unrealistic and unrewarding cultures and subcultures, such as anarchic or extremely restricting societies, destroy morale and promote behavior disorder.

In general, those who have pondered the problem, whether modern living has adversely affected mental health, are inclined to believe that contemporary sociocultural stresses are greater than the ones of the past. Erich Fromm eloquently maintains that alienation of persons from themselves, from others, and from the product of their work is greater in a market-oriented society than ever before.[45] It is true that industrialization, mechanization, and urbanization have created new and specific stresses,[32] resulting in boredom, disregard for one's individuality, and the loneliness of the modern metropolis. Kenneth Keniston believes that our highly successful society asks for much, offers little, and thus increases alienation.[71] Rapid social change is probably another significant stress of modern living. By the time an individual adjusts, the scene of modern living has changed radically and new coping reactions become necessary. If no adjustment occurs and an individual develops a behavior disorder, we speak of culture shock. This is particularly evident in behavior disorders of immigrants.[120] Alexander Mitscherlich wonders whether the emerging fatherless society may be responsible for a corrosion of values, which may be as malignant as the unrealistic and infantile attitudes produced by authoritarian societies.[99] The new freedom embodied in the possibility of selecting one's occupation, one's spouse, and one's identity may also have created new stresses. Although some modern stresses seem to be greater than ever before, we must not underestimate our new knowledge and ability to diagnose and to help; only a generation ago, any remedy for many diseases, behavior disorders, and social problems was out of the question.

The Course of Behavior Disorders

The concept of a natural course of a disorder is more applicable to diseases in the narrower sense of the word than to the broad spectrum of behavior disorders. In any case, the psychiatrist studying the natural course of a disorder must scan a field extending far beyond the therapeutic relationship itself; he otherwise makes unwarranted, unsupported etiological deductions. In concentrating on the course of a disorder, he may also discover those factors that keep the patient "ill," and from a therapeutic point of view, these may be more important than those that first made him "ill." Conceptually, it would be a mistake to assume that recovery is a turning about of a pathogenic process; rather, it may be a new "equilibrium." The course of a disorder is conditioned by a number of factors beyond the original conditioning and precipitating factors. On the face of it, "recovered" patients differ; some seem to reinstitute old patterns; others seem to find new revisions. Yet, from the viewpoint of epidemiology and etiology for the assessment of therapeutic effectiveness, the question of characteristic courses is critical and requires meticulous study which examines factors that determine and lie behind statistical trends and clinical impressions.

Influential events operating during the course and remission of a disorder can more easily be directly observed than the beginnings. This vantage point does not, however, remove puzzling and paradoxical problems; for example, improvements when a patient is transferred, for economic reasons, from a superbly staffed private institution to an understaffed public institution. Both traumatic and favorable events produce benign or pathological responses, depending on how they are experienced and interpreted. A punishment that is experienced consciously or unconsciously as deserved may result in improvement, and a promotion experienced as undeserved may be followed by a depression. Karl Menninger underscores some of the factors that influence the course of a disorder:[97] secondary gains, a self-destructive attitude, an unfavorable environment, and conscious and unconscious resistance to treatment are handicaps; a favorable environment with the capacity and opportunity for loving relationships, a constructive attitude, and what one calls in everyday language the will to recover, are assets. Two related, though vague, psychobiological assets should be emphasized: a toughness of fiber and an integrative power—a capacity for repair that undoubtedly has many roots. Unfortunately, we are still ignorant of the appropriate time base (weeks, years) in which behavior change can be expected to occur with or without treatment. We will conclude this overview of causes and courses of behavior disorders with a brief word of caution by Pierre Janet: "With a little interpretation, displacement, dramatization, and elaboration in conjunction with the lack of critical faculty, anything in the world can be generalized, anything can be made into an element of everything." [66]

NOTES

1. Nathan Ackerman, "Interpersonal Disturbances in the Family," *Psychiatry*, 17 (1954), 359.
2. Robert F. Bales, *Interaction Process Analysis* (Cambridge: Addison Wesley, 1950).
3. Jack D. Barchas and Daniel X. Freedman, "Brain Amines: Response to Physiological Stress," *Biochemical Pharmacology*, 12 (1963), 1232.
4. Walter Ritter von Bayer, Heinz Häffner, and Karl Peter Kisker, *Psychiatrie der Verfolgten* (Berlin: Springer Verlag, 1964).
5. Frank A. Beach, "A Review of Physiological and Psychological Studies of Sexual Behavior in Mammals," *Physiological Review*, 27 (1947), 240.
6. P. K. Benedict and I. Jacks, "Mental Illness in Primitive Society," *Psychiatry*, 17 (1954), 377.
7. Bruno Bettelheim, "Individual and Mass Behavior in Extreme Situations," *Journal of Abnormal Social Psychology*, 38 (1943), 417.
8. William H. Bexton, W. Heron, and T. H. Scott, "Effects of Decreased Variation in the Sensory Environment," *Canadian Journal of Psychology*, 8 1954), 70.

9. Wilfred R. Bion, *Experiences in Groups* (New York: Basic Books, 1961).
10. Francis Board, H. Persky, and D. A. Hamburg, "Psychological Stress and Endocrine Functions," *Psychosomatic Medicine*, 18 (1956), 324.
11. Morton D. Bogdanoff and E. H. Estes, "Energy Dynamics and Acute States of Arousal in Man," *Psychosomatic Medicine*, 23 (1961), 23.
12. Jan A. Böök, *A Genetic and Neuropsychiatric Investigation of a North-Swedish Population* (Basel: Karger, 1953).
13. Murray Bowen, "A Family Concept of Schizophrenia," in Don Jackson, ed., *The Etiology of Schizophrenia* (New York: Basic Books, 1960).
14. Mary A. B. Brazier, "The Electrical Activity of the Nervous System," *Science*, 146 (Dec. 11, 1964), 1423.
15. Warren M. Brodey, "On Family Therapy," *Family Process*, 2 (1963), 281.
16. Eugene B. Brody, "Psychologic Tension and Serum Iodine Levels in Psychiatric Patients without Evidence of Thyroid Disease," *Psychosomatic Medicine*, 11 (1949), 70.
17. William E. Bunney, Jr., and E. L. Hartmann, "Study of a Patient with 48-hour Manic–Depressive Cycles, I. An Analysis of Behavior Factors," *Archives of General Psychiatry*, 12 (1965), 611.
18. William E. Bunney, Jr., E. L. Hartmann, and J. W. Mason, "Study of a Patient with 48-hour Manic–Depressive Cycles, II. Strong Positive Correlation between Endocrine Factors and Manic Defense Patterns," *Archives of General Psychiatry*, 12 (1965), 619.
19. Dorothy T. Burlingham, *Twins* (New York: Universities Press, 1952).
20. William Caudill, "Cultural Perspectives on Stress," *Symposium on Stress* (Washington, D. C.: Army Medical Service Graduate School, 1953).
21. William Caudill, *The Psychiatric Hospital as a Small Society* (Cambridge: Harvard University Press, 1958).
22. Elie A. Cohen, *Human Behavior in the Concentration Camp* (New York: Norton, 1953).
23. Lee J. Cronback and Goldine C. Gleser, *Psychological Tests and Personnel Decisions* (2nd ed.; Urbana: University of Illinois Press, 1965).
24. Henry P. David and Helmut von Bracken, eds., *Perspectives in Personality Theory* (New York: Basic Books, 1957).
25. John Marcell Davis, W. F. McCourt, and P. Solomon, "The Effect of Visual Stimulation on Hallucinations and Other Mental Experiences during Sensory Deprivation," *American Journal of Psychiatry*, 116 (1960), 889.
26. Geoffrey Dean and H. D. Barnes, "The Inheritance of Porphyria," *British Medical Journal*, 2 (1955), 89.
27. José M. R. Delgado, "Free Behavior and Brain Stimulation," in Carl C. Pfeiffer and John R. Smythies, eds., *The International Review of Neurobiology*, Vol. 6 (New York: Academic Press, 1964).
28. José M. R. Delgado, W. W. Roberts, and Neal E. Miller, "Learning Motivated by Electrical Stimulation of the Brain," *American Journal of Physiology*, 179 (1954), 587.

29. William C. Dement, "The Effect of Dream Deprivation," *Science*, 131 (1960), 1705; and 132 (1960), 1420.
30. William C. Dement and N. Kleitman, "The Relation of Eye Movements during Sleep to Dream Activity," *Journal of Experimental Psychology*, 53 (1957), 339.
31. Wesley Dingman and M. B. Sporn, "Molecular Theories of Memory," *Science*, 144 (1964), 26.
32. Leonard J. Duhl, ed., *The Urban Condition* (New York: Basic Books, 1963).
33. Joseph W. Eaton and Robert J. Weil, *Culture and Mental Disorders* (Glencoe, Ill.: The Free Press, 1955).
34. Alfonso Esobar, ed., *Feedback Systems Controlling Nervous Activity* (Mexico City: Sociedad Mexicana de Ciencias Fisiologicas, A.C., 1964).
35. Edward V. Evarts, "Effects of Sleep and Waking on Activity of Single Units in the Unrestrained Cat," in G. E. W. Wolstenholme and Maeve O'Connor, eds., *CIBA Foundation Symposium on the Nature of Sleep* (Boston: Little, Brown, 1961).
36. Henri Ey, "Hughlings Jackson's Principles and the Organo-dynamic Concept of Psychiatry," *American Journal of Psychiatry*, 118 (1962), 673.
37. Hans J. Eysenck and D. B. Prell, "The Inheritance of Neuroticism," *Journal of Mental Science*, 97 (1951), 441.
38. Robert L. Faris and Henry W. Dunham, *Mental Disorders in Urban Areas* (Chicago: University of Chicago Press, 1939).
39. Max Fink, "Quantitative EEG in Human Psychopharmacology: Drug Patterns," in Gilbert H. Glaser, ed., *EEG and Behavior* (New York: Basic Books, 1963).
40. Daniel X. Freedman, "Psychotomimetic Drugs and Brain Biogenic Amines," *American Journal of Psychiatry*, 119 (1963), 843.
41. Daniel X. Freedman and Charles W. Gardner, unpublished data.
42. Daniel X. Freedman and Nicholas J. Giarman, "Brain Amines, Electrical Activity and Behavior," in Gilbert H. Glaser, ed., *EEG and Behavior* (New York: Basic Books, 1963).
43. Sigmund Freud, "Group Psychology and the Analysis of the Ego" [1921], *Standard Edition*, Vol. 18 (London: Hogarth Press, 1959).
44. Sigmund Freud, "Introductory Lectures on Psychoanalysis, I and II [1916–1917]," *Standard Edition*, Vols. 15–16 (London: Hogarth Press, 1961).
45. Erich Fromm, *The Sane Society* (New York: Rinehart, 1955).
46. Ernest Furchtgott, "Behavioral Effects of Ionizing Radiations: 1955–1961," *Psychological Bulletin*, 60 (1963), 157.
47. Joaquin M. Fuster, "Effects of Stimulation of Brain Stem on Tachistoscopic Perception," *Science*, 127 (1958), 150.
48. Ralph W. Gerard, "Neurophysiology: Brain and Behavior," in Silvano Arieti, ed., *American Handbook of Psychiatry*, Vol. II, pp. 1620–1638 (New York: Basic Books, 1959).
49. Arnold Gesell and Catherine S. Amatruda, *Developmental Diagnosis* (New York: Paul B. Hoeber, 1947).

50. Nicholas J. Giarman and Daniel X. Freedman, "Biochemical Aspects of the Actions of Psychotomimetic Drugs," *Pharmacological Review*, 17 (1965), 1.
51. J. L. Gibbons, "Electrolytes and Depressive Illness," *Postgraduate Medical Journal*, 39 (1963), 19.
52. Herbert Goldhamer and Andrew W. Marshall, *Psychosis and Civilization* (Glencoe, Ill.: The Free Press, 1953).
53. Douglas Goldman, "Specific Electroencephalographic Changes with Pentothal Activation in Psychotic States," *Electroencephalography and Clinical Neurophysiology*, 11 (1959), 657.
54. Roy R. Grinker, Julian Miller, Melvin Sabshin, Robert Nunn, and Jum C. Nunnally, *The Phenomena of Depression* (New York: Paul B. Hoeber, 1961).
55. Roy R. Grinker and John P. Spiegel, *Men under Stress* (Philadelphia: Blakiston, 1954).
56. Roger Guillemin, "Hypothalamic Factors Releasing Pituitary Hormones," in Gregory Pincus, ed., *Recent Progress in Hormone Research*, Vol. 20 (New York: Academic Press, 1964).
57. Geoffrey W. Harris, "The Upjohn Lecture of the Endocrine Society: Sex Hormones, Brain Development and Brain Function," *Endocrinology*, 75 (1964), 627.
58. John A. Harvey, A. Heller, and R. Y. Moore, "The Effect of Unilateral and Bilateral Medial Forebrain Bundle Lesions on Brain Serotonin," *Journal of Pharmacology and Experimental Therapeutics*, 140 (1963), 103.
59. Eckard H. Hess, "Imprinting in Birds," *Science*, 146 (1964), 1128.
60. August B. Hollingshead and Lawrence Z. Freedman, "Social Class and the Treatment of Neurotics," in *The Social Welfare Forum* (New York: Columbia University Press, 1955).
61. August B. Hollingshead and Fredrick C. Redlich, *Social Class and Mental Illness* (New York: John Wiley, 1958).
62. Davenport Hooker, "Reflex Activities in the Human Fetus," in R. G. Barker, S. J. Kounin, and H. F. Wright, eds., *Child Behavior and Development* (New York: McGraw-Hill, 1943).
63. David H. Hubel and T. N. Wiesel, "Receptive Fields, Binocular Interaction and Functional Architecture in the Cat's Visual Cortex," *Journal of Physiology*, 160 (1962), 106.
64. Don D. Jackson, "A Critique of the Literature on Genetics of Schizophrenia," in Don D. Jackson, ed., *The Etiology of Schizophrenia* (New York: Basic Books, 1960).
65. Don D. Jackson, "The Question of Family Homeostasis," *Psychiatric Quarterly* (Supplement, Part I), 31 (1957), 79.
66. Pierre Janet, quoted in T. A. Ross, ed., *An Introduction to Analytic Psychotherapy* (New York: Longmans, Green & Co., 1932).
67. Irving L. Janis, *Air War and Emotional Stress. Psychological Studies of Bombing and Civilian Defense* (New York: McGraw-Hill, 1951).
68. E. Roy John and K. F. Killam, "Studies of Electrical Activity of Brain dur-

ing Differential Conditioning in Cats," *Recent Advances in Biological Psychiatry*, 2 (1960), 138.

69. Franz J. Kallmann, "The Genetics of Mental Illness," in Silvano Arieti, ed., *American Handbook of Psychiatry*, Vol. I, pp. 175–196 (New York: Basic Books, 1959).
70. Franz J. Kallmann, "Psychogenetic Studies of Twins," in Sigmund Koch, ed., *Psychology: A Study of a Science*, Vol. 3 (New York: McGraw-Hill, 1959).
71. Kenneth Keniston, "Alienation and the Decline of Utopia," *American Scholar*, 29 (1960), 1.
72. Seymour Kety, "Chemical Boundaries of Psychopharmacology," in Seymour M. Farber and Roger H. L. Wilson, eds., *Man and Civilization: Control of the Mind* (New York: McGraw-Hill, 1961).
73. K. P. Kisker and L. Strötzel, "Soziologisch-psychologische Voraussetzungen und methodische Probleme einer psychiatrischen Familienforschung," *Fortschritte der Neurologie-Psychiatrie*, 29 (1961), 477.
74. Nathaniel Kleitman, *Sleep and Wakefulness* (Chicago: University of Chicago Press, 1963).
75. Ernst Kretschmer, *Physique and Character* (New York: Harcourt, Brace, 1926).
76. Howard D. Kurland, "Steroid Excretion in Depressive Disorders," *Archives of General Psychiatry*, 10 (1964), 554.
77. Paul F. Lazarsfeld and Hans Zeisel, *Die Arbeitslosen von Marienthal* (Leipzig: Hersel, 1933).
78. Alexander H. Leighton, *My Name Is Legion* (New York: Basic Books, 1959).
79. Paul V. Lemkau, "The Epidemiological Study of Mental Illnesses and Mental Health," *American Journal of Psychiatry*, 111 (1955), 801.
80. Kurt Lewin, *Field Theory in Social Science* (New York: Harper, 1951).
81. Theodore Lidz, *The Family and Human Adaptation*. Three Lectures (New York: International Universities Press, 1961).
82. John C. Lilly, "Mental Effects of Reduction of Ordinary Levels of Physical Stimuli on Intact Healthy Persons," *Psychiatric Research Reports*, No. 5 (Washington: American Psychiatric Association, 1956).
83. Robert Lifton, *Thought Reform and the Psychology of Totalism* (New York: Norton, 1961).
84. Robert B. Livingston, "Some Brain Stem Mechanisms Relating to Psychosomatic Functions," *Psychosomatic Medicine*, 17 (1955), 347.
85. Rudolph M. Loewenstein, *Christians and Jews, a Psychoanalytic Study* (New York: International Universities Press, 1951).
86. Konrad Lorenz, *Pas sogenannte Böse-zur Naturgeschichte der Aggression* (Wien: G. Barotha-Schoeler Verlag, 1963).
87. Oliver H. Lowry, J. V. Passonneau, F. X. Hasselberger, and D. W. Schulz, "Effect of Ischemia on Known Substrates and Cofactors of the Glycolytic Pathway in Brain," *Journal of Biological Chemistry*, 239 (1964), 18.

88. Alexander R. Luria, *The Role of Speech in the Regulation of Normal and Abnormal Behavior* (New York: Pergamon Press, 1961).

89. Malcolm F. MacDonnell and J. P. Flynn, "Attack Elicited by Stimulation of the Thalamus of Cats," *Science*, 144 (1964), 1249.

90. Paul D. MacLean, "Contrasting Functions of Limbic and Neocortical Systems of the Brain and Their Relevance to Psychophysiological Aspects of Medicine," *American Journal of Medicine*, 25 (1958), 611.

91. Horace W. Magoun, "An Ascending Reticular Activating System in the Brain Stem," *Archives of Neurology and Psychiatry*, 67 (1952), 145.

92. Robert B. Malmo and W. W. Surwillo, *Sleep Deprivation: Changes in Performance and Physiological Indicants of Activation*, "Psychological Monographs," 74, No. 15 (1960).

93. John W. Mason, "Plasma 17-Hydroxycorticosteroid Levels during Electrical Stimulation of the Amygdaloid Complex in Conscious Monkeys," *American Journal of Physiology*, 196 (1959), 44.

94. Roger K. McDonald, "Problems in Biologic Research in Schizophrenia," *Journal of Chronic Disease*, 8 (1958), 366.

95. Roger K. McDonald and V. K. Weise, "The Excretion of 3-Methoxy-4-Hydroxy-mandelic Acid in Normal and in Chronic Schizophrenic Male Subjects," *Journal of Psychiatric Research*, 1 (1962), 2.

96. Jack Mendelson, P. Solomon, and E. Lindemann, "Hallucinations of Poliomyelitis Patients during Treatment in a Respirator," *Journal of Nervous and Mental Disease*, 126 (1958), 421.

97. Karl A. Menninger, *The Vital Balance* (New York: Viking Press, 1963).

98. R. P. Michael and J. Gibbons, "Interrelationships between Neuropsychiatry and the Endocrine System," *International Review of Neurobiology*, 4 (1961).

99. Alexander Mitscherlich, *Auf dem Weg zur Vaterlosen Gesellschaft* (Munich: Piper, 1963).

100. William Offenkrantz and A. Rechtschaffen, "Clinical Studies of Sequential Dreams," *Archives of General Psychiatry*, 8 (1963), 497.

101. James Olds and P. Milner, "Positive Reinforcement Produced by Electrical Stimulation of Septal Area and Other Regions of Rat Brain," *Journal of Comparative and Physiological Psychology*, 47 (1954), 419.

102. Benjamin Pasamanick and A. M. Lilienfeld, "The Association of Maternal and Fetal Factors and the Development of Mental Deficiency," *Journal of the American Medical Association*, 159 (1955), 155.

103. Neil J. Peterson, "Imprinting and Operant Conditioning," *Journal of Comparative and Physiological Psychology*, in press.

104. Carl C. Pfeiffer, L. Goldstein, H. B. Murphree, and E. H. Jennéy, "Electroencephalographic Assay of Anti-Anxiety Drugs," *Archives of General Psychiatry*, 10 (1964), 446.

105. Martin L. Pilot, *Psychosomatic Disorders in Monozygous Twin Pairs*, ("*Proceedings of the 3d World Congress of Psychiatry*," Vol. 1 [Montreal, 1961]).

106. Gregory Pincus, H. Hoaglund, H. Freeman, F. Elmadjian, and L. P. Romanoff, "A Study of Pituitary-Adrenocortical Function in Normal and Psychotic Men," *Psychosomatic Medicine*, 11 (1949), 74.

107. Karl H. Pribram, A. Ahumada, J. Hartog, and L. Ross, "A Progress Report on the Neurological Processes Disturbed by Frontal Lesions in Primates," in J. M. Warren and K. Akert, eds., *Symposium on the Frontal Granular Cortex and Behavior* (New York: McGraw-Hill, 1964).

108. Floyd Ratliff, "Interaction and the Detecton and Enhancement of Contours," in Walter A. Rosenblith, ed., *Sensory Communication* (New York: John Wiley, 1961).

109. A. Rechtschaffen and L. Maron, "The Effect of Amphetamine on the Sleep Cycle," *Electroencephalography and Clinical Neurophysiology*, 16 (1964), 438.

110. Fredrick C. Redlich, "Der Bewusstseinsverlust beim Cerebralen Insult," *Deutsche Zeitschrift für Nervenheilkunde*, 143 (1937), 251.

111. Lorrin A. Rigs, F. Ratliff, J. C. Cornsweet, and T. N. Cornsweet, "The Disappearance of Steadily Fixated Visual Test Objects," *Journal of the Optical Society of America*, 43 (1953), 495.

112. Eli Robins and I. P. Lowe, "Quantitative Histochemical Studies of the Morphogenesis of the Cerebellum, I—Total Lipid and Four Enzymes," *Journal of Neurochemistry*, 8 (1961), 81.

113. Martha E. Rogers, A. M. Lilienfeld, and B. Pasamanick, "Prenatal and Paranatal Factors in the Development of Childhood Behavior Disorders," *Acta Psychiatrica Neurologica, Scandinavica*, Suppl. 102 (1955).

114. David Rosenthal, ed., *Genain Quadruplets* (New York: Basic Books, 1963).

115. Mark R. Rosenzweig, D. Krech, E. L. Bennett, and M. C. Diamond, "Effects of Environmental Complexity and Training on Brain Chemistry and Anatomy: A Replication and Extension," *Journal of Comparative and Physiological Psychology*, 55 (1962), 429.

116. Burton S. Rosner, William R. Goff, and Truett Allison, "Cerebral Electrical Responses to External Stimuli," in Gilbert H. Glaser, ed., *EEG and Behavior* (New York: Basic Books, 1963).

117. Hal E. Rosvold and M. K. Szwarcbart, "Neural Structures Involved in Delayed-Response Performance," in J. M. Warren and K. Akert, eds., *Symposium on the Frontal Granular Cortex and Behavior* (New York: McGraw-Hill, 1964).

118. Vernon Rowland, "Steady Potential Shifts in Cortex," in Marie A. B. Brazier and Mary Agnes Barhiston, eds., *Brain Function* (Berkeley and Los Angeles: University of California Press, 1963).

119. Joseph J. Schildkraut, G. L. Klerman, R. Hammond, and D. G. Freind, "Excretion of 3-Methoxy-4-Hydroxymandelic Acid (VMA) in Depressed Patients Treated with Antidepressant Drugs," *Journal of Psychiatric Research*, 2 (1964), 257.

120. Carlos A. Seguin, "Migration and Psychosomatic Disadaptation," *Psychosomatic Medicine*, 18 (1956), 404.

121. Charles Shagass, M. Schwartz ,and M. Amadeo, "Some Drug Effects on Evoked Cerebral Potentials in Man," *Journal of Neuropsychiatry*, 3, Suppl. 1 (1962), S49.

122. William H. Sheldon, S. S. Stevens, and W. B. Tucker, *The Varieties of Human Physique* (New York: Harper, 1940).

123. William H. Sheldon and Stanley S. Stevens, *The Varieties of Temperament* (New York: Harper, 1942).

124. Eliot T. O. Slater, *Psychotic and Neurotic Illnesses in Twins* ("Medical Research Council Special Report Series," No. 278 [London: H. M. Stationery Office, 1953]).

125. Frederick Snyder, "The New Biology of Dreaming," *Archives of General Psychiatry*, 8 (1963), 381.

126. Solomon H. Snyder, J. Axelrod, R. J. Wurtman, and J. E. Fischer, "Control of 5-Hydroxytryptophan Decarboxylase Activity in the Rat Pineal Gland by Sympathetic Nerves," *Journal of Pharmacology and Experimental Therapeutics*, 147 (1965), 371.

127. R. W. Sperry, "The Great Cerebral Commissure," *Scientific American*, 210 (1964), 42.

128. John P. Spiegel, "New Perspectives in the Study of the Family," *Marriage and Family Living*, 16 (1954), 4.

129. Leo Srole, Thomas S. Langner, Stanley T. Michael, Marvin K. Opler, and Thomas A. C. Rennie, *Mental Health in the Metropolis: The Midtown Manhattan Study* (New York: McGraw-Hill, 1962).

130. Hans Lucas Teuber, "Some Alterations in Behavior after Cerebral Lesions in Man," in Allan D. Bass, ed., *Evolution of Nervous Control from Primitive Organisms to Man* (Washington, D. C.: American Association for the Advancement of Science, 1959).

131. William H. Thorpe, *Learning and Instinct in Animals* (Cambridge: Harvard University Press, 1956).

132. Nikolaas Tinbergen, *The Study of Instinct* (Oxford: Clarendon, 1951).

133. Richard M. Torack and Russell J. Barnett, "The Fine Structural Localization of Nucleoside Phosphatase Activity in the Blood-Brain Barrier," *Journal of Neuropathology and Experimental Neurology*, 23 (1964), 46.

134. James S. Tyhurst, "Individual Reactions to Community Disaster," *American Journal of Psychiatry*, 107 (1951), 764.

135. W. Lloyd Warner and P. S. Lunt, *The Social Life of a Modern Community* (New Haven: Yale University Press, 1941).

136. W. Weinberg, "Mathematische Grundlagen der Probandenmethode," *Zeitschrift Indust. Abstamm. und Vereb.* 48 (1927), 179.

137. James M. A. Weiss, "Suicide: An Epidemiologic Analysis," *Psychiatric Quarterly*, 28 (1954), 225.

138. Louis Joylon West, H. H. Janszen, B. K. Lester, and F. S. Cornelisoon, "The Psychosis of Sleep Deprivation," *Annals of New York Academy of Science*, 96 (1962), 66.

139. Alan Wheelis, *The Quest for Identity* (New York: Norton, 1958).
140. Roy W. Whitman, M. Kramer, and B. J. Baldridge, "Which Dream Does the Patient Tell?" *Archives of General Psychiatry*, 8 (1963), 277.
141. Torsten N. Wiesel and D. H. Hubel, "Effects of Visual Deprivation on Morphology and Physiology of Cells in the Cat's Lateral Geniculate Body," *Journal of Neurophysiology*, 26 (1963), 978.
142. Katharine Wolf, "Observations of Individual Tendencies in the First Year of Life," in Milton J. E. Senn, ed., *Problems of Infancy and Childhood* (New York: Josiah Macy, Jr., Foundation, 1953).
143. Lyman C. Wynne, I. M. Ryckoff, J. Day, and S. I. Hirsch, "Pseudo-mutuality in the Family Relations of Schizophrenia," *Psychiatry*, 21 (1958), 205.
144. William C. Young, R. W. Goy, and C. H. Phoenix, "Hormones and Sexual Behavior," *Science*, 143 (1964), 212.

CHAPTER SEVEN

The Psychiatric Interview and Examination

◆ This chapter will orient the beginner to techniques of interviewing and examining patients and of organizing and recording the data obtained. Young psychiatrists, as ducklings who take to water after they crack their shells, are immediately launched into work with patients, but good interviewing can hardly be learned from a "cookbook" outline. Carefully supervised clinical experience and listening both to one's own recorded interviews and to recordings of experienced clinicians will be more helpful in mastering interviewing techniques.[25]

The art and science of conducting a good interview, obtaining a useful history, and making pertinent clinical observations during the interview are psychiatry's most basic and important tools. During the interview, the clinician makes certain observations, which in some cases are supplemented by psychological tests; these procedures constitute the psychiatric examination. Neither psychiatrist nor patient is a passive object; each reacts reciprocally. The psychiatric interview is a highly sensitive and personal instrument, not a programmed inquisition; and there is no reason to believe (at this time) that it can be replaced by mechanical processing of data obtained through questionnaires or psychological measurements.

Psychiatric and Medical Anamnesis and Examination

The methods of psychiatric interview and examination traditionally are patterned after the medical anamnesis and physical examination. In organic medicine, a history or anamnesis, that is to say, an exploration of what the patient remembers, is first made. It usually includes the chief complaint, the present illness, the past illness, and a review of systems. History-taking is followed by a physical examination, the application of various clinical procedures, and by laboratory tests. The anamnesis with the components of chief complaint and present illness was taken over in early psychiatric practice. The past history was divided into a personal history, and a family history; to the physical examination a mental status examination was added. In addition to the physical, clinical, and laboratory procedures, the patient was given a number of psychological tests. In general, this psychiatric approach was as orderly and systematic as the approach in general medicine; unfortunately, it was by no means as productive. This traditional or conservative approach to the psychiatric history and examination still is used in many institutions and is also recommended in most psychiatric textbooks, although its extraordinary rigidity is offensive to many psychiatrists, and to sensitive patients as well. It is not theoretically based and fits the contours of the human personality much as the iron virgin of medieval torture fitted the human body. Essentially, it was designed to classify patients with severe mental illnesses at a time when there was, in fact, no real treatment. These patients were mostly of the lower classes, on whom the psychiatrists—perceived as formidable authority figures—felt free to use what some psychiatrists call the "robust approach."

This general method has endured tenaciously, and there are several reasons why psychiatrists have clung so stubbornly to it. One reason is that students like a structured approach to "objective" data that can be learned quickly, even mechanically; they master it easily and become able to write a comprehensive record. Many older psychiatrists emphasize the importance of this and complain that the younger generation has lost the ability to write a good psychiatric history. The field, however, has become very complex; the newer dynamic and the older descriptive psychiatry have not mixed well, and it is not as easy nowadays to write a psychiatric case history as it was a generation ago. To be sure, it would be convenient if we could provide systematic exercises for the beginner, as in scales for music students, but in a field dealing directly with all the complexities of human personality there are no props. A poor system is no substitute for the skillful practice of a difficult art and science. Another reason for the psychiatrist's conservative approach has been his pervasive tendency to shape his own methods after medical precepts. Nonetheless, psychiatric and medical methods of observation can be strikingly different.

(1) A function of the psychiatric interview is to determine certain difficulties and problems of a person (what Harry Stack Sullivan called the headaches in living[32]), rather than the characteristics of a possibly existing disease. (2) Psychiatric observation is focused heavily upon the interview, as most of the data about mental status are there obtained; hence, the objective examination, comparable to the physical examination, is less important and less rigidly defined. (3) In the psychiatric interview, psychological, social, and cultural data are stressed for obvious reasons; in the medical history, the data obtained are predominantly biological. (4) The importance of a reciprocal relationship between interviewer and patient is emphasized. Psychiatrists are specifically and acutely aware of being participant-observers. They also know that important social and personal relationships and roles have conscious, preconscious, and unconscious aspects. (5) Although all medical examinations must endeavor not to be noxious, the psychotherapeutic intent of the psychiatric interview must be particularly stressed. More often than not, the first psychiatric interview is really the first psychotherapeutic hour.

The Modified Psychiatric Interview

Such considerations as these have led many psychiatrists to veer away from the procrustean methods of the traditional examination. In the interest of more flexibility, modifications of the traditional method have emerged. A knowledgeable and humane psychiatrist can work well with any approach, especially if he modifies it in his own individual way. Yet the traditional method is so inadequate, that Jules V. Coleman ironically states, "Nothing of importance except the patient as such and the problem of his treatment is left out." [6]

Modifications of the traditional examination have come variously from psychoanalysis, psychology, social work, and child psychiatry. Psychoanalysis has undoubtedly contributed most. Freud expressed dissatisfaction with the conventional interview.[10] Many psychoanalysts have made original contributions to the interview; among them are the lively descriptions by Theodore Reik,[26] Felix Deutsch's use of free association in the anamnesis,[7] and the writings of Jacob E. Finesinger.[8] Karl Menninger devoted a book, the most thorough of its kind, to the psychiatric case study,[22] and made further important contributions to clinical methodology in his study of the diagnostic process.[21] For one of the most stimulating discussions of the interview we are indebted to Harry Stack Sullivan.[32] Child psychiatrists were most prone to disavow the traditional approach and develop their own methods. It simply is not possible to proceed in a meaningful interview with a child by following a prepared schedule; the child must feel comfortable and understood, and must trust the therapist. The relaxed and unconventional approach is well exemplified by play therapy.

Significant practical contributions to the change in approach have come from social workers, who were seriously concerned with the development of specific interviewing skills.[11] David Riesman drew attention to the importance of social factors in all types of interviews.[27] Carl R. Rogers,[28] analyzed the clinical content of interviews in the framework of his system of psychotherapy. Jurgen Ruesch and Gregory Bateson provided psychiatry with a general statement about communication, which is of fundamental importance for interviewing.[29] Detailed linguistic analyses of speech were carried out by L. A. Gottschalk,[13] J. Jaffe,[15] and Robert E. Pittenger.[24] A. E. Scheflen[30] analyzed gestures. The important contributions of linguistics and kinetics were critically reviewed by G. F. Mahl.[19]

Distilled from all these contributions, some new modifying principles emerged. (1) Psychiatrists became sensitive to the voice of the unconscious. Conscious data and utterances were seen as only part of the picture; it was necessary to keep in mind the existence of powerful unconscious forces during any meaningful exploration or intervention. (2) Psychiatrists became cognizant that data of the psychiatric interview and examination are obtained in a relationship.[32] The former narrow emphasis on so-called facts and data was not sufficient; data and facts had to be interpreted in the context of the psychiatrist–patient relationship. (3) Interviews and examinations are not purely diagnostic, but therapeutic.

Pursuing these points, Merton M. Gill, R. Newman, and Fredrick Redlich recorded and analyzed a series of interviews of psychiatric patients and made an attempt to formulate underlying assumptions. The reader is referred to the details of their discussion and examples.[12] More than others in the field, these authors have minimized the diagnostic point of view and herein lie the strength and the weakness of the approach delineated in *The Initial Interview in Psychiatric Practice*. The only type of therapy following the initial interview that these authors consider is exploratory psychotherapy; and, perhaps more accurately, the book should bear the title, "The Initial Interview in Analytic Psychotherapeutic Practice." What follows in this chapter is a consideration of a more universal approach as demanded by the practice of general psychiatry.

The Initial Consultation

General remarks: In a psychiatric consultation a socially approved professional healer[9] with a certain type of training and competence meets a person who, according to somebody's judgment, is in need of his services. Without his socially approved status the healer could do very little for his patients; they would not even come to him. The identity of this professional person is not entirely specific; the services cover a considerable range of activities; and the judgment of whether psychiatric services are in order depends on certain medical and psychological considerations as well as socioeconomic and cultural circumstances. The patient is rarely aware of the intricacies of the situation: the meeting, therefore, needs structuring. Much of the structure of the consultation derives from the general rules that govern the encounter of a therapist and a patient. The reasons for the patient's seeing the psychiatrist, varied but not infinite, are broadly defined by what the culture considers abnormal behavior. The patient must be entitled to the psychiatrist's services either by certain social arrangements or by his payment for services, except for emergency situations. Physicians expect, and are entitled to, cooperation from patients and their families to the best of their abilities; but many severely disordered patients neither can, nor wish to, cooperate, and even mildly disturbed patients may not be able to cooperate well. Families of patients also may not be helpful, and this can have a decisive influence on the interaction of the patient with the therapist. The patient and his family should not, of course, expect a cure or improvement from the initial consultation, but they have a right to expect a serious effort by the professional person to help within the framework of his mission. No formal contract is entered into between psychiatrist and patient, but an implicit covenant is established between them. In most cases, the psychiatrist's primary aim is to help the patient; in some cases, he works in order to help the patient's family, a hospital or dispensary, school, court, employers, or the "community." Such dual and multiple allegiances may create conflicts.

The patient is expected to consider the psychiatrist not only as trustworthy but competent, if anything constructive is to come of the encounter. It is important for the psychiatrist to hold in mind his own involvements, which must fundamentally shape the interview: the need to make a living, to help, to learn, to investigate, or to perform specific tasks to be considered later.

All these considerations apply to the first interview (also called the admission interview, the intake interview, or the initial interview or consultation). In such a consultation the psychiatrist assesses the patient's problems in order to help the patient take the next step. Some psychiatrists speak of a diagnostic interview, but a therapeutic orientation in the first encounter is of vital importance. Typically, the first interview is an extraordinary condensation, into one short hour, of the problems and experiences of the past. To appreciate what has happened, and is happening now, is a fascinating task that requires great skill and sensitivity.

Goals of the Psychiatric Interview

The following goals are pertinent: (1) *Rapport and empathy.* Two strangers meet in a particular context and get acquainted. Each must offer something to the other; they must establish meaningful contact, and they should like each other, or at least appreciate some human qualities in each other. C. D. Aring pointed out that it is not sympathy and compassion that count, but empathy: the ability to understand, to put oneself into the patient's place, yet to retain one's objectivity.[2] Switching back and forth from objectivity to empathic identification is required. The psychiatrist, more than any other specialist, must rely on his ability to introspect and assess his own reactions to the patient. He hardly has gadgets and tools but he *is*, in fact, his most important instrument. (2) *Psychosocial assessment and medical diagnosis.* Psychiatrists must obtain a relevant sample of information about certain psychosocial and physiological difficulties of the patient, information that enables them to make a diagnosis and an assessment of the patient's personality. Many consultations have the stamp of both medical and psychosocial approaches; in others, depending upon the problem, the information that is sought will be predominantly psychosocial. Not all procedures need to be carried out in all cases. Clinical judgment, the division of professional labor, the exigencies of time, and socioeconomic conditions will together determine what is important and possible and guide a selective procedure. The experienced examiner, sensitive to the psychological and social dynamics of his patient, interacts with him in an unstructured and flexible fashion. In this first hour, he is also alert to the possibilities of organic illness in general and to brain disease in particular. If cues of somatic illness or cerebral deficit present themselves, he may have to shift from a freewheeling approach and pursue such cues in detail, as physicians are generally trained to do. However, if brain disease or organic illness exists, it must not be assumed that all search for psychosocial cues will be abandoned.

Our approach is, in part, determined by implicit theories, which vary with the individual clinician.

We again emphasize, however, that regardless of theoretical orientation, the clinical psychiatrist's job is, at bottom, quite practical. Essentially, the psychiatrist, the patient, and the patient's family want to know what is wrong and what can be done about it. Yet it is also true that the psychiatrist's theoretical allegiance will determine to considerable extent what he is looking for and what he finds. An existentialist, say, will explore life's meaning for the patient; a psychoanalyst, his unconscious conflicts; a biologically oriented psychiatrist, his organic illness and constitution. Yet all of them must be concerned with the ultimate goal: (3) *Help and cooperation.* Gill, Newman, and Redlich wrote of the reinforcement of the wish for psychotherapy,[12] and this surely can be extended to apply to any kind of psychiatric help. Just what kind is needed will be determined by the psychiatric examination. We want the patient and his family, whenever possible, to cooperate in the psychiatrist's endeavor; and the clinician can begin to foster this cooperation during the first interview by demonstrating to the patient what a sensitive and skillful interviewer can do together with the patient, and by reinforcing the patient's desire to cooperate in whatever therapy is best for him.

To admonish the psychiatrist-in-training to be polite and considerate with his patients is something of an insult. His courtesy must go a bit deeper than Amy Vanderbilt's. Lawrence S. Kubie[18] describes some of the unconscious dimensions of politeness in an article, "Say You're Sorry," in which a child patient talks to his therapist only after the latter apologizes for an insult. An effort must be made to hold the psychiatric examination in a setting that is as comfortable as possible for the patient (no klieg lights, even if we film some interviews and examinations!). Psychiatric examinations must be private; not all hospital personnel seem to understand this. Concern for the patient's comfort—like the psychiatrist's technique—must not be ostentatious; it should be so natural that neither the psychiatrist nor the patient is aware of any particular technique. Even under the best of circumstances, to achieve this takes time, effort, and experience.

There are a few general rules for the interview in addition to the foregoing somewhat trite admonitions. Menninger aptly remarked that once a patient gets to a psychiatrist, the next move is up to the psychiatrist.[21] For the psychiatrist, to talk too much and to ask too much is as bad as to sit before the patient like an idol and intimidate him in the first hour by an endless silence. On the other hand, the psychiatrist cannot escape, or help the patient to escape, uncomfortable topics just to be "nice." The interview should be a meaningful and absorbing experience both for the psychiatrist and the patient.

The first interview should not be contrived as stressful; the patient should not get too upset. Franz Alexander and T. M. French speak of evoking a maximal emotional charge,[1] but it may be preferable to think of facilitating an optimal emotional charge. In any case, an interview ideally should be a highly significant experience for the patient. Advice should be used very sparingly, whatever the theoretical allegiance of the psychiatrist. Casual humor may have a modest place in an initial interview, but the razor-sharp edge between humor and sarcasm, as Ernst Kris implied,[17] should be kept in mind. The interviewer should be ever flexible and sensitive to the moods of his patients; rigidity is often the hallmark of a poor interview. In one instance, reported in *The Initial Interview in Psychiatric Practice,* a psychiatrist, during a specialty board examination, began the interview by asking the patient whether he was a full-term baby. And at the end of the thirty-minute ordeal, the patient, entirely sensitive to the psychiatrist's problem, wished him good luck in his examination. In another case, the psychiatrist, having grossly misunderstood the teachings of non-directive therapists, which recommend that therapists be attuned to their patients' feelings, kept repeating the last phrase the patient said; the result was a completely stilted and ineffective encounter. There is certainly no harm in asking a direct question, and often much can be learned by both physician and patient from a healthy respect for concrete details; omissions and commissions become more meaningful and vivid thereby. Nonetheless, the search for detail must be tempered by tact and available time. The patient's curiosity can be elicited but he is not to be badgered. On some occasions, psychiatrists also have to answer questions, instead of replying mechanically, "Now I wonder why you asked me that." At times, of course, this latter may be precisely the right reply, because a psychiatric interview is not simply a conversation, nor the completion of a schedule to obtain or give factual information; it is also an exploration of the patient's feelings and reflections.

We want to learn a good deal from the initial consultation. What was the patient's path to the psychiatrist? What are his psychosocial problems, and how do they bother others? Is illness involved? Does the patient suffer from a brain or other physical disease? Are the troubles more personal, or environmental? How did they develop? What is the patient's ability and motivation to do something about them? How can the therapist help him? To be sure, these are many and difficult questions; only rarely, after prolonged study (not just after one short hour), will we be able to answer all of them fully.

Sequence of the First Consultation

It is convenient to have certain basic data about the patient, such as address, telephone number, date of birth, place of birth, education, religion, occupation, marital status, occupation of parents and spouse, name of the nearest relative, and also the name of the referring person. Such information immediately provides some important socioeconomic cues and permits one to move promptly *in medias res*. Such a schedule, filled out in the patient's handwriting, may provide valuable clues for a psychiatrist with a knowledge of graphology.

The *opening phase* of the consultation consists of three elements: (1) the ordinary rituals and greetings of a first meeting; (2) the expert and unobtrusive observation of the patient; and (3) the introduction of the theme of the meeting by certain initial statements. Two customary questions in the opening phase are: "What's troubling you?" and "What brings you here?" The first few words and sentences of the patient are often of particular significance; it pays to ponder over them.

The *middle phase* is a freewheeling and unhurried inquiry, to which most of the interview is devoted. There are no prescribed topics, no schedules, no special questions, and no tricks—nothing but our sensitive concern with the patient, what is wrong with him, and what can be done about it. This is the time to tune in with the third ear, as Theodore Reik put it;[26] there may never be another chance like it. The psychiatrist should focus on the patient's words; his mood; what he says and what he does not say; but he should also feel free to interrupt, ask questions, and clarify. The first interview is a time for conscious clarification, rather than for interpretation of the unconscious. This is a useful differentiation made by E. Bibring.[4] If there are important diagnostic cues pointing to organic illness and cerebral deficit, the unstructured approach is not indicated, and an anamnesis resembling the conventional medical approach then is in order. The student will learn when to use one or the other only through experience.

The third, or *end*, phase of the first interview involves a casual inventory of what has been communicated. This, in fact, goes on throughout the interview; but at the end, the psychiatrist should in effect ask himself what it was all about, what specific information he still must obtain in order to come to some decision about the next step. This does not necessarily mean that he should ask questions, but he may decide to do so. He may inquire, for instance, about any attempts at treatment that have been undertaken previously. (It is quite embarrassing to advise authoritatively a procedure that has been tried before and failed.) There may be a need to fill in certain gaps for the patient's benefit. The second concern in the end phase is to make proper arrangements for the next step, and there is always a next step, whether or not it is treatment. There ought to be a definite closing; patient and psychiatrist should come to as clear and practical an understanding as possible—including arrangements about time—of future meetings. One cannot always be definite, but an effort should be made to be explicit about the schedule of therapy, cost of treatment, and the basic obligations of the patient and therapist.

Having described the first interview, we should hasten to add that such a typical interview rarely takes place. It is always modified by specific events and by such considerations as: (1) the motivations and expectations of the patient; (2) the professional identity of the psychiatrist; and (3) personality variables of psychiatrist and patient.

Motivations and Expectations of the Patient

A patient comes to a psychiatrist for myriad reasons and circumstances. Is the patient fully or dimly aware that he has difficulties? Does he admit or deny them? What is the patient's concept of his difficulties? Does he categorize them as organic illness; mental or emotional illness (whatever that may be); a slight nervousness; poor relations with one or many persons; failures and frustrations in important aspects of living; deviations from cultural norms, which make him feel guilty; or possibly a general lack of fulfilment and feelings of disgust or forlornness? The psychiatrist will do his best to find out what these difficulties are, and in the course of doing this he ought to ask himself: What does the patient think I can do for him? Does he expect a diagnostic consultation or therapy? Does he have any idea what psychiatric therapies are? Does he want comfort and reassurance, a prescription of medicine, shock treatment; or is he reasonably prepared for the long pull of intensive psychotherapy? What is his concept of a psychiatrist and of the imaginary or real purpose of the consultation? Conscious and unconscious experiences of past and present influence the patient's conceptions. The development of transference requires time and positive reinforcement; it is rarely strongly evident in the first session. Who sent the patient? Did he come of his own will after long and painful deliberations, or at the spur of the moment? Did family members, friends, or employers prevail upon him to take the step, or was he forced or tricked into the psychiatrist's office? Did he come because he is considered dangerous to himself or others? Does his job, marriage, status in the community, or his liberty depend on the consultation? Of one fact we may be sure: the patient seeks a response of recognition on some level approximate to his current need—perhaps of the spot he is in, the struggle he is having, his wish for a change, his desperation or courage, his efforts, his hunger for warmth, and his loneliness.

Professional Identity of the Psychiatrist

By professional identity, we mean the concept the psychiatrist has of himself as a professional person; the concept embodies the role that society assigns to him. Psychiatrists usually stress their professional role as physicians, with its many social and economic advantages. Recently, however, with the preponderance of psychosocial problems and psychotherapeutic techniques in psychiatric practice, this medical identity has been shaken in some members of the profession. It also should be mentioned that the public is not at all clear about the role of the psychiatrist. Different persons, social classes, and cultures have assigned him different roles. Many, even in the more educated groups in the United States, are not certain that psychiatrists are physicians.

Beginning with the first consultation, the relationship between psychiatrist and patient will be influenced by the professional identity and role of the psychiatrist. Does the psychiatrist consider himself a specialist who detects signs and symptoms of diseases and then prescribes therapy based on sound theoretical and empirical principles, as physicians are supposed to do? Or does he conceive of his role as an "educational" counselor who helps the suffering person to identify the cause and nature of his suffering and helps him to learn new ways of solving his problems? Or does he consider himself a sage, holding the answers to many problems of living? In our opinion, the psychiatrist must strive to maintain a dual identity: that of a physician with interest and competence in the diagnosis and treatment of organic illness, and that of a special educator and investigator who explores severe psychosocial difficulties, reconstructs the predisposing and precipitating events, and helps his patients with problems of living. There is, of course, a danger here; such a dual orientation may lead to identity diffusion or to a deliberate restriction of professional identity.

Personalities of Psychiatrist and Patient

The third set of variables, and perhaps the most important, focuses on the personalities of therapist and patient and on the nature of the latter's disorder. Obviously, interviews with highly educated or intelligent persons will be unlike interviews with mentally deficient, deteriorated, and illiterate persons. Interviews will also vary, depending on whether patients are psychologically sensitive or obtuse, and verbally proficient or incompetent. Certainly, they will not be the same with children or senile patients; and they will also be influenced by whether patients are in contact with reality, or are autistic, depressed, manic, anxious, or at ease. All this is self-evident; what is less appreciated is that interviews vary as a function of the personality of the interviewer. Although, in theory, techniques should eliminate such differences, in psychiatry they never do so completely. All psychiatrists, and particularly good ones, retain a very definite personal note in their techniques. Actually, if attempts are made to eliminate this personal note, a very stilted and ineffective style may result. Characteristics of the psychiatrist that interfere with therapy ought, of course, to be altered or eliminated; yet, the changes must not do violence to the basic characteristics of his personality. One consequence of this is that not all therapists can treat all types of patients. It is important to recognize one's idiosyncrasies and utilize one's particular assets. During the period of learning, students must concentrate on these difficulties and work with patients who are troublesome in these terms.

It is important that in such work the student psychiatrist appreciate the existence or the traces of his infantile aggressiveness and sexual needs. Often, this is worked through in the course of the analytic therapy of the student, but this is not the only method. To a certain extent, it can be done by careful supervision. The successful therapists have the opportunity to select those patients whom they can help most, and thus maximize their successes.

We have already mentioned that psychiatrists must not have pervasive and crippling neuroses; these result in scotomata, which prevent effective diagnostic and therapeutic work. In any case, the self-observant, introspective psychiatrist should early school himself to notice whether he is too passive, too aggressive, too seductive, bored, or out of touch with a given patient, or with all patients.

Interviews with Highly Disturbed Patients

Some patients, such as the blocked catatonic, the mute, hysterical, excited, confused, retarded, and depressed patient, or those with severe organic deficit, cannot participate in the type of interview we have described. Repeated, persistent, and sensitive efforts must first be made by the therapist to gain the confidence of the patient and to establish contact with him before there is any attempt to obtain anamnestic material. It is important, however, to keep in mind that many such patients not only understand what is going on around them, but are particularly aware of the preconscious and unconscious nuances of the therapist's behavior. Although they may not be able coherently to label their perceptions, and they may respond with withdrawal; nonetheless, they tend to detect covert aggression, rejection, and seductiveness very easily. To interview very agitated, hostile, or aggressive patients may take considerable courage and directness. Sometimes the presence of a third person or the use of sedating and tranquilizing drugs is advisable if the therapist fears the patient may be assaultive.

Interviews with Patients' Relatives

The success of psychiatric treatment more often than not depends on effective contact with family members. This has long been known by social workers; psychiatrists who all too often neglect this direct contact with family members and friends discover this later. Contact with the family can be uncomfortable and difficult, and in some schools of therapy—for instance, psychoanalysis of adults in private practice—it is strictly avoided. Psychoanalysis emphasizes reconstruction from the patient's utterances rather than independent reconstruction. It also fosters activity on the part of the patient rather than outsiders to rebuild his relationships with his own past and present. In general psychiatry, however, contact with relatives, though occasionally confusing, is usually enlightening—and often essential. The patient must know that the psychiatrist is seeing members of his family. Seeing family members separately in consultation may raise difficult problems of confidentiality and loyalty, bothersome to those physicians who are unclear about their mission. A simple way out is to see family members and the patient together, but this is not always feasible, nor is it uniformly advisable. It is best to inform the patient about what the psychiatrist and family members discuss and, more important, why and how such discussions occur.

Whatever method the psychiatrist chooses, it should be his candid intent to act in the patient's best interests and to do so with discretion, tact, and firmness. If he communicates his intent to the patient; if he is firm rather than arbitrary; honest rather than manipulative; authoritative rather than authoritarian and omniscient; he generally will win—and merit—the patient's trust when he consults the family members. Often, the interview with family members takes more skill and tact than the interview with the patient. Most relatives are defensive about their roles in the patient's illness, and the psychiatrist feels less at ease with them than in the situation where the psychiatrist–patient relationship is clearly established. Obtaining information from relatives must be as therapy-oriented as the interview with the patient. The psychiatrist must bear in mind that this does not mean that relatives have to be treated; perhaps some must be, others not.

Interviews with family members, friends, and associates of patients may be conducted by another psychiatrist; most often it is a function of the psychiatric social worker, who has developed high skills in carrying out such procedures. Very valuable information can be obtained by these mental health workers, who may make their inquiries in the patient's home and work environment. Unfortunately, psychiatric social workers have become increasingly reluctant to do this; like psychiatrists, they rarely see the patient in his own setting or life situation. To integrate the diagnostic therapeutic work of the social worker with the work of the psychiatrist is an important, complex, and difficult task. Roles in the integration are relatively better established in child psychiatric practice than in work with adults. In some clinics, social workers have come routinely to do the so-called intake interview. Psychiatric opinion about this practice is mixed; some consider this a good way to use such skilled and highly trained interviewers. As a rule, social workers like it because it gives them a powerful position in the structure of an outpatient clinic. Whenever social workers carry on casework with family members, the psychiatrist should assist them by explaining, supporting—and understanding—the social worker's role in the treatment.

Technique of the Psychiatric Examination

The recorded systematic observation of the patient's behavior, including certain tests of the patient's psychological functions, are known as the psychiatric examination, and also as the psychological or mental status. Today, it is apt to be less formal than it used to be, and a more natural and practical part of the total psychiatric consultation. We have warned against a stereotyped interview, and we are equally wary of a stereotyped psychological status. The endless variety of human traits and habits must be recognized; and on that account we recommend the use of a wide variety of approaches in psychiatric examination. The determinant is the problem that is encountered whether it is a psychotic person; a neurotic patient, with minor and sensitive problems of adjustment; a child; a senile person; a mental defective; or a patient with psychosomatic problems. From the very beginning, the psychiatrist's inquiry will take different routes with each of these.

We have noted that most of the information underlying the psychological status comes from the psychiatric interview. Only repeated observations and a good history will enable the clinician to separate enduring qualities of the personality from transient manifestations of behavior. It can, and often should, be supplemented by observations by other mental health workers who are in contact with the patient. The nurse and psychiatric aide, who have a continuing contact with the hospitalized psychiatric patient, will be able to provide valuable observations. Pertinent data about patients are obtained by clinical psychologists during the formal and standardized observations and from inquiries referred to as psychological tests.[20] These standardized clinical procedures are discussed more fully in Chapter 8.

There are three sources of data the psychiatrist obtains directly: (1) the observations of the patient's behavior during the first and subsequent interviews, and in other situations if such opportunities exist (Ian Stevenson and William M. Sheppe, Jr., rightly feel that we overrate the first examination[31]); (2) scrutiny of the content of the interview; and (3) in certain cases, a series of simple tests. In general, we try to focus on the very personal, specific, idiosyncratic, or unique characteristics of the patient. Observations of the patient's appearance and characteristics of his communication give us basic information. The first glimpse of a person's face, clothing, speech, gestures, and the observation of his behavior during the social ceremony of greeting and seating, are as important for the psychiatrist as for writers and pictorial artists, politicians, diplomats, businessmen (and presumably for such nonprofessional experts on human nature as headwaiters, bartenders, and possibly fortune tellers and confidence men). A keen power of observation is a much-needed quality in psychiatry. The wise and astute "private eye," investigating in behalf of the patient's dilemma, is far more to the point than the headiest philosophies.

We can usually determine, without asking many questions, whether a patient is oriented or confused, depressed or elated, in contact or autistic, and whether or not he has disturbances of consciousness. From clinical observation, we also learn whether he is a mature person who can handle a social situation, and particularly the interview, with reasonable competence and judgment; or whether he is regressed, acts out aggressively or sexually, or has withdrawn from reality. Yet these "objective" observations are enormously enhanced if they are integrated with the observations and inferences from a scrutiny of the interview. To rely only on observations of nonverbal behavior (one might speak of "veterinarian's psychiatry") would be absurd, as anyone can testify who has seen patients whose language he could not understand. We depend heavily on verbal and written communication and have to integrate these messages with the nonverbal cues. Thus, we weigh interview behavior and our information of behavior outside the room; and we ask questions.

In the past, much more than now, psychiatrists were concerned with a superficial and ritualistic scrutiny of intellectual functions. In certain patients with innate or acquired deficit, such concern is of central importance, yet we have become less formal in our inquiry into intelligence and its application in everyday life. Most statements about intelligence, orientation, attention, memory, coherence, and organization of thought increasingly tend to be derived from an evaluation of the patient's history, occupation, and social performance; upon his conduct in the interview; and upon his own way of evaluating problems, including his illness and his treatment.

If a patient speaks intelligently and gives a coherent story, we surely do not have to ask whether he knows where he is and what the date is, or ask him to subtract serials of seven from 100. We are usually able to detect gross defect of intelligence without such crude, strange, and insulting questions. It is possible to check on memory, attention, and retention by asking about events that can be ascertained objectively, such as the patient's age, how long he has been in the hospital, when he was admitted, and by mentioning one's own name to the patient and casually checking later whether he can recall it. Hendrickson *et al.* recommended assuming that mental functions are intact until there is very good reason to doubt this.[14]

If there is likelihood of disturbance in these areas, a more detailed inquiry into intellectual deficit, thought disorders, and memory disturbance is justified. Occasionally, especially when no psychologists are available, psychiatrists may decide to administer some simple psychological tests, particularly the paper-and-pencil variety which are easily interpreted, though of limited value. One brief test of intelligence suitable for psychiatric patients is the Preliminary Test of Intelligence; it is easy to score and correlates well with the standard intelligence tests. Items include: (1) *Vocabulary:* define saucer, temperature, immune, infallible. (2) *Arithmetic:* (a) How many are 3 apples and 4 apples? (b) If a man drives his automobile 160 miles in 4 hours, what is his average rate of speed? (c) A man receives $20.00 interest from a savings account in a bank; if the rate of interest is 2% how much money does he have in the bank? (3) *Comprehension:* (a) Why do we wear clothes? (b) Where is the sun in the middle of the night? (4) *Similarities and Differences:* (a) chair and table; (b) pity and sympathy. Scoring criteria may be found in the original article describing the test.[16]

Under the impact of psychoanalysis the interest of psychiatrists has shifted somewhat from the cognitive aspects of behavior to those of drive behavior (rarely observed directly), affect, and control. Hallucinations and delusions are no longer considered solely as manifestations of disturbed thinking, but of a much more sweeping disturbance involving affect and control. Basic mood (ranging from sadness to euphoria), appropriateness of affect, ambivalence, and the manifestations of the basic emotions, such as anxiety and fear, shame, anger, and guilt, are in the center of our inquiries. To recognize the subtle and varied forms of these emotions is essential. To pay attention to a sighing inspiration or the imperceptible clenching of a fist may be as important as the observations of the great symptoms that intrigued Charcot and Emil Kraepelin.

With such considerations, we leave the lower order of observations and find ourselves at the higher levels of systematization, classification, and dynamic formulation. As much as we recommend an effort to separate observation from inferences and theory, we stress that the kind of observations made will depend to appreciable extent on the theoretical orientation of the observer. All psychiatrists, regardless of their school, try to make sense of their observations and discover meaning in their interactions. To tap one's own preconscious responses—one's intuition—in this search for meaning is one of the basic methods of psychoanalysis and dynamic psychiatry.

One more word about the problem of objectivity. As psychiatrists are, in a sense, their own instrument and get important cues from their own "subjective" feelings, the type of objective rigor that is demanded in the natural sciences is neither feasible nor desirable in many phases of psychiatry. This subjectivity, however, does not dispense with the necessity for an operational approach.[5]

Our procedures should be made as explicit as possible. We should specify the source of our knowledge—those observations and inferences made in clinical observation, testing, recording, and classifying. We should supply "for instances" and be as specific as possible, both about the particular patient and our descriptive language.

Physical Examination

One of the most important tools of all physicians is the physical examination. We will use this tool, just as we use other medical methods when they are indicated. It is obvious that a physical examination is necessary whenever there is the slightest suspicion of illness. A physical examination may also provide the psychiatrist with important psychological information. The patient's cooperation; anxiety; feelings of shame and secretiveness; or exhibitionism and seductiveness may be quite revealing. It is prudent that male psychiatrists carry out physical examinations of female patients, particularly pelvic examinations, in the presence of a female assistant.

As the function of the central nervous system is of special relevance, the neurological findings obtained in a general physical examination, or in a special neurological examination, are particularly important. Techniques of such examinations are found in diagnostic manuals and in textbooks of neurology and need not be described here.

In examination of patients with intellectual deficit, disturbances of memory and attention, aphasias, agnosias and apraxias, a thorough neurological examination is essential. To differentiate general intellectual deterioration from the deficit produced by aphasias, agnosias, and apraxias is not an easy task. We state the essentials of examination of aphasic, agnosic, and apractic patients in Chapter 16.

Often the patient is referred to the psychiatrist by another physician who has carried out a thorough and competent examination, and repetition may not be necessary. Obviously, a physical examination should not be carried out simply to impress the patient with the fact that the psychiatrist is a "touching doctor" and not merely a "talking doctor," as Menninger puts it.[21] To put a patient through such an inconvenience for this purpose would not be suitable. It may be important, however, to convince certain patients by examination that they are not physically ill. In this respect, it should be kept in mind that repeated physical examinations, even if they yield no positive findings, will tend to reinforce the patient's belief that, after all, there is something physically wrong with him. Psychiatrists should also be thoroughly aware that physical examinations and laboratory procedures can create some anxiety in many normal persons, and even more in the majority of psychiatric patients.

Many psychiatrists do not carry out physical examinations; many have lost the skill to do them. They justify their avoidance of the physical examination by stating that others are more competent to do them, or that the examination will disturb the budding transference. The first reason may be valid; the second is dubious. Whether or not the psychiatrist will perform a physical examination depends to some extent on the psychiatrist's professional identification: if he sees himself primarily as a psychological healer, he will not. In our opinion, general psychiatrists ought to see themselves as physicians, which is, of course, what they were trained to be. In hospital practice, psychiatrists are generally required to give physical examinations. The ordinary way out for the psychiatrist in office practice is to refer patients who require a physical examination to internists and general practitioners. And, when psychiatrists find that their medical skills are getting rusty, this may be the right thing to do. If the psychiatrist does not pay attention to organic illness, however, some serious mistakes are bound to occur. Often, the factors of professional time and availability may dictate who carries out the physical examination; the important thing is that it get done whenever necessary.

Discussions of laboratory tests and their significance will be found in appropriate texts and manuals. The psychiatrist ought to be familiar with the most important tests because he may find himself in situations where he must request such tests, and understand their relevance, particularly in any collaboration with other physicians. The use of certain simple tests, such as blood count, urinalysis, and liver-function tests, has become routine in patients who receive certain tranquilizers and antidepressants. Psychiatrists should be particularly aware that some procedures, such as electroencephalographic, radiological, and basal-metabolism, and particularly lumbar-puncture examinations, involve considerable inconvenience for the patient. These procedures may evoke a good deal of anxiety, and appropriate explanations before and after them are most important.

The Psychiatric Record

TAKING NOTES We agree with Menninger, who remarks that a lot of nonsense has been said about taking notes.[21] Most psychoanalysts recommend that notes not be taken during the interview. Many competent psychiatrists have a flexible attitude about note-taking. No one advocates behaving like a court stenographer, and with some patients any note-taking is a mistake. Most patients accept unobtrusive and casual note-taking; with some practice it is possible to develop a method that distracts neither the writer nor the patient, yet permits brief notes that can be elaborated later into a fuller record. It is also the exceptional patient who is seriously disturbed by sound recording, or even filming. It goes without saying that the patient's permission for sound recording or filming must always be obtained; and one should also be alert to the possibility that, to a minimal extent, the patient and the therapist may, even if not self-consciously, be talking for the record.

THE CONTENT OF THE PSYCHIATRIC RECORD Psychiatric records vary greatly. Private practitioners, particularly those with an analytic-psychological orientation, may write running accounts, beginning with a first interview and ending with the last one. It is important to note not only what the patient does and says, but also what the therapist does and says. These records may be interspersed with the therapist's thoughts and recommendations. A separation of "facts" and "opinions" is important throughout the record. To keep good records is an arduous task; there is also a strong inner resistance in most of us to the writing of a full record, and there are some who find that a few brief notes suffice to recall relevant sequences of material.

Institutions usually demand records to their own taste, and there is little a resident or student can do about it. Unfortunately, a rigid and obsolete outline for recording clinical interaction can be a serious obstacle to learning and also to research. It has often been said that a "complete" record is necessary for research, but even the most complete records, unless specially designed for certain specific purposes, are not suitable for research. In the early sixties, several attempts have been made to devise a record that will lend itself to analysis by computers; [3] and it is conceivable that this will become the record of the future. Such a record requires highly categorized information, which, as we know too well, is very difficult to obtain in psychiatry. Yet, there are some segments of the psychiatric record that lend themselves to such treatment. Since narrative records, as we use them at present, have serious limitations for many research purposes, a computer record would be a desirable achievement, assuming it does not supplant the rich and live data, which our good records currently contain. Much depends on what we wish to do with such records. For therapeutic purposes, since therapy constitutes an on-going process of selection and structuring, it may be more expedient to tailor the record to the needs of the therapist; many therapists learn to recall and record data at the end of the day, or after the hour. For research and statistical, as well as medical–legal purposes, more general and rigorous record-keeping is required. When records represent a communication to a community of therapists, as in a hospital, a disciplined approach is essential. We find that the sooner one trains himself for adequate recording, the less onerous the task.

COMPONENTS OF THE RECORD The elements of the conventional case record are (1) the initial consultation, (2) progress notes, (3) final summaries, and (4) discharge note.

(1) *Report of the initial consultation.* The importance of this interaction warrants a detailed and at times near-verbatim report. It will also include data about the patient from other sources, such as the referring person and family members, if such reports are contributory. It must contain the reason for seeing the patient and under what circumstances this occurred. Key topics will be the chief complaint, present illness, and previous treatment, although a sketch of the present life situation and main events of the past should be noted, if such information is obtained. The record should include a brief statement of the patient's psychological status; a fuller record of psychological observations may have to be based on prolonged contacts. (An outline for a description of psychological status is suggested below under final summaries.) Physical examination and laboratory tests should be recorded if they are relevant. Contemplated procedures and plans for treatment need to be discussed. The length of the consultation report may vary a great deal; it must, however, provide a clear statement of the basic issues involved and give a responsible *summary,* which permits others to understand the nature of the problem and the reasons for the decisions that were taken.

(2) *Progress notes.* Progress notes are the backbone of the psychiatric record. In the past, they were an appendage to a hospital record, a bulky history obtained in the first days and weeks. The initial history loomed like a hydrocephalus on an atrophic body; little followed in subsequent notes because, typically, there was little progress or treatment. The emphasis now is on treatment and progress, hence on progress notes. Material should not be

limited to interactions between therapist and patient but should also include reports of other mental health workers: the nurse, psychologist, social worker, and occupational therapist. After the patient has spent some time in the hospital, a supplementary statement about diagnosis and treatment should be made, unless nothing can be added to the discussion of these topics in the report of the initial consultation. The time when such a statement is made may vary according to whether the patient is in a "slow" institution, where long-term therapy is planned, or in a "fast" service in a busy general hospital, where he is seen in consultation or brief therapy.

(3) *Final summaries and formulations.* This section of the record should contain: (a) a clear statement of the circumstances and reasons for admission and a summary of the initial consultation; (b) summaries of the psychological status, relevant physical findings, and psychological and laboratory tests; (c) summaries of the history of the present disorder, the family and sociocultural history, chronological life history, and the present life situation; (d) summary of progress notes; and (e) final notes consisting of diagnostic and prognostic formulation, results of therapy, and disposition at time of discharge.

SUMMARY OF PSYCHOLOGICAL STATUS A more casual description is preferable to the time-worn mental status with its high degree of formality, artificial categories, and stilted phraseology. It should be kept in mind that concrete and apt literary descriptions, not embellishments on the data, are still superior to our most objectively scientific accounts. Attempts to describe fully and accurately have led to the formation of multiple rating scales, most of them designed by psychologists, but only very few are used by psychiatrists. There is no doubt that such efforts must continue; in the meantime, however, until they become more manageable, we must rely on rather simple schemes of description. For the beginner, a few pointers are given below:

Describe appearance, dress, facial expression, gestures, voice, and manner of speaking. Pay attention to the individual characteristics as they reveal themselves in the budding relationship with the therapist. What does the patient communicate by his behavior, and how does he respond to our communications?

Scrutinize the interview and state your primary inferences about affective behavior: mood (euphoria, sadness, apathy); predominance of certain emotions (anxiety, specific fears, guilt, shame, anger, expression of hostility, destructiveness); self-destructiveness and self-neglect; display of erotic and sexual behavior (exhibitionism, seductiveness); or of dominant or submissive behavior; or of dependent needs. What are the devices for controlling such emotions and drives? The patient's self-evaluation and self-esteem? His specific aptitudes? What is the patient's general intelligence? Any evidence of a general or specific intellectual deficit? Disturbance of logic and syntax as revealed in speech and writing? Is the patient confused, disoriented, or is the general level of consciousness impaired? Are there gross defects in memory and recall? What are the patient's judgment and reality-testing? His participation in social, recreational, and occupational activities. His attitude toward his disorder and treatment? His insight and capacity for insight? His relationship to the therapist and his capacity for a relationship in therapy? At what junctures and on what topics do his behavior patterns shift, become disrupted, and how? What is the pace, pressure, consistency, and intensity of these significant behavioral patterns?

HISTORY OF THE PRESENT DISORDER This should begin with the chief complaint in the patient's (or other informant's) words. Following the chief complaint, state the development of the present illness in chronological order. Many patients cannot state a definite period when their difficulties started. In any case, past disorders as well as therapeutic interventions should be described in chronological order. Most of the material of this section will be derived from the first few interviews. It is well to consider: (1) changes in interpersonal relationships; (2) signs and symptoms of changes in intellectual and personality functions; (3) general changes in the physical and psychosomatic sphere, particularly output of energy, disturbances of sleep, disturbances of food-intake and elimination, changes in sexual function; (4) attempts to solve problems and conflicts (devices of adjustment, and psychological and somatic therapies).

THE FAMILY HISTORY In this section of the summary important members of the patient's family should be described, indicating the source of material and reporting significant interpersonal relationships. Describe the social, economic, ethnic, and religious background of the family and the family's status in the community. The outstanding characteristics and values of the family and its key members deserve mention. Mention important genetic patterns. The sketching of a genealogical table with birth order is recommended. The therapist thereby has a map pointing to events that had inevitably to be significant to the patient, what he had to contend with in his family; the deaths, separations, and illnesses occurring around the patient when young, or even preceding him, may be useful information for reconstructing developmental influences, and a briefly annotated genealogical chart conveniently contains such data.

CHRONOLOGICAL LIFE HISTORY This should be a *chronological* account of important life events. Such a biography is preferable to the artificial segmentation of the old-fashioned psychiatric history. The Meyerian life chart is still quite suitable for this purpose.[23] It may be written in terse style, following the statements of date and age in each instance, but should convey an overall impression of the patient's development. Again, this section will reflect the therapist's experience and maturity to a great extent; the experienced clinician will discern which events are important and will be able to convey a meaningful description of the patient's development through the record of data. It is not the universal but the specific experience that shapes a person's fate; no guide can substitute for the therapist's knowledge and intuition in arriving at a clearly discerned life history and its significance for the patient's psychiatric disorder.

For the beginner, it might be of some value to consider a few points that have been of some, though greatly varying, importance in the genesis of psychiatric disorder. It is crucial not to follow this outline slavishly as a guide to history-taking, but rather to incorporate the relevant points in the life chart. It matters little whether some of these points are not covered, as long as they are not important for the patient's problem.

SOME IMPORTANT POINTS IN THE PERSONAL HISTORY *Infancy.* Date and place of birth; mother's condition during pregnancy; full-term birth? Type of delivery; congenital defects; health in infancy; time of teething, walking, talking, and toilet training. Describe the setting and emotional climate in which the patient was raised, and his acceptance and care as an infant.

Childhood. Diseases, convulsions; mental development; neurotic symptoms, such as night terrors, sleep-walking, temper tantrums, finickiness, bed-wetting. Characterize relationship to parents, particularly of the Oedipal triangle, and to siblings; discipline and emotional climate in childhood. Were there illnesses, separations, or changes of status of significant adults? If so, how did the family react?

Educational history. Performance and expectations in school, favored subjects, failures; neurotic and antisocial symptoms; relationship to teachers and peers; crucial events during secondary and higher education; adult education.

Occupational and social history. Age when starting work; important job experiences in chronological order; performance; reason for change; reason for choice of job and job satisfaction; economic and occupational success or failure; social status and social aspirations.

Social and cultural interest. Relationships to peers, friends; community activities; hobbies and leisure activities; religious activities; ethical orientation and philosophy of life.

Sexual and marital history. Sexual information and experiences in childhood and adolescence; biological and psychosocial events in puberty and adolescence; menarche and menstrual history; masturbation, onset and frequency; petting and necking; premarital sex life, courting; marital adjustment and compatability; separations and divorces; pregnancies and abortions; potency and orgasm. Describe type and frequency of sexual relations; use of methods of birth control; extramarital relationships; sexual deviations; general attitudes to sexuality.

Involution and old age. Physical signs and symptoms of the menopause; socioeconomic changes; general physical and psychological decline; failures and other stresses in old age.

Medical history. Given in detail and chronological order: illnesses; accidents; treatments; attitude to illness and treatment; hypochondriasis; denial of illness; degree of cooperation with physicians, nurses, and so forth. What are the patient's eating, sleeping, and toilet habits? State also how the patient uses or abuses alcohol, nicotine, and drugs.

The Personal History logically leads to the *Present Life Situation.* Under this heading the patient's current occupational, educational, cultural, social, and sexual activities should be briefly summarized. One should get a clear impresssion of how the patient lives and what he does; in some cases, a brief description of the typical day of the patient might be indicated.

(4) *Discharge note.* This note consists of a final discussion of diagnosis, treatment, and recommendations at the time of discharge. *Final Diagnostic and Therapeutic Formulations.* A description of the diagnosis states the following: (1) description of the disorder; (2) severity and duration; (3) precipitating stresses; (4) predisposition. If no clear diagnosis can be made (which occurs not infrequently and lies in the nature of many behavior disorders), the differential diagnosis should be discussed and procedures stated, which may help to clarify the situation. If several senior staff members disagree on the diagnosis, the disagreement should be stated. Many psychiatrists in the United States are not inclined to argue about descriptive diagnoses; they are mainly concerned with understanding dynamic and genetic patterns (what M. Levine calls the dynamic and genetic diagnosis), predictions, and planning of treatment. What is the conflict? What are its conscious and unconscious determinants? What solutions have been tried? What dynamisms are involved? What are the epigenetic patterns in the case? What gains and what losses does the disorder cause? And, most of all, what therapy is recommended, and what are the patient's assets and handicaps when he becomes involved in treatment? Finally, there should be some assessment of the effect of such therapy.

Abstracts of the Psychiatric Record

Abstracts of the record usually consist of the previously mentioned summaries, and are often requested by other hospitals, physicians, social agencies, insurance companies, lawyers, and courts. They may vary greatly in length and may have to be written at any time during the patient's contact with the therapist; in teaching institutions they are often required for the purpose of an orderly case presentation. In most instances, the patient (or, when the patient is unable to do this, responsible family members) should give written permission, except in emergencies, and when records are subpoenaed, to supply such information. A number of states have no statute of privileged communications; and for this reason, physicians must be particularly conscientious in safeguarding the interest of the patient.

A complete interview is not necessarily a good interview; this statement is not an invitation to imprecision or lack of organization in formulating the data gleaned in an interview. Students should not be expected to stick compulsively to an outline. The record should reflect the activities of the writer; it should not determine the activities. The writing of a psychiatric record is an artistic and scientific endeavor. Such a record reflects interviewing, diagnostic, and therapeutic skills that have to be learned during a lifetime of clinical experience.

NOTES

1. Franz Alexander and T. M. French, *Psychoanalytic Therapy* (New York: Ronald Press, 1946).
2. C. D. Aring, "Sympathy and Empathy," *Journal of the American Medical Association,* 167 (1958), 448.
3. P. G. S. Beckett and R. Senf, "Methodological Problems in the Electronic Processing of Psychiatric Data with Examples from a Follow-up Study," *Psychiatric Research Reports,* 15 (1962), 133.
4. E. Bibring, "Psychoanalysis and the Dynamic Psychotherapies," *Journal of the American Psychoanalytic Association,* 2 (1954), 745.
5. Percy W. Bridgman, *The Way Things Are* (Cambridge: Harvard University Press, 1959).
6. Jules V. Coleman, "The Teaching of Basic Psychotherapy," *American Journal of Orthopsychiatry,* 17 (1947), 622.
7. Felix Deutsch and William F. Murphy, *The Clinical Interview* (New York: International Universities Press, 1955).
8. Jacob E. Finesinger, "Psychiatric Interviewing I. Some Principles and Procedures in Insight Therapy," *American Journal of Psychiatry,* 105 (1948), 187.
9. Jerome D. Frank, *Persuasion and Healing* (Baltimore: Johns Hopkins Press, 1961).
10. Sigmund Freud, "Fragment of an Analysis of a Case of Hysteria [1905]," *Collected Papers* (New York: Basic Books, 1959), Vol. III, pp. 13–148.
11. A. Garrett, *Interviewing: The Principles and Methods* (New York: Family Welfare Association of America, 1942).
12. Merton M. Gill, R. Newman, and Fredrick C. Redlich, *The Initial Interview in Psychiatric Practice* (New York: International Universities Press, 1954).
13. L. A. Gottschalk, G. C. Gleser, and G. Hambidge, Jr., "Verbal Behavior Analysis," *Archives of Neurology and Psychiatry,* 77 (1957), 300.
14. W. J. Hendrickson, R. H. Coffer, and T. N. Cross, "The Initial Interview," *Archives of Neurology and Psychiatry,* 71 (1954), 24.
15. J. Jaffe, "Language of the Dyad. A Method of Interaction Analysis in Psychiatric Interviews," *Psychiatry,* 21 (1958), 249.
16. M. Keller, I. L. Child, and Fredrick C. Redlich, "Preliminary Test of Intelligence," *American Journal of Psychiatry,* 103 (1947), 785.

17. Ernst Kris, "Ego Development and the Comic," *International Journal of Psycho-Analysis*, 19 (1938), 77.
18. Lawrence S. Kubie and H. A. Israel, "Say You're Sorry," *Psychoanalytic Study of the Child*, 10 (1955), 289.
19. G. F. Mahl, "Exploring Emotional States by Content Analysis," in Ithiel deSola Pool, ed., *Trends in Content Analysis* (Urbana, Ill.: University of Illinois Press, 1959).
20. R. G. Matarazzo, J. D. Matarazzo, G. Saslow, and J. S. Phillips, "Psychological Test and Organismic Correlates of Interview Interaction Patterns," *Journal of Abnormal Social Psychology*, 56 (1958), 329.
21. Karl A. Menninger, *A Manual for Psychiatric Case Study* (New York: Grune and Stratton, 1952).
22. Karl. A. Menninger, *The Vital Balance* (New York: Viking Press, 1963).
23. Adolf Meyer, *Psychobiology: A Science of Man* (Springfield, Ill.: Charles C Thomas, 1957).
24. Robert E. Pittenger *et al., The First Five Minutes: A Sample of Microscopic Interview Analysis* (Ithaca, N.Y.: Martineau, 1960).
25. Fredrick C. Redlich, John Dollard, and R. Newman, "High Fidelity Recording of Psychotherapeutic Interviews," *American Journal of Psychiatry*, 107 (1950), 42.
26. Theodore Reik, *Listening with the Third Ear* (New York: Farrar, Straus, 1948).
27. David Riesman, "Some Observations on Interviewing in a State Mental Hospital," *Bulletin of the Menninger Clinic*, 23 (1959), 7.
28. Carl R. Rogers, *Client-Centered Therapy* (Boston: Houghton Mifflin, 1951).
29. Jurgen Ruesch and Gregory Bateson, *Communication, the Social Matrix of Psychiatry* (New York: Norton, 1951).
30. A. E. Scheflen, "Communication and Regulation in Psychotherapy," *Psychiatry*, 26 (1963), 126.
31. Ian Stevenson and William M. Sheppe, Jr., "The Psychiatric Interview," in Silvano Arieti, ed., *The American Handbook of Psychiatry*, Vol. I, pp. 215–234 (New York: Basic Books, 1959).
32. Harry Stack Sullivan, *The Psychiatric Interview* (New York: Norton, 1954).

CHAPTER EIGHT

Psychological Tests in Clinical Psychiatry

Roy Schafer

Purpose of Psychological Tests

In modern clinical psychiatry, psychological tests are used to help clarify diagnosis, identify basic inner conflicts and impairments of function, and assess major assets for coping with inner conflicts and with the surrounding world. They are particularly sensitive to disruptions of thought, affect, and action associated with incipient or borderline psychosis, and with the various organic syndromes. Tests are also used to help assess changes in personality organization and mental efficiency resulting from psychological and physical therapies. They have been applied to children as early as the preschool years and to adults during senility. They have been used with populations of normal subjects for such purposes as vocational counseling, personnel selection, and assessment of student adjustment; and they have been employed in research on many problems in developmental, clinical, social, and experimental psychology and psychiatry.

In the clinical situation, it is best as a rule that the tests be administered early in the work with the patient. Also, many psychological examiners prefer to know at most only the general aspects of the patient's presenting problem and such biographical data as age, education, familial status, and occupation. Working with such limited data, they are able to arrive at a relatively independent or uncontaminated appraisal of the patient and at the same time formulate the findings in a pertinent fashion. When integrated with the interview material, these findings assist the therapist in planning treatment, giving advice, and making disposition. They assist him by throwing light on basic themes running through the initial interviews and by calling attention to strengths, impairments, defenses, or malignant trends not readily discernible in one or a few interviews. In certain well-compensated borderline cases and in acute, severely regressed schizophrenics, even many interviews may not clearly define the type and strength of internal factors making for illness and health, or regression and progression.

Psychological tests derive a great deal of their effectiveness simply from being relatively standardized procedures. By "standardized" is meant that the examiner presents the same tasks to each patient and presents them in essentially the same way. Of course, there is some allowance for variation in the conduct of the testing appropriate both to the patient's emotional state and intellectual level and to the circumstances of testing, such as its being conducted in a clinic, school, or court. Thus, the examiner keeps his contribution to variation in the test situation to a minimum.

Also, by presenting carefully selected and more-or-less unfamiliar tasks to the patient, he is able to bypass much of the patient's wittingly or unwittingly well-rehearsed, stereotyped, and therefore obscuring versions of his past and present experience and behavior. Consequently, he is able to ascribe most of the individual trends in the responses to factors internal to the patient, factors that are characteristic of the patient's responses to problems in general. He is usually in an excellent position to compare one patient with others and to describe distinguishing features of the patient's personality, his problems, and his problem-solving behavior. Some patients produce far more revealing responses than others, of course, but in all cases the psychologist attempts to work out as full a cross-sectional picture of the patient's personality as possible. This picture may then be synthesized with what is known about the patient's history so as to highlight developmental arrests, persisting crises, and latent trends of significance.

The prevailing psychodiagnostic practice is to administer several tests to each patient. The tests most frequently used are the Rorschach Test, the Thematic Apperception Test, and the Wechsler Adult Intelligence Scale. These three tests consitute a basic test battery, which, in most cases, provides a broad and representative sample of the patient's functioning under a variety of challenging conditions.[30] These conditions range from abstract intellectual problems and visual-motor tasks to creative acts of imagination and spontaneous self-expression. These tests also represent the basic types of problem presented by almost all commonly used psychological tests. Much of the following discussion will, therefore, be organized around them. Later parts of the chapter will describe some other tests, including a widely used personality questionnaire and tests specially devised or used for detecting and estimating the extent of mental deficit associated with organic brain damage. Scholastic aptitude and achievement tests, and tests used in vocational counseling and placement will not be discussed; they play no direct role in clinical psychodiagnosis. Lee J. Cronbach has reviewed tests of this type.[7]

Interpreting Ink Blots: The Rorschach Test

The Rorschach Test is the best-known and most widely used of the projective tests. It is called a projective test for the following reason: it presents the patient with relatively ambiguous, unformed, and unorganized material and requires him to organize it and invest it with meaning; in so doing, he inevitably "projects" or expresses basic and enduring inner tendencies, which determine his individual pattern of thought, feeling, and behavior.

The Rorschach Test was developed more than forty years ago by the Swiss psychiatrist and psychoanalyst Hermann Rorschach.[27] It consists of ten white cards, on each of which is a bilaterally symmetrical ink blot. Five of the ink blots are shades of gray and black; two include a few red areas in addition; and three are multicolored. The patient is asked to tell what each ink blot might look like. Whenever he asks for more specific instruction, he is told, "It is up to you"; or "Whatever you wish." He is allowed, if he so proposes, to interpret parts of each ink blot separately. He may turn the cards and look at them from any angle. Ordinarily, he may take as long as he wishes and may give as many responses as he wishes. His responses are recorded as close to verbatim as possible, and his reaction times are noted. Nonverbal expressive acts are recorded at their time of appearance.

For the patient, it is somewhat like finding meaningful representations in clouds. It is a test of imagination (though not a test of whether he has an imagination or not, as some patients assume). Rather, it brings out *his kind of imagination;* its relative freedom as regards emotion, originality, playfulness, and faithfulness to reality; certain aspects of its predominant content; and its moments of disruption under the pressure of anxiety and guilt. For, although imagination often serves to master anxiety and guilt, it may operate in the opposite way to increase anxiety and guilt, as by touching on certain difficult personal themes; and thereby it may bring about its own curtailment, fragmentation, or impoverishment. Through a person's imagination we can study those of his drives, emotions, and fantasies that are pushing toward expression, together with the defenses and controls by which he habitually attempts to suppress or regulate them. His values and prejudices may become apparent, along with his idealized and derogated images of himself and others. Anxious and guilty preoccupations with sex, his body, his anger, and his dependency needs may all be thrown into sharp relief.

The patient's Rorschach Test responses are scrutinized from four vantage points: their scores, their dynamic content, their adherence to logical, realistic organization and communication, and their context of expressive behavior. Major diagnostic conclusions are ordinarily based on the convergence or fitting together of evidence seen from these four vantage points.

(1) *The scores.* Each response is scored with regard to a number of its aspects, the most significant of which are: (a) its location on the ink blot (that is, its utilizing the entire ink blot, a large detail, a tiny detail or a white space); (b) its determinants (that is, its basis in the form, color, shading, or apparent kinesthetic qualities of the area in question, or some combination of these); and (c) its objective accuracy (that is, its gross or fine congruence with the actual contour of the ink blot or its vagueness or arbitrariness).

Patterns of overemphasis and underemphasis highlighted by the scores point to significant personality characteristics. For example, if the patient gives many responses and a very high proportion of these are inaccurate or vague, it is likely that his contact with reality is seriously disturbed by severe anxiety, psychotic regression, or both. If he overemphasizes color as a determinant of his responses, and if he uses colored areas with relatively little regard for their form, it is likely that he is an emotionally volatile, possibly impulsive individual; whereas if he uses colors frequently but always with very careful regard for their forms, he is likely to be a compliant, overconsiderate person. If he rigidly attempts to interpret every minor detail and to produce many responses thereby, he is likely to be a perfectionistic, overmeticulous person. Actually, interpretation of score patterns is far more complex than these examples suggest. It is the *configuration* of many scores and of the other aspects of the record and the test battery that ultimately determines the precise interpretation of any single score pattern.

(2) *The dynamic content.* The dynamic content of the responses may bear on such central themes of human existence as aggression (for instance, percepts involving bombs exploding, animals fighting, weapons, or blood); dependency needs (for example, food, emaciated creatures, or Santa Claus); guilt (for instance, angels and devils); sex; fear; and the like. Any persistent, perceptually arbitrary, emotionally intense, or imaginatively extreme emphasis on one of these basic themes, particularly when it tends to exclude or overshadow others, indicates that the implied dynamic trend plays a major part in the patient's present functioning and illness. As with the scores, it is the configuration of dynamic themes that is the matrix for interpretation of any one theme.

(3) *Disruption of thought organization and communication.* This becomes evident when responses are narratively elaborated far beyond anything that is perceptually justified; when two or more responses absurdly fuse into each other; or when the wording of responses becomes notably cryptic, illogical, or confused. For example, an objectively amorphous ink-blot area may be arbitrarily seen as a highly articulated figure engaged in a specific, complex action; a simple nondescript profile of a face may be seen as filled with specific and intense emotion and may even then elicit feelings of fear or excitement; an area that looks both like blood and an island may be seen as "a bloody island"; an area at the top of a blot may be called the North Pole simply because it is at the top. It is psychotic patients from whom conspicuous and frequent disruptions of this sort are expected.

(4) *Test behavior.* This aspect includes the patient's behavior and attitudes toward the test, the tester, and his own test responses. These may range from euphoria and grandiosity to dejection, hopelessness, and helplessness. The patient may be belligerent, seductive, pedantic, impulsive, restless, listless, ingratiating, suspicious, and so on.

In recent years, the tendency has grown among some clinical psychologists to emphasize test behavior and dynamic content and to minimize scores and patterns of thought organization. Even though in some cases this approach may contribute sufficient basic information to yield useful test reports, it often leads to serious errors of description and diagnosis. One reason for this is that test behavior and content are subject to transient fluctuations of the patient's mood, initiative, and rapport; in contrast, formal aspects of the patient's responses typically reflect modes of function of many years' duration and are, therefore, relatively stable. The formal characteristics are also relatively safe from conscious manipulation, because the patient ordinarily has no idea of their significance and specific implications.

Ignoring the scores in particular has been encouraged by the negative and contradictory results obtained in research studies purportedly testing the validity of their significance.[7] On the whole, however, these studies have been inadequate tests of validity, for they have not been based on configurational analysis of scores carried on in relation to other aspects of the record; and, in addition, the validating criteria, such as success in school or on the job, or response to psychotherapy, have often been poorly chosen, poorly defined, or poorly scaled.

At the same time, numerous well-designed studies have been reported that have established meaningful correlations between Rorschach scores and significant personality features; for example, those reported by Seymour B. Sarason.[28] Robert R. Holt and his co-workers, using a combination of new and modified scores, have demonstrated how Rorschach results may be used to predict subjects' responses to regression-inducing experiences such as sensory isolation, hypnosis, and taking LSD.[17] Nevertheless, it also remains correct to say that the general value of the test scores has been established through the work of experienced and competent professionals with many thousands of patients. This is the same way that the general value of psychotherapy has been established.

Major comprehensive discussions of the Rorschach Test will be found in the writings of David Rapaport *et al.*,[25] Bruno Klopfer *et al.*,[20] Samuel J. Beck,[2] and Roy Schafer.[31] The *Journal of Projective Techniques* carries many reports of research using the Rorschach Test.

The Thematic Apperception Test

The Thematic Apperception Test (TAT) was developed in the 1930's by Henry A. Murray and his co-workers at the Harvard Psychological Clinic.[23] It consists of a series of black-and-white pictures, which are presented to the patient one at a time with the request that he make up a story around each. The story is to include events leading up to the depicted situation and an outcome. The thoughts and feelings of the characters may also be asked for and, in the case of some pictures which are very fanciful, the patient may be encouraged to "let his imagination go" as much as possible.

The typical TAT card depicts one or more individuals in a situation of emotion or conflict. There is considerable ambiguity in the stimuli, however, in that indications about the background and future of the situation are absent, and in many cases the conflicts and emotions depicted are not clear. In some cases, not even the sex or age of a character is well defined. At the extreme, one of the stimuli is a blank card, for which the patient is to make up the picture as well as the story.

The following are some examples of the pictures: a pensive, sad, or frustrated boy sitting before a violin on a table; a somewhat distressed elderly woman looking into a room; a woodcut depicting a gaunt, wretched, or wicked old man standing amidst chaotically represented gravestones; the heads of two persons apparently embracing; a disturbed man standing with his back to a bed in which a woman is lying limp and with her breasts exposed. The range of pictures touches more or less directly on situations of sexual or aggressive conflict, love, intimacy, fear, aspiration, depression, anger, guilt, loneliness, dependency, rejection, and other kinds of common, strong, and intimate human experience.

Some of the pictures are shown to all patients, regardless of age and sex. Others are specifically for males or for females; some are specifically for adults. As many as twenty pictures may be shown, although in practice, in order to save time, only eight to twelve pictures are likely to be used.

Like the Rorschach Test, the TAT is considered a projective technique. To tell stories, the patient must create new detail in the past and future; because of the ambiguity and incompleteness of the pictures, he must create much of the present. Also, he will ordinarily take up the motivations, thoughts, and feelings of the characters. In filling in all these gaps, he will inevitably draw on his characteristic expectations in life, his actual patterns of interpersonal relationship, and his dominant fantasies.

To illustrate the variety of response available to the patient, we may consider the first card, depicting the boy and the violin. The boy may be seen as sad, frustrated, sullen, or pensive. If sad, it may be because he has been forced to practice against his will, or because he has tried to play and has failed. If he has been forced to practice, it may be because he had wanted to be outdoors playing with the other boys, or because he had felt inadequate to the task. If forced, he may submit or rebel. If he submits, he may ultimately learn to play well or poorly. If he rebels, he may do so indirectly or directly; if directly, by persuasion, verbal attack, or by smashing the violin. The possibilities can be spun out virtually endlessly. Empirically, we do encounter ever new variations on these themes. The same is true for most of the other pictures. Experience and research have amply supported the projective or self-expressive nature of the patient's choice and development of themes.

Of course, the TAT stories are not taken literally by the examiner. Interpretation is a matter of complex inference and comparison, as in interviews. When, for example, in a story told about Card 1, the parents have forced the boy to practice the violin, the examiner does not assume that this or something quite like it has really happened. When, however, the patient repeatedly refers throughout the test to parents or authority figures imposing their will on a character with whom he appears to be identified, it is likely that he views relationships as a matter of struggles between domineering persons and submissive or rebellious ones; that internally he is pulled in contrary directions; and that, depending on how he tells the stories, in his overt behavior he is likely to emphasize one or more of these poles of power relationships.

Thus, in interpreting the TAT, one inspects the entire series of stories for characteristic identification figures, goals, obstacles, and affects, as well as patterns of relationship. One asks whether the characters are repeatedly successful, failing, helpless, pessimistic, sad, optimistic, happy, aggressive, conciliatory; or are threatened by others, afraid of themselves, aiming at great success, establishing lonely islands of security, and the like. The interpreter recognizes, too, that different facets of the patient's self may be divided among several characters. For example, the stories of one patient may repeatedly refer to conflict between, on the one hand, the central figure who is pursuing apparently natural goals and pleasures, and with whom the patient appears to be primarily identified; and, on the other hand, persons representing strict morality. The interpretation may be that these forbidding figures are chiefly embodiments of the strict conscience or superego *within* the patient and not actual persons. In another instance, a young male patient may be preoccupied with the psychology of the female figures in his stories; this might reflect an unconscious fantasy of himself as pleasurably and anxiously girlish, and, at the same time, it may express his attitudes toward actual young women and his beliefs about them.

In addition, the examiner watches for perceptual distortion; elaboration of pictorial detail, or introduction of feelings inappropriate to the picture; odd verbalizations and logical and emotional *non sequiturs*; all of these may indicate thought disorder. As in the Rorschach situation, the patient's test-taking attitudes and behavior are also observed and analyzed.

While scoring systems have been established by various investigators, the TAT stories are usually interpreted in a flexible, clinical manner. The examiner attempts to follow whichever themes emerge conspicuously, much as an interviewer or therapist interprets while listening to a patient.

Recent general discussions of this test have been presented by Morris I. Stein[32] and William E. Henry;[16] Rapaport *et al.*[25] is also a useful reference. Again, the *Journal of Projective Techniques* is a source of many research reports involving the TAT; for example, a recent study by Brian Welch *et al.*[40] illustrates the study of manic–depressive disorders with the TAT.

The concept of a thematic apperception test lends itself to many variations. Special sets of pictures have been prepared for young children,[3] adolescents,[33] Negroes,[35] and, in connection with numerous research projects, for dynamic trends of special interest, such as the handling of aggression and attitude toward the feminine role. In one study, the pictures dealt with patterns of relationship among hospital personnel.[6] One variation allows the patient freedom of choice in introducing some figures into the pictures from a supply of cut-out figures.[39] Another is a series of sketches of a dog and his family depicting various aspects of infantile psychosexuality and interpersonal relationship;[5] in this test—the "Blacky test"—the freely told story is in each case supplemented by answers to specific questions concerning the wishes and defensive attitudes of the characters.

Another variation, used in studying the psychology of humor, as well as in psychodiagnostic work, is the Mirth Response Test developed by Jacob Levine and Fredrick Redlich.[21] It consists of a series of funny cartoons. Inasmuch as each cartoon bears on a significant emotional situation, the patient's spontaneous mirth responses, as well as his understanding of and attitudes toward the cartoons, may be used to define areas of strong inner conflict and of relative security. Some variations on the TAT are entirely verbal in nature, such as one in which conflict situations are described and the patient is asked what the central characters then do in each instance and what their reasons are for so doing.[29] Although many of its variations have been shown to be clinically sensitive, the TAT itself continues to be by far the most widely used test of this sort.

The advantage of using the TAT along with the Rorschach Test lies in its closeness to the language, imagery, and behavior of daily life. Where the Rorschach Test indicates broad patterns of functioning and general areas of conflict, the TAT suggests specific forms of social behavior, specific attitudes and expectations, specific types of persons with respect to whom certain conflicts and security feelings exist. The Rorschach Test is considerably less "structured" than the TAT in that its stimuli and instructions are more ambiguous; consequently, it usually reflects deep trends of fantasy and anxiety more clearly than the TAT. The TAT results can be relatively restricted by defensive clichés and adherence to "proper" social form. As a rule, however, the TAT has considerable evocative power.

Miscellaneous Projective Techniques

Two of the more popular supplementary projective techniques are the Draw-a-Person Test and the Sentence Completion Test. There are several versions of each of these tests. What follows describes one common form of each.

In the Draw-a-Person Test, the patient is given a pad of paper and a pencil and simply asked to draw a person. All details, such as sex and position, are left up to him, except that he is encouraged to draw a complete figure. Upon completing his drawing, he is asked to draw a picture of a person of the opposite sex. Interpretation of the drawings takes into account both formal and content characteristics. Formal characteristics include the size of the figures, the sequence and relative size of the sexes, placement on the page, the degree of articulation and detail, and distortions, pressure of the pencil, fastidiousness of execution, and the like. Content features include unusual emphasis on, avoidance of, or distortion of specific parts of the body, or apparel, action, or posture. It will be noted, for example, whether the face is emphasized more than the rest of the figure; whether discomfort is evident while rendering the hands or the genital or breast areas; and whether the facial expression tends to be hostile, withdrawn, or seductive.

Some interpretative approaches to drawings are highly symbolic and intuitive, and there is controversy as to their theoretical justification. There are also conflicting research claims as to their validity. It does appear, however, that perceptive and intuitive clinical psychologists who have worked intensively with drawings are able to infer leading personality features and problems with impressive accuracy. The same seems to be true of almost any test situation.

The Sentence Completion Test requires the patient to complete a number of sentences. The sentence beginnings, as in TAT cards, pertain to a wide variety of emotionally significant human experiences and relationships. Typical sentence beginnings are: "I never———"; "If my mother only had———"; "Most girls———"; and so forth. The patient is encouraged either to respond very spontaneously or to finish the sentence in the way that best expresses his thoughts and feelings. Typically, the sentence completions are analyzed according to their content, although their formal characteristics may be diagnostic of major defenses and controls, and of thought disorder. The same is true of any verbalization in a standardized situation. The principles of Sentence Completion interpretation do not differ fundamentally from those used in the TAT. Actually, this type of test stands midway between the TAT and the Word Association Test, to which we shall now turn briefly.

Historically, the Word Association Test is perhaps the first projective test of any significance, particularly as used early in this century by the subsequently famous psychoanalyst, Carl Jung.[18] Later, Luria did some highly imaginative research with word associations as indicators of conflict, in the early days of the Soviet Union.[22] In the Word Association Test, a list of words is called out one at a time, and the patient is asked to respond to each in turn with one other word, the first that comes to mind, no matter what it is. The word list includes such words touching on likely areas of conflict as *love, hate, father, mother, intercourse, breast,* and *suicide.* The examiner inspects the responses for delay in reaction time, atypical content, emotional expression, relevance to the stimulus word, and so forth.

On the whole, the Word Association Test has not worked out as a very sensitive instrument for detecting and illuminating *distinctive* areas of conflict in the individual case. The emotionally charged words tend to elicit some degree of disturbance of response from most patients. This test has, however, been found useful in detecting certain forms of thought disorder and major defensive tendencies.[25] It is little used, especially compared to the

Sentence Completion technique, which itself is often used in lieu of the TAT because it takes much less time. Considerable sacrifice of depth and subtlety is usually the price paid for this convenience in time, however. The *research* potential of the Word Association type of instrument has not been sufficiently appreciated.

There are numerous other projective tests of interest. They, along with the Rorschach, TAT, and other tests discussed in this chapter, have been discussed at greater length in Harold H. Anderson and Gladys L. Anderson[1] and in Arthur Weider.[39]

Intelligence Tests

Intelligence testing is the pioneer form of today's psychodiagnostics. Its formal history extends back to 1904, when the French psychologist Alfred Binet, in collaboration with Theodore Simon, arranged a group of thirty tests or problems in order of difficulty and was able to differentiate normal and feeble-minded children by their performance on these problems. A later version of this instrument, known as the Binet-Simon Test, was adapted for use in the United States by Lewis M. Terman in 1916 and has become widely known as the Stanford-Binet. It was revised by Terman and Maud A. Merrill in 1937 and again in 1959.[34] It comprises a wide variety of questions, problems, and puzzles. They are arranged on a series of levels of increasing difficulty. The test yields a score that may be used to compare one person's level of achievement with that of his average age-mate. His score may be expressed as a Mental Age in years and months, or as an I.Q., which is essentially the ratio Mental Age/Chronological Age × 100. For example, if a seven-year-old child obtains a Mental Age of eight years, then his I.Q. is 114, which is just another way of saying that he passes as many items on the intelligence test as the average child of eight, or that in his mental development he is about a year ahead of his average age-mate of seven.

As intelligence testing became a well-established practice, examiners learned to note and interpret individual patterns of passes and failures, as well as distinctive and self-expressive test responses and test behavior. For example, some patients are weak on items requiring social judgment, though strong on items requiring visual-motor skills; some patients attack problems impulsively and with low frustration tolerance; others are circumspect and persevering; and so on. Thus, the intelligence test began to be used as a *personality test* as well as a psychometric technique, and its clinical usefulness was thereby greatly increased. For example, it became possible to distinguish low-level performance, reflecting truly limited endowment and development, from low-level performance based on psychosis, severe anxiety, or negativism in patients whose premorbid intelligence was average or higher.

Yet, as a clinical and psychometric instrument the Stanford-Binet has a number of shortcomings. (1) Having been standardized on children and adolescents, it is not well suited for the testing of adults, though it has been used extensively for this purpose. (2) Because *on the average* there is no significant increase in the number of Stanford-Binet items passed by persons beyond the age of fifteen years, the examiner is forced to act as if mental development stops at a Mental Age of fifteen years. Consequently, fifteen has been used as the chronological age in computing the Stanford-Binet I.Q.'s of all persons older than fifteen. This procedure ignores the obvious observations that certain mental abilities continue to develop beyond the age of fifteen, and that some abilities, such as are involved in learning new material, decline progressively with advancing age. Thus, the type of items used in the intelligence test and the method of scoring it create gross artifacts. (3) The Stanford-Binet is overweighted on the side of verbal items, especially on the higher age levels. It thereby often penalizes patients whose main assets are perceptual or motoric rather than verbal; and it is often not an adequate instrument to study visual-motor impairments in certain patients. As a result, the Stanford-Binet must often be supplemented by a nonverbal test of intelligence—a time-consuming and inexact procedure. (4) The Stanford-Binet consists of varied items arranged according to age levels, with little or no continuity in the type of item from one age level to the next. It thus offers no possibility of establishing an individual's range in any one intellectual area or of quantitatively comparing his level of achievement in different areas. Basically, it limits the examiner to thinking of intelligence in global terms only.

A new type of intelligence test was called for. It had to be one that systematically took into account that intelligence is not a unitary trait, but comprises a variety of such functions as judgment, concept-formation, planning ability and anticipation, concentration, visual-motor speed and organization, and availability of vocabulary and information. It had to be standardized on adults. Its I.Q. scores had to compare adults with their age-mates and not with a hypothetical fifteen-year-old. It had to include equivalent amounts of verbal and nonverbal material and equivalent I.Q. scores for over-all achievement in both areas. It had to be organized in subtests composed of relatively homogeneous items, each sampling one type of cognitive functioning, with the items arranged in their order of increasing difficulty, and each subtest yielding a score directly comparable to the other subtest scores. Thus, equal weight would be given to the different major areas of intelligence.

Such a test appeared in the late 1930's in the form of the Wechsler-Bellevue Scale. It was developed by David Wechsler, who, in recent years, has revised his test in collaboration with the Psychological Corporation and has published it under the name of the Wechsler Adult Intelligence Scale, or WAIS.[37, 38] The WAIS comprises eleven subtests: Information, Comprehension, Arithmetic, Similarities, Digit Span, Vocabulary, Digit Symbol, Picture Completion, Block Designs, Picture Arrangement, and Object Assembly. The first six subtests make up the verbal part of the test and are used to derive a verbal I.Q.; the latter five, the performance part and performance

I.Q. All subtest scores taken together yield a total I.Q. The various subtests appear to tap the variety of intellectual functions mentioned above.

In clinical practice, the patient's performance is assessed in several ways. First, the over-all level of his intelligence is appraised in order to help estimate, however roughly, the level of functioning that may be reasonably expected of him at work and in his family and community. In addition to guiding the determination of current impairment and considerations of disposition, this appraisal may bear on the intensiveness and subtlety of the psychotherapy to be prescribed. For example, ordinarily, an above-average I.Q. appears to be required for psychoanalysis.

Second, the patterning of assets and deficiencies in the different intellectual functions tapped by the subtests is appraised. This is done partly because different patterns of subtest scores may yield the same I.Q., just as different *styles* of problem-solving in any one subtest may still result in the same subtest score being obtained. The pattern of scores may suggest particular forms of neurosis or psychosis, as well as the presence or absence of specific intellectual assets for work and social adaptation. It has been found, for example, that on the average, schizophrenics tend to have a wider dispersal of their subtest scores and, hence, of their current abilities, than non-schizophrenics.[25]

Third, the content of responses, and the manner of responding and of dealing with success and failure are observed and analyzed. On the questions of information, for example, highly intellectualistic obsessional neurotics tend to give lengthy pedantic responses; emotionally labile, naïve hysterics tend to give impulsive and uncertain responses; reckless psychopaths tend to make wild guesses and to improvise pretentious and often absurd specific detail. Martin Mayman *et al.* have summarized a general rationale and set of interpretative principles for Wechsler's intelligence test.[1]

There is probably as much misunderstanding and abuse of the I.Q. as of any psychological concept or measurement yet advanced in psychology. A number of cautions are therefore indicated:

(1) The notion of a fixed I.Q. for any individual should be held with reservations. It is, for example, not rare for a young child's I.Q. score to increase or decrease significantly in the course of time. Also, it is commonly observed in clinical practice that a patient's over-all level of functioning may be lowered significantly, *though only temporarily*, by anxiety, distractibility, apathy, negativism, confusional trends, overmeticulousness, or impulsiveness. Fortunately, it is often possible for the experienced tester to make a gross estimate of the extent of the patient's impairment as well as of his level of intellectual functioning under optimal conditions. He does this by inspecting the pattern of passes and failures within each of the subtests and by referring to certain of the subtest scores, which as a rule are significantly less vulnerable to the impact of psychological disorders. Each I.Q. is thereby considered in relation to the patient's developmental level and total state at the time of testing.

(2) It must be borne in mind that an I.Q. score is at best approximate. It indicates a range, such as dull, average, or superior, within which a given individual usually functions. Small differences in I.Q. scores among individuals are, therefore, meaningless; and the same individual who may function brilliantly in certain types of situations may function dully in others, perhaps as a reflection of interfering anxiety and defensive restriction of ego functioning. It is not rare, for example, for intellectually gifted persons to be relatively weak on nonverbal subtests as a result of the combination of a value bias against manual skills and feelings of inadequacy and anxiety in the sphere of action as opposed to verbalization and reflection.

(3) No single test taps all the capacities that promote adaptation and accomplishment in the varied aspects of life. Special talents, such as those involved in the arts and in interpersonal skills, may not be tapped by the intelligence test or reflected in the I.Q. score at all.

(4) The total score on one intelligence test, whether it be a Mental Age, an I.Q., or something else, should never be compared *without qualification* with the score on another test, for the reason that the range of possible scores tends to vary from one instrument to another, and the distribution of scores within that range may also vary. Scores of 140 on the Stanford-Binet, the WAIS and the Army General Classification Test are not exactly comparable with one another, for example. This is especially true in the case of very high or very low scores. Nevertheless, it is useful to know that the general trend in intelligence test construction has been to set up the scale of scores, so that the average is around 100; the upper limit of the range for mental deficiency is placed at around 70 (marking off approximately the lowest 2 per cent of scores obtained in the general population); and the lower limit of the range for the very superior at around 130 (marking off the highest 2 per cent of scores).

(5) There are undoubtedly different types or organizations of intelligence, so that if two individuals obtain the same total I.Q. score, this in itself is not a basis for expecting them to function on the same level in all intellectual areas.

(6) Motivational and attitudinal factors may make a significant difference in the actual accomplishments of which different individuals with the same I.Q.'s are capable. A well-organized, dedicated "plugger" with an I.Q. of 115 can get through college; an inefficient, unmotivated student with the same I.Q. may flunk out of high school.

A responsible and competent psychologist usually will convey in his reporting of intelligence test results such details, implications, and reservations as will enable colleagues to be maximally objective in using these results. It is nevertheless surprising how often one encounters uncritical use of I.Q. scores, even among experienced and sophisticated psychiatrists.

In recent years, Wechsler has also brought out the Wechsler Intelligence Scale for Children, or WISC.[36] It covers the age range five to fourteen; the WAIS covers the age range from fifteen on. The WISC is organized and scored in the same manner as the WAIS. It is increasingly popular and may ultimately replace the Stanford-Binet, except in the testing of children or mental defectives with a Mental Age between two and five, an age range covered by the Stanford-Binet.

There are also tests that have been devised to estimate the level of intelligence or general maturity of children even during the first years of life. The famous Gesell scales are an example.[10] The long-range stability of the scores obtained from infants is not great; and the predictive value of the infant scales cannot be considered very good in the individual case. Because such factors as maturation, motivation, conflict, and mental stimulation are always influential, even the scores of preschool children appear to be only very grossly predictive of future levels of function.

There are numerous group forms of intelligence tests such as those used in schools and in the armed forces. There are also numerous short forms of intelligence tests, which are useful in giving a quick estimate of general intelligence level. Naturally, these variations on the full and individually administered intelligence test sacrifice much psychodiagnostic as well as psychometric sensitivity and accuracy. A general survey of the varieties of individual and group, and child and adult intelligence tests may be found in Cronbach[7] and Weider.[39]

The Diagnostic Questionnaire

In clinical practice, the most widely used diagnostic questionnaire is the Minnesota Multiphasic Personality Inventory or MMPI.[41] It comprises 504 statements about each of which the patient is to say whether it is mostly true of him, not mostly true of him, or something about which he can render no judgment. The items cover many personality traits, social behaviors, subjective experiences, and symptoms. A few of the statements are: "I am happy most of the time"; "I am sure I get a raw deal from life"; "I wish I were not so shy"; "It makes me uncomfortable to put on a stunt at a party even when others are doing the same sort of things"; "I have used alcohol excessively."

The 504 statements were selected from an original list of over a thousand. In the standardization of the test, the original list was administered to a large number of normal subjects and psychiatric patients. By statistical analysis of their answers, it was possible to single out those items that more or less successfully identified patients with one or another known diagnosis. For example, sixty items were responded to by depressive patients in a certain way with significantly high frequency compared to the normal control group. These sixty items were then defined as the Depression Scale. Once the Depression Scale had been established, each new patient's Depression score was the sum of Depression Scale items he answered in the "typical" depressive way.

In this way, nine diagnostic scales were derived: Hypochondriasis, Hysteria, Depression, Psychopathic Deviate, Hypomania, Schizophrenia, Paranoia, Psychasthenia (obsessive and compulsive reaction), and Masculinity–Femininity. In addition, some supplementary scales were derived to help estimate the patient's tendency to minimize or maximize his maladjustment tendencies, and his tendency to present his character in an exaggeratedly honorable light. Scores on these supplementary scales help assess the validity and trustworthiness of the other scores.

It should be noted that it is not assumed that the patient's response to each item is necessarily true of him. Rather, it is ascertained whether and to what extent the *way* he answers the questions, that is, his verbal behavior in the test situation, corresponds to the way the typical members of various clinical groups answer these same questions. If, for example, he answers certain questions the way hysterics tend to, even if some of these questions have little to do with hysteria as such, and if these are the very questions and answers that successfully differentiated the standardization sample of hysterics, then he will score high on the Hysteria Scale and will be likely to have noteworthy hysterical characteristics, among others.

In practice, the interpretation of the MMPI scores has become a subtle matter requiring intensive experience. Typically, it is the *profile* of scores on *all* the scales that is interpreted. A variety of meaningful profiles has been identified. Also, it is possible to predict from the profile not only diagnosis but certain leading personality traits. In addition, numerous new scales have been established by further statistical analyses of responses given by groups of subjects with one or another distinctive personality characteristic. Scales for social introversion, manifest anxiety, prejudice, social dominance, and ego strength are examples.

Because it yields simple scores with relatively high reliabilities, and because it can be applied to an infinite variety of clinical, occupational, and other groups, the MMPI has been an exceedingly popular research instrument. In the first fifteen years after its appearance in 1940, 689 separate publications appeared on this test. Many of these define or apply new scales, such as those just mentioned. General surveys of the test and its applications have been presented by Starke R. Hathaway and Paul E. Meehl,[15] and W. Grant Dahlstrom and George Schlager Welsh.[8] A briefer presentation than these may be found in Weider.[39]

Fundamentally, the derivation and clinical use of this test is entirely empirical. No basic theory of personality is involved. By its nature, the test limits the psychologist to inferences based upon a pattern of numbers that are the end results of complicated processes about which he has no information. The test lacks the suggestiveness and subtlety of projective tests in which, step by step, the response process in a complex situation may be observed and analyzed. On the whole, process analysis is exceedingly difficult to quantify or otherwise validate so that champions of the MMPI approach have come forward to stress the advantage of the relatively more mechanical, objective, and "actuarial" interpretation of MMPI profiles. The issue, however, is not simply one of ease of objective research and quantitative accuracy of diagnosis and prediction. Those more identified with projective testing stress the closeness they achieve to the prevailing content, mechanisms, and organization of the patient's subjective experience. They attempt to observe and conceptualize phenomena much closer to those dealt with by the psychotherapist.

Other well-known diagnostic questionnaires, such as the one by Robert Bernreuter, have been surveyed by Cronbach.[7]

Detecting Brain Damage: The "Organic" Tests

Numerous tests have been constructed or used to help detect brain damage and to estimate the severity of its effects on functioning. Only a few representative tests of this sort can be covered here. In skilled hands, the WAIS and the Rorschach Test are usually able to do the gross diagnostic job by themselves; and these tests will also be referred to in what follows. It will be helpful to consider the "organic" tests under headings designating the diagnostic deficits usually encountered in cases of actual brain damage.

Impaired conceptual thinking. Patients with brain damage more or less lose the capacity for abstract conceptual thinking. As described by Kurt Goldstein,[11] this impairment has a number of aspects. In severe cases objects, persons, or events can be related to each other only in terms of *concrete situations* in which they might be encountered. Individual properties cannot be abstracted in thought and considered apart from other properties of the same object; for example, that an object is red or round or metallic cannot be considered securely in isolation from its other properties and its concrete meaning or function. *Hypothetical thinking,* the consideration of the merely possible, or the dealing with abstractions apart from their correspondence with concrete reality, is impaired. Also, the ability to *analyze* phenomena into their elements and to *synthesize* elements into a total concept or object is reduced; for example, one will detect impaired ability to analyze and synthesize designs in such a way as to be able to duplicate them with small blocks. Even where an abstract concept appears to have been attained or retained, it cannot be handled flexibly in relation to other concepts pertaining to the same objects or phenomena; in other words, the ability to *shift* from one abstract conceptualization to another is lost; and, in the light of this observed rigidity, even the retained abstract concept cannot be considered to reflect unimpaired conceptual thinking.

One subtest of the WAIS, Similarities, is a test of verbal concept-formation. In it the patient is asked to say how a pair of objects or actions are alike or similar; for example, an orange and a banana, a table and a chair, wood and alcohol, praise and punishment. The abstract conceptual response to the first is ordinarily "fruit," to the second "furniture," and so on. Intermediate between concreteness and abstractness are responses stressing specific actions which may be carried out with these objects or specific physical properties they have in common; for example, in the case of the orange and the banana, "you eat them both" or "both have peels." When the patient is extremely concrete, he cannot conceive of objects as being alike or similar; they are either identical or different. The patient may know in a limited sense that both an orange and a banana have peels and can be eaten; and yet he may well insist that they are not alike, remaining bound to the total concrete objects in his appraisal. That is to say, their differences in shape, color, and texture or their totality as objects will dominate his thought. At best, such a patient may tie objects together in terms of a concrete situation, saying, for example, that an orange and a banana may be found in a fruit store, or that you sit in a chair when you eat at the table.

The understanding and explanation of *proverbs* is also usually impaired. Obviously, proverbs are highly abstract formulations even though cast in the form of concrete images.

The Color-Form Sorting Test is another test that investigates impairment of conceptual thinking. It consists of twelve forms: four squares, four triangles, and four circles. One of each of the shapes is colored red, one blue, one green, and one yellow. The patient is asked to divide the objects into groups that belong together. If he succeeds in sorting them according to color or shape and can verbalize the concept, he is then asked to divide them in a different way. If he cannot shift, he is offered certain standardized cues to help him, in order to aid the tester to assess the extent of his difficulty. Many patients with brain damage cannot make even one sorting, let alone two. In their first or second sorting, they often try to construct geometric patterns of different or similar shapes or colors. Sometimes they can only sort the objects according to color and shape simultaneously.

The Vigotsky Test is a much more complicated form of the Color-Form Sorting Test. The typical organic patient is virtually helpless in solving this problem. This test is of limited diagnostic usefulness, however, inasmuch as it is also very difficult for many non-brain–damaged individuals.

Another test, one of intermediate conceptual complexity, is the Object Sorting Test. This consists of over thirty commonly encountered objects, such as real and toy silverware, real and toy tools, smoking equipment, pieces of paper, corks, and the like. In the first part of the test, the patient is asked to put with one specified item at a time all of the others that belong with it and then to verbalize the concept he used. He is asked, for example, to put with the real fork, the real pipe, or the toy tool everything else he thinks belongs with it. This part of the test assesses relatively independent concept-formation. In the second part of the test, the examiner puts groups of objects before the patient and asks him to try to say why they can all belong together. For example, the tester presents a group of red objects, paper objects, tools, rectangular objects, and the like. Here, it is more a matter of grasping conventional, ready-made concepts, than of conceptualizing independently.

The typical intact adult individual of average or better than average intelligence will present more-or-less abstract conceptual groupings and conceptualizations in both parts of the test; he may fail a few difficult items altogether or offer concrete conceptualizations on them. In contrast, the responses of the typical brain-damaged patient will be almost entirely concrete. He may appear to do well on some of the items, if he has retained the notion of grouping according to material or function; but he will manifest his impairment in his difficulty in shifting from this type of conceptualization to any other. Also, he is likely to be unable to deal with the reappearance of the same object in several groupings. For instance, in the second part of the test, a ball is included in four separate groupings: the red objects, the round objects, the rubber objects, and the toys. The patient will probably persist in regarding it concretely as a ball or, at best, cling to one of its conceptual properties, such as its material. This test is also useful in detecting schizophrenic thought disorder.[25, 30]

Impaired conceptual thinking is evident almost invariably in the Rorschach Test. There, the patient may be unable to conceive of giving alternate interpretations to the same areas; in fact, he will tend to think that each ink blot is a real picture or a diagram of something specific. In so thinking, he will manifest his inability to think hypothetically or to shift from one possibility to another. As a result, he will often perseverate with the same response throughout the test; he will fail some or many of the cards; and he will have difficulty abstracting and using the colors, shadings, and other properties of the blots in a flexible manner. Throughout, he is likely to be more or less perplexed and to complain of feelings of inadequacy and helplessness.

Impaired Memory and Learning Ability

Severe impairments of memory and learning ability are commonly encountered in organic patients. One test often used in this connection is the Wechsler Memory Scale. Although relatively crude in its design, standardization, and scoring, this test nevertheless reflects memory impairment both quantitatively and qualitatively. It includes items of "orientation" and "mental control" of the sort used in the traditional psychiatric diagnostic examination. These items ask the patient to tell where he is, and the day, month, and year of this examination; to recite the alphabet; to count backward by ones and forward by threes; and so forth. The test also includes a digit-span subtest; immediate recall of two short stories; recall of abstract geometrical designs; and recall of pairs of words, some of which are meaningfully related to each other, and some not. Most reliably, it is on story recall, memory for designs, and memory for the paired words that the brain-damaged patient falls down. As regards his impaired capacity for hypothetical thinking, it is noteworthy that he will have particular difficulty learning the pairs of words not meaningfully related to each other, such as "cabbage-pen." What he remembers of the geometric designs is likely to be highly oversimplified and fragmentary. He may fail completely to remember one or both of the stories.

Wechsler designed this test to yield a Memory Quotient (M.Q.) that would be roughly comparable to the I.Q. The calculation of the M.Q. takes account of the fact that there is normally a progressive decline in memory efficiency (as measured by tests) beginning in the third decade of life. The M.Q. is not, however, a sensitive measure in itself, for it may not reflect severe and diagnostic impairments that occur on one or two subtests only.

Lapses of memory may be observed in all the tests used. For example, in the Information and Vocabulary subtests of the WAIS, in the Rorschach Test, and in the TAT, the patient may manifest fluid thinking; that is, he may lose track of his train of thought and of what he has already said, and he may thereby juxtapose fragments of response with no regard for their logical or emotional incompatibility.

Impaired Visual-Motor Organization

There are a variety of ways in which visual-motor organization may be studied. One of the most popular is some form of the block designs test. The Block Designs subtest of the WAIS will serve as an example. In this test, the patient is required to assemble colored cubes in such a way as to reproduce ten designs of increasing complexity. Each design is presented in less than life-size on separate pages of a booklet. Some of the designs require four blocks and some nine. There is a time limit for each item, and there is bonus credit for speedy solutions of the difficult items.

In attempting to match the designs, the clear-cut organic patient will encounter difficulty early in the test, perhaps beginning with the very first item. He may be concerned that the design in the booklet is smaller in size than the design he will make with his blocks; he may be concerned with the absence of dividing lines on the pictured design, because this does not correspond with the lines formed by the juxtaposed edges of his blocks; he may be unable to analyze the pictured designs into their components and will accordingly be limited to making no attempt or arbitrary attempts; he may construct a rotated version of the design; and he may experience difficulty in the motor execution of his attempted solution. He may solve some of the problems only after exceeding the generous time limit. In these difficulties, he will therefore indicate not only problems of visual-motor coordination, but problems of conceptual thinking (analysis and re-synthesis of the designs and difficulty with similarity rather than identity of reproduction), and of spatial orientation (the correct position of the blocks).

One test often used to assess visual-motor organization is the Bender Visual-Motor Gestalt Test.[4] In this test, the patient is presented with a series of cards, one at a time, on each of which is a relatively simple geometric figure. He is to copy each figure on a sheet of paper. The first card shows a circle flanked by a diamond, with one corner of the diamond touching the edge of the circle; the second card shows a series of dots in a straight line; a later design shows three sides of a rectangle and a snaky line passing it by and just touching one of its corners.

In this test, the patient must obviously be able to retain his orientation in space, and execute dots, straight lines, and curves with good control; arrange to have lines cross or just touch; and move his pencil to and from his body, from left to right or right to left, and at various angles to his body, often reversing direction in the course of a continuous movement. Because of his impaired visual-motor organization and the associated tendency to be disoriented in space, and because of his impaired ability to grasp visual patterns (just as he can hardly, if at all, grasp abstract verbal concepts), the severely organic patient encounters considerable difficulty. He may rotate the figures, misplace them, and perseverate in making the series of dots; he may be unable to execute dots and may substitute loops, which, developmentally, are primitive versions of dots; he frequently takes an exceedingly long time to make the figures and then only by dint of very slow sketching and repeated erasing.

The Draw-a-Person Test, referred to earlier in connection with projective tests, is also pertinent in regard to visual-motor functioning. Despite his taking great pains, the brain-damaged patient is likely to draw a highly primitivized, incomplete, tentative, and sometimes almost unrecognizable human figure—one that is in some ways similar to those produced by preschool children. This impaired performance indicates, in particular, the conceptual as well as visual-motor primitivization of his body image.

Problems of Differential Diagnosis

Several problems of differential diagnosis in regard to brain-damaged patients must be mentioned. First, the tests are progressively less clearly diagnostic the lower the premorbid I.Q. of the patient: persons of low intelligence are not only generally uncertain in dealing with the test materials but specifically show a great deal of concreteness of thought and crudeness of execution.

Second, many schizophrenic patients also show marked concreteness of thinking; this is particularly likely when the schizophrenic manifests the complex and still little-understood personality changes that we call "deterioration." It is true, however, that many schizophrenic patients show tendencies toward overabstract thought, and also show tendencies toward fantastic elaboration of morbid content in imagery and language, thus enabling a differential diagnosis to be made from the ordinarily earthbound, colorless, and perplexed organic condition. Most helpful of all in this differential diagnosis is a subtle difference that an experienced examiner can usually detect. The difference is that the organic patient appears to be steadily struggling to respond in terms of simple external reality, whereas the schizophrenic patient appears at least partly lost in, or committed to, his internal, morbid, fantastic world, and to his projections of this world onto the environment. Even so, certain schizophrenics, who were originally of low intelligence or who have shown a marked mental decline, are difficult to differentiate from organic patients.[14] These problems are also discussed in chapters 14–16.

A third differential diagnostic problem is that one cannot count on the same pattern of impairment showing up in each patient with brain damage. In certain cases, the conceptual impairment will be the most striking; in others, the visual-motor impairment will stand out, and so on. Thus, a rigid set of "signs" that applies to all patients and all tests in the battery cannot be established. Perhaps the only consistent finding is a qualitative one that pervades the test results; namely, the concreteness of thought below the level of functioning that may reasonably be expected from the patient.

Finally, differential diagnosis within the realm of brain damage is, at present, difficult. In this area, valuable research still needs to be done. The investigations of Ralph M. Reitan[26] are notable in this regard.

Despite the difficulties mentioned, tests are often strikingly sensitive to subclinical impairments of function. Thus, mild toxic reactions or residual effects of shock treatment may be discerned, if not in quantitative impairments, then in pervasive slight traces of concreteness and confusion. Tests may thus serve an important function in many neurological examinations.

Discussions of these and other tests for identifying and measuring organic deficit will be found in Weider.[39] Goldstein and Martin Scheerer[12] have presented impressive and careful research with conceptual tests and Zygmunt A. Piotrowski's early paper on the Rorschach Test responses of organic patients[24] is still a major reference. Research results obtained with conceptual tests of schizophrenics have been presented by Jacob S. Kasanin[19] and Rapaport *et al.*,[25] among many others. Ward C. Halstead's extensive research with a battery of varied tests[13] must also be mentioned.

Collaboration of Psychiatrist and Psychologist

Referral for testing is indicated whenever there is a question of differential diagnosis within or between the neurotic disorders and psychotic disorders, and also where brain damage and mental deficiency are in question. Although the test findings do not always lead to unequivocal diagnostic conclusions, they can be counted on to contribute significant evidence bearing on the alternative possibilities. Referral for psychological testing is also indicated whenever it seems necessary to arrive in a short time at a formulation of the organization and dynamics of the patient's personality. The test report may confirm, amplify, amend, and in some cases apparently contradict the initial clinical impressions. The need to assess change during or after a course of treatment is a third indication for testing. Finally, appraisal of the patient's intellectual level may also be carried out most accurately with the help of tests.

One of the chief indications for the use of psychological tests stems not from clinical practice but from research questions. Tests have been used fruitfully in many psychiatrically oriented research projects. Some of these uses have been referred to above.[4, 6, 9, 12–15, 17, 19–21, 24–29, 40] The addition of test findings to those obtained by interview and behavioral observation will no doubt continue to round out research into important questions concerning the structure and mechanisms of the different psychogenic, psychosomatic, and neurological disease entities; the assessment of personality and personality change; and the crucial patterns of relations among group members (including family groups and therapist–patient groups).

A number of typical problems that come up in the *clinical* collaboration of psychiatrist and psychologist-as-psychodiagnostician will be discussed briefly.

(1) *Referral:* It is wisest for the psychiatrist to refer a patient for testing with a statement of the questions he hopes to have answered and to let the psychologist decide on the tests to be used to help answer these questions. Psychodiagnosis is a subtle and complex matter. There are few psychiatrists who have studied and worked with the tests sufficiently to have expert opinions as to the techniques to be employed. Also, it is often advisable to discuss the referral with the psychologist in advance, in order to be sure that testing is appropriate to help answer the questions. Sometimes, for example, a patient may be referred for testing because a therapeutic or administrative impasse has developed; and the solution of the problem may not require more test-derived information about the patient at all. Certain questions with major administrative aspects, such as degree of suicidal risk, readiness for discharge from the hospital, and even the type of therapy indicated, are usually essentially beyond the power of the tests to answer. However, the test results may add to the general understanding of the patient's present condition in these instances and thus contribute to ultimate decision-making.

(2) *Apparent contradictions:* From time to time, psychological test results appear to contradict the clinical impression of the patient. The most frequent instance of this is when the tests indicate schizophrenic features in a patient who manifestly appears to present a neurosis or a character disorder. Assuming a competent psychological appraisal, it is best in such instances to maintain suspended judgment as to the correctness of one or the other impression, for the tests often prove to be right in the long run, even though at other times no evidence is forthcoming to support them. Part of the problem in such instances may lie in differing definitions of schizophrenia, particularly as to its boundaries, or in differing attitudes toward the use

of diagnostic labels. In any case, the core of a good psychological test report will be a description of the patient's patterns of functioning; the diagnostic formulation will really be no more than an attempt to summarize the implications of this description in terms of one or another of the conventional diagnostic labels.

(3) *Assessment of change:* Psychological tests, when repeated during or after a course of therapy, often show less change than expected in patients who appear to have made substantial clinical improvement. This result may be partly a consequence of the fact that the appraisal of change through tests is a relatively unexplored field for research; significant indications of change may be simply overlooked. Part of the explanation undoubtedly is that a good psychodiagnostic evaluation is concerned essentially with basic, deeply ingrained, pervasive modes of function. Qualitative alterations of these modes, so-called character change, are not ordinarily significantly involved in therapeutic progress. Personality changes that occur appear to be primarily quantitative, some already existing trends increasing in strength and others decreasing. In many instances, it appears to make a very big difference in social behavior and adaptation whether the strength of certain impulses, anxieties, guilt feelings, or defenses has been reduced, and whether the tolerance of certain tendencies, such as the sexual, affectionate, and self-assertive, has increased. Relatively small quantitative changes in psychological test patterns often appear to be correlated with significant changes in the clinical picture, which seems to support the view that small quantitative changes may be sufficient for significant behavioral change. The successful therapist should not, therefore, look for massive changes in the test results, though in certain instances, as in the lifting of depression or a severe anxiety state, or the subsiding of an acute psychotic break, a fuller and richer personality picture may be evident in the tests, where before it had been obscured by constricted or bizarre responsiveness.

Certain irrational stresses and strains in the interdisciplinary collaboration of psychiatrist and psychologist have been discussed elsewhere.[31] On the whole, a professional collaboration based on mutual respect, frankness, and knowledge of each other's special skills, and a common frame of reference and set of concepts concerning diagnosis and personality, constitute an excellent foundation for achieving a high degree of accuracy in the assessment of patients.

NOTES

1. Harold H. Anderson and Gladys L. Anderson, eds., *An Introduction to Projective Techniques and Other Devices for Understanding the Dynamics of Human Behavior* (New York: Prentice-Hall, 1951).
2. Samuel J. Beck, *Rorschach's Test* (New York: Grune & Stratton, 1944–1952), 3 vols.

3. Leopold Bellak, *The Thematic Apperception Test and the Children's Apperception Test in Clinical Use* (New York: Grune & Stratton, 1954).
4. Lauretta Bender, *A Visual-Motor Gestalt Test and Its Clinical Use* (Research Monograph No. 3 [New York: American Orthopsychiatric Association, 1938]).
5. Gerald S. Blum, *The Blacky Pictures, Manual of Instructions* (New York: Psychological Corp., 1950).
6. William A. Caudill, *The Psychiatric Hospital as a Small Society* (Cambridge: Harvard University Press, 1958).
7. Lee J. Cronbach, *Essentials of Psychological Testing* (2nd ed.; New York: Harper, 1960).
8. W. Grant Dahlstrom and George Schlager Welsh, *An MMPI Handbook: A Guide to Use in Clinical Practice and Research* (Minneapolis: University of Minnesota Press, 1960).
9. Seymour Fisher and Sidney E. Cleveland, *Body Image and Personality* (Princeton, N. J.: Von Nostrand, 1958).
10. Arnold L. Gesell and Catherine S. Amatruda, *The First Five Years of Life* (New York: Harper, 1940).
11. Kurt Goldstein, *The Organism* (New York: American Book Company, 1939).
12. Kurt Goldstein and Martin Scheerer, *Abstract and Concrete Behavior*, "Psychological Monographs," Vol. 53, No. 2, 239 (1941), 1.
13. Ward C. Halstead, *Brain and Intelligence: A Quantitative Study of the Frontal Lobes* (Chicago: University of Chicago Press, 1947).
14. Eugenia Hanfmann and Jacob Kasanin, *Conceptual Thinking in Schizophrenia* ("Nervous and Mental Disease Monograph Series," No. 67 [New York: Nervous and Mental Disease Publishing Company, 1942]).
15. Starke R. Hathaway and Paul E. Meehl, *An Atlas for the Clinical Use of MMPI* (Minneapolis: University of Minnesota Press, 1951).
16. William E. Henry, *The Analysis of Fantasy* (New York: John Wiley, 1956).
17. Robert R. Holt and Joan Havel, "A Method for Assessing Primary and Secondary Process in the Rorschach," in Maria A. Rickers-Ovsiankina, ed., *Rorschach Psychology* (New York, John Wiley, 1960).
18. Carl Jung, *Studies in Word-Association* (London: Heinemann, 1918).
19. Jacob S. Kasanin, ed., *Language and Thought in Schizophrenia* (Berkeley: University of California Press, 1944).
20. Bruno Klopfer *et al.*, *Developments in the Rorschach Technique* (Yonkers-on-Hudson, N. Y.: World Book Co., 1954), 2 vols.
21. Jacob Levine and Fredrick Redlich, "Intellectual and Emotional Factors in the Appreciation of Humor," *Journal of General Psychology*, 62 (1960), 25.
22. Alexander R. Luria, *The Nature of Human Conflicts*, translated by W. Horsley Gantt (New York: Liveright, 1932).
23. Henry A. Murray, *Explorations in Personality* (New York: Oxford University Press, 1938).
24. Zygmunt A. Piotrowski, "The Rorschach Inkblot Method in Organic Disturb-

ances of the Central Nervous System," *Journal of Nervous and Mental Disease,* 86 (1937), 525.

25. David Rapaport, Merton M. Gill, and Roy Schafer, *Diagnostic Psychological Testing* (Chicago: Year Book, 1945), 2 vols.
26. Ralph M. Reitan, *The Effect of Brain Lesions on Adaptive Abilities in Human Beings,* unpublished manuscript from the department of neurology, Indiana University Medical Center (1959).
27. Hermann Rorschach, *Psychodiagnostics,* translated by Paul V. Lemkau and B. Kronenberg (New York: Grune & Stratton, 1942).
28. Seymour B. Sarason, *The Clinical Interaction* (New York: Harper, 1954).
29. Helen D. Sargent, *The Insight Test, a Verbal Projective Test for Personality Study* (New York: Grune & Stratton, 1953).
30. Roy Schafer, *The Clinical Application of Psychological Tests* (New York: International Universities Press, 1948).
31. Roy Schafer, *Psychoanalytic Interpretation in Rorschach Testing* (New York: Grune & Stratton, 1954).
32. Morris I. Stein, *The Thematic Apperception Test* (rev. ed.; Cambridge, Mass.: Addison-Wesley, 1955).
33. Percival M. Symonds, *Adolescent Fantasy* (New York: Columbia University Press, 1949).
34. Lewis M. Terman and Maud A. Merrill, *Measuring Intelligence* (New York: Houghton Mifflin, 1959).
35. Charles Eugene Thompson, *Thematic Apperception Test, Thompson Modification* (Cambridge, Mass.: Harvard University Press, 1949).
36. David Wechsler, *Wechsler Intelligence Scale for Children* (New York: Psychological Corp., 1949).
37. David Wechsler, *Manual for the Wechsler Adult Intelligence Scale* (New York: Psychological Corp., 1955).
38. David Wechsler, *The Measurement and Appraisal of Adult Intelligence* (Baltimore: Williams and Wilkins, 1958).
39. Arthur Weider, ed., *Contributions toward Medical Psychology* (New York: Ronald Press, 1953), Vol. 2.
40. Brian Welch, Roy Schafer, and Cynthia F. Dember, "'TAT' Stories of Hypomanic and Depressed Patients," *Journal of Projective Techniques,* 25 (1961), 221.
41. George Schlager Welsh and W. Grant Dahlstrom, eds., *Basic Readings on the MMPI in Psychology and Medicine* (Minneapolis: University of Minnesota Press, 1956).

CHAPTER NINE

Diagnostic Process and Nosology

The Meaning of Diagnosis

Any scientific discipline requires systematic observation, recording, and classifying of its pertinent information. In medicine, these procedures are called *diagnosis.* By means of the diagnostic process, physicians attempt to determine the nature of the disease with which they are confronted and also to distinguish one disease from another. The diagnostic process involves stressing relevant data, eliminating irrelevant information, and arriving at a conclusion that is pertinent to the case at hand. In essence, these are scanning, eliminating, and matching procedures in which physicians have developed unusual skills. The underlying empirical and logical principles are by no means simple. In psychiatry, diagnoses of individual patients as well as systems of nosology are not natural systems but instead depend on a variety of theoretical assumptions.

It is clear that only if two or more cases have anything in common can we make meaningful statements about them or propose any systematic intervention; if each case is idiosyncratic, no diagnosis as such is possible, and treatment remains crudely empirical. In a sense, each case is unique but commonly shares a sufficient number of patterns with some others to be a member of a class of cases. Diagnosis enables clinicians and scientists to communicate effectively with each other about their cases and compare one case with another.

Diagnosis and Therapy

The process of abstraction inherent in the diagnostic process entails the hazard of reductionism. This cannot be overemphasized. In our need to systematize and compare, we often go too far; a living patient may become a colorless case, a concept, or a label. One method of avoiding overreduction is to ask ourselves the seemingly naïve but crucial question: diagnosis for what? Classifications shift, as they should, according to the major purpose for which we classify, for example, etiology, prognosis, research, institutional management, or therapy. Obviously, we diagnose to satisfy our need for systematic scientific presentation, but, pragmatically, physicians diagnose to obtain guidelines for treatment. Diagnosis is implicitly and explicitly in the service of therapy; it provides the necessary focus for therapeutic intervention. Years ago, when psychiatrists functioned primarily as shipping clerks and storekeepers for the insane, they needed a different diagnostic system from that required today, now that a rational form of treatment is beginning to emerge. We agree with Karl Menninger that diagnosis and therapy cannot be separated from each other, any more than psychiatric history-taking can be separated from psychiatric examination.[14] However, we would even go further, by explicitly asserting that diagnosis must be highly differentiated if treatment is highly differentiated. If but one type of treatment is recommended, as in early Rogerian counseling, diagnostic differentiation is unimportant. If highly differentiated methods of treatment are available, as in the modern therapy of infections, they are invariably matched with equally differentiated diagnostic methods. A major reason for the lack of emphasis on a highly differentiated descriptive diagnostic classification in the United States—and a corresponding emphasis on dynamic individuation—is the fact that a highly individualized psychotherapy has become such an important therapeutic instrument here. Yet, the purposes for which classifications are made should be kept in mind. One purpose, aside from the ever-present demands of therapy, is to sharpen the physician's perceptions and to challenge him to discriminate and discover. Through working with patients in analytic therapy, we have found, and have come to focus on, features of behavior (for example, identity, transference) which were, of course, missed by earlier classifiers. We do not believe psychiatry has yet adapted to the newer orders of information, nor sifted out those modern concepts and operations that are relevant for diagnosis. Today, some psychiatrists who believe that everything can be treated by one method abhor diagnostic distinctions as intruding upon the encounter of one human with another. However, a developed sense both of descriptive diagnosis and of diagnosis through evidence gathered in therapeutic interactions—an investigative attitude—is increasingly required for the sound development of a scientific psychiatry.

Diagnosis is in the service of therapy, but the word therapy is in itself ambiguous and covers many types of intervention; for instance, we include under the term (wrongly, to be sure) the segregation and incarceration of persons who are considered to be dangerous and undesirable. Some of our broader diagnostic labels (for example, psychosis) serve to a certain extent the purpose of facilitating such segregation. This again shows that diagnostic and therapeutic activity must be viewed not only in professional and scientific terms, but also in a wide psychosocial context. Criteria for hospitalization have changed; a quite "sick" patient today may be maintained outside an institution, depending in part on practical circumstances and in part on the possible social consequences of his behavior, rather than the severity of his particular symptoms.

Two different psychiatric diagnostic approaches may be distinguished. The clinical diagnosis of the individual patient is a psychiatric formulation, which weighs the relevant descriptive and etiological data pertinent to the therapeutic planning for this patient (and no other). The second type is a research and epidemiological diagnosis, permitting the comparison of populations of cases.

Semantic Confusion

The language of psychiatry is an overelaborated professional jargon, confused and confusing. There are so many points of view, so many schools, so many national differences that very few diagnostic concepts mean one and the same thing to all psychiatrists. Common diagnostic terms, as schizophrenia, psychopathic personality, psychosis, neurosis, and the like, mean different things to different psychiatrists; and to some, these terms mean nothing whatsoever. If one and the same behavior disorder is called an anxiety reaction in the U.S.A., vegetative dystonia in Germany, and neurasthenia (with the connotation of cerebral exhaustion) in the U.S.S.R.; and if it is recognized that these terms denote the same phenomenon, communication is still possible, and data about similar events may be compared. Leaders in our field are uncomfortably aware of our semantic troubles. Jules H. Masserman chastises psychiatry for the clumsy use of psychiatric words and compares it to the use of astrological terms in modern astronomy.[13] Another critic, Thomas S. Szasz, rightly chides us for the use of panchreston—words that explain everything.[26] However, the problem is by no means only a question of terminology; the terminology reflects our lack of empirical knowledge and, in some instances, a certain disregard for principles of logic. At bottom, our task is one of observation, of alert matching and comparison of clinical phenomena. Historically, of course, this has always been the task; but with an appreciation of what is constant and what is variable in behavior, or what is primary and secondary, we can now hope for a more informed diagnostic approach.

The use of appropriate diagnostic labels is of importance to the expert, but it is also important to the lay person, and care must be taken that lay persons do not become confused by psychiatric terminology. Difficulties often arise when patients misunderstand the diagnostic labels used by their therapists.[18] For example, a patient with a mild reactive depression is told he is suffering from a depression; he promptly looks up the word in a medical dictionary and forthwith assumes he is suffering from a severe disorder. Patients have a need, as do their therapists, to label their troubles, but without help they are rarely equipped to handle the labels psychiatrists offer them, explicitly or inadvertently. At times, patients attach highly individual labels to themselves and become known by these trademarks, which serve, in a family group or hospital, as identifying devices to themselves and to others. A patient persistently complains to one and all that he has "no feelings" and becomes known by his own term, "the hollow man." This is the "lay diagnosis," the explanation by which he and the group recognize his illness.

Classes and Types of Disorder

The logical rules for diagnosing are quite clear; one pigeonhole for every disorder and no overlap between them. As Carl G. Hempel elegantly puts it, the classes must be mutually exclusive and jointly exhaustive.[8] The diagnostic scheme must not cover up our ignorance; the individual diagnosis must be valid and reliable. Validity means that the terms correspond to demonstrably real phenomena. The term agoraphobic, for instance, refers to a person who suffers from a pathological fear of open places; such persons exist—it is a valid term. The term *passive-aggressive* personality designates a person who uses his excessive passivity in a hostile manner. This term is also valid but much more difficult to delineate reliably; how passive and how hostile must a person be to deserve this label? Diagnosis must be reliable and must permit a high level of agreement among observers; and this, as H. H. Strupp and J. V. Williams have shown,[25] is often not the case. The need for operational definitions of diagnostic terms has already been mentioned (see Chapter 7). We must define diagnostic concepts in terms of the elementary operations that lead to them. For example: What do you specifically observe that constitutes "passive-aggressive" behavior? Put simply, we must be able to give instances and make clear how we know what we assert.

Hempel pointed out that many phenomena that we describe cannot be grouped into classes but rather comprise types.[8] Members of a class have characteristics that differentiate them clearly from members of another class; for example, cats from dogs; liver diseases from pulmonary diseases; or, getting closer to psychiatry, a behavior disorder associated with general paresis from a behavior disorder associated with brain tumor. Types, on the other hand, are hypothetical constructs; we assume their existence and know that, in reality, concrete phenomena only approximate them. Between two types there may be an infinite number of transitional phenomena or "border states"; or there may be some definite clustering around the "ideal" type, a finding which often gives the semblance of the existence of classes.

At our present level of knowledge, it seems that we have great difficulty grouping into classes those behavior disorders that are not caused by organic lesions. When we speak of an anxiety reaction, for instance, we mean that anxious behavior is judged to be excessive, extreme, important or striking, and that it is, in any case, in the foreground of our observations; in a different patient it may be mild and occur only rarely. There is, however, no one who has never experienced anxiety. Accordingly, "diagnosis" becomes a matter of quantitative measurement, which at present in most cases is neither feasible nor practical. In practice, we are quite satisfied to designate as an anxiety reaction an extreme type without any pretense of attempting exact measurement. This type, however, can only be differentiated by approximation from other, less anxious types. Most psychiatric diagnoses, then, with the exception of some organic reactions, are typological diagnoses. In time, as we acquire a greater ability to describe or measure significant behavioral variations of a population, we will become much less concerned with types, a trend that is currently noticeable in the biological sciences.

Diagnosing Diseases and Behavior Disorders

In organic medicine, we differentiate between the *subjective symptoms,* for example, the patient's reports about pain or about other experiences, which he describes in the course of a clinical history, and *objective signs* noted during physical examination. In examinations of human behavior, the difference between signs and symptoms, and between objective behavior and experience, is less clear. If a patient reports an anxiety attack, do we view it as a symptom? Or, if we observe it, does it become a sign? It is advantageous to view them both as significant items of behavior and also to record any similarities and incongruities between verbal accounts and observed behavior that may be of diagnostic and therapeutic significance.

We have already stated that it is preferable to speak of behavior disorders rather than of mental, emotional, or psychological illness. Psychiatrists, of course, are concerned with many aspects of organic disease: with brain diseases that cause behavior changes; with the so-called psychosomatic diseases, which are influenced by or possibly caused by emotional factors; and, finally, with behavioral reaction to general illness and injury. Notwithstanding such relations and interactions, the concepts of abnormal behavior and demonstrable organic pathology should not be confused.

That the coding of input, or response to stress, or capacity to adapt must be biologically mediated, and that some yet-to-be-discovered tissue mechanisms may be wholly or partially accountable for certain disorders, is not at issue. More basic is the fact that many persons with behavior disorders are cast into the sick role. First and last, we are concerned with troublesome and inept behavior. Whether behavior disorder is the best term remains to be seen. In any case, it is a broader term than disease, and whatever the causes of disorder, the disordered *behavior* remains an essential category for description, correlation, and analysis.

The tendency of psychiatry to see behavior disorders as diseases is not surprising. Psychiatry is a child of medicine, and our medical training has strongly influenced our basic terminological concepts. Such words as *neurosis* and *psychosis,* resembling medical diagnostic terms with their Greek endings, have perpetuated the tradition that underlies both our language and orientation. Persons suffering from behavior disorders are said to be "ill"; they are called "patients"; they are referred for "treatment"; they are admitted to hospitals and clinics; and, all too often, they are put into beds whether they need bed rest or not. Thus, all behavior disorders are still referred to by most psychiatrists as "mental illness." The implications of the sick role have not sufficiently penetrated our thinking. Whether all persons suffering from behavior disorders without brain disease should enjoy the advantages of the sick role—and assume the burden of its disadvantages as well—is an open question that cannot be answered by a general statement. (See Chapter 5.) The impairment of function which the core groups of behavior disorders show is, without question, a real handicap in those relationships in which responsibility and reliability are expected; persons with such disorders are, of course, compelled, by their inability to sustain normal obligations, to move into some situation in which they exempt themselves from expected functions.

The disease concept in psychiatry has been severely criticized by Szasz, who holds that mental illness has become a myth, much as the witches and evil spirits, which at one time were supposed to explain certain types of deviant behavior.[26] Szasz ridicules psychiatric diagnostic efforts by comparing them to the efforts of a blind policeman directing traffic on a superhighway. Yet, the tendency to equate behavior disorder and illness to some degree has worked as a positive force for the development of a scientific psychiatry; otherwise, the term could not have been kept alive for so long. Before the behavioral sciences were sufficiently developed, this concert of disease permitted an objective and scientific approach to behavioral deviations. Sigmund Freud made his fundamental discoveries about the neuroses by approaching them initially from the vantage point of a medical and biological tradition. In both illnesses and behavior disorders, we discern noxious or stressful stimuli, and defensive and restitutive responses. The stresses may be more than the organism can handle, with faulty function as the result. Such considerations have induced George L. Engel to use a unified concept of adaptation for health and disease in psychiatry and general medicine.[4] Of course some psychoses (for example, febrile delirium) are physical illnesses or, more precisely, manifestations of physical illness. In its broad biological meaning, the concept of illness led to models by which we understand aspects of behavior disorder, for example: levels of integration of mental function (introduced by John Hughlings Jackson to explain behavior in cerebral lesions); or the role of defensive efforts in leading to symptom formation; and the damaging secondary consequences of symptoms that follow models of the inflammatory process and the unfortunate consequences of reparative processes, as in scar formation.

The assertion that disease is a "myth" can lead to a conception of the malfunctioning evident in behavior disorder that is equally as mythological as the misapplication of the disease model. Metaphorically, we all may be players strutting upon a stage; but if we are all simply playing a role, we still need to investigate how the casting came to be, and why it is that sick roles are not easily interchanged. The questions at the heart of the problems of differentiating the multiple factors leading to behavior disorder, and the relationship between biological and psychosocial factors, cannot be abolished by a semantic sleight-of-hand. It should also be remembered that there is no great harm in using the handy and familiar words, ill and sick (how awkward it would be to say "behavior disordered") as long as we know that mental, emotional, or behavioral illness is not identical with physical illness.

Diagnosing Psychosis and Neurosis

These are some time-honored diagnostic concepts in psychiatry; actually, these terms are so universally accepted that we conveniently forget the embarrassing fact that it is very difficult to define them. The term *psychosis*—in different contexts—has been reserved for severe and sweeping disturbances of the higher mental functions; the student will have no difficulty recognizing these, even if our formal definitions are unsatisfactory. In the *neuroses*, the higher mental functions are relatively unimpaired. Freud devoted an article to the psychoanalytic differentiation of psychosis and neurosis. In psychosis, he thought the disturbance lay in a rift between ego and the environment; in neurosis, the conflict was between id and ego, the latter representing the pressures of the outer world and the superego.[6] In this article, Freud stressed the internalized and conflictual nature of neurosis and the more severe and overt impairment of adaptive and ego-functions in psychosis. Yet, empirically it is sometimes difficult to draw a sharp line between psychosis and neurosis. Further, theoretical distinctions are not absolute; neurotics have adaptive problems, and psychotics have conflicts; both conditions impair reality-testing, though in different degrees. From a social point of view, the difference between psychotic and neurotic can be reduced to a difference of the psychiatric sick role, which we have already discussed. For psychotics, the sick role is often mandatory; the extent to which the sick role is extended to neurotics and sociopaths is far from settled, either in the minds of experts or the general public.

The validity and usefulness of the concepts of neurosis and psychosis, and their differentiation, were questioned by Karl M. Bowman,[3] Fredrick C. Redlich,[22] and others. Clearly, severity of the disorder is not a completely satisfactory criterion. Some disorders we label neuroses; for example, certain obsessive–compulsive neuroses, may be severe, socially disabling, and resistive to treatment. Some schizophrenic reactions, which we call psychoses, may be relatively mild and transient; others may not interfere too seriously with many aspects of everyday living. In the face of constantly changing facilities and techniques of treatment, it seems unrealistic to create a rigid compartmentalization of severe and mild disorders. The best and possibly the only differentiating criterion is the fact that in psychosis the higher mental faculties, which permit us to recognize and evaluate the inner and outer world, are more deeply impaired than in neurosis. In any case, these broad diagnostic categories all too frequently force us to assume the existence of "borderline" cases. The sharp boundary between neurosis and psychosis is undoubtedly spurious, and one wonders why we have clung to these terms so tenaciously. Pierre Janet suggested that their usefulness lies in social and legal applications; [9] in legal usage, however, the terms psychosis or insanity have more often obscured than illuminated the crucial issue of responsibility for socially undesirable behavior. We believe that the elimination of the terms psychosis and neurosis would create terminological progress. But we cannot hope that fundamental terminological change will be achieved rapidly and, in any case, not by dictate. Eugen Kahn proposed a long time ago to drop the term neurosis, with little success.[10] In this book, the word *psychosis* is used somewhat loosely but sparingly as a one-word term for severe behavior disorders with impairment of the higher mental processes; the term *neurosis* is retained for a broad grouping of, generally speaking, milder personality disorders.

Our efforts to "pigeonhole" are more justified in dealing with behavior disorders with demonstrable physical etiology than in the case of behavior disorders without such pathology, such as the neuroses and sociopathies. Whether the "functional psychoses," the schizophrenias and the manic-depressive psychoses can be rigorously delineated and classified is an open question. These disorders were differentiated according to their symptomatology and course by Emil Kraepelin; [11] this attempt was considered one of the outstanding contributions of the "great classifier." Yet, the longer we study these disorders, the less we are convinced that current views of their diagnostic boundaries are correct. Today, we are almost as hard put to set the boundaries between some of these psychoses and the neurotic reactions, as we are to delineate the fuzzy distinction between the normal and the neurotic. Nonetheless, the core disorders can be identified before they merge into shades of gray. Some psychiatrists view normality, neuroses, and psychoses as comprising a continuum of behavioral states, but the drastic consequences of certain inputs in severe psychosis and the usually profound disruption in function suggest a discontinuity—a discretely different organization. In one sense, a continuity is evident in that all these conditions constitute different levels or states of organization of homologous behavioral operations. Perhaps an apt analogy is water and ice: these are consequentially different states of the identical material, each state involving qualitative as well as quantitative differences; only a small temperature decrease near the freezing point is consequential for a change of state from water to ice; the effect of the same input at a higher temperature would be unapparent. Too often, however, we seem to be moving in slush!

Nosological Approaches

All nosological approaches are admixtures of *etiological* and *symptomatic* points of view. Even if the etiological considerations predominate, as is the case with the American Psychiatric Association classification,[1] descriptive considerations crop up in all subclasses. Since our knowledge of the etiological factors in behavior disorders is quite undeveloped, it is not surprising that the lacunae of the system must be filled in by descriptive detail. E. Stengel concludes rightly that the coexistence of etiological and symptomatic points of view is necessary and should not bother us unduly.[24] The shift of interest from descriptive to dynamic considerations came with the impact of psychoanalysis; it was assumed that insight into unconscious conflict helps the patient, and this assumption moved our diagnostic interest from phenomenological description to the dynamic formulation of such conflicts and their genesis. It followed that the mere word *descriptive* wrongly gained the derogatory connotation of an old-fashioned approach—a sterile inventory of an ancient check list of odd behavior—whereas anything that was *dynamic* came to be regarded as superior and progressive!

Clinical and Statistical Approaches

Clinicians employ a variety of methods to achieve a reduction of variables and to stress the most relevant ones. They rely to a certain extent on deductive theoretical approaches, but for the most part they depend on the broad empirical knowledge derived from the observation of all kinds of patients and problems of living. The good clinician exploits in full measure such undefinable qualities as intuition and empathy. In psychiatry, there are relatively few pathognomic signs that permit a diagnosis. When asked how they arrive at a diagnosis, psychiatrists are often at a loss to answer. They do not wish to be secretive or authoritative, but the operations leading to a diagnosis are intuitive as well as empirical and logical; often, it is the context in which the abnormal behavior occurs that impresses the diagnostician, and although it is possible to do so, this is difficult to objectify. Those diagnoses that do stem from intuitive processes must, of course, be defended within the framework of descriptive, empirical science and logic; this goes without saying. And the fact is that the intuitive diagnosis frequently predicts the nature, extent, and tractability of the impairments a patient is apt to experience.

During the last few decades, there has been, in general medicine, an increasing reliance on objective methods and particularly on a great variety of laboratory procedures. A multitude of findings has accumulated, which cannot be reduced clinically to a few common denominators, and this has required the introduction into medicine and psychiatry of sophisticated statistical methods, such as factor analysis and other multiple-correlation techniques. Psychologists and others have used such techniques to demonstrate basic characteristics of clusters of behavioral phenomena in psychiatric disorders.[5, 27] In general, psychiatrists have not paid enough attention to the efforts of these "tough-minded" scientists, possibly because the subtlety of clinical diagnosis often is lost in the statistical meat grinder. Whether the primary data fed to the statisticians and computers are truly adequate and "primary" is probably at the heart of the dissatisfaction with these procedures. Most "elements" of behavior have a variety of different meanings, depending on their context; and it requires laborious work to specify items for quantification. Henry A. Murray,[19] Timothy Leary,[12] and Ernst Prelinger and Carl N. Zimet [20] used aptly descriptive, dynamic, and epigenetic variables and have provided us with complex systematic approaches to diagnosis. Roy R. Grinker has demonstrated that a well-trained clinical group can reliably specify objectifiable behavioral items which are relevant to clinical material, for example, in depression or anxiety.[7] The results of these time-consuming investigations have so far not been extensively used in practical clinical work, but they have impressed us both with the enormous complexity of personality diagnosis and the feasibility of employing objective techniques for clinical research purposes.

Comprehensive Diagnosis

A variety of approaches is necessary to deal with a wide spectrum of behavior disorders, ranging from brain diseases to psychogenic disorders. In principle, these diagnostic approaches can be grouped into biological, psychological, and sociological categories. Formulations, psychodynamic and epigenetic summaries of the patient's problems and traits, are gradually replacing the old one-word diagnoses in many American psychiatric centers. Whether one or the other of these approaches predominates depends on the nature of the individual diagnostic problem, as well as on the orientations of the individual clinician and his institution. The replacement of the old label diagnosis by a broader formulation has led some to contend that American psychiatry is not interested in behavioral description and diagnosis. We hold that this accusation is not correct. In part, the charge is directed at an overly exclusive focus on psychodynamic and psychogenetic mechanisms, on inferences about unconscious conflict and development while explicit historical and behavioral data and concurrent information from relatives and friends are ignored. Such exclusiveness impairs perspectives in assessing the patient, but this is simply bad psychiatric practice. The fact is that the pragmatic American psychiatrist has not been satisfied with labels, which all too often do not fit the package and do not predict the behavior in which he is interested. At times the parsimony of a single diagnosis leads to distortion. In general, we remain closer to the data by making a biological diagnosis and a psychosocial diagnosis: these, if knowledge permits, may be integrated. The use of diagnostic formulations is preferred because one-word labels never do justice to the complex facts of psychiatry, to the mixtures of coping ability, symptoms, disorganization, persisting immaturity, and potential for regression and new learning, which we try to assess in each patient. In addition, during the last decades psychiatrists have also become explicitly interested in the social events surrounding each behavior disorder. The "natural history" of psychotic disorders, once restricted to shifts in symptomatology, was observed largely within the singular confines of an asylum and now appears ready for new and more comprehensive study.

Modern psychiatry is not interested, as it used to be, in dealing with stable states, but with dynamic processes. These processes often defy any abstraction other than apt description. The dynamic and multifactorial approach, incidentally, is not only characteristic for psychiatry but also gaining importance in general medicine. In summary, we consider diagnostic formulation, or a comprehensive diagnosis of an individual patient, a scientifically and therapeutically sound procedure.

Why then are one-word categories used at all? The reason, apart from medical conservatism, is psychiatry's need not merely to characterize the behavior disorders of the individual patient but of populations of patients. One-word diagnoses, in contrast to diagnostic formulations, are not subtle, complex, or precise enough for clinical work (and never will be), but they are potentially useful in epidemiological work and public health planning; and it should be pointed out that some labels, of course, are better, and more defensible, than others. The labels designating behavior disorders associated with cerebral and known genetic diseases, for example, are relatively precise. In contrast, such labels as schizophrenia or depression, and the broad designations of psychosis and neurosis, have a relatively low degree of validity and reliability. Admittedly, this has implications for our therapeutic and scientific activities. Perhaps a more enlightened psychiatry of the future will scorn our diagnostic attempts as much as we scorn those of our forebears in the Middle Ages and antiquity.

Current Systems of Epidemiological Classification

Emil Kraepelin's system of classification, revised over the years in the seven editions of his classical textbook of psychiatry,[11] was based on etiological, symptomatological, and prognostic principles. He referred to his nosological entities by such terms as disorder (German: *Störung*) but also insanity and mental diseases. He assumed the existence of classes of disorders that could be clearly recognized and delineated. In his "provisional" classification, Kraepelin differentiated disorders associated with brain diseases and disorders produced by psychological causes. In the first group he included: mental disorders produced by brain trauma; disorders produced by cerebral diseases; mental disorders caused by poisoning, including alcoholism and other addictions; mental disturbances in infections, with a separate section for syphilitic diseases; arteriosclerotic, senile, and presenile insanities; dementia praecox; epilepsy; and manic–depressive insanity. The psychologically caused diseases are divided into four groups. In the first group, psychological traumatic factors are of prime importance; it includes nervous exhaustion, "fright neurosis," psychogenic depression, induced insanity, prison psychosis, and traumatic neurosis. In the second and third groups, constitutional "endogenous" factors are most important. The second group includes hysteria and paranoia. A special constitutionally deviant group forms the third group and includes nervousness, impulsive insanity (poriomania, kleptomania, and so forth), and sexual deviations. These disorders, again, are differentiated from the fourth group, consisting of erethitic, weak, odd, and rigid psychopaths; liars and swindlers; and enemies of society. Idiots, imbeciles, and morons comprise the last group in Kraepelin's classification. From the very beginning, Kraepelin's formulations were criticized by many of his leading contemporaries, especially by Karl Bonhoeffer,[2] whose distinction between exogenous and endogenous psychoses is still recognized by many European psychiatrists. As psychiatric therapy was virtually nonexistent in Kraepelin's day, there is little reference in his work to the therapeutic implications of the diagnostic classes; there is also no consideration of social data because, like most of his colleagues, Kraepelin studied patients in the isolation of the traditional psychiatric institutions of his time. Kraepelin had prognostic criteria strongly in mind, and surely a nosology with prognostic value has merit. However, our actual ability to prognosticate in the individual case is reminiscent of the old king who was able to identify a witch by boiling her in a stewpot and tasting the broth. Kraepelin's terminology sounds strange and archaic, but it must not be overlooked that his system has become the matrix of most subsequent classifications and that his influence, in spite of his shortcomings, has remained strong.

J. E. Meyer reviewed the current schemes of nosology of behavior disorders.[17] These schemes reflect, as one would expect, the basic theoretical points of view of their authors. A system devised by Karl Kleist and his student, Karl Leonhard, is based on the assumption of localizable cerebral dysfunction. The Scandinavians, Erik Essen-Moeller, Gabriel Langfeldt, and Erik Stromgren, have slightly modified the Kraepelinian system and adapted it to their epidemiological interests. Henrious C. Rümke's complex classification and the Russian classification show strong links to Kraepelinian ideas. The systems of Kurt Schneider in Germany; of L. van der Horst in Holland; and of Henri Ey and Pierre Pichot in France contain both phenomenological and etiological points of reference. Adolf Meyer's classification of *ergasias*, a Greek word for reaction types, is virtually forgotten today. Meyer's use of the concept of mental illness as reactions to the life situation, however, has been of lasting importance.[16] Recently, existentialist psychiatrists have questioned current systems of classification but have not devised any approach to replace the old schemes for communication within the profession. The same can be said, as we shall see, about psychoanalysis.

Freud, who contributed most to the undermining of the Kraepelinian system, never explicitly attacked it. He was somewhat contemptuous of the academic diagnostic approach and not interested in it, but he used Kraepelin's classification because there was none better. His own early departures in diagnostic differentiation, such as between actual neurosis, transference neurosis, and narcissistic neurosis, never became popular. In general, psychoanalysts have been markedly uninterested in classification. Sandor Rado devised a diagnostic scheme which has not been widely used.[21] Ernst Kris once expressed the idea to us that diagnoses should be based on the use of the prevalent defense mechanism, for example, identifiers, deniers, projectors, and the like; but the idea was not developed further.

Karl Menninger is the one contemporary psychoanalyst who has been seriously concerned with problems of classification. He takes a stand for a unitary concept of mental disease, of the sort which has been advanced over the last hundred years by a number of psychiatrists.[15] Menninger regards mental illness as a failure of adaptation to stresses: the emergency devices required may be painful, cumbersome, or handicapping and may themselves require treatment. Mental diseases are seen as varying in intensity but not in their essential character. Menninger assumes that, depending on capacities of the ego to adapt, progressive stages of "dysorganization" result, manifesting themselves in five levels of "dyscontrol." In a major publication he describes these five levels: nervousness, neurosis, naked aggression, psychosis, and, finally, malignant anxiety and death. We agree with many of Menninger's points: in his emphasis on describing stresses and the patient's behavior in mastering stresses or failing to do so; in his recommendations to describe syndromes but not to set up artificial classes, and to avoid reification. Yet Menninger creates a new classification with new artifacts, such as including addiction with neuroses and organic brain syndromes and epilepsies with naked aggression. In our opinion, a unitary concept for all behavior disorders, including those caused by brain diseases, is apt to oversimplify. It tends to settle for holistic pseudo-knowledge without tapping the complex and manifold data that will eventually lead to our understanding of the causes, mechanisms, and goals of deviant behavior.

The Quest for a Simple Scheme

The Psychiatric Division of the World Health Organization commissioned Stengel to examine the problem of an international classification.[23] Stengel stresses that a prerequisite for a truly satisfactory classification would be a far-reaching agreement on basic concepts and theories, an agreement that is unlikely at present. He states that an unpretentious beginning might be made, however, by adopting a relatively simple scheme such as the one recently presented by J. E. Meyer.[17] This author recognizes neurotic and sociopathic reactions, schizophrenias, affective disorders, various cerebral syndromes, and mental deficiency. Such a scheme, even if not universally accepted, seems simple enough to permit conceptual translation into other simple schemes. However, the simplicity itself may lead to faulty abstractions. Paradoxically, then, our schemes are either too complex or too simple; and in any case, they rarely fit the data.

Apart from the efforts of individual authors, two schemes of classification deserve to be mentioned: the Psychiatric Section of the International Statistical Classification of Disease (ISCD)[28] and the classification of the American Psychiatric Association (APA).[1] The ISCD has found little favor with international psychiatry. It has been considered unmanageable, incomplete, complicated, incoherent, and inconsistent. The ISCD is being used in the United Kingdom, Finland, New Zealand and Thailand; British psychiatrists in general find it unsatisfactory.[23] The American Psychiatric Association classification is the product of a hard-working committee, which was headed by the late George N. Raines. Because it is the only diagnostic classification widely used in the United States, we are reporting it in some detail. *The Diagnostic and Statistical Manual, Mental Disorders,* published by The American Psychiatric Association, offers the following nomenclature.

DISORDERS CAUSED BY OR ASSOCIATED WITH IMPAIRMENT OF BRAIN TISSUE FUNCTION

ACUTE BRAIN DISORDERS

Disorders Due to or Associated with Infection

Acute Brain Syndrome associated with intracranial infection. *Specify infection*

Acute Brain Syndrome associated with systemic infection. *Specify infection*

Disorders Due to or Associated with Intoxication

Acute Brain Syndrome, drug or poison intoxication. *Specify drug or poison*

Acute Brain Syndrome, alcohol intoxication.
Acute hallucinosis
Delirium tremens

Disorders Due to or Associated with Trauma

Acute Brain Syndrome associated with trauma. *Specify trauma*

Disorders Due to or Associated with Circulatory Disturbance

Acute Brain Syndrome associated with circulatory disturbance. (*Indicate cardiovascular disease as additional diagnosis.*)

Disorders Due to or Associated with Disturbance of Innervation or of Psychic Control

Acute Brain Syndrome associated with convulsive disorder. (*Indicate manifestation by Supplementary Term.*)

Disorders Due to or Associated with Disturbances of Metabolism, Growth or Nutrition

Acute Brain Syndrome with metabolic disturbance. *Specify*

Disorders Due to or Associated with New Growth

Acute Brain Syndrome associated with intracranial neoplasm. *Specify*

Disorders Due to Unknown or Uncertain Cause

Acute Brain Syndrome with disease of unknown or uncertain cause. (*Indicate disease or additional diagnosis.*)

Disorders Due to Unknown or Uncertain Cause with the Functional Reaction Alone Manifest

Acute Brain Syndrome of unknown cause.

CHRONIC BRAIN DISORDERS

Disorders Due to Prenatal (Constitutional) Influence

Chronic Brain Syndrome associated with congenital cranial anomaly. *Specify anomaly*

Chronic Brain Syndrome associated with congenital spastic paraplegia.

Chronic Brain Syndrome associated with Mongolism.

Chronic Brain Syndrome due to prenatal maternal infectious diseases.

Disorders Due to or Associated with Infection

Chronic Brain Syndrome associated with central nervous system syphilis. *Specify as below*

Meningoencephalitic
Meningovascular
Other central nervous system syphilis

Chronic Brain Syndrome associated with intracranial infection other than syphilis. *Specify infection*

Disorders Associated with Intoxication

Chronic Brain Syndrome associated with intoxication.

Chronic Brain Syndrome, drug or poison intoxication. *Specify drug or poison*

Chronic Brain Syndrome, alcohol intoxication. *Specify reaction*

Disorders Associated with Trauma

Chronic Brain Syndrome, brain trauma, gross force. *Specify.* (*Other than operative*)

Chronic Brain Syndrome associated with brain trauma.

Chronic Brain Syndrome, brain trauma, gross force. *Specify.* (*Other than operative*)

Chronic Brain Syndrome following brain operation.

Chronic Brain Syndrome following electrical brain trauma.

Chronic Brain Syndrome following irradiational brain trauma.

Disorders Associated with Circulatory Disturbances

Chronic Brain Syndrome associated with cerebral arteriosclerosis.

Chronic Brain Syndrome associated with circulatory disturbance other than cerebral arteriosclerosis. *Specify*

Disorders Associated with Disturbances of Innervation or of Psychic Control

Chronic Brain Syndrome associated with convulsive disorder.

Disorders Associated with Disturbances of Metabolism, Growth or Nutrition

Chronic Brain Syndrome associated with senile brain disease.

Chronic Brain Syndrome associated with other disturbance of metabolism, growth or nutrition (Includes presenile, glandular, pellagra, familial amaurosis)

Disorders Associated with New Growth

Chronic Brain Syndrome associated with intracranial neoplasm. *Specify neoplasm*

Disorders Associated with Unknown or Uncertain Cause

Chronic Brain Syndrome associated with diseases of unknown or uncertain cause (Includes multiple sclerosis, Huntington's chorea, Pick's disease and other diseases of a familial or hereditary nature.) *Indicate disease by additional diagnosis*

Disorders Due to Unknown or Uncertain Cause with the Functional Reaction Alone Manifest

Chronic Brain Syndrome of unknown cause.

MENTAL DEFICIENCY*

Disorders Due to Unknown or Uncertain Cause with the Functional Reaction Alone Manifest: Hereditary and Familial Diseases of This Nature

Mental deficiency (familial or hereditary).

- Mild
- Moderate
- Severe

Disorders Due to Undetermined Cause

Mental deficiency, idiopathic.

- Mild
- Moderate
- Severe

* Include intelligence quotient (I.Q.) in the diagnosis

DISORDERS OF PSYCHOGENIC ORIGIN OR WITHOUT CLEARLY DEFINED PHYSICAL CAUSE OR STRUCTURAL CHANGE IN THE BRAIN

PSYCHOTIC DISORDERS

Disorders Due to Disturbance of Metabolism, Growth, Nutrition or Endocrine Function

Involutional psychotic reaction.

Disorders of Psychogenic Origin or without Clearly Defined Tangible Cause or Structural Change

Affective reactions.
- Manic depressive reaction, manic type
- Manic depressive reaction, depressive type
- Manic depressive reaction, other
- Psychotic depressive reaction

Schizophrenic reactions.
- Schizophrenic reaction, simple type
- Schizophrenic reaction, hebephrenic type
- Schizophrenic reaction, catatonic type
- Schizophrenic reaction, paranoid type
- Schizophrenic reaction, acute undifferentiated type
- Schizophrenic reaction, chronic undifferentiated type
- Schizophrenic reaction, schizo-affective type
- Schizophrenic reaction, childhood type
- Schizophrenic reaction, residual type

Paranoid reactions.
- Paranoia
- Paranoid state

Psychotic reaction without clearly defined structural change, other than above.

PSYCHOPHYSIOLOGIC AUTONOMIC AND VISCERAL DISORDERS

Disorders Due to Disturbance of Innervation or of Psychic Control

Psychophysiologic skin reaction. (*Indicate manifestation by Supplementary Term*)

Psychophysiologic musculoskeletal reaction. (*Indicate manifestation by Supplementary Term*)

Psychophysiologic respiratory reaction. (*Indicate manifestation by Supplementary Term*)

Psychophysiologic cardiovascular reaction. (*Indicate manifestation by Supplementary Term*)

Psychophysiologic hemic and lymphatic reaction. (*Indicate manifestation by Supplementary Term*)

Psychophysiologic gastrointestinal reaction. (*Indicate manifestation by Supplementary Term*)

Psychophysiologic genito-urinary reaction. (*Indicate manifestation by Supplementary Term*)

Psychophysiologic endocrine reaction. (*Indicate manifestation by Supplementary Term*)

Psychophysiologic nervous system reaction. (*Indicate manifestation by Supplementary Term*)

Psychophysiologic reaction of organs of special sense. (*Indicate manifestation by Supplementary Term*)

PSYCHONEUROTIC DISORDERS

Disorders of Psychogenic Origin or without Clearly Defined Tangible Cause or Structural Change

Psychoneurotic reactions.
- Anxiety reaction
- Dissociative reaction
- Conversion reaction
- Phobic reaction
- Obsessive compulsive reaction
- Depressive reaction
- Psychoneurotic reaction, other

PERSONALITY DISORDERS

Disorders of Psychogenic Origin or without Clearly Defined Tangible Cause or Structural Change

Personality pattern disturbance.
- Inadequate personality
- Schizoid personality
- Cyclothymic personality
- Paranoid personality

Personality trait disturbance.
- Emotionally unstable personality
- Passive-aggressive personality
- Compulsive personality
- Personality trait disturbance, other

Sociopathic personality disturbance.
- Antisocial reaction

Dyssocial reaction
Sexual deviation (*Specify supplementary term*)
Addiction
Alcoholism
Drug Addiction

Special symptom reactions.
Learning disturbance
Speech disturbance
Enuresis
Somnambulism
Other

Transient Situational Personality Disorders

Transient situational personality disturbance.
Gross stress reaction
Adult situational reaction
Adjustment reaction of infancy
Adjustment reaction of childhood
Habit disturbance
Conduct disturbance
Neurotic traits
Adjustment reaction of adolescence
Adjustment reaction of late life

NONDIAGNOSTIC TERMS FOR HOSPITAL RECORD

Alcoholic intoxication (simple drunkenness).

Boarder.

Dead on admission.

Diagnosis deferred.

Disease none.

Examination only.

Experiment only.

Malingerer.

Observation.

Tests only.

The nomenclature limits itself to disorders of mental functioning; it does not include neurological diagnoses. The scheme uses the term disorder to designate groups of related syndromes. Each group is subdivided into reactions. Mental disorders are divided into two large classes: disturbances of mental functioning resulting from cerebral impairment and disorders that are the result of general difficulty in adaptation. It is recognized that cerebral behavioral reactions may also be associated with psychotic and neurotic reactions that are not the result of the cerebral impairment. Mental deficiencies are called primary when no cerebral impairment exists and secondary when the mental deficiency is the result of impairment. The mental deficiencies are characterized according to severity by the designations mild, moderate, and severe. The acute and chronic brain disorders are rigidly separated and differentiated in great detail according to the etiology of the cerebral syndrome.

The disorders of psychogenic origin, or without clearly defined physical cause or structural change in the brain, are subdivided into: psychotic disorders; psychophysiologic, autonomic, and visceral disorders; psychoneurotic disorders; personality disorders; transient situational personality disorders; and a group of "nondiagnostic terms for hospital record." In the psychotic "psychogenic" subgroups, we find many very detailed types of manic-depressive, psychotic-depressive, schizophrenic reactions, including the schizo-affective types. Involutional psychotic reaction, although grouped with the psychogenic reactions, is considered to be caused by disturbance of metabolism, growth, nutrition, or endocrine function. Psychophysiologic reactions, somewhat to our amazement, are listed as due to disturbances of innervation or of psychic control. The psychoneurotic group includes anxiety reaction; a split of hysterical reactions into dissociative reactions and conversion reactions; phobic; obsessive-compulsive; depressive; and "other psychoneurotic reactions." The personality disorders include character neuroses, sociopathic disturbances (including sexual deviations, alcoholism, drug addiction) and such varied syndromes as learning disturbance, speech disturbance, and somnambulism. In the group of transient situational personality disorders, we find such listings as transient situational personality disturbances, gross stress reactions, and various adjustment reactions according to phases of life. The strangest group is "nondiagnostic terms for hospital record," which contains such odd listings as boarder, dead on admission, malingerer, and so forth.

The APA classification is an ambitious scheme. Stengel refers to it with faint irony as an example of the democratic process, which offers something for everyone.[23] It reinforces, like all major systems of classification, a trend to reification and artificiality and contains many diagnostic oddities. The scheme is exhaustive, but also so cumbersome that for most epidemiological research a certain reduction and condensation of entities is necessary. One of the valuable features of the APA classification is the opportunity to list precipitating and predisposing factors; severity; chronicity; and prognosis.

Since no satisfactory, universally accepted classification exists and since all systems of classification necessarily suffer from an inherent rigidity, we believe that this book should not slavishly follow official schemes. In the clinical section of this book, we present a simple and informal scheme of classification. The neuroses, an inclusive term for symptom neuroses, character neuroses, and sociopathies, are grouped together as primarily psychogenic behavior disorders in Chapter 12. Psychosomatic diseases, in which psychogenic factors play a decisive but variable role, make up Chapter 13. Schizophrenias and affective psychoses are discussed in chapters 14 and 15; they are viewed, generally speaking, as behavior disorders of unknown etiology. Chapters 16, 17, and 18 deal with cerebral syndromes associated with behavior disorders. Mental subnormality (Chapter 19) is dealt with separately, in recognition of this field as an important subspecialty. The same applies to behavior disorders in childhood and adolescence (Chapter 20). Behavior disorders in old age (Chapter 21), addiction (Chapter 22), and alcoholism (Chapter 23) are heterogeneous groups, presented in individual chapters for practical reasons. In following such an outline, we were obviously guided more by didactic needs than by taxonomic compulsion. A certain arbitrariness as to what to include in the different syndromes is, at our present state of knowledge, unavoidable; it does not matter so long as the listing is complete. We grant the reader that a bad system is worse than no system at all; but, at the least, we must have a framework for epidemiological work and for discussion of individual patients. We hope we have sufficiently emphasized that the boundaries of behavior disorders are fluid, that border states abound, and that we must beware of false generalizations and reifications.

NOTES

1. *American Psychiatric Association Diagnostic and Statistical Manual for Mental Disorders* (Washington, D.C.: American Psychiatric Association, 1952).
2. Karl Bonhoeffer, "Die exogenen Reaktionstypen," *Archiv für Psychiatrie und Krankheiten*, 58 (1917), 58.
3. Karl M. Bowman and M. Rose, "A Criticism of the Terms 'Psychosis,' 'Psychoneurosis' and 'Neurosis,'" *American Journal of Psychiatry*, 108 (1951), 161.
4. George L. Engel, *Psychological Development in Health and Disease* (Philadelphia: Saunders, 1962).
5. Hans J. Eysenck, *The Structure of Human Personality* (London: Methuen, 1953).
6. Sigmund Freud, "Neurosis and Psychosis" [1924] *Standard Edition* (London: Hogarth Press, 1961), Vol. 19.
7. Roy R. Grinker *et al.*, *The Phenomena of Depressions* (New York: Paul B. Hoeber, 1961).
8. Carl G. Hempel, "Problems of Taxonomy and Their Application to Nosology and Nomenclature in the Mental Diseases," in Joseph Zubin, ed., *Field Studies in the Mental Disorders* (New York: Grune & Stratton, 1961).
9. Pierre Janet, "The Relation of the Neuroses to the Psychoses," A *Psychiatric Milestone* (New York: Society of the New York Hospital, 1921).
10. Eugen Kahn, *Psychopathic Personalities* (New Haven: Yale University Press, 1931).

11. Emil Kraepelin, *Psychiatrie. Ein Lehrbuch für Studierende und Ärzte, 7. Aufl.* (Leipzig: Barth, 1915).
12. Timothy Leary, *Interpersonal Diagnosis of Personality* (New York: Ronald Press, 1957).
13. Jules H. Masserman, "Language, Behaviour and Dynamic Psychiatry," *International Journal of Psycho-Analysis*, 25 (1944), 1.
14. Karl Menninger, A *Manual for Psychiatric Case Study* (New York: Grune & Stratton, 1952).
15. Karl Menninger, *The Vital Balance* (New York: The Viking Press, 1963).
16. Adolf Meyer, *The Collected Papers of Adolf Meyer*, Eunice Winters, ed. (Baltimore: Johns Hopkins Press, 1950).
17. J. E. Meyer, "Problems of Nosology and Nomenclature in the Mental Disorders," in Joseph Zubin, ed., *Field Studies in the Mental Disorders* (New York: Grune & Stratton, 1961).
18. Rafael Moses and D. X. Freedman, " 'Trademark' Function of Symptoms in a Mental Hospital," *Journal of Nervous and Mental Disease*, 127 (1958), 448.
19. Henry A. Murray, *Explorations in Personality* (New York: Oxford, 1938).
20. Ernst Prelinger and Carl N. Zimet, *An Ego-Psychological Approach to Character Assessment* (New York: The Free Press of Glencoe, 1964).
21. Sandor Rado, *Psychoanalysis of Behavior: Collected Papers* (New York: Grune & Stratton, 1956).
22. Fredrick C. Redlich, "Some Sociological Aspects of the Psychoses," in *Theory and Treatment of the Psychoses* (St. Louis: Washington University Studies, 1956).
23. Erwin Stengel, "Classification of Mental Disorders," *Bulletin of the World Health Organization*, 21 (1959), 601.
24. Erwin Stengel, "Problems of Nosology and Nomenclature in the Mental Disorders," in Joseph Zubin, ed., *Field Studies in the Mental Disorders* (New York: Grune & Stratton, 1961).
25. Hans H. Strupp and Joan V. Williams, "Some Determinants of Clinical Evaluations of Different Psychiatrists," *Archives of General Psychiatry*, 2 (1960), 434.
26. Thomas S. Szasz, "The Problems of Psychiatric Nosology," *American Journal of Psychiatry*, 114 (1957), 405.
27. J. Richard Wittenborn and Fred A. Mettler, "Practical Correlates of Psychiatric Symptoms," *Journal of Consulting Psychology*, 15 (1951), 505.
28. *World Health Organization Manual of the International Statistical Classification of Diseases, Injuries and Causes of Death* (Geneva: World Health Organization, 1957).

CHAPTER TEN

General Principles of Psychiatric Treatment: I *The Psychosocial Therapies*

Behavioral Change and Goals of Therapy

A significant trend in modern psychiatry is the increasing importance of therapy in practice and research. An astonishing number of new (and sometimes not so new) therapeutic theories and techniques are proposed. The therapeutic enthusiasm of the younger psychiatrists is startling, perhaps almost frightening, to the older psychiatric generation, with its more conservative view about the immutability of human nature. Today, the unpardonable sin in most psychiatric circles is not that of opposition either to psychological therapy or to the somatic approaches but rather to speak of the general limitations of *any* therapy to effect behavior changes. Extreme positions are advanced: some psychiatrists propose to treat nearly every form of human suffering. Needless to say, an indiscriminate approach may be harmful to patients and detrimental to the prestige of the profession.

A broad and implicit social agreement provides the framework within which community, patient, and therapist regulate their transactions. To require therapeutic attention, behavior disorders must be considered significant by the patient, his community, and the therapist; that is, they must be judged to be at certain levels of severity. Judgments about severity vary, depending upon the social context in which the disorder occurs. The accepted reason for enlisting psychiatric help in an Indonesian jungle is not the same as in Westport, Connecticut, a sophisticated community of 22,000 where about thirty psychiatrists stand ready to help. There is little disagreement about the need for treating problems that are clearly severe, but there is discussion among therapists about the need to help with less severe problems, and about the question of just where the cutoff point should be. But even in the case of a relatively mild problem, there must be agreement that it is a true or significant psychiatric problem. In general, psychiatrists, even in a well-staffed community, should deal with minimal disorders only to prevent serious disorders or if such deviations indicate deeper disturbances, which are, perhaps, obvious only to professional observers.

Patterns of psychiatric practice shift constantly, and in any specific instance there is room for disagreement among the major parties involved. Thus, what the community refers to the psychiatrist may be considered by him a problem for welfare services or educational reform; what the psychiatrist sees as an instance for therapeutic intervention may be thought by the family or community to be a matter for social discipline; or the family may want the psychiatrist to induce conformity in a person whom the psychiatrist diagnoses as being responsibly in conflict with familial values rather than suffering a neurosis. Nevertheless, there is a general consensus concerning the major classes of behavior disorders that warrant psychiatric attention.

The psychiatrist was not always the knight valiant going forth into the community to slay the dragons of mental illness. It is true that in medical-legal situations in civil and military life, the psychiatrist has long been employed as a rather direct agent of social control. But more recently in an extension of traditional public health work, he has entered the community as one of a number of experts acting to ameliorate or shift current social practice. In both instances, he may bring a special regard for the primary interests of the patient as he is related to his community, a regard derived from his experience in mediating the reciprocal needs of patients and families in more traditional therapeutic situations. The psychiatrist certainly knows that, in general, personal or social influences can profoundly temper the intensity and consequences of a behavior disorder. In applying this knowledge to a new context, he encounters special problems of social psychiatry, which can be better understood when the nature, intent, and limits of traditional psychiatric therapy have been appreciated. The hope is that the special viewpoints of psychiatry can bring to the established field of social welfare and community organization more than the mantle of medical authority; but it is not at all clear that this will be possible.

What are the changes in behavior that, under favorable circumstances, therapy will bring about? At a time when all psychiatric troubles were viewed as diseases with specific signs and symptoms, this question could be answered without much difficulty. Behavioral change meant the disappearance or amelioration of the signs and symptoms that brought the patient into therapy. Certainly, in a number of behavior disorders associated with brain diseases, in the psychosomatic disorders, and also in some of the functional psychoses and the symptomatic neuroses that resemble diseases, it is enough to describe behavioral change in terms of alteration of symptoms. However, psychiatrists are dealing to an increasing extent with character neuroses and sociopathies; what does change mean in these cases? What are the goals of psychiatric therapy? The behavioral change must certainly be extensive and not trivial, and this requirement brings us to the consideration of the widely misunderstood concept of cure in psychiatry.

Cure is a medical concept, which denotes complete restoration of function and return to complete well-being. Physicians properly speak of cure after an infection is successfully treated, or cancerous tissue is completely removed. They use the term symptomatic cure when deficiencies are controlled to the extent that overt signs and symptoms disappear completely, although the underlying disease process persists. There are true cures in psychiatry; this is quite evident in successfully treated symptomatic psychoses and in some organic deficit states.

As a rule, however, the use of the term cure in psychiatry is not appropriate. Surgeons can make bacteria and pus disappear by proper treatment, but behavior does not disappear; it only changes. A certain inertia and constancy is inherent in personality. Our patients, no matter how successfully treated, do not lose all their aggression; all their passivity; all their sexual infantilism; all their anxieties; nor do they lose their most general style of experiencing and approach. One can lose one's symptoms but, hopefully, not one's individuality. Thus, in many cases in psychiatry, the term cure is not applicable: we speak, instead, of improvement or restoration to a prior state of functioning, which may be far from perfect.

Some of the most influential schools of psychiatric therapy, and particularly of psychotherapy, are not overendowed with modesty. Sigmund Freud, very early in his career, searched for methods that would produce more lasting and less "superficial" results than was then possible with the use of suggestion and simple hypnosis. In later years, Freud became less concerned with therapeutic change and saw the distinctive merit of his method as a radical and deep exploration of behavior. Notwithstanding such views, most psychotherapists influenced by Freud have wished to produce a realignment of psychological forces to enable their patients to enjoy life more fully, solve their tasks more efficiently, and become better human beings. But who can tell what a better human being is or ought to be? Certainly, psychiatrists cannot claim such omniscience and are obliged to accept the values of a collective social system as guidelines. In highly individualistic cultures, self-actualization or self-realization is seen as the goal of certain psychotherapies. The goal of realizing one's human potential is encountered in Buddhism, particularly in the practices of Zen Buddhism, which fascinated and stimulated Karen Horney, Erich Fromm, and Alan Watts. Self-actualization as a therapeutic goal is, of course, quite different from the more modest aims of medical therapy. In any case, whether psychiatrists try to help patients to suffer less and enable them to inflict less suffering on others; or whether their aim is to help their patients to actualize themselves, the behavioral changes, whether "subjective" or "objective," should be defined in rational and operationally verifiable terms. There is no place in psychiatry for mystical, irrational, or suprarational approaches. We do not deliver people from evil, nor are we supposed to give meaning to their lives, although after successful therapy life may well be more meaningful. Finally, the old medical adage—to cure few, to improve many, and to comfort most—also holds in psychiatry even if such limited goals are belittled by some.

Basic Types of Psychiatric Therapy

Strictly speaking, psychiatric therapy refers to biological and psychosocial methods of treatment, which are based on scientific evidence. If this definition were taken literally it would exclude not only those interventions which plainly are keyed to unscientific beliefs or assumed magic and supernatural forces, but also commonsense methods and the many therapies which are based on vaguely formulated and poorly tested theories. And not much would remain, because there are very few truly scientific therapies in our field. Thus, as we try to help our patients we must keep in mind that the problem of rationale for therapy, whether organic or psychological, is still in a primitive state; caution and admission of ignorance, as well as tolerance for daring new ideas, must guide the judicious therapist. Furthermore, in psychiatry as well as in other medical specialties, the qualities of a therapist depend not only on technical knowledge but also on certain important human qualities. With increased knowledge, technical competence will become more important and more clearly definable; yet the human qualities of the therapist will never be unimportant in a field where suffering, trust, and confidence are involved.

A classification of psychiatric therapies may be based on the phenomenological description of treatments or on a differentiation of underlying principles and theories. The latter is troublesome, because theories are often only implied and not clearly and specifically developed. More often than not, practices do not conform neatly with the stated theories; this is true even in the most elaborated therapies, although such an incongruity is generally not admitted. The most fundamental distinction can be made between the somatic therapies and the psychotherapies. *Somatic therapies*, also called organic and biological therapies, consist of various chemical, hormonal, and physical measures, which directly or indirectly affect the brain and through their cerebral action produce or inhibit behavioral changes. In a few instances, such therapies are fairly specific, for example, for general paresis, pellagra psychosis, cretinism, galactosemia, and the like. Most organic therapies have evolved empirically, with no sound theoretical basis. Some organic therapies, as well as many psychotherapies, owe their results to the so-called placebo effect and, strictly speaking, are not really organic therapies. *Psychotherapies*, or more correctly the *psychosocial therapies*, are behavioral methods that influence the total behavior of the patient with the intent of producing increased well being and improved psychological and social performance. In what follows, different types of psychosocial therapies and organic therapies will be, for didactic reasons, discussed in separate sections and as abstractions. Therapeutic transactions with patients, regardless of the method or combination of methods used, are, however, never abstractions.

The Psychosocial Therapies

The psychotherapies produce behavior change largely through verbal and symbolic techniques in a professional relationship between a socially approved healer and a suffering person. The technique must be based on some scientific rationale to deserve the designation of psychotherapy; it cannot be a mystical or magical procedure, although it seems that many suffering persons are helped by such procedures. In a beautifully written little book, *The Power within Us*, Nuñez Cabeza deVaca describes how shipwrecked Spanish sailors in the seventeenth century were forced to cure sick Indians by their prayers. After some spectacular successes, the Spaniards became convinced of their own miraculous power. The role of faith and enthusiasm operating in the therapist is not as yet well explained, but unquestionably it is a crucial factor. Supervision helps the therapist to monitor his own responses, which are mobilized by the therapeutic situation. Of course, a general belief system is more comforting for physicians than confidence in *this* specific observation but skepticism about *that* one; it is obviously difficult to sustain an investigative attitude in this field. Recently, a number of psychiatric investigators have become interested in the explanation of techniques used in religious conversion, faith healing, and thought reform, phenomena which are related but different in aim and method from psychotherapy.[48] The critical effects of "personality," the impact of the physician as a person dealing with the patient whose defect or need creates a special dependence, still remain to be investigated. Freud pointed to the major and overriding role of transference and suggestion and the cure through "love." Since comfort and aid are so largely mediated through persons, we should expect the doctor–patient relationship to be sustained by irrational as well as rational wishes and needs for personal attention. No other motivational dimension has a longer or more extensive history of reinforcing and shaping behavior. The patient who follows the doctor's "orders" is not just obeying a regimen but following the doctor's lead; the physician's attitudes, confidence, and approach are in part imitated and identified with. This dependency and willingness to be "good" for the doctor (or need to rebel) occurs in all of medicine, including psychiatry. The need to be heard, seen, and looked after, if not rescued, is basic, then, to bringing doctor and patient together and is as crucial to the transaction as the ailment that is the occasion for it.

Psychotherapeutic techniques must enable the patient to correct his pathological and undesirable habits and help him replace them with useful and gratifying attitudes and behavior. In large measure, the culture defines these patterns of behavior. Put simply, psychotherapists treat misfits, a harsh but correct term used by Alexandra Adler.[1] To view psychotherapy essentially as a learning process puts it into the broad category of educational methods. Yet it differs from ordinary educational experiences in these important aspects: the nature of the behavior disorders that require such intervention is so severe that society usually grants the recipient the sick role; the psychological healer has the special status of a therapist; the subject matter for the patient's learning is the self, a person's private and basic patterns of response. In view of the latter consideration, the model of parental function in fostering growth and development seems the educational mode most closely related to therapy.

The psychotherapies may be conveniently divided into analytic and directive-suppressive techniques. Some proponents of the analytic techniques maintain that improvement is caused by the emergence of new insights as the result of interpretation of highly charged experiences that were unknown or unconscious. Other proponents of analytic techniques maintain that the central event is a patient–therapist relationship, which permits the communication of significant emotional experiences. Both elements certainly occur in actual therapy, but most therapists stress either one or the other of these principles. The explicitly directive and suppressive therapies are referred to at times by the derogatory term superficial; the patient's experience, however, may be far from superficial, since very powerful emotional reactions may take place in directive therapy. All therapies involve support and direction; the "directiveness" in any therapy consists of the basic rules of procedure and the specific response the therapist chooses to make or omit. All therapies involve "learning"; the so-called behavior therapies are usually individualized therapies involving a relationship in which conditioning theory and techniques are employed.

Jerome D. Frank believes that all psychotherapy can be explained by a common underlying principle: the suggestive power of the socially sanctioned therapist.[21] This notion was previously advanced by Freud, who felt, however, that only psychoanalysis makes an honest effort both in theory and practice to elucidate the role of suggestive power by analyzing it in the phenomenon of transference. Frank,[21] Hans J. Eysenck,[18] and others assume that all psychotherapies work equally well, but, in our opinion, no adequate comparative studies have been carried out. A lively debate on the results of psychotherapy has been under way.[18] The fact that different patient populations become hidden under monolithic diagnoses, that different skills are obscured by the assumption that all therapists of a given training are equally able, and that equally able therapists proceed in different ways makes objective evaluations most difficult.

Psychotherapy also may be divided into individual therapies and group therapies. The latter have recently become more important, not only because they permit larger numbers of patients to be reached, but also because a number of authors maintain that these therapies are more powerful than individual therapies. Much of the therapy in institutional settings is, wittingly or unwittingly, a form of group therapy.

The clearer the indications for psychotherapy, the better off the therapist and patient will be. Generally speaking, habits that are learned can be unlearned or, at least, not employed. Psychotherapists should not lose sight of the fact that there are many human problems that are determined by economic, social, cultural, and legal processes, which essentially are not accessible to psychotherapy. Insofar as therapy is a mode of exercising influence toward facilitating behavior change, it should be kept in mind that procedures inducing change and etiological factors producing disorder are not necessarily directly related.

There is agreement that psychotherapy is the method of choice for the treatment of character neuroses and symptom neuroses. There is much less agreement as to whether the psychosomatic diseases, the schizophrenias, and manic-depressive reactions should be treated by psychotherapy. It cannot be denied, however, that there are reliable, experienced therapists who are able to treat successfully some patients with psychosomatic diseases, schizophrenias, and depressive behavior disorders. In the United States, psychotherapy of schizophrenias and depressions is rather widely practiced and is described in some detail in the clinical section of this book. Psychotherapists have also tackled a variety of sociopathies, with results ranging from moderate success to failure. As a general rule, it is felt that younger patients do better than older patients who have more rigidly established habits. Ideally, we should prefer to treat children, but this presupposes treating their families too. Early adulthood, when the young individual establishes his own existence and identity, is an important and useful time for treatment. There is general agreement that high motivation of patients and relative absence of gains from the disorder are important prerequisites. When a suffering patient truly wants to rid himself of his troublesome symptoms and habits, he is highly motivated for therapy. If a person makes others suffer but is unaware of his own pain (or is highly invested in his own pleasure, as in the sociopathic reactions, addictions, and some perversions), he is less likely to benefit from psychotherapy. The inability to check antisocial impulses makes psychotherapy more difficult. An unfavorably harsh reality situation may render psychotherapy impossible. Motivation for psychotherapy may be increased by skilful maneuvers of the therapist. This is particularly important in delinquent patients whose initial motivation may be quite low (or nonexistent). Good intelligence and psychological-mindedness, often expressed by a certain verbal ability, are important prerequisites in insight-producing psychotherapies.

Not only the goals but also the methods, and actually the very existence of psychotherapy, depend upon the culture that has produced it. Although systematic techniques of altering human behavior from child-rearing to opinion-molding are as old as mankind, the systematic approach of psychotherapy is the product of a scientific psychology. Such an approach did not simply spring from the brain of a genius but is directly linked to the general scientific and social advances of the nineteenth and twentieth centuries. In certain areas of human problems, a scientific approach is gradually replacing religious and philosophical approaches. Even more specifically, it is possible to explain why certain psychotherapies exist in certain cultures and not in others. The reasons why psychodynamic therapy, for instance, seems to flourish more in the United States than in other countries have been mentioned in Chapter 1. The less scientifically founded a therapy, the more it will depend on the reinforcing factors of a cultural milieu. At present, no psychotherapy, even the most advanced, is based on pure scientific evidence, but rather on a mixture of scientific realism and prescientific beliefs. Therefore, the flourishing of a given therapy depends on existing affinities between general cultural values and the implied values of that therapy.

As would be expected after the relatively brief and rapid development of psychotherapies, the field is in a confused state; this can be bewildering for the student and induces many therapists to stick religiously to a particular school; they prefer some guidelines to a completely unstructured situation. Such a need for a frame of reference does not, of course, stem only from the needs of the therapist for theory. To work with patients requires structure, and even ritual cannot be entirely dispensed with. It may be that some patients are helped primarily by finding a sympathetic listener in a well structured context. The therapist has to be a socially approved healer with specific knowledge and techniques and not just a well-meaning neighbor. Although in good psychotherapy ritualistic qualities tend to be unimportant, it will take time for rituals to become rational techniques, for belief to mature into testable theory, and for the many schools to give way to a generally accepted pattern of practice, as we have witnessed in certain areas of organic medicine. In an introductory text, no thorough survey, comparison, or meaningful critique of the various therapies and their techniques is possible; the present discussion will be limited to a brief description of some basic characteristics of the main approaches.

Classical Psychoanalysis

The technique of classical therapeutic analysis is very complex and does not lend itself to brief presentation. Freud believed that the future will attribute far greater importance to psychoanalysis as the science of the unconscious than as a therapeutic procedure. Yet he thought of psychoanalytic treatment as *primus inter pares* for those disorders that can be reached by it, primarily the milder neuroses, character disorders, certain sexual inhibitions and perversions, and depressions. He was doubtful about the therapy of schizophrenia and paranoia, although some of his students were more optimistic. The aim of psychoanalysis is to replace unconscious acts by conscious acts or, as Freud put it later: "Where there was id, ego shall be." [26] Hans W. Loewald wrote that the patient who comes to analysis for help is led to self-understanding by the understanding he finds in the analyst.[50] The basic aim is to produce in the patient a profound insight in the relationship of his infantile neurosis to his present way of life and particularly to its faulty aspects.

Classical psychoanalysis is characterized by the utilization of the basic concepts of transference and resistance and the uncovering of unconscious factors in behavior and its development. *Transference* means the movement toward the analyst of emotionally charged behavior which had been previously displayed to key figures such as parents and siblings. In every successful analysis, a so-called transference neurosis develops; that is, the analysand reexperiences or demonstrates in the analysis certain aspects of his infantile neurosis. In clear or masked form, he tries, in characteristic maneuvers, to achieve with the analyst what he once wanted from significant persons in his life. He demonstrates core conflicts and wishes thereby, and through this communication the patient's style and difficulties are more convincingly dealt with because they are evident and present. The therapist may also transiently develop a transference reaction to the patient; this is termed *countertransference*. The success of therapeutic analysis depends to a considerable degree on the therapist's perception and handling of these transferences. By *resistance* is meant the patient's unconscious maneuvers to block uncovering of the unconscious processes and to defend himself against the anxiety of change or insight. The psychoanalytic method relies on *interpretation* of the unconscious components in the patient's conflicts as seen in his current life; his dreams; in the specimens of his behavior toward the analyst encountered in resistance and transference within the analytic hour; and in his memories of childhood.

Patients are asked to associate freely rather than to give deliberate and rational accounts; they must learn to suspend their usual criticism and editing in order to attend to the order and meaning of their inner life. To a muted and limited extent, expected responses are inhibited, and the usual expectations governing reciprocal human relations are suspended during the hour. *Free association* essentially means full and unedited reporting of mental events, including seemingly trivial or obnoxious details. The patient will let his thoughts and wishes be verbally expressed; the analyst will listen, clarify, and interpret, but, unlike a friend or parent, he will not directly gratify. The patient may also be asked to make an effort to check certain pathological impulses outside of the analytic hour. The term *abstinence rule* refers both to such restraint and to the relative suspension of ordinary rewards and punishments—no patting on the back and no berating—during the analytic hour. Thus, the usual conventions and responses that surround goal-directed behavior, including behavior directed toward need satisfaction, are dispensed with, permitting a regression and the emergence of private thoughts, wishes, and fantasies. The interpretation of dreams, parapraxias, symbolic acts, and—most of all—the patient's transference and resistance are the basic method of psychoanalysis. The patient connects his inner life and his private and unconscious wishes with his behavior and the conflicts and goals evident in his conduct. Freud called the analysis of dreams the royal road to the unconscious.[25] Dreams are interpreted as attempts at wish-fulfillment of infantile instinctual wishes and their recurrences in the frustrations of everyday living. The task of the analyst and patient is to decode the language of the dream and gain insight into the dreamer's unconscious conflict.

Karl Menninger focuses on the *regression* that patients invariably undergo in the process; the analyst remains not passive but neutral, or nonjudgmental, in attitude, and, as far as external behavior goes, deliberately unresponsive and socially uninvolved with the patient.[54] The analyst's responsiveness and his collaboration with the patient are solely in the work of interpreting, reconstructing, and clarifying patterns that become evident to patient and therapist. Psychoanalysis is an active and not a passive emotional experience for therapist and patient alike. The use of the couch is an ingenious device but not essential for analysis. In many adolescents and a few other patients the use of the couch is not indicated. Emotional intensity is not identical with vigorously acting out one's emotions; indeed, the latter is not tolerated in classical psychoanalysis. Psychoanalysis demands relative self-control and a capacity for self-reflection, and patients incapable of following the "abstinence rule" are not suited for classical psychoanalysis.

Psychoanalytic treatment is a lengthy procedure. Sessions are usually held four to five times a week, and each lasts for a short hour. In spite of attempts to shorten the treatment, analyses have become longer; it is not unusual for an analysis to last hundreds of hours over a period of many years. Analysis is essentially an educational process; it is a second education of adults and also of children and is supposed to correct the consequences of the traumas and faults of the primary education. It allows the individual to pay attention to the interconnections of his internal and private sensations and feelings. With the support of the analyst, the patient can update his earlier and private modes of experience and see himself and others with some new perspective. An enormous amount of material has to be worked through in a slow, patient, repetitive fashion. It is the patient's reformulation and freedom to choose that is sought, not the adoption of the analyst's values, a point that sharply differentiates analysis from conversion. After a successful analysis, the patient will take with him the ability to introspect (not ruminate) with candor and to apply such insights, when necessary, to life problems. Hopefully, he will no longer be a stranger to himself but rather in charge of his reserves and tolerant of his limitations.

A number of Freud's students, and some very outstanding ones, modified Freud's original methods of treatment. Among them were Franz Alexander and Thomas M. French[4] who, by stressing the so-called principles of flexibility and corrective emotional experience, created a bridge between psychoanalysis and the analytic psychotherapies. In the field of child analysis and also in the analysis of adults, considerable modifications were introduced by

Melanie Klein.[43] More important than any other development is the current emphasis on *character analysis* of persistent maladaptive patterns of behavior.

Current criticism of psychoanalysis focuses on the relation of theory to technique, on the results with classical methods in comparison with other methods, and on concern over the cost and social inaccessibility of psychoanalytic therapy. The benefits derived from the classical method in paving the way for the development of all insight-oriented psychotherapies have been very great.

The Therapies of Adler, Jung, and Rank

Alfred Adler as well as Sigmund Freud made it quite clear that the theories of psychoanalysis and individual psychology are very different;[2] this proposition applies also to therapy. Followers of Adler use a therapeutic dialogue with their patients during which they clarify the patient's concept of his life pattern and try to influence the patient to give up his neurotic motives, replacing them with a less neurotic and more socially acceptable pattern. There is more emphasis on future goals than on past conflicts. Victor Frankl, who at one time subscribed to Adler's school of individual psychology, has taken over the concept of life pattern and meaning of life from Adler.[22] In Adlerian therapy the patient's inferiority complexes, masculine protests, and other overcompensations are emphasized. As Adlerians do not recognize unconscious conflicts, transference, or resistance, there is little endeavor to explore unconscious instinctual strivings and defenses. This therapeutic approach is relatively short and, if one can judge by the writings of Alfred Adler and his students, rather unsophisticated. Still, much of what Adler has said has been absorbed into today's general armamentarium for therapy, and Adler now gets little credit for it.

Carl Gustav Jung has written little about therapy,[41] and his influence on techniques of treatment is small, both in this country and in Europe. Jung's complex mysticism and his emphasis on the innate and archaic do not lend themselves to therapeutic activity. Yet psychotherapy of neurotics and schizophrenics has been taught in the Jungian Institute in Zurich. Jungian analysis is an interpretative therapy using the concepts and symbols revealed by folklore, myth, and the dream and its dark and archaic symbols in order to aid self-understanding. Compared with classical analysis, the Jungian procedure is relatively short. Jung emphasized the concept of self-actualization as an aim of therapy long before existentialist therapies and neo-Freudians embraced this goal and before Western intellectuals discovered Zen Buddhism.

Otto Rank had a strong influence on psychiatric social work through the so-called functional school of social work but was largely ignored by psychiatric therapists. His contributions, an emphasis on the therapeutic relationship and its temporal finiteness, and the dramatic impact of setting time limits, have found their way into the general current of psychotherapy.[65] Theodor Reik, a very insightful student of Freud, left the classical movement, although his teaching of therapy did not essentially differ from Freud's basic views.

The Neo-Freudians

The so-called neo-Freudians, Karen Horney, Erich Fromm, and Harry Stack Sullivan, had a strong therapeutic orientation and a definite impact on the current therapeutic scene in the United States. Fromm has rather definite notions about an ideal of man and pressed his efforts to mold patients to attain such goals of self-actualization and growth.[28] In contrast to most other analytic therapists, Sullivan had a strong interest in hospital psychiatry and particularly in schizophrenia. In general, the neo-Freudians analyze the patient–therapist relationship, the patient's adaptation to his environment, and the development of his maladaptive social patterns. The principal difficulties of the patient, however, are viewed not so much as unconscious conflicts between instinctual and adaptive strivings of the patient but more as faulty characterological responses to his basic anxiety, or as faulty and distorting "dynamisms" and security operations. In terms of techniques, neo-Freudians are rather active in the therapeutic role. The students of Horney use techniques that are quite similar to classical analysis, such as reliance on interpretation of dreams, parapraxias, and transference.[37] The staples of the more superficial therapies (as Ruth Monroe puts it)[55] were also used by Sullivan when they seemed necessary. An appealing fusion of Freudian and Sullivanian ideas on therapy has been presented by Frieda Fromm-Reichmann.[29]

One might say about classical analysis as well as its modifications that there is currently a trend toward an analysis of defenses, adaptations and an emphasis on the here and now. It would appear that today's analysts are more comfortable and familiar with the psychic terrain explored by several generations of workers and hence are more flexible in emphasizing whatever aspect of behavior is relevant to the task at hand. The tendency to find a problem one is looking for, such as the manifestation of instinctual forces in dreams, thoughts, and symptoms (id analysis), and make this an exclusive focus in therapy seems obsolete. The existence of instinctual activity, in any event, is not a problem but a fact of life; the therapist must discern whether or not the pattern of gratification is a problem for the patient and, concretely, how and when it is.

Therapists who have not learned the value of self-critique and analysis of their own motives and problems (which should not be a morbid self-mortification), nor learned to appreciate that judgment can be clouded by unrestrained indulgence of one's need to cure, to rescue, and to make everything right, will be tempted to simplify life and promulgate nostrums rather than inquiry. In spite of many schools and the contentious criticisms that fly between them, there seems to be a unifying trend and a greater scientific realism in current analytic therapy. The crucial differences between these approaches and schools in all probability cannot be appreciated in what they say *about* what they do; rather, the student will find he must translate the jargon of talking about therapy into concrete experiences.

Psychoanalysis and Analytic Psychotherapy

Is there a real difference between psychoanalysis as a therapy and so-called analytic or dynamic psychotherapy? Opinions on this point are divided. Freud compared pure analysis to gold and the psychotherapies to alloys.[27] Merton M. Gill and other proponents of classical analysis state that there is a definite difference between the two.[30] Only a procedure that makes the analysis of transference and resistance the main procedure should be called psychoanalysis; one might add that psychoanalysis also must aim to explore unconscious conflicts and uncover infantile amnesia. By necessity, such therapy is lengthy; its endeavor is a total analysis of the patient's personality and development. Psychoanalysts refrain as much as possible from any active molding of the patient other than to induce him to analyze competently.

Nonetheless, there are analysts who feel that all psychotherapy must rest on analytic sciences of behavior and that analytic psychotherapy and psychoanalysis cannot be rigidly separated.[44] Franz Alexander, who contributed to the flexibility of psychoanalysis and the richness of psychotherapy, doubted that a real distinction could be made.[3] Certainly all analytic therapists permit some degree of transference to develop and interpret transference and resistance as well as dreams, parapraxias, defenses, and symptoms, and their dynamic and genetic meaning. Frequency of interviews and length of treatment do not necessarily differentiate psychoanalysis and psychotherapy.[11] It is not unlikely that the differentiation is made, at least in part, for social reasons, to protect the guild of analysts' professional need for identity. We believe there is one genuinely differentiating feature: true psychoanalysis is as much an exploration and investigation as it is a therapy. Freud certainly felt this was the case, and Karl Menninger has expressed similar ideas.[54]

Brief Analytic Psychotherapy

To distinguish between brief and long psychotherapy is far from profound, but it is of practical significance. Although prolonged dynamic psychotherapy has supplied us with most of the concepts used in psychotherapy today, and although it requires a great deal of time to help certain patients, only brief therapy will enable us to reach the masses of suffering people who are in need of psychotherapy. Just what is brief analytic psychotherapy? John Dollard and his co-workers defined it as a therapy that may last from six to thirty hours.[15] We do not feel, however, that a meaningful distinction can be set by time limits. We report the "blitz therapy" of a patient who has been helped significantly in a few minutes.

A lawyer whose wife was hospitalized in a psychiatric institution was referred to one of the authors by the wife's psychiatrist. When the patient arrived, he was asked why he was sent; he replied that his wife's doctor had told him that it was he who was making his wife ill. When he was asked to explain how he had done this, he said he couldn't say because he didn't know. The therapist then inquired if he had asked his wife's doctor for an explanation, and he replied that he had not. It was then suggested that he had better see the wife's doctor again, and then call for another appointment. The therapist never heard from the patient again, but had a furious telephone call from the referring psychiatrist, who asked what the therapist had told the husband. A year or so later, a physician friend of the husband asked the therapist what he had done for the husband. Before his talk with the therapist, he had been guilt-ridden, depressed, and nasty to himself and others; afterward, he seemed congenial, self-assured, and behaved toward his wife in a more realistic fashion. Evidently, the five minutes he had spent with the therapist triggered a more realistic attitude and an increase in his self-esteem, or helped to consolidate an attitude which was silently developing.

Psychoanalysts have labeled such rapid successes transference cures. Explanations of the transference cure state that they occur because the patient loves his therapist, identifies with his wishes, or wants to resist uncomfortable depth therapy.[45] Essentially, transference implies the ability to invest in others, to shift and modify behavior directed toward the search for love and satisfaction and self-esteem; in analysis, the infantile sources and repetitive patterns of this human tendency are observed and discussed with the aim of allowing transference to be less compelled, more under the organization of reality satisfactions, less driven by infantile needs. It is likely that most "cures" by psychotherapy are in part cures through love, that is, they use the power of attachments and the wish for gratification in order to modify behavior and achieve self-mastery. The power of conversion must lie in similar internal changes based on love of a supreme being or a leader, which then facilitates reorganization of attitudes and behavior. Instantaneous "cures" may also occur in rare cases where a realistic solution of the person's problems and needs is ingeniously found.

Some analysts have viewed brief therapy as a diminutive of classical analysis. The concepts are identical; differences consist only of a change in emphasis and quantity.[11] In a lively section of his introductory text, Kenneth M. Colby describes how he utilizes the concepts of transference, resistance and of dynamic genetic interpretations of unconscious and conscious processes in brief psychotherapy. A somewhat similar approach was taken earlier by Felix Deutsch[14] and the Balints,[5] who focused on certain specific and circumscribed problems that trouble the patient but retained the classical psychoanalytic stance. Dollard, F. Auld, and A. M. White, in their description of brief therapy, attempted to explain brief psychotherapy through principles of analytic theory and learning theory.[15] Both therapist and patient learn; the patient is able to learn if the therapist becomes a reliable love object and the therapeutic atmosphere is permissive. The patient learns to sift out unrealistic from realistic fears. He learns to label his frustrations and conflicts and thus becomes able to learn new and more adaptive responses. The application of what he learns must occur in real life, not merely in the therapist's office. Some psychoanalysts have stated that the concepts of classical analysis do not really fit the processes of brief psychotherapy, and they grapple with the problem of formulating more appropriate concepts. Roy R. Grinker maintains that the transactional theory has definite therapeutic applications and is, as a frame of reference, superior to the traditional use of the analytic concepts of transference, resistance, and regression.[33] He feels that the fostering of a transference neurosis and the extensive interpretation of unconscious material of dreams and infantile regression is not necessarily advantageous to the progress of therapy. It is more important, in his opinion, to dwell on social configurations and on the explicit and implicit relationship to the therapist who functions as a helping participant-observer. The chief topic is the patient's anxiety and related feelings: if proper communication ensues, the patient is able to change.

Direct and meaningful communication in a dramatic dialogue is the essence of Jules V. Coleman's active approach.[12] Action does not mean direction but rather responsiveness and interaction. Coleman feels that bantering or ridiculing lightly and good-naturedly is an effective approach for the affectionate communication of insight. Such communication helps patients of all types and backgrounds to escape from their desperate isolation. As we understand him, Coleman is not interested in descriptive diagnosis; in his view problems differ according to the dynamics of the patients and require specific sensitivity of communication. Motivation does not matter; patients may be considered motivated as long as they come to the therapeutic hour. The doctor is to be receptive and ready to offer relevant service to those who come for it and ready to terminate it when the patient has received some restoration of function. The therapist is to support but not infantilize the patient and should have confidence in self-restorative trends in the patient. Coleman's approach is pertinent, but we disagree with his complete de-emphasis of descriptive diagnosis; in our opinion, patients differ in their suitability for therapy and also (and significantly) in their degree of motivation for treatment. The chief research problem here is still to identify the characteristics, the strengths, and the motivations of the different populations who come for help. All of psychiatry has the task of describing behavior and conditions for its change in order to discover principles by which behavior is organized and factors that lead to psychopathology. We have also noticed that the good-natured humor of banter can often degenerate into unsuitable sarcasm and may serve only the sadistic and omnipotent needs of some inexperienced therapists. Nevertheless, it is astounding to see how quickly young therapists learn under such auspices as compared with ordinary methods. Ordinarily, in trying to teach all the various aspects of human behavior which we encounter, we can easily confound and confuse the beginner who, after all, must learn to be relevant and realistic. Proper communication as the essence of therapeutic process was also stressed by the late Hellmuth Kaiser.[42] This therapist saw the essence of neurosis as an inability to communicate properly; he became convinced that it is not insight and interpretation by the therapist, but the ability to communicate that has healing power. We agree that the dynamic psychotherapist and his patient must communicate. But what do we communicate about? In our opinion, the content of such communication is an attempt to help the patient to gain insight into the dynamics of his current problems and their genesis.

Rogers' Client-Centered Therapy

Carl Rogers and his students developed a therapeutic technique that has become quite influential with psychologists but has been largely ignored by psychiatrists.[66] Rogers sees the essence of the therapeutic process in a definitely structured, permissive relationship that allows the "client" to gain an understanding of himself to a degree that enables him to take positive steps in his new orientation. The therapist simply reflects the client's feelings; by doing this consistently, he helps the client to change his self-image and to exchange his lack of self-esteem for a positive regard. Gradually, the patient regains a new freedom; he grows emotionally and gives up his immature behavior. Rogers objects to any attempt to direct, suggest, prescribe, or even to interpret. He feels that what he used to call the nondirective viewpoint places a high value on the individual rights and the dignity of the client. He believes that individuals have the right to select their goals and will do this wisely if their self-esteem is increased and if they have an opportunity to grow emotionally. It is obvious that Rogers and his students have dealt largely with relatively mature individuals in student-counseling centers and not with the much sicker population that many psychiatrists treat. Any diagnosis was irrelevant for Rogers, who advocated only one type of treatment. Psychiatrists, however, as all physicians, use many different approaches for many different disorders. They also believe they have the right and duty to make decisions whenever this is necessary for their regressed and disabled patients. In spite of these differences, we feel that Rogers and his students have made some very valuable contributions, not only through the development of a therapy, but also through the painstaking recording and analysis of their therapeutic interviews.

A Common Brand of Dynamic Psychotherapy

Apart from the feuds centering on loose or rigid theories and pseudoprecise or vague techniques of current schools, there is a distinct trend toward the practice of a common-ground analytic psychotherapy. This therapy, with its many diversifications, is being taught increasingly to novices in some of the outstanding North and South American training centers and is also beginning to be advanced in a few European centers. It is usually referred to as *dynamic psychotherapy,* a term, which, as we have mentioned before, is not very satisfactory. Patients are seen in a fifty-minute hour in private offices, outpatient clinics, and hospitals, with usually one to three sessions a week, extending over months or years. Many psychotherapists feel such treatment should not be free but that patients should pay for it according to their abilities, a view that was first advanced by some psychoanalysts but has been challenged by many others.[51]

Most psychotherapists prefer to work primarily with a highly motivated patient, yet one must remember that those with low motivation often need help most desperately. It is generally felt that the patient's motivation is important in this type of therapy, but it is commonly agreed that motivation may be facilitated by appropriate techniques, for example, creating a permissive relationship with a stable and loving therapist who provides opportunity for identification, or demonstrating to the patient that the therapist acts exclusively in the patient's interest. It is often forgotten, even by analysts, that what Rogers calls an attitude of unconditional positive regard for the patient, and other measures that maximize security and confidence, are essential if one person is to confide in another. Such regard and support does not mean unconditional agreement or the inability to tolerate differences of view; the therapist's "alliance" with the patient is not with the patient's delusions or symptoms but with his integrity, his individuality as a person with predicaments, and his assets for the struggle to survive and to grow. Motivation is increased most of all when the patient notices that he is being helped.

In dynamic psychotherapy, the adult patient and therapist usually sit opposite each other and talk. It is recommended that the therapist talk less than the patient. There are good reasons for this: first, the procedure is designed to provide optimal emotional discharge, discovery, and self-knowledge for the patient and not for the therapist; second, there are also many problems to which the therapist cannot contribute. When therapists talk too much, they are apt to speak nonsense. Topics are mostly the emotions of the patient, his anxiety and depressive feelings, and his guilt and shame, of which he may be unaware or only dimly aware. These topics arise through his telling of thoughts and experiences and reporting ongoing feelings, not as an abstract discourse; reflection about recurrent problems in which shame or anxiety arise is different from a patient talking as a textbook and not from his authentic, specific experience. The therapist helps through economic interpretation of preconscious conflicts and clarification of conscious problems. He, in effect, teaches the patient to make correct observations and formulations increasing the patient's awareness and helping him to differentiate what is real from what is unreal and what can be changed from what cannot.

Interpretations and clarifications that are nontheoretical, specific, and concrete are not only helpful but also demonstrate the competence of the therapist and thus increase the therapist's chance to help. As G. L. Klerman once remarked, the therapist makes the obvious explicit. In a permissive relationship, the patient may begin to feel, say, and understand what was not consciously felt and understood before. In a relationship with a benign authority who is on the patient's side (in the sense that the therapist consistently has the patient's best interests at heart), the patient may find the courage to take the first steps in learning new responses and trying out new attitudes.

The *early phase* of psychotherapy has been described briefly in Chapter 7. It is not confined to one single hour. Essentially, during this opening phase the therapist and patient find out whether they can relate to one another and like each other well enough to "travel" together for awhile; most importantly, the therapist tries to determine whether the patient can profit from this type of relationship. In this phase, the therapist scans the main problems with which he can help in a limited period of time and determines what his strategy should be. It may be to await developments; it always should be based on cues from the patient and not solely on the psychiatrist's abstract rules. During the *main phase*, the principal problems are tackled. Techniques and underlying principles of dealing with them are far from clear. Whether permissiveness, support, a liberating relationship, an increase in self-esteem, catharsis, insight, or an increased capacity for self-learning are the decisive factors of the psychotherapeutic process is not known at present. In all likelihood, all these factors in some combination are responsible for change; we believe that sensitive accepting, listening, and timely interpretation are the main tools. Rarely does the patient's problem yield to a first assault but rather requires patient and repetitive working through. When some insight is reached in the therapeutic session, it has to be applied in real life.

The *terminal phase* prepares the patient for termination, which, to a certain extent in dynamic psychotherapy, as well as in analysis proper, in many respects is arbitrary and occurs when returns are markedly diminishing for patient and therapist.[16] In brief therapy, of course, only a very limited range of problems, maybe only one problem, hopefully a crucial one, may be dealt with. The best criterion for termination is the patient's and therapist's agreement that the patient can, from a certain point on, proceed on his own power. Many therapists set a date for termination at some juncture in the therapy; this is often arrived at through mutual agreement. The therapist may frequently encounter intensified symptoms and various attempts to continue the treatment, to reassert childish needs to cling and be dependent and these attitudes can be interpreted. Nor is it true that the patient who leaves with anger or reluctance has not been helped. Similarly, it is not necessary to prolong termination with ritualistic preparations.

The therapist also may abruptly terminate or cling to the patient because he somehow feels inadequate or irritated or cannot tolerate the growing independence of his once needy patient. One of the most regular phenomena we encounter in the teaching of psychotherapy is the beginner's emotionality—his countertransference—when he is engaged in listening to his patient and to the voice of his own unconscious. It is invariably present and is manifested by anxiety, anger, sexual arousal, boredom, and a host of maneuvers, which on scrutiny appear irrational and not in the interest of therapy. To recognize such emotional reactions and to enable the psychotherapist to overcome them was one of Freud's great merits. In some cases, mere clarification and support by a supervising teacher may achieve this; in others, nothing short of psychoanalysis of the therapist will do. Every student of psychotherapy (and even every highly skilled therapist) must deal with such emotional difficulties, and every teacher of psychotherapy must assist the student in this task. As we continue investigating the psychotherapeutic process, an art mastered by few in the past, it is becoming an applied science with specified rules and techniques that can be learned by many.

Directive and Supportive Psychotherapies

In these therapeutic approaches, systematic attempts are made to change the patient's attitude and behavior by inducing him to accept the assumptive systems of the therapist.[21] Techniques such as advice and suggestion, active help, praise, and exhortation are used in everyday life and, more often than not, help not at all in the deeply ingrained difficulties about which psychiatric patients complain. To promise any success, such techniques must be not only very powerful but also employed by strongly authoritative healers. The suffering persons must have absolute confidence in them, a confidence that is reinforced by successes but not significantly shaken by failures. The techniques essentially are: (1) Direct suggestion, persuasion, advice, and intellectual guidance. (2) Various verbal and nonverbal "magical" procedures, which are most important in primitive medicine but by no means negligible in modern practice. (3) Praise and exhortation, which reinforce or inhibit certain types of behavior; these may be used by therapist or therapy group, but the latter's influence is usually much more powerful. Group acceptance or rejection of an individual, depending on his behavior and effort, is one of the strongest motivations and is effectively used in such directive therapeutic groups as Alcoholics Anonymous and in Synanon, a self-help group of drug addicts. (4) Manipulation of the physical and social environment, particularly of persons in positions of influence to the patient, for example, parents of children in treatment. The prescriptions of rest, diversification of work, change of environment, sexual abstinence or gratification, and the like, also fall within this category. Of importance, however, is arousing the patient's hope, willingness, and fervent desire to participate in improvisations and exercises. Hence, emotional arousal is an essential part not only of the analytic but also of the directive and suggestive therapies.

Directive therapies are widely practiced but rarely well taught. At present, in the United States, very few write about such techniques,[71, 72] although undoubtedly a great deal of directive, suggestive therapy is going on all the time. Procedures that place so heavy an emphasis on magic power and the therapist's personality have little appeal to a younger generation that is repelled by magical procedures and attracted by rational therapy. Yet, in the hands of some therapists, these techniques work. And in some quarters, one can see a swing of the pendulum, a growing intrigue with mystical experience and rejection of emotionally relevant rational approaches (such as analysis of the transference). Directly coercive techniques, such as frightening patients out of their symptoms and habits, may be harmful. An eight-year-old boy with nocturnal enuresis was told by his family physician: "Your little wee-wee will be burnt off with electricity if you don't quit wetting the bed." The boy promptly stopped bed-wetting, but developed nightmares and a marked general passivity and dependency that lasted for years. Some theoretical assumptions for directive therapies have been supplied, but most directive psychotherapists do not utilize them.

Certain therapies are close to directive therapies, although not properly in this category. One is the so-called *anaclitic therapy,* which S. Margolin described and used.[52] This is a therapy that focuses on the anaclitic or dependent needs of a patient and provides, in a planned fashion, emotional support, warmth, and protection; the concepts are expressed in psychoanalytic language. Anaclitic therapy has been used successfully by Erich Lindemann in the therapy of patients with ulcerative colitis.[49] *Conditioning* therapies are referred to in numerous Russian papers and texts, but until recently Western texts have seldom specified how these techniques are used.[17] Joseph Wolpe[77] has described a technique he calls psychotherapy by reciprocal inhibition. He proposes to inhibit fear of aggression by teaching the patient to use aggressive response and inhibits anxiety related to sexual functions by coaching his patients to carry out sexual functions only when they are pleasurably aroused. Wolpe also uses relaxation exercises and hypnotic techniques. He claims to have striking successes with his method, which essentially is based on a Pavlovian model. Wolpe's psychotherapy by reciprocal inhibition is based on the notion that the link between anxiety and the anxiety-provoking stimulus can be weakened if an anxiety-antagonistic response is evoked at the same time. The patients are trained to relax and are then presented with the anxiety-provoking stimuli in a graded series; the next stimulus is presented only when the preceding one can be imagined or experienced without anxiety. Analytic psychotherapy is viewed as a non-systematized technique utilizing such principles of learning. Other learning theorists, as discussed in Chapter 3, recommend "extinguishing" maladaptive patterns, such as by "punishing" stuttering (or making the patient notice his behavior) and rewarding the adaptive response (normal speech). Another example of a conditioning therapy is the treatment of enuretics by a simple apparatus that rings a bell when the bed sheets are moistened by the patient's voiding in his sleep; the patient awakens immediately and, of course, stops urinating. After a number of such trials, the patient is conditioned to awaken without enuresis.

D. Ewen Cameron and his co-workers[9] evolved a therapy called psychic driving. It consists of exposing the patients to highly charged praising (positive) or critical (negative) statements—if possible his own utterances—from morning to night over periods of weeks and months. The hospitalized patients have to listen to 250,000 to 500,000 repetitions. As patients find this procedure intolerable, they are prepared for acceptance of treatment with tranquilizing drugs. In general, this treatment is far too drastic even for the intractable and desperate patient for whom Cameron recommends it, and it has not found wide acceptance in spite of reported successes.

It appears to us that the virtue of some of the more inventive and pragmatic conditioning and "teaching" therapies lies in the notion that explicit steps may be required and that when the student does not learn, the teacher —not the student—has failed to present these steps at the proper intervals. There is a practical emphasis on behavior that many analytic therapists overlook but which good teachers employ in guiding students. However, whether conditioning therapy takes sufficient account of motivational and transference factors is not clear. It may be that certain behaviors, such as phobias and stuttering, which are in themselves easily "demonstrated" to the patient, lend themselves to such treatment more than the more internalized disorders. In any event, where complex disorders are treated by any therapy, the problem is to identify the factors that influenced behavior change, and these are not revealed by what the therapist calls his work—whether analysis, conditioning, or learning.

A number of very old techniques such as the training practiced by Yogas for thousands of years also fall into the category of directive techniques. These techniques involve elaborate breathing and postural exercises that enable the subject to relax and to gain amazing control over vegetative functions. Western psychiatrists have rarely used approaches of this kind, although some have been proposed, for example, the autogenic training advocated by J. H. Schultz.[69] The same is true for Edmund Jacobson's relaxation therapy,[39] and for the massage and various types of body manipulations recently revived by the followers of Wilhelm Reich. Finally, we should mention explicit and practical interventions, the management of situations or crises, which often is, if not directive, manipulative. The imaginative doctor, whatever his theoretical orientation, may respond to a patient with a question, a remark, or an "arrangement" (a referral; a termination; a prescription to rest; or encouraging the patient to avoid a stressful visit; a request for a conference with the family; and so forth), which effectively shifts the balance of pathogenic forces.

Hypnosis

Hypnosis, a trancelike condition that has been used for scientific and therapeutic purposes, can be produced in about 20 per cent of the population. The very simplicity of the technique invites abuse and therapeutic application by unauthorized, unethical, and uninformed persons, who often apply it when such use is not indicated and possibly dangerous. For this reason, and because it has been praised as a panacea, hypnosis has a dubious reputation in the United States, and the American Psychiatric Association found it necessary to publish a warning statement. It was recommended that hypnosis be used for analgesic and sedative purposes only by those who have qualified knowledge in psychopathology and diagnosis; and that it be taught in medical schools, presumably in departments of psychiatry, but not in isolated courses. In the hands of authorized personnel, hypnosis has value as an experimental procedure and, to a limited degree, as a therapy. There are two types of therapeutic hypnosis: (1) directive or authoritative hypnosis, in which the patient is ordered to give up a symptom or attitude; and (2) cathartic hypnosis. Josef Breuer and Sigmund Freud were the first therapists to use cathartic hypnosis to induce their patients to search for hidden memories. Freud later abandoned the procedure when he recognized that many patients could not be hypnotized and decided that depth psychological exploration was more feasible in patients who were not in a state of trance.

Hypnosis has a superficial similarity to sleep; however, electroencephalographic findings clearly differentiate the two states. As a matter of fact, actual sleep may be superimposed on the trance state by hypnotic suggestion. The similarity to sleep derives from the far-reaching relaxation that may occur during hypnosis. Reduction of anxiety and tension may accompany such relaxation if this is suggested to the patient. On the other hand, anxiety, rage, guilt, and shame may also be produced and increased during hypnosis. Statements have been made that intellectual powers may be increased during hypnosis, but what is actually possible is only the removal of inhibitions and the mobilization of what was consciously not accessible. That is, inaccessible memories may be obtained or sharpened, and after reduction of anxiety and inhibition rote-learning may improve. Another widely held assumption maintains that hypnotized subjects may be induced to commit crimes. There is, however, no evidence that unethical behavior that is not latently present can be invoked,[6] although inhibitions can be lowered and undesirable motivations can be evoked.

The mechanisms involved in the hypnotic state are unclear, although there are many theories, which have been reviewed by Lewis R. Wolberg, a judicious proponent of therapeutic hypnosis.[75] Some of the most important theories are Jean Martin Charcot's theory that hypnosis is an artificial dissociative state; the Pavlovian theory that views a hypnotic trance as a state of cortical inhibition; Clark Hull's suggestibility theory; and Martin T. Orne's theory,[60] which sees hypnosis as a form of play-acting to please the hypnotist. Gill and Margaret Brenman consider hypnosis as a form of selective regression, which is induced by sensory deprivation and the establishment of an archaic oral-dependent relationship of the hypnotized subject to the hypnotist.[31]

Technique: There are many ways to produce hypnotic trance. A simple procedure consists of placing the subject or patient in a comfortable supine position in a quiet room. The hypnotist repeats in a monotonous voice that the patient is becoming sleepy and wishes to close his eyes. Some hypnotists ask the subject to gaze at an object held close in front of the patient's eyes; the forced convergence of the eyes actually promotes such a desire. Others suggest that outstretched hands will feel light or heavy, and this promotes a "dissociative attitude"—that is, a sensation or movement which somehow occurs but without self-direction. Once the patient closes his eyes, he usually falls into a state of trance, which is rarely very deep during the first session. Further suggestions of motor acts or of drowsiness ensue. During the trance, he will comply with the commands of the hypnotist; if commands are to be carried out after the hypnotic trance, we speak of *posthypnotic suggestion*. Therapeutic trance should not exceed one hour. The patient should be asked to awaken promptly and without any feelings of fatigue or malaise. During hypnotic sessions (especially where there is not an established working relationship of patient and therapist), a third person should be present or in a nearby room to protect the therapist from any accusations of improper behavior, and, in any event, written consent for the procedure is advisable.

Indications: Hypnosis may be used to reduce psychological and muscular tension and subjective discomfort in a wide variety of psychiatric and somatic conditions. It has been used as an anesthetic in surgical and obstetrical patients, in intractable pain of terminal patients, and in many psychosomatic disorders such as prolonged hiccoughs and unbearable itching. Hysterical amnesia and hysterical conversion symptoms can be readily relieved by hypnosis in most cases, but the symptoms typically recur shortly in an identical or modified form. Wolberg warns of the extensive use of authoritative hypnosis and sees the usefulness of the method more in cathartic hypnosis, often in combination with analytic therapies.[74] Whether a revival of cathartic hypnosis on a large scale is justified seems dubious, but limited applications by some experienced practitioners seem to work. In the hands of an experienced therapist, the danger of occurrence of hysterical states in a hypnotic trance that gets out of hand is slight. To treat a patient by hypnosis who can be helped more efficiently by other organic or psychological methods is a serious mistake.

Related to cathartic hypnosis or hypnoanalysis is the use of sedative and hypnotic drugs to help the patient to obtain catharsis and re-experience painful, forgotten, and distorted memories, which previously could not be mastered. Such narcoanalysis, with the aid of intravenous sodium pentothal or sodium amytal, was successfully used by Roy R. Grinker and John P. Spiegel [34] in patients with combat neuroses; its use in civilian practice is limited. LSD-25, Psilocybin, and mescaline are currently being used by some workers in this way, especially with alcoholics and character problems.

Existentialist Therapy

Existentialist psychotherapy is the most recent newcomer on the scene. Existentialist psychiatrists are a rather heterogeneous group, and it is impossible to write about their therapy as if it were a unified approach. There is, at times, the inescapable impression that they are primarily unified by their antagonism to classical psychoanalysis and traditional general psychiatry. Yet this is an oversimplification, because the Swiss existential therapists, Medard Boss, Hans Knöpfel, and some others, are relatively close to psychoanalysis. Many of the leaders of existentialist psychiatry have not been truly interested in therapy, and relatively little has actually been written about existentialist therapy. Rollo May explains this by the disinclination of existentialists to deal with technique.[53] Existential psychiatrists who do not think in terms of pathology but in terms of modes and conditions of existence are also opposed to a concept like cure. Only diseases can be cured, not human existence. As existentialist psychiatrists are opposed to compartmentalization, most of them do not recognize the unconscious or any process of treatment that makes the unconscious conscious. Many of their statements about therapeutic goals and methods are so vaguely broad that they are difficult to apprehend. Victor Frankl stresses that neurotic patients lack meaning in their lives. The so-called *noogenic neurosis* is a life without meaning; Frankl conceives of the therapeutic task as a way of giving meaning to patients.[22] In his logotherapy he tries to discover such meaning by a method of Socratic discussion. At first, Frankl conceived of logotherapy as a complement to other methods, but one now gets the impression that it is a somewhat unspecific approach in its own right. We consider it a fundamental error to regard the primary task of psychotherapy as the giving of meaning; [57] this is a task for philosophers and theologians. It may happen, of course, that patients will find meaning after successful therapy. With Allen Wheelis, we are inclined to think that psychotherapy cannot be a substitute for a Weltanschauung and that such a quest is bound to lead to disappointment.[73]

Boss, who tried to combine psychoanalytic technique with Heideggerian philosophy,[6] is one of the few existentialist psychiatrists who have specifically written about treatment. It is very difficult to evaluate Boss's approach, because for anyone who is not thoroughly acquainted with Heidegger's existentialism, the language and concepts are quite obscure. In general, existential therapists have interpreted existence in holistic terms. The concepts of man's freedom to choose; the need to commit oneself; to grasp one's existential anxiety; the need to appreciate one's forlornness over the finiteness of existence; the need to give life meaning; and the need to understand man's limitations are important and recurrent topics. Existentialism, and probably existential therapy, has aroused interest primarily among the more philosophically inclined therapists and patients; on the European Continent, the movement has gained broader acceptance than in the United States.

The Group Therapies

Group therapy is characterized not only by the fact that a number of patients with behavior disorders is treated instead of an individual but also by its use of group influences. As individual therapy, it attempts to decrease isolation, increase self-esteem, solve identity problems, and reach new and better adaptive responses. An increasing number of psychiatrists is becoming convinced of the value of the method and considers group therapy, and in particular family therapy, one of the most important psychiatric therapeutic advances in midcentury. A group represents a powerful vehicle for structuring and reinforcing behavior; the emotion that is elicited, as anyone reflecting on family experience knows, is intense, and the opportunity for learning about oneself by acting in the company of others and through the response of others is optimal. In terms of intensifying and eliciting response on the one hand, and modifying such emotional response, on the other, the properly structured group experience is, perhaps, more vivid than the transference neurosis slowly fostered in psychoanalysis.

Until recently, the greatest advantage of group therapy was seen simply in the fact that more patients could be treated by this method than by individual therapy. The therapeutic use of group influences by faith healers and in shrines and spas over all the world is very old. Joseph Hersey Pratt, a physician of Boston, was the first deliberately to use therapy with groups in a medical setting. The genius of Paul Schilder recognized the value of group therapy early and extended psychoanalytic principles to group therapy. Other pioneers were S. R. Slavson, Trigant Burrow, and R. Dreikurs. Austen Riggs lectured to his patients occasionally over loudspeakers. Modern analytic group therapies have become prominent since World War II; they are being described and explored by S. H. Foulkes,[20] L. Grinberg, M. Langer and E. Rodrigué,[32] Florence B. Powdermaker and Jerome D. Frank,[64] and others.

TYPES OF GROUP THERAPY Group therapy, as individual psychotherapy, may be divided into directive and analytic therapy. Directive group therapy has a limited place in psychiatry; the use of lectures with group discussion, as in Pratt's original method, has fallen into disuse. Much current work in Western countries is based on combined principles of psychoanalysis and group dynamics. It permits not only very relevant observation but also therapeutically controlled social interaction and recognition of the self through the response of others.

An interesting form of group therapy is psychodrama, which was developed by Jacob L. Moreno.[56] The technique consists of the spontaneous enactment of emotionally charged topics, conflicts, and relationships in the real or fantasy life of the patients. The therapist functions as a stage director; the patient or principal actor is supported by other persons, patients, and therapists, the so-called alter egos, and also by the group of spectators. The role of the therapist-director is to initiate action and also to integrate and interpret meanings. However, as in all analytic group therapy, the main emphasis rests on the productivity and creativity of the patients. The procedure, much akin to play therapy, yields rich and fascinating clinical material and is impressive when personally demonstrated by Moreno. Yet it has been taken up by others only to a limited degree; seemingly, there is considerable resistance to this creative technique.

STANDARD TECHNIQUES OF GROUP THERAPY Many techniques have been described for the variants of analytic group therapy; some group therapists, especially those influenced by the Tavistock Clinic, focus almost entirely on group interactions; others pay almost as much attention to a member's accounts as they would in individual therapy. All group therapists recognize the importance of the group leader, even in so-called leaderless therapeutic groups. In some training centers, students of group therapy are required to join didactic groups as "patients" before they lead group sessions. Group therapies are carried out in outpatient clinics, hospitals, and, rarely, in private practice. Comfortable seating around a table or in a living room is preferable to a classroom arrangement. The size of groups varies; the group dynamics of small groups of six to eleven members, which in our opinion are optimal, are, of course, very different from those of large groups.

There has been some difference of opinion as to whether the group should be heterogeneous or homogeneous.[38] Too much heterogeneity may hinder the therapeutic effectiveness of the group. Generally, it is difficult to combine patients with severe psychoses and those with mild neuroses or persons of appreciably different levels of intelligence. Differences in social status must be considered; still, the de-emphasis of social position or social success may be of some help in the therapeutic process. It is useful to have members of both sexes in the group. Apart from family groups, adults and children are not customarily put into one group. Uniting of adolescents with adults has been found helpful by some therapists.

Discussion should be as free as possible, and the competent group therapist is skilled in promoting this. Most groups work with one therapist; sometimes a second professional person is introduced into the group as an observer. The roles of observer and therapist should be well structured. Qualifications of the group therapist are similar to those of an individual therapist. In particular, he should be capable of satisfactory peer relationships and have little need of authoritative behavior or of recognition.[64] He exerts his influence through direct methods and also through group practices and customs, which he helps to establish. He responds, clarifies, and interprets behavior and relationships but in general is active only when the group becomes confused, helpless, or inactive over a long period. The essence of the group discussion is that everyone is heard; everyone's feelings are expressed; and everyone in the group "works." The group may function at various levels of depth, but no subject is "too hot to handle." If possible, once a group is formed, new members are not to be added. The termination of the group has similarities with the resolution of individual therapy, except that the criteria are even more complicated because the progress of therapy with the different members of the group will not be the same. Group members learn to proceed under their own power, and eventually there is a diminishing return; this is the most important criterion for termination. A. Wolf introduced a technique in which group members have alternate sessions by themselves;[76] such exercises in independence also help in the problems of group resolution.

Whether group or individual therapy is superior is an unanswerable question. In certain settings, as in industrial organizations, schools, the armed forces, hospitals, and prisons, where natural groups already exist, group therapy is of demonstrable value. In general, the less educated and the lower classes do relatively well in groups; resistance to group therapy is strongest in the upper and middle classes but it is by no means insurmountable. Some patients do better in individual therapy; others, in group therapy. Those who know both methods tend to feel that group therapy mobilizes stronger emotions; it facilitates the direct observation of social interaction by all members rather than stressing learning through observing the transference. Escape, resistance, identificaton, displacement, projection, and generalization can be demonstrated very clearly. A controlled acting out of the group and therapeutic measures to control such acting out often have a very powerful impact on the patients. Last but not least, it should be noted that not only differences in the "talents" and inclinations of patients exist but also that there are differences among therapists. Some therapists take more easily to group therapy and seem more effective with this approach; others are inclined to individual work. With some patients, a double-barreled approach combining individual and group techniques may be successfully employed; this may enhance pertinent observations that can be a basis for new learning and revised attitudes.

One of the most important applications of group therapy is its use in hospitals, where it can be conducted as formal group therapy or in fostering constructive group influences by encouraging patients and staff to assume jointly responsibilities in what the pioneer in this field, Maxwell Jones, called the therapeutic community: [40] the establishment of patient governments and of joint patient-staff meetings. Nea M. Norton, Thomas P. Detre, and Henry G. Jarecki [58] used family therapy with small groups consisting of the hospitalized patient and key members of his family and also with large groups made up of all patients of the same therapist and the members of their families. The larger groups numbered twenty to thirty members and also included social workers, occupational therapists, and nurses. Such combinations of group therapies with groups of patients, groups of relatives, and groups of relatives and patients together is referred to as multidimensional group therapy.[85] Such group therapies provide, apart from involvement of all affected, opportunities to effect changes in the self or others that are vivid and visible.

Hospitalization and Milieu Therapy

In Chapter 1, the emergence of the modern psychiatric hospital was briefly described, with some attention to the changing concepts about the use of hospitalization for psychiatric patients. Indications for hospitalization are today more clearly defined than formerly, and, in general, we are less inclined to hospitalize psychiatric patients. We hospitalize patients for the following reasons: (1) to remove the patient from unbearable pressures of his environment that make therapy difficult or impossible; (2) to carry out diagnostic and therapeutic procedures that are not feasible outside the hospital; or (3) to protect and treat the patient who is dangerous to himself and others in the community. There are patients who face such odds in their natural social environment that only a new controlled therapeutic environment can provide the conditions for positive behavioral change. In this modern sense, for some patients at least, hospitals are still asylums or, as we prefer to call them today, therapeutic communities.

Psychiatry hardly uses the complicated diagnostic procedures that only the modern general hospital can provide. Psychiatric therapies in hospitals are rarely highly specialized technical procedures but constitute, rather, a very well-organized therapeutic milieu, which teaches the patient, and in some cases his family as well, to live better. They ought to be, as Charles Burlingame realized some time ago, not retreats but institutes of living. In such a setting, individual therapy, even if it is as frequent as one hour a day (never on Sundays, of course!), will be supplemented by group therapies and will benefit from patients' interactions, not just with psychiatrists, but with all mental health workers and, last but not least, with other patients. In such a setting, the patient learns the role of patienthood,[47] that is, to work on his problems in a sheltered environment for a limited period of time. We know, of course, that there are failures. Some patients cannot return to their natural communities; a few, because our therapeutic knowledge is insufficient; others, because good therapy is not available; and some, because biological and social odds are stacked against them. For some, what is euphemistically called continuous care may be necessary, but such necessity is becoming rarer. We do not wish to give the impression that we overvalue psychosocial therapies and minimize biological therapies. In hospitals, particularly, with their large populations of patients with psychotic depressions, schizophrenias, and behaviors associated with brain diseases, biological therapies are gaining in importance. Yet the therapeutic milieu of the modern psychiatric hospital is of prime importance. Harry A. Wilmer, who sensitively described the therapeutic milieu, stresses that the effectiveness of the milieu depends to a large degree on the attitudes of the psychiatric and administrative staff and their interaction with the society of patients.[14] A stable and reliable atmosphere must be created in which patients can learn to replace their inadequate responses with appropriate responses. The professional personnel must take a stand concerning the degree to which they wish to let patients take responsibility for living and learning in the modern mental institution. In many institutions the professional staff has encouraged patients to form a patient council or patient government. Such an organization may present the patients' interests and permit them to participate in the conduct of hospital affairs. Patient governments help the patients to assume responsibility and are considered therapeutically desirable even if they function in varying degrees only as "puppet governments."

Occupational therapy has the goal of socializing patients by providing them with skills, enhancing their self-esteem, and countering the disintegrating forces of idleness in mental hospitals.[19] Recreational therapy aims to gratify patients by meaningful play and to enhance their creative activities. Today, there is a tendency to prescribe occupational and recreational therapy according to specific dynamic needs of the patient and to make these therapies more realistic; the traditional basket-weaving is being replaced by serious individual training for skills and jobs. Vocational counseling and educational extension courses are also becoming parts of the therapeutic program. These efforts have been designed to meet specific patients' needs and not the maintenance requirements of the institution; what used to be called industrial therapy was really forced labor. In general, patients' needs have become more important than the esthetic or useful qualities of the finished product. Preparation for the type of work (including schoolwork), which the patient must take up when he re-enters the community, is becoming an important consideration in programing rehabilitation. Another advance consists of recognizing and utilizing the artistic and creative potential in patients by such activities as painting and sculpturing[57] and music.[61]

There are many reasons why patients and their families object to hospitalization: high cost; depriving the patient of his earning power; social stigma; and the fact that hospitalization may elicit even more conscious and unconscious anxiety, guilt, and shame than psychiatric therapy in general. The occurrence of such emotions in the patient and his family must not, however, deter the therapist from incisive intervention when it is necessary. A psychiatrist's reluctance to send a patient to a hospital may be a disservice to the patient and his family, for whom this resource may be of decisive benefit as well as a temporary relief. It is necessary, of course, to hospitalize the relatively rare patient who is destructive or self-destructive, but the indication to hospitalize dangerous patients is still frequently misused: hospitalization should not be an incarceration that deprives the patient of his freedom, his civil rights, and his chance of real help. Hospitalization may represent punitive or self-punitive behavior by the patient and his family or the therapist; we must be alert to such a possibility.

While there is a justified tendency today to hospitalize psychiatric patients for the shortest possible time, some patients need prolonged treatment, particularly some children and adolescents in a psychiatric school or hospital setting; or others require permanent confinement to an institution. In any event the modern trend is not to let patients become regressed and asocial. Of course the avoidance of regression at all cost, could become a harmful fad. In all good psychosocial therapy, a certain degree of controlled and temporary regression is bound to occur. Further, the nature of some of the available long-term hospital experiences is such that the patient can, through group living and psychotherapy, attain a deep and thorough understanding of the way he relates to others and can emerge with a more stable basis for social adjustments and gratification. With the growth of easily available treatment in psychiatric wards in general hospitals and in state and private institutions, and with day hospitals, "hospitalizing" and rehospitalizing the patient becomes a *phase* in a continuing program of treatment, not a "disposition." With a patient-centered treatment program comprised of varied facilities for a patient, rather than an institution-centered program, into which the patient must be fitted, hospitalization need not be a stigma, a punishment, or an abandonment. Rather, we hope to be able to use whatever treatment resource is practical for an ongoing problem; and the therapeutic utility of the hospital for the patient, rather than "severity of illness," is the best criterion for a decision. It should be remembered that these innovations aim to keep the family and community engaged with the patient, just as we attempt to aid the patient to be able to learn how *and* when to engage with them.

Rehabilitation

Attempts to restore patients who have suffered from diseases and accidents to their normal occupational and social functions are referred to as rehabilitation. In psychiatry, a clear differentiation of rehabilitation from therapy and from efforts at prevention of recurrence is not possible. Physical rehabilitation is of little concern in psychiatry; occupational, educational, and social rehabilitation should be, from the very outset, a part of the treatment process. The *open hospital* may be defined as a setting that has never become separated from the community and where efficient efforts can be made more easily to rehabilitate the patient in his community. For some patients, particularly if hospitalization is prolonged, it is beneficial to spend only the day or the night in the hospital. Such *day-or-night hospitals* have been developed in a number of centers in America and Europe. Another approach to rehabilitation is the so-called *halfway house.* This essentially is an open hospital and day center, an institution within the community to which patients from ordinary psychiatric hospitals are transferred; the setting permits and encourages work, participation in community activities, and also provides psychiatric therapy and a certain measure of shelter. In combination with industrial relocation centers, such units have been successfully used in Great Britain. J. Bierer finds the development of patient's clubs also therapeutically valuable.[7] In the United States, Abraham Low founded an organization of discharged patients, Recovery, Inc., not dissimilar from Alcoholics Anonymous, which has some promise along similar lines.

Psychiatric patients of the lower classes meet special difficulties in returning to their families after hospitalization. However, once they are in the community, there is no relationship between successful posthospital adjustment and social class.[23] In recognition of this, new and more vigorous efforts by social workers and psychiatrists to facilitate such adjustment have been made in "aftercare" clinics and home care units.

Prevention

Although this word occurs frequently in the vocabulary of psychiatrists, the fact is we have little knowledge of how to prevent mental disorders and little evidence of effective action. Prevention, like treatment, must be based on precise knowledge of etiological variables. When such knowledge exists, prevention becomes possible; if not, it remains wishful thinking or wild application. We agree with Gerald Caplan,[10] however, that research about prevention and experimentation with preventative methods are most important.

In the public-health literature, primary, secondary, and tertiary prevention are distinguished. *Primary prevention* seeks to eradicate diseases and disorders by eliminating their causes and stopping their spread. *Secondary prevention* essentially means early diagnosis and therapy to prevent further development of symptoms. *Tertiary prevention* refers to limitation of disability in patients with irreversible pathology and to initiation of rehabilitation. In our opinion, the terms secondary and tertiary prevention are not appropriate; they are therapeutic endeavors. Most preventive measures are of a psychosocial nature; some of the most effective methods are biological. Control and elimination of etiological agents have resulted in the marked reduction of general paresis, pellagra, or the bromide psychoses and the mental deficiences associated with galactosemia and phenylketonuria. Public health programs that reduce accidents and the use of industrial poisons obviously will also reduce those disorders that are so caused. The problem of preventive reduction of psychoses caused by habit-forming drugs, a much more complicated problem, is dealt with in chapters 22 and 23.

Prevention through genetic control is successful to a very limited degree. The large-scale attempts to control mental diseases genetically under National Socialism were barbaric and utterly unscientific. There is rarely enough compelling evidence to justify compulsory sterilization, or even legal prevention of marriage. Sterilization is indicated only in a very limited number of conditions, as in a few hereditary psychoses like Huntington's Chorea, or in certain familial cases of mental deficiency; schizophrenics are a small problem in this respect, because they rarely have a large number of children. Indications are by no means purely biological; assessment of social factors is important, and it is better to rely on voluntary cooperation and agreement than on state laws. Benjamin Pasamanick[63] pointed to the importance of prevention of trauma during pregnancy and takes the position that such prevention will diminish the incidence of some behavior disorders. The problem of therapeutic abortion is discussed in Chapter 24.

A number of techniques promise prevention of difficulties resulting from separation and emotional deprivation. We will later take up such techniques as natural childbirth or obstetrical psychoprophylaxis, the rooming-in program, and more reasonable approaches to feeding and toilet training of infants (in Chapter 25). There are many other changes in the child-rearing of preschool children that are based on an increased scientific and realistic understanding of conscious and unconscious needs of parents and children.[24] The years of late adolescence and young adulthood, before the most important decisions about marriage and occupation are made, and before children are on the scene, are probably the crucial years for preventive measures, such as counseling on interpersonal relations of individuals and sensitivity training of groups. As these practices may find broad application they may tend to prevent behavior disorders. We are, however, only at the very beginning of such endeavors. It is also the psychiatrist's responsibility to take a lead in public adult education about matters of mental health and behavior disorders, about which the public knows all too little. Elaine Cumming and John H. Cumming have demonstrated and reported the difficulties of such endeavors.[13]

So-called secondary prevention or early diagnosis and appropriate action are particularly important in the psychoses. The early diagnosis of neuroses is not easy, because patients do not consult psychiatrists at this stage; for early diagnosis we must rely on general practitioners of medicine, teachers, ministers, and others. Early treatment is likewise difficult, because motivation is lacking. Unfortunately, human beings are willing to seek help for their emotional problems only when the water is up to their necks. Lawyers, ministers, educators, and particularly practitioners of medicine are in a good position to prepare patients in a realistic fashion for the need and nature of a psychiatric consultation or admission to a psychiatric hospital. They can diminish the anxiety, guilt, and shame of the patient and his family and also realistically prepare those involved for some of the necessary social and economic arrangements. Many behavior disorders are recognized and dealt with in their incipient stage by workers in social agencies. It is of great importance, therefore, that these workers are well trained to deal with such problems and receive help, whenever it is indicated, from a consultative relationship with psychiatrists. Services, exemplifying prevention, have been set up in Amsterdam by A. M. Querido. In a network of clinics, public health agencies and social agencies, he established teams that promptly visit patients with psychiatric emergencies at their homes.[46] One professional in such teams may obviate the need for fifty hospital beds! Principles of tertiary prevention have been discussed already in the section on rehabilitation.

Evaluation of Psychosocial Therapies

There is a critical need for the careful, objective appraisal of all psychiatric therapies.[70] The psychosocial therapies in particular have not been thoroughly evaluated. In any case, there is no "hard-nosed" documentation of their effectiveness. There are very few comparisons of treated and untreated cases.[68] Certainly, there is a need for adequate long-term catamnestic studies, such as the follow-up studies by P. O'Neal, J. Bergman, J. Schafer, and L. Robins,[59] which showed that untreated sociopaths who appeared in children's courts developed serious difficulties as adults. In most cases, evaluations are made by the therapist himself, who is bound to be a subjective optimist and inclined to overestimate his successes and deny his failures. In the literature,[36] there are surprisingly few reports of failures. We are apt to consider therapy as successful because it exists; possibly, Frank is right when he says that all therapies do some good or they would disappear.[21] Indeed, it is remarkable that many of our major psychotherapies have "survived" for a long time, presumably on the basis of convincing detailed case reports and an "appealing" rationale rather than on the basis of hard evidence. Our inability and unwillingness to evaluate psychosocial therapies cannot be simply explained by man's incurable gullibility or by a lack of scientific sophistication. Evaluation of any therapy, and particularly of psychosocial therapy, is a complex problem.[45] Qualitative evaluation alone is scientifically not satisfactory, and quantitative evaluation presents very difficult methodological hurdles. We either oversimplify our approach or consider more variables that we can manipulate, and we then maintain that the complexities of psychosocial therapy defy evaluation. Criteria, such as discharge from a hospital or clinic, and the crude differentiations into cured, improved, or unchanged that are used so often have little value for a scientific assessment of behavior change. They depend largely on certain social interactions in the institution and community. Furthermore, if evaluation of the effectiveness of one or another kind of psychotherapy is undertaken, it should be recalled that the therapist—whatever he labels his therapy—may consequentially differ in his behavior and interventions from his colleagues of similar persuasion. Even when hospital discharges are used as a criterion of improvement, these are the subject of very different interpretations. Some writers attribute the increase of discharges from hospitals in recent years to drugs, others to social and occupational rehabilitation.

As long as psychiatrists thought they treated clear-cut symptoms of well-defined diseases, the matter was relatively simple (that is, the symptoms were or were not seen to disappear). Today we have begun to appreciate the complexity of normal and abnormal behavior and are less simplistic. An appealing approach was suggested by M. B. Parloff, H. C. Kelman, and J. D. Frank[62] who recommended the following broad criteria for the evaluation of psychotherapy: comfort, self-awareness, and social effectiveness. In further evaluating therapeutic "results" our interests have increasingly focused on behavior change. If this approach advances we will be describing the patient's specific modes of interpreting input and organizing to cope with it. Changes in these behavioral parameters may be grossly evident only in certain negative features—behaviors the patient no longer resorts to in particular crises, the diminished attention he pays to persisting symptoms, the ease with which he masters what for him were once psychologically insuperable obstacles. If growth and development have anything to do with behavior change, the assessment of change—especially in the neuroses—must be based on accurate inventory by multiple judges of prior techniques by which the patient coped; it will take much work to identify, survey, and give proper weight to these consequential factors. A catalog of diagnoses, symptoms, and complaints may not be sufficiently precise to assess behavior change, and a listing of the patient's psychodynamic mechanisms may be too general to be useful. Finally, differences in modes of experience and functioning may have to be tested over appropriately long periods of time and in objective behavioral test situations. The conceptual and methodological work required is clearly challenging.

In any case, psychiatrists have had to recognize that behavioral change is the result of many factors.[67] It is hoped that more realistic and sophisticated evaluations will gradually be introduced, which will increasingly consider the complexities of behavior disorders, of the psychosocial therapies, and of behavior change and permit selection rather than "survival" of the fittest therapy. As the concepts and methods of the psychosocial therapies become more scientific through clinical research and experimentation, not only evaluation, but also prediction of results should become possible. The relatively simpler problems of evaluation of the organic therapies and particularly of drug therapies will be discussed in Chapter 11, which is devoted to the organic therapies.

NOTES

1. Alexandra Adler, *Guiding Human Misfits* (New York: Macmillan, 1938).
2. Alfred Adler, *The Individual Psychology of Alfred Adler* (New York: Basic Books, 1956).
3. Franz Alexander, *Psychoanalysis and Psychotherapy* (New York: Norton, 1956).

4. Franz Alexander and Thomas M. French, *Psychoanalytic Therapy* (New York: Ronald Press, 1946).
5. Michael and Enid Balint, *Psychotherapeutic Techniques in Medicine* (Springfield, Ill.: Charles C Thomas, 1962).
6. Theodore X. Barber, "Antisocial and Criminal Acts Induced by Hypnosis," *Archives of General Psychiatry*, 5 (1961), 301.
7. Joshua Bierer, *The Day Hospital* (London: Lewis, 1951).
8. Medard Boss, " 'Daseinsanalysis' and Psychotherapy," in Jules H. Masserman and Jacob L. Moreno, eds., *Progress in Psychotherapy*, Vol. 2; p. 156 (New York: Grune and Stratton, 1957).
9. D. Ewen Cameron, L. Levy, and L. Rubenstein, "Effects of Repetition of Verbal Signals upon the Behaviour of Chronic Psychoneurotic Patients," *Journal of Mental Science*, 106 (1960), 742.
10. Gerald Caplan, *Principles of Preventative Psychiatry* (New York: Basic Books, 1964).
11. Kenneth M. Colby, *A Primer for Psychotherapists* (New York: Ronald Press, 1951).
12. Jules V. Coleman, "Banter as Psychotherapeutic Intervention," *American Journal of Psychoanalysis*, 22 (1962), 69.
13. Elaine Cumming and John H. Cumming, *Closed Ranks* (Cambridge: Commonwealth Fund, 1957).
14. Felix Deutsch, "The Associative Anamnesis," *Psychoanalytic Quarterly*, 8 (1939), 354.
15. John Dollard, Frank Auld, and Alice M. White, *Steps in Psychotherapy* (New York: Macmillan, 1953).
16. Marshall Edelson, *Ego Psychology, Group Dynamics and the Therapeutic Community* (New York: Grune and Stratton, 1964).
17. Hans J. Eysenck, ed., *Behavior Therapy and the Neuroses* (Oxford: Pergamon, 1960).
18. Hans J. Eysenck *et al.*, "The Effects of Psychotherapy," and discussion, *International Journal of Psychiatry*, 1 (1965), 97.
19. Gail S. Fidler and Jay W. Fidler, *Introduction to Psychiatric Occupational Therapy* (New York, Macmillan, 1958).
20. Siegmund H. Foulkes, *Introduction to Group Analytic Psychotherapy* (London: Heinemann, 1948).
21. Jerome D. Frank, *Persuasion and Healing* (Baltimore: Johns Hopkins Press, 1961).
22. Viktor E. Frankl, "The Concept of Man in Psychotherapy," *Pastoral Psychology*, 6 (1955), 16.
23. Howard E. Freeman and Ozzie G. Simmons, *The Mental Patient Comes Home* (New York: John Wiley, 1963).
24. Anna Freud, "Observations on Child Development," in *Psychoanalytic Study of the Child*, Vol. 18 (New York: International Universities Press, 1951).
25. Sigmund Freud, "The Interpretation of Dreams" [1900], *Standard Edition* No. 5 (London: Hogarth Press, 1955).

26. Sigmund Freud, "New Introductory Lectures on Psychoanalysis" [1933], *Standard Edition* No. 22 (London: Hogarth Press, 1964).
27. Sigmund Freud, "Lines of Advance in Psychoanalytic Therapy" [1919], *Standard Edition* No. 17 (London: Hogarth Press, 1957).
28. Erich Fromm, *The Sane Society* (New York: Rinehart, 1955).
29. Frieda Fromm-Reichmann, *Principles of Intensive Psychotherapy* (Chicago: University of Chicago Press, 1950).
30. Merton M. Gill, "Psychoanalysis and Exploratory Psychotherapy," *Journal of the American Psychoanalytic Association*, 2 (1954), 771.
31. Merton M. Gill and Margaret Brenman, *Hypnosis and the Related States* (New York: International Universities Press, 1960).
32. Leon Grinberg, L. J. Alvarez de Toledo, *El Grupo Psicológico* (Buenos Aires: Editorial Nova, 1959).
33. Roy R. Grinker, *Psychiatry and Social Work; a Transactional Case Book* (New York: Basic Books, 1961).
34. Roy R. Grinker and John P. Spiegel, *Men under Stress* (New York: Blakiston, 1945).
35. Josef P. Hes and S. L. Handler, "Multidimensional Group Psychotherapy," *Archives of General Psychiatry*, 5 (1961), 70.
36. Paul H. Hoch, "Aims and Limitations of Psychotherapy," *American Journal of Psychiatry*, 112 (1955), 321.
37. Karen Horney, *New Ways in Psychoanalysis* (New York: Norton, 1939).
38. Walter W. Igersheimer, "Analytically Oriented Group Psychotherapy for Patients with Psychosomatic Illnesses," *International Journal of Group Psychotherapy*, 9 (1959), 71.
39. Edmund Jacobson, *Progressive Relaxation* (Chicago: University of Chicago Press, 1938).
40. Maxwell Jones, *The Therapeutic Community* (New York: Basic Books, 1953).
41. Carl Gustav Jung, *Collected Papers on Analytic Psychology*, translated by Constance E. Long (New York: Moffat, Yard, 1922).
42. Hellmuth Kaiser, "The Problem of Responsibility in Psychotherapy," *Psychiatry*, 18 (1955), 205.
43. Melanie Klein, *New Directions in Psychoanalysis* (New York: Basic Books, 1961).
44. Robert P. Knight, "An Evaluation of Psychotherapeutic Techniques," *Bulletin of the Menninger Clinic*, 16 (1952), 113.
45. Lawrence C. Kolb, "Psychotherapeutic Evaluation and Its Implications," *Psychiatric Quarterly*, 30 (1956), 579.
46. Paul V. Lemkau and Guido M. Crocetti, "The Amsterdam Municipal Psychiatric Service," *American Journal of Psychiatry*, 117 (1961), 779.
47. Daniel J. Levinson and Eugene B. Gallagher, *Patienthood in the Mental Hospital* (Boston: Houghton Mifflin, 1964).
48. Robert J. Lifton, *Thought Reform and the Psychology of Totalism* (New York: Norton, 1961).

49. Erich Lindemann, "Psychiatric Problems in Conservative Treatment of Ulcerative Colitis," *Archives of Neurology and Psychiatry*, 53 (1945), 322.
50. Hans W. Loewald, "On the Therapeutic Action of Psychoanalysis," *International Journal of Psychoanalysis*, 41 (1960), 16.
51. Sandor Lorand and W. A. Cansole, "Therapeutic Results in Psychoanalytic Treatment without Fee," *International Journal of Psychoanalysis*, 39 (1958), 59.
52. Sydney Margolin, "On Some Principles of Therapy," *American Journal of Psychiatry*, 114 (1958), 1087.
53. Rollo May, "Contributions of Existential Psychotherapy," In R. May, E. Angel, and H. F. Ellenberger, eds., *Existence* (New York: Basic Books, Inc., 1958).
54. Karl Menninger, *Theory of Psychoanalytic Technique* (New York: Basic Books, 1958).
55. Ruth L. Monroe, *Schools of Psychoanalytic Thought* (New York: Dryden, 1955).
56. Jacob L. Moreno, "Fundamental Rules and Techniques of Psychodrama," in Jules H. Masserman and Jacob L. Moreno, eds., *Progress in Psychotherapy* (New York: Grune and Stratton, 1958), 3.
57. Margaret Naumberg, *Schizophrenic Art* (New York: Grune and Stratton, 1950).
58. Nea M. Norton, Thomas P. Detre, and Henry G. Jarecki, "Psychiatric Services in General Hospitals. A Family Oriented Definition," *Journal of Nervous and Mental Disease*, 136 (1963), 475.
59. Patricia O'Neal, John Bergman, Jeannette Schafer, and Lee Robins, "The Relation of Childhood Behavior Problems to Adult Psychiatric Status. A 30 year Followup Study of 262 Subjects ," in J. Gottlieb and G. Tourney, eds., *Scientific Papers and Discussions* (Washington, D.C.: A.P.A. District Branch Publication, February 1960), 99.
60. Martin T. Orne, "The Mechanisms of Hypnotic Age Regression: An Experimental Study," *Journal of Abnormal and Social Psychology*, 46 (1951), 213.
61. Peter Ostwald, *Soundmaking: The Acoustic Communication of Emotions* (Springfield: Charles C Thomas, 1963.)
62. Morris B. Parloff, Herbert C. Kelman, and Jerome D. Frank, "Comfort, Effectiveness, and Self-Awareness as Criteria of Improvement in Psychotherapy," *American Journal of Psychiatry*, 111 (1954), 343.
63. Benjamin Pasamanick and A. M. Lilienfeld, "Association of Maternal and Fetal Factors with Development of Mental Deficiency," *Journal of the American Medical Association*, 159 (1955), 155.
64. Florence B. Powdermaker and Jerome D. Frank, *Group Psychotherapy* (Cambridge: Harvard University Press, 1953).
65. Otto Rank, *Will Therapy and Truth and Reality* (New York: Alfred A. Knopf, 1945).
66. Carl R. Rogers, *Counselling and Psychotherapy* (New York: Houghton Mifflin, 1942).

67. Melvin Sabshin and J. Ramot, "Pharmacotherapeutic Evaluation and the Psychiatric Setting," *Archives of Neurology and Psychiatry*, 75 (1956), 362.
68. George Saslow and A. D. Peters, "A Follow-up Study of 'Untreated' Patients with Various Behavior Disorders," *Psychiatric Quarterly*, 30 (1956), 283.
69. Johannes H. Schultz and Wolfgang Luthe, *Autogenic Training* (New York: Grune & Stratton, 1965).
70. Ian Stevenson, "The Challenge of Results in Psychotherapy," *American Journal of Psychiatry*, 116 (1959), 120.
71. William B. Terhune, "Re-education in the Treatment of Psychoneuroses," *Hawaii Medical Journal*, 15 (1956), 541.
72. F. C. Thorne, "Critique of Recent Developments in Personality Counseling Theory," *Journal of Clinical Psychology*, 13 (1957), 234.
73. Allen Wheelis, *The Quest for Identity* (New York: Norton, 1958).
74. Harry A. Wilmer, *Social Psychiatry in Action; a Therapeutic Community* (Springfield, Ill.: Charles C Thomas, 1958).
75. Lewis R. Wolberg, *Hypnoanalysis* (New York: Grune & Stratton, 1945).
76. Alexander Wolf, "The Psychoanalysis of Groups," *American Journal of Psychotherapy*, 3 (1949), 525.
77. Joseph Wolpe, *Psychotherapy by Reciprocal Inhibition* (Stanford: Stanford University Press, 1958).

CHAPTER ELEVEN

General Principles of Psychiatric Treatment: II *The Organic Therapies*

The Pharmacological Therapies

Both unwarranted enthusiasm and cynicism concerning the use of drugs for psychiatric disorders are far from new. Bromides, paraldehyde, and barbiturate sedatives were introduced in medicine between 1857 and 1903; opiates (once said to have an almost specific effect on the treatment of agitated depression) and belladonna have a long history; and rauwolfia was used in India as early as 1000 B.C. In only a few decades, most of the older drugs have been replaced in importance, first in the 1930's by insulin and metrazol therapy, then by electroconvulsive therapy, followed by lobotomy, and, today, by a number of newer psychotropic compounds.[39] Chlorpromazine and reserpine were introduced in 1952 and 1953 because of their tranquilizing effect in the psychoses; they produced "sedation" without hypnosis and, surprisingly, demonstrated a link of extrapyramidal systems with an array of effects on excitement, mood, cognition, and perception. In 1957, iproniazid came into use as an antidepressant. The psychotropic drugs were originally investigated for their effect on blood pressure, temperature, allergic reactions, or bacteriostatic actions and were only incidentally found to have behavioral effects. But following their introduction, loud hosannas were heard: mental hospitals were being rapidly emptied. The facts, of course, were not this startling, and the slight trend toward increased discharge rates had preceded the advent of drugs. There is undoubtedly much to be learned from events in this era: from the large population of drug users, who hoped drugs would relieve tensions of everyday living, and from the adherents of a strict psychogenic view of etiology, who underwent momentary crises of faith with the vision of years of intricate psychodynamic explanations being negated by the simple application of neurochemicals. It seems evident that the experience of normal emotions is man's link to civilized relationships and that the capacity to experience some tension, love, mourning, and grief is necessary for reliable psychological strength. From all that can be appreciated about the organization of psychobiological systems, it would appear that major human problems of living and learning will neither be "solved" nor dissolved by chemicals. The organization of neurochemical systems will, however, differentially alter the conditions under which behavior can be structured and restructured and will partially determine the pattern, direction, and intensity of behavioral sequences.

It now is apparent that chemotherapy has (1) a major place in the treatment of the major psychoses, especially the schizophrenias and, to a lesser extent, the severe depressions; (2) a much less secure and as yet unclear place in the treatment of neuroses and sociopathic and situational reactions. If we take stock of where we stand, it is evident that at the basic science level these developments have led to an increased momentum of research, a development far more welcome than its descriptive name, "neuropsychopharmacology." Drugs have not only provoked research into the bases for the array of observed effects, but have been used as tools for study of the social and biological processes that influence the organization of behavior. They have been applied to studies of normal and disturbed behavior,[79, 83] in both its subjective and objective aspects. In animals,[3, 79] research has been conducted on the effects of drugs on maturation; learning; memory; drive (fear, hunger, sex); punishment;[3] deprivation; reward; social behavior; adaptation to stress; neuroendocrine and autonomic patterns; motor activities and their associated electrophysiology and neurochemistry. One inescapable fact is that the control of biological sequences underlying the organization of behavioral processes has been brought more closely into the realm of molecular specificity. There was hope that the newer compounds might eventually lead to an understanding of the pathophysiology of some behavior disorders since the drugs either resemble or influence the metabolism of endogenous substances, which, in unexplained ways, influence mood and behavior.[34] The few but sometimes surprising biochemical links with neurobehavioral mechanisms that have already been established emphasize our ignorance of what may lie ahead in research. Through work stimulated by the psychotropic compounds, "organicists" have been compelled to become less naïve about how it is that behavior could be linked with biochemical and neural mechanisms, and behavioral scientists have become aware that the statement that bodily processes affect behavior is not an empty formalism; rather, they have been endowed with new tools for manipulating different and differentiated behavioral states.[25]

Impact of Drugs on Clinical Psychiatry

How are we to view the impact of these drugs on clinical psychiatry? They have changed our definition of psychiatric patients and psychiatric treatment; treatment is not now coextensive with hospitalization. A severely ill psychiatric patient need not be a hospitalized patient, and a patient who visits a clinic a few times a year may well be a severely ill patient who may or may not require periods of hospitalization. In this newer trend of practice, drugs have played a key role. It is obvious that patients on a regimen of drugs for as much as ten years have not been deprived of their intellect, their relation to their surroundings, their imagination, their ability to be anxious, to experience human emotions, to grow, to grieve, or to be sexually gratified. The language with which drug effects are discussed by patient and therapist, however, is misleading: the statement that drugs "do" something or "produce" an effect is best translated (though awkwardly), "Drugs lead to conditions that (for example) make sedation or excitement highly probable." The tranquilizing drugs can sedate without impairing ready arousal; apparently they can relax overinhibited behavior (as in mute and withdrawn patients) without producing "release" behavior and can "restrain" hyperactivity without inducing coma or arrest of respiratory muscles. No amnesia or confusion occurs, as with shock therapy, nor have the drugs induced that blind impulsiveness and social carelessness characteristic of lobotomized patients. The problem of drug withdrawal and addiction has, with some exceptions, been minimal, and the death rate and risk has been small. Dose effects can be tailored for the individual case, and undesirable drug effects usually can be controlled; these are generally temporary and "reversible" with drug withdrawal.

In controlled clinical studies, the drugs clearly have an almost specific ameliorative effect on the majority of severely disturbed patients. On the other hand, there is no evidence that they "cure"; certainly, they do not compel the sick patient to become well. One can see here a loose analogy to the situation with infectious diseases: the impact of specific chemotherapeutic agents changed the picture of the course, danger, cure, and prevention of infectious diseases. Some disorders were specifically cured; some relatively untouched, infectious diseases certainly were not generally abolished; and some new problems emerged. Bacteriostatic agents, on the other hand, could suppress only a few infections, allowing repair processes to take effect. The psychotropic agents might be viewed as having an impact midway between these. In dampening the intensity of internal disorganizing forces, they have facilitated the impact of all those "non-drug" factors that operate to enhance therapeutic effects. They have made effective patient management easier. In hospital settings, behavioral improvement and diminution of bizarre and regressed performance can lead to better attention, which is also better received. For schizophrenic patients, the drugs may have partially succeeded in specifically arresting a malignant course, facilitating their adaptation to a community. If we consider the total range of psychotic populations, the efficacy of pharmacotherapies has not been matched even by psychological therapies in highly staffed hospitals. Properly given and taken, the drugs may well be a factor in preventing or delaying relapses and initial hospitalization.

These conclusions derive both from clinical judgment and an assessment of a number of studies. For example, John M. Davis reviewed over four hundred drug studies[18] and found an overwhelming preponderance of results, which showed that in psychotic populations tranquilizing drugs have an effect greater than barbiturates or placebo; these effects transcend factors related to setting or to social and "non-drug" influences. Even when studies clearly prejudiced in favor of drugs were rejected and when such factors as adequacy of design and quantitative methods, size of sample, and duration and dose of drug were analyzed for their effect on outcome, Davis had to conclude that a degree of efficacy in psychotic populations was clearly and objectively demonstrated. The collaborative studies of the Veterans Administration[61] similarly showed drugs superior to placebo and a similar evaluation of controlled studies in chronic schizophrenia has been reported by Jonathan O. Cole and colleagues at the Psychopharmacology Service Center of the National Institute of Mental Health.[15,17] In an elegantly designed study of effects of three different phenothiazines in acute schizophrenics in nine hospitals, private and public, this group found that the drugs, although differing in patterns of side effects, were equally effective and, over a short period, far superior to placebo; long-term evaluations of treatment outcome in acute disorders are still required. All schizophrenic symptoms, not simply the so-called target symptom of overactivity, were improved. This has been the general experience in controlled studies: thought disturbance, paranoid symptoms, social withdrawal, and the like are as favorably influenced as agitation.

The trend for certain antidepressant drugs in highly controlled studies is similar; the drug clearly tends to be superior to placebo in both acute and chronic severe depression.[16] In one major study, electroshock therapy was rated superior to the drugs in psychotic depression,[43] an area where matching of subpopulations requires further research in order to evaluate the "where, when, how, and why" for one rather than another organic treatment. In the schizophrenic psychoses, relapse is more probable with withdrawal of the drug (occurring more rapidly when staff and patients are aware of the withdrawal and more slowly when they are not).[68]

There is, further, some evidence that drug therapy coupled with intensive treatment of psychotic patients in the community can obviate the necessity for their hospital treatment.[59] David M. Englehardt *et al.*[27] have published results that epitomize studies of discharged patients; drug treatment with a potent phenothiazine (chlorpromazine) is more effective than treatment with a less potent drug (promazine) or placebo in preventing or delaying relapse and hospitalization. None of these studies negates the notion that bias and the physician's expectation affect the therapeutic process; rather, such studies seem to tap a more fundamental process closely related to the patient's capacity to sustain a level of organization sufficient for coping with the usual range of daily demands. These studies establish a range of effectiveness for the major tranquilizers and antidepressants in the very severe acute and chronic disorders, when the criteria for effectiveness are established by objective assessments of *scoreable* behavior. It should be remembered, especially with chronic disorders, that base rates and expectancy of relapse must be carefully established before the ameliorative, preventive, or curative effects of these drugs can be finally determined.

Evidence for the effectiveness of the major or minor tranquilizers in the neuroses and psychosomatic disorders is far less convincing. Symptoms of acute anxiety and of panic may be clearly ameliorated either by astute patient management (the major ingredient of which is a simple and firmly structured approach with receptive listening and the opportunity to learn) and/or with non-phenothiazine tranquilizers such as chlordiazepoxide (Librium) and its congeners, or meprobamate (Equanil, Miltown), much as bromides and barbiturates traditionally were used: occasionally if underlying depression is diagnosed, amitryptiline (Elavil) or imipramine (Tofranil) are employed.

Evaluation of Drug Studies

The clinician must be prepared to evaluate the professional literature critically, yet therapy involves the application of arrays of facts in particular contexts. This is true for all therapies, including drug therapies. The greatest body of objective knowledge of the effects of therapy has been obtained in drug evaluation; but objective studies of drug effects alone do not and cannot provide an automatic program for prescribing for the individual patient nor provide a comprehensive description of mode and mechanism of action. Thus, in applying objectively derived facts to the patient, the physician assesses a wide range of information; he not only identifies the presence of behavior pathology and evaluates the individual patient's ability to cope with stress, but also assesses the degree of such pathology and the conditions that dampen or exacerbate pathological acts. Clinical responsibility and judgment are indispensable requisites in using these drugs.

Such judgment must include an assimilated knowledge of the actual conditions from which objective facts were derived. Without knowledge of the facts of clinical life in a variety of settings, with different patient populations one would be handicapped in evaluating the meaning of the results.[22] Obviously, Veterans Hospital patients represent a different population than state or private hospital patients; further, patients differ in their phase of illness as well as in the way their culture evaluates and responds to it. Population variables also influence side effects; Karl Rickels, for example, found that an outpatient population and a medical clinic population of psychiatric patients differed markedly in the nature of their side effects, the medical clinic group showing a preponderance of somatic side effects.[70] As yet, the dimension of personality has not clearly been shown to differentiate drug effects in behavior disorders, but G. L. Klerman, A. DiMascio, M. Greenblatt, and M. Rinkel [56] and J. M. von Felsinger, Louis Lasagna[29] and H. K. Beecher have distinguished personality traits that differentiate drug effects in normal populations; a brilliant clinical study by G. J. Sarwer-Foner[74] indicated that severely disturbed individuals with a great fear of passivity and a special need for activity to maintain controls reacted adversely to the restraint induced by tranquilizing drugs.

The nature and adequacy of rating scales also must be considered. What is being evaluated, and how and by whom must be judged by the reader; for example, chronic schizophrenic patients who are scored as less "withdrawn" on a rating scale may also, if the design permits one to score the actual range of behaviors, be more suspicious and hostile. Who makes the ratings or judgments is likewise important; it has been found that nurses and attendants may appreciate a different category of behavior change in the ward than the physician. Experimental design and controls must be critically evaluated. The student should become able to distinguish controls superficially introduced for decoration from those that control factors essential to the question being investigated. "Double-blind" control procedures are useful for hypothesis verification, but these can be misleading if one did not take into account the base-line variability of a population or the events occurring in a real clinical investigation: unforeseen circumstances can arise, which, in effect, break the code; patients do not take the drug or they hide it; they distinguish the drug by taste or physiological response; the staff may pick up clues, which identify either the drug or the placebo. It is important to know something about the basic pharmacology of the drug and its clinical use; there are many instances of drug studies that employ what the experienced clinician knows to be an inadequate dosage, with inadequate indications for the use of the drug, and with an inadequate period of medication. Finally, astute clinical investigation, carried on with the same spirit of skeptical inquiry which is supposed to characterize the controlled study, can raise and refine major problems for study and elucidate the basis for major findings that emerge from "hard" research.

Problems of Drug Classification

It is simply a matter of convenience to assign a single effect to a single drug; and attempts to classify drugs are, perhaps, most useful in that they illuminate our basic problems about conceptualizing neurobehavioral processes. Most antihistaminics (from which the phenothiazine tranquilizers were originally developed) have, among other actions, local anesthetic, anticholinergic, and adrenergic blocking properties. Ascriptions of convenience (tranquilizer, energizer) describe the desired but not the inevitable nor sole effect of the drug. Antidepressant compounds that inhibit monoamine oxidase (MAO, an enzyme inactivating some amines that influence brain excitability) were first called psychic energizers, because, rather than directly stimulate, they appeared to "prime the pump"; for example, monkeys showed more reactivity (rather than spontaneous activity) during periods of waking but deeper sleep during normal sleeping periods.[20] Yet, mood changes in humans often seem to follow initial changes in psychomotor activity; some patients are more active but still depressed. That this activity or reactivity represents more psychic energy is highly dubious, even as a poetic metaphor. In any event, these "energizers," among a number of complex pharmacologic effects, potentiate some sedatives and narcotics (because of the inhibition of liver enzyme systems associated with the biotransformation of these drugs) as well as the cardiovascular effects of certain amines and of amino acids incorporated through the diet (in such foods as herring and cheese).

The term "tranquilizer" denotes "antianxiety" effects (the hopeful synonym, ataractic, wistfully denotes "peace of mind"). Since behavioral effects can be demonstrated on a wide range of symptoms in schizophrenia, Cole and others[17] have suggested reviving the term "antischizophrenic" or "antipsychotic" compounds. But this is not really satisfactory; the demonstrated effectiveness of these drugs in objective clinical studies does not mean that any instance of psychosis, in any of its varied phases, is responsive to drugs, nor that drug treatment in each instance of psychosis is sufficient to erase the psychosis and restore normal function. Another approach notes that the most dramatically evident effect of the drugs is to calm and restrain excessively agitated and manic behavior; since this can be seen in widely different diagnostic groups, it was suggested that the drugs be classified according to their effect against "target symptoms." But this proposal overlooks the specific effects of the phenothiazines on the gamut of schizophrenic symptoms from withdrawal to hyperactivity. In fact, in manic-depressive disorders, the phenothiazines are of moderate value only in the manic phase; and in the agitation of delirium tremens they are less effective than other classes of drugs. It may be speculated that if a core of processes having to do with intensity in behavior is in some sense dampened, this might account for the shift in the range of schizophrenic symptoms such as hallucinations, withdrawal, mutism, and seclusiveness; but this unitary view does not explain the absence of clear effects in some highly stressful but nonschizophrenic disorders. Thus, these attempts at classifying merely revive a recurrent problem in psychiatry; namely, that the specific organizing (or disorganizing) processes underlying the different psychiatric syndromes are only partially appreciated. We often cannot adequately detect or describe the underlying processes, and yet we know that similar "target" symptoms can be differently constructed. Therefore, neither a "disease process" nor a "target symptom" approach is sufficiently comprehensive for classification, although both approaches contain a considerable amount of clinical truth. Finally, the neural link of brain systems influencing behavior and basic vegetative and mood processes is impressive and has served as a basis for classification:[19] J. Delay *et al.* viewed the phenothiazines as "neuroleptic" drugs, which stimulated central neural elements; he classified them into (1) psycholeptic drugs (phenothiazines), which produce extrapyramidal effects as well as behavioral sedation; (2) psychoanaleptic or antidepressive drugs; and (3) psychodysleptic or psychotomimetic drugs.

Basic Pharmacologic Principles

No drug is limited solely to effects upon behavior. Every drug acts to inhibit, facilitate, replace, alter, or compete with special and ubiquitous cellular mechanisms that normally regulate body chemistry. Mechanisms of drug *action* expressed in biochemical terms should be differentiated from mechanisms of drug *effect*. What we observe as an effect is arrived at through a number of pathways and the interaction of a number of systems. No drug acts directly upon behavior, and no behavioral pattern can be entirely determined by drug action. Behavior, whether that of an isolated organ or of an organism, is influenced by the surrounding conditions; in the case of psychotropic compounds, these are psychosocial conditions.

However drugs are classified, mechanisms of drug effect must be described with consideration of cellular actions, interactions among cellular systems, their status *prior* to drug administration, and the contingencies prevailing during the period of drug action. Aside from dose and time parameters and route of administration of a drug (which often can produce different drug effects), the *setting* in which the drug is given is a potent factor in the mechanism of drug effect. Sodium amytal, in sedative dosage, will produce a cheerful intoxication when taken with a congenial group; when given in a therapeutic situation it has hypnotic properties. It was used for "narcosynthesis" because of the ease with which painful memories and traumatic experiences could be related while the patient was "intoxicated" under the drug.[45] Although called "truth serum," it did not in fact produce a compulsion to confess; experiments showed that unless individuals were quite neurotic, they could lie beautifully while under the influence of the drug.[69]

The *attitude* of the physician giving a drug is a variable of considerable importance for *any* therapeutic activity; and Thomas P. Detre,[21] Michael H. Sheard,[77] and others have indicated that a disparaging approach by the physician can impair the effectiveness of a drug; the clinical effectiveness of drugs differs according to the attitude of the doctor. The patient's expectations when he comes to a physician are also important. In general, the "rules of the game," which are implicit between the doctor and the patient, what both expect and believe they are together for, structure the dialogue and influence and channel what can ensue. All physicians are aware of the *placebo effect*,[51] which, fundamentally, is based upon these implicit and explicit psychosocial factors. Stewart Wolf and Harold G. Wolff[87] and others have shown the role of the physician's attitude on physiological processes; one physician had the effect of increasing the flow of HCl in patients and another an effect of systematically decreasing it. The pill-giving ritual, although important, must not be overestimated, and one must stipulate the condition and the duration of placebo effects as well as population factors; the mechanism of placebo effects that do occur also requires study. Although many attempts have been made to define a "placebo personality," [60] there are no "pan-placebo reactors." The condition being treated with placebo is important; in the treatment of pain, where anticipation has been shown both experimentally[46] and clinically to be a crucial factor, placebo effects are routinely demonstrable.[8] In psychosis, as has been indicated, they are of far less consequence, though not insignificant. Drugs such as LSD-25 appear to enhance responsiveness to certain psychosocial elements in a setting; drugs such as chlorpromazine might be described as selectively shifting the range of cues to which an organism readily responds.

Perhaps the most important factor in psychopharmacology is the *prior state*, and there are many examples of the importance of this factor. For an excited, maniacal patient, the required dosage of sodium amytal is often large enough to produce dangerous respiratory problems for a normal person. This drug "alerts" the patient in catatonic stupor, whereas amphetamine may produce sleep.[24,26] In normal subjects, marked postural hypotension can be observed twenty-four hours after a single dose of chlorpromazine, but this is not so frequently the case in schizophrenic patients who in general seem to adapt more readily to the autonomic effects of tranquilizing drugs.[58] Since apparently identical effects can be achieved either by stimulating or depressing opposing neural systems, labeling a drug as "stimulant" or "depressant" will not necessarily describe the operative mechanism. The prior balance of such agonist-antagonist neural subsystems may be a critical factor in drug idiosyncracy. Thus, in some children and in some predisposed adults, excitement rather than sedation occasionally can be seen with barbiturates. The delicate control over these linked behaviors is interesting, since it requires only a slight molecular alteration in the thiopental molecule reliably to produce excitement. Sex can be a factor: women are thought to be somewhat more responsive to phenothiazines, and there may be differences in the various extrapyramidal side effects between the sexes.

The critical consideration related to prior state is the definition of the psychopathology of the population. The safest assumption is that the schizophrenic patient is a different psychobiological organism. Thus, it may not be useful to study effects of drugs in normals in order to predict response in patient populations. As a matter of clinical fact, "calming" a normal person with a phenothiazine is vastly different from treating an excited catatonic and, generally, far less effective. Insufficient attention has been given in the behavioral sciences to "norms" for what might be considered different organisms or organismic states. This can have important clinical consequences: for example, the antidepressant compound iproniazid was first tested on a population of schizophrenic patients and, of course, not found to be useful. Without the concept that individual states make a difference, we would be unable to account not only for drug idiosyncrasy and allergy but for the role of side effects. These differ both with individuals and with molecular structure. It is still to be determined whether or not some individuals are better "suited" for one drug than another (for example, chlorpromazine rather than an "alerting" phenothiazine such as triflupromazine) even though in large populations such differences as yet have not been objectively substantiated.[65]

Mode of Drug Action

Every drug has multiple sites and mechanisms of action; and specific molecular configurations, even among compounds that are related, can lead to great or slight differences of effects. In general, psychoactive drugs induce periods of neurochemical and neurophysiological change—certain states in which the range and category of inputs which normally influence behavior will be shifted. Specification of these factors and ranges of input and output constitutes the definition of the "action" of a drug. This is by no means a satisfactory generalization; but without it, the nature of the problem of mechanism of action is misunderstood. We will canvass general problems relevant to mode of action of these drugs, the specific pharmacology of which must be pursued in relevant texts and reviews.[85]

Mode of Drug Action: Neurobehavioral Studies

Reserpine and the phenothiazine compounds have been the most extensively studied at the neurochemical, neurophysiological, and behavioral levels. New compounds are typically screened with a series of laboratory tests and observations with animals. These include a search for drug-induced catalepsy and for taming effects in aggressive animals; action against the rage produced in rats by septal lesions; and a survey of motor and autonomic effects.[52] The ability of animals to perform with motor skill but not to overrespond to the signals usually indicating pain and danger (that is, not to be overaroused through fear and overanticipation) is sought through tests of the effects of drugs on conditioned avoidance and conditioned suppression. Yet no suitable analogue for schizophrenia has been devised in animals,[28] and since it is also difficult to induce depression in animals reliably (although reserpine has been so employed),[82] there is some dissatisfaction with these screening procedures. Finally, drugs are tested in terms of their effects on various limbic, midbrain, and reticular systems. The vast number of pathways in these systems makes it safe to state only that many tranquilizing compounds variably influence the thresholds for arousal in components of these systems. There appear to be a number of different pathways whereby desired drug effects are achieved. Action on systems that process and filter input could provide a period of delay prior to response, an interposition that would be important in psychiatric disorders; for example, influences on pathways from the cortex to the activating systems may play a role.[55]

Mode of Drug Action: Biochemical Studies

Discrete biochemical explanations alone cannot comprehensively account for drug effects. Still, a number of neurochemical processes relevant to drug action have been identified. The old concept that a cell is little more than a bag filled with a random mixture of enzymes has been replaced by the picture of subcellular ultrastructure. Psychotropic compounds have stimulated efforts biochemically to map and evaluate cellular components in terms of their role in neural function. The perivascular glial cells interposed between blood and neurone probably serve as a specialized exchange station analogous to an extracellular space; as a part of the blood-brain barrier, this may be a site of action for drugs. The quantity of drug administered is far greater than the amount that actually penetrates these various membranes finally to arrive at the critically active receptor sites. The neurone includes a network of internal membranes and channels ("endoplasmic reticulum") with small granule-containing vesicles and larger mitochondria distributed throughout the intervening areas of cytoplasm. Mitochondria consist of highly organized enzyme complexes integrated into an enclosed system of infolded membranes, an arrangement permitting the efficient trapping of energy released during the oxidation of intermediates derived from glucose upon which the brain is dependent. Phenothiazines can inhibit electron transport and uncouple this energy system from oxidative phosphorylation, but the over-all level of adenosine triphosphate (ATP) in the brain after chlorpromazine may actually even increase. In general, drug effects have not been elegantly explained in terms of these metabolic changes or enzymatic effects. A more dynamic approach has been to link oxidative phenomena with graded states of neuronal activity; chlorpromazine most sensitively inhibits the *transition* from resting oxidative states to states of high activity in both brain slices and isolated mitochondria.[2]

In the general attempt to link physical-chemical phenomena to bodily and behavioral response, there has been a focus upon critical transducer sites such as the synapse. This site of information transfer contains, in addition to mitochondria, minute synaptic vesicles, which are thought to be storage sites allowing for the efficient release *or* retention of neurohumors. A neurohumor is a diffusable metabolite, which can act either as a synaptic transmitter or a substance that modifies the environment in which the transmitter acts. Among those substances for which there is some evidence implicating a central neurohumoral action are serotonin, norepinephrine, dopamine, gamma-amino-butyric acid (believed to be inhibitory), and acetylcholine; only acetylcholine has received a degree of experimental support as a true central synaptic transmitter, although other elements in the brain are clearly selectively responsive to a range of agents. There are also correlations between behavioral states and changes in concentration of acetylcholine, such as a rise in total brain acetylcholine during both sleep and the sedation induced by a number of drugs. In contrast, anticholinergic compounds with psychotomimetic activity (for example, scopolamine, or piperidyl glycollates such as Ditran) reduce brain acetylcholine levels.[41]

Current interest in the biochemical basis for psychotropic drug action is focused on the various amines. These are remarkably active biological substances, which in minute quantities can induce physiologic response in a wide range of tissues. They are synthesized and inactivated in brain and at the central synapse are thought to act at least as modulators. Along with their associated enzymatic machinery, they are selectively localized in subcortical nuclei, which are said to subserve consciousness and its affective and motor expression. For example, metabolism of dopamine, almost exclusively concentrated in the corpus striatum, has been linked to extrapyramidal disorders. There are many "schemes" or notions, based on complex studies (usually of peripheral nerve), which attempt to explain how these drugs work. Many drugs and substances structurally related to these indole or catechol amines are considered to act by interfering with their "life cycle," that is, with the transport of their precursors; their synthesis in the cytoplasm; their uptake binding, release, and reuptake in substructures; and their inactivation.[34] In experimental phenylketonuria, the amino acid phenylalanine has been shown to compete (probably at the cell wall) with the serotonin precursor for transport into the cell, resulting in lower brain levels. Within the cell, the amines are taken up and retained in vesicles and organelles, and it is postulated that there are two intracellular reservoir pools; one, close to the synaptic receptor in the nerve ending and easily released by sympathomimetic amines and drugs (tyramine, amphetamine) and a larger, deeper lying pool, in which release leads to destruction of the amines rather than attachment to the receptor.[5] An amine is inactivated by enzymes—or functionally inactivated by retention in the various pools or binding to various substances. Reserpine markedly lowers brain amine levels apparently by releasing the amines from the granular material (of both pools) and by preventing amine storage; the effects are not hypertensive since the amine is destroyed. In contrast, the psychotomimetic drug LSD-25 and its active congeners (as well as an extreme environmental stress or toxic doses of amphetamine) can induce intracellular binding of brain serotonin and a fall of norepinephrine. Monoamine oxydase (MAO) inhibitors may cause hypotension even though actual levels of norepinephrine are increased; alone, such inhibitors do not produce a *functional* excess of norepinephrine. The greater quantities of undestroyed amine are packed in the intracellular pools and appear ready, so to speak, to be released in small or large quantities by appropriate endogenous chemicals; with an excess of tyramine, for example, there are potent hypertensive effects. The hypotension may be due to the production and the storage in the easily released pool of "false transmitters" (octopamine), amines that are inactive at the receptor, which are synthesized in the presence of the inhibitor.[57] In any event, more than MAO inhibition is involved in the effect of these drugs. Chlorpromazine, perhaps through its membrane stabilizing properties, blocks the cellular uptake of exogenous amines and the reuptake and recirculation of intracellular amines thereby exposing amines more rapidly either to metabolism or to the receptors; because the drug also blocks the receptor, the over-all effects are hypotensive. The antidepressant imipramine has similar effects (shunting the amines to different metabolic paths), but the receptor is not blocked and in fact is somehow "sensitized" to the unbound amine. It is interesting that both categories of antidepressant drugs do not seem entirely to be "directly" acting; where they show an activation effect in clinical depression, this may depend in part on the status of endogenous amines, the effects of which they markedly enhance. Accordingly, the prior neurobehavioral state and the prior functional status of brain amines in depression may be one significant factor in the antidepressant effect of these drugs.

Whereas it is a fact that psychotropic drugs act on the traffic of brain amines at various subcellular sites and that alterations of amine metabolism are associated with certain excited or sedated states, it is not clearly established how the amines affect neural function. In peripheral systems, where norepinephrine acts as a transmitter and serotonin as a neuromodulator, it is clear that they alter the threshold for stimulation of certain organs. Such effects of serotonin (on the gut, for example) depend on a prior state—upon the balance and level of ongoing stimulation. Some, but not all, of the central effects of serotonin tend to be of a sedative nature, and certain of these effects may involve cholinergic receptors; excesses of norepinephrine may be crudely associated with certain excitatory states and deficiencies with certain states of exhaustion and sedation.

Thus, from the available data, it may be speculated that the amines normally regulate and buffer certain states of central excitation and that when the biochemical equilibria of the amines are disturbed, intensified maladaptive responses to normal excitation can occur.[4] If genetic or stress-induced impairment of the binding and release of brain amines occurs in clinical disorder, the human would be at a chemical disadvantage in handling life stresses, and drugs would then be helpful in compensating for these effects. Many notions remain to be tested. Although the metabolic products of these drugs do not adequately explain their action, the pattern of urinary metabolites of the endogenous amines may eventually provide data accounting for individual differences in drug response.[12] The possibility for this lies in the fact that psychotropic drugs directly or indirectly influence the pathways for amine binding, release, and metabolism. Drugs may also block or induce enzymes, alter physical-chemical properties of membranes and receptor substances, and influence ion flux and metabolic processes and thus directly or indirectly influence neural function. At this juncture, the psychiatrist can only be alerted to the fact that biochemical regulations of overinhibited or overaroused behavior exist and they partially comprise the mechanisms through which psychotropic drugs act.[13]

Mode of Drug Action: Clinical Studies

Mechanism of drug action can be described at various levels, and although it is more important for the clinician to be aware of the practical indications for the use of the drug, attempts have been made to formulate the basis for their action at a descriptive level. Thus, the drugs seem to raise the threshold for arousal to signals of pain or mental anguish. They produce a delay or indifference[86] to certain categories of input and, as one of our hypomanic patients put it, permit him to regulate the pace at which internal events occur. The result of these effects on processes related to intensity is to shift mental states so that a better level of organization can emerge. For both the antidepressant and the tranquilizing drugs, a "split" between motor activities and mood and mental functions can, at times, be seen; many observers note that psychomotor changes can precede the changes in mood, affect, and general organization. This implies a dissociation, although a mild one, and one that may serve integrative purposes. Perhaps for the psychotic, any dissociation or delay between input and response is organizing rather than more confusing.

The occurrence of extrapyramidal symptoms shows that the modulation and regulation of motor activity is involved in the action of drugs, but it is also argued that the actual clinically manifest symptoms must occur for the drugs to have a clinical effect. This is doubtful; rather, the symptoms are evidence of the close link of the drugs with neural systems (from the caudally located emetic center to the limbic system),[33] which are linked (behaviorally) to perception, attention, and the arousal and dampening of affect. Consideration of all these factors, neural, chemical, experiential, physiological, psychomotor, and psychopathological, are relevant as a comprehensive psychopharmacology of the psychotropic compounds is developed.

The Use of Drugs in Therapy

A compendium of complete pharmacotherapy can be found elsewhere, but the following principles emphasize the major characteristic drugs and their use. The physician must assess the phase and stage and intensity of the disorders with which he deals. He should, in giving the drug, collaborate with the patient and, most importantly, continue to stay in touch with him. He should treat each patient as an occasion for an individualized investigation, carefully monitoring the patient's responses (especially side effects) to the drug while restraining himself from senseless changes of drugs or dosage regimen. During the treatment, he will assess the utility of the drug in the patient and entertain alternative explanations of drug effect. Most importantly, he will distinguish between long-term effects of the drug and immediate effects. There usually is a lag between drug withdrawal and disappearance of behavioral effects; the fact that metabolites of phenothiazines may persist for months does not explain this lag, and patients do vary widely in the rapidity with which relapse occurs. In other words, the use of drugs in psychosis is not to be governed solely by the immediate presence or absence of one or another behavioral effect. The physician should not stop giving the drug (any more than he would start giving the drug) without scrutinizing the adequacy of the dosage schedule or without assessing whether his idiosyncratic motives are interfering with his professional judgment. Many young psychiatrists feel their omnipotence and usefulness is threatened by the drug (a magical view both of themselves and of drug action). If a patient improves, they often wish symbolically to celebrate this with the patient by removing him from a regimen that has been helpful and that, at the time of withdrawal, shows no indications of *not* continuing to be helpful. Yet many patients, as soon as they feel better with or without drug treatment seem remote from any influence that would help them to learn new patterns, and the physician knows that such patients may simply get into similar trouble again later on. In a suitable situation, such patients may or may not be given drugs; this depends on clinical indications as to whether or not a degree of insight, new learning, or deep personality change appear to be possible *and* whether the drug therapy appears essential for this patient to maintain his basic intactness and organization. In psychotic patients, the drugs usually facilitate therapy. Of course, the drugs should not be used when their psychological effects are clearly more disruptive than helpful. The treatment aim and plan also affect the way in which drugs are used; for many schizophrenic out-patients, a brief visit at weekly or monthly intervals allowing an assessment of medications and a supportive focus on overall life adjustment (without any attempts to probe into motives or responses to the complexities in daily life) is a common and practical therapeutic regimen. Such treatment programs may be extended in various ways, utilizing vocational and other treatments as experience with community clinics accumulates. When the physician does not focus *with* the patient upon underlying motivations or exploration of symptoms, this does not mean he disregards them or is ignorant of their presence; rather, such treatment regimens are pragmatically designed to respond both to what the patient requires and what the circumstances permit. The therapist's attitude about conducting a treatment, his attitude—both about the limits of his right to influence the patient's way of life and his obligation to apply the knowledge he does have—is critical. Whether insight therapies or supportive and milieu therapies are used, the therapist prescribing medication should be able to act with the confidence to which he is entitled by virtue of his authentic knowledge about drugs, their effects, and the rationale for their use in behavior disorders. He should not be distracted by spurious issues of power, by irrational fears of unduly influencing patients or whatever; rather he knows better than the patient, knows how to proceed and treat, and, for that reason, he is licensed to help the patient. This does not preclude listening, investigating, and assessing with the patient the various responses to drug treatment and the motives underlying various resistances and fears of pharmacotherapy as these arise during treatment. It is, after all, only through his personal influence and mode of exercising it that the physician can proceed to foster a collaborative treatment. The psychiatrist's authority does not require that he be a despot, a policeman, or a reformer; it does entail responsive and responsible application of medical and psychological knowledge within the limits of the doctor–patient relationship.

Only through experience with a few compounds in adequate dosage and with investigation in the manner described can a physician develop experience that sharpens judgment and leads to cogent decisions in the individual case. In general, the psychiatrist should wonder why he is *not* using drugs in the treatment of a psychotic patient; why they are not, to some extent, helpful; and why, in view of the objective data, the patient should not continue to take drugs.

The Phenothiazines

The various drugs of the phenothiazine group (see Figure 11–1) are derivatives of phenothiazine obtained by various substitutions at positions 2 and 10.

The most important and representative drug of the phenothiazine group is chlorpromazine. It was developed from substituted phenothiazines (such as promethazine or Phenergan) with strong antihistaminic properties. In general, these compounds tend to dampen a number of compensatory activities evoked by stress; the sympathetic compensatory response to hypotension is blocked, and once body temperature is lowered the drug tends to stabilize that state by blocking brain stem sites. Chlorpromazine was first used by A. Deschamps and H. Laborit as an auxiliary in artificial hibernation. Jean Delay and P. Deniker, in 1952, were the first to report on its use in the therapy of schizophrenia and other psychoses with psychomotor agitation; and in North America, Heinz Lehmann pioneered in identifying its effectiveness. Chlorpromazine has since been used more extensively and investigated more thoroughly than any other phenothiazine. Apart from differences in dosage (usually called potency, which is not synonymous with efficacy) and side effects, the other phenothiazines have very similar therapeutic effects. Numerous rearrangements of the molecule have produced interesting compounds, some with tranquilizing and others with antipruritic or anti-Parkinsonian effects. Generally, the three-carbon chain (at R_1) is found in the psychoactive phenothiazines and various substituents on this chain and at Position 2 constitute the chief molecular rearrangements. These are sometimes grouped

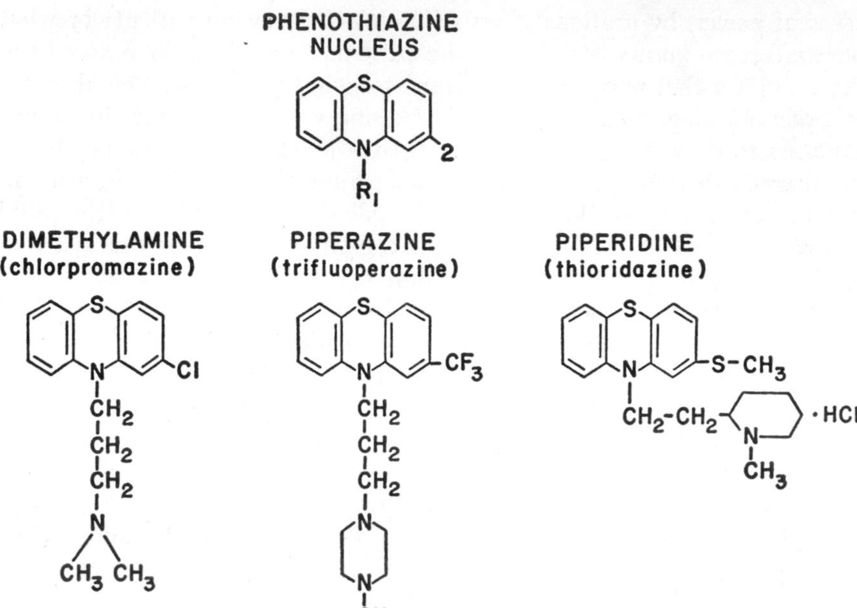

Figure 11–1.

into: (1) A piperazine group characterized by a piperazine ring in the carbon side chain such as fluphenazine or Prolixin and trifluoperazine or Stelazine (both of which have a CF_3 at the 2-position), and prochlorperazine or Compazine, thiopropazate or Dartal, and perphenazine or Trilafon, each with a Cl at the 2-position. (2) The chlorpromazine model group is characterized by a three-carbon side chain with a dimethylamine group at R_1 and is represented by chlorpromazine or Thorazine or Largactil (Cl at 2), triflupromazine or Vesprin (CF_3 at 2), and promazine or Sparine (H at 2). (3) A piperidine group may be attached to a carbon chain at R_1 and is represented by mepazine or Pacatal and thioridazine or Mellaril in which a thiomethyl group appears at Position 2. Chlorpromazine has adrenergic blocking effects; on initial administration it produces a fall in blood pressure from 20 to 40 mm. Hg. It has antiemetic effects and usually increases appetite and constipates; over time, patients will usually show a gain in weight. The drug has a marked sedating and tension-reducing effect in animal and man, and during the first days of therapy it can produce a somnolence that usually disappears.

INDICATIONS The phenothiazines are effectively used in all non-depressive psychotic states, particularly in the schizophrenias. The drugs have been useful in symptomatic psychoses with excitation and psychomotor agitation. Severe and prolonged delirium tremens responds better to paraldehyde or chlordiazepoxide. We see little indication for its use in the majority of neurotic states. In the management of acute manic or catatonic excitement, either electroshock, sodium amytal intravenously given, or the administration of parenteral chlorpromazine can be of value. These drugs have been used (without impressive results) with autistic children and are employed for certain impulse disorders in adult and pediatric psychiatry. Hyperkinetic disorders in children, on the other hand, have been more successfully treated with amphetamine and its derivatives.

SIDE EFFECTS AND COMPLICATIONS Nasal congestion and flushing, galactorrhea and polyuria and oral-pharyngeal moniliasis (rarely), and occasionally contact dermatitis and hyperglycemia are seen. Major complications are: (1) A *neurological syndrome* resembling Parkinsonism with a decrease in spontaneous motility, muscular rigidity and tremor, masklike face, and cogwheel rigidity of the extremities. Various forms of dyskinesia result, resembling dystonia, torsion spasm with choreiform, ballistic and myoclonic symptoms; oculogyric crises (occasionally); and trismus and akathisia (inability to sit, a motor restlessness and impulsion to move, usually of the feet but also of the hands). Parkinsonian symptoms, and especially akathisia, can be treated by anti-Parkinson agents, but it is important to recognize that patients may feel they are getting worse or refer these bodily changes to psychological symptoms, thereby finding motives for their inability to stop moving. A few instances of persistent dyskinesia have been noted, generally in older persons who did not initially receive anti-Parkinson drugs. Occasionally, abdominal wall rigidity masquerading as a "surgical abdomen" baffles the unwary practitioner. Drug fever is sometimes observed; in general, if rare or bizarre metabolic and endocrine side effects are encountered, it should be recalled that hypothalamic mechanisms are influenced by these drugs. Apart from active seizure states, there is no contraindication to their use in brain syndromes, but adjunct anti-Parkinson drugs are not advisable in these cases. (2) *Cardiovascular effects* are important. Tolerance usually develops to the postural hypotension that may follow oral or parenteral doses; however, neurocirculatory collapse is observed with initial doses and is serious. The hypotension may be less frequently encountered with the newer derivatives. When shock is encountered, the patient should be kept warm and the lower extremities elevated. Oxygen and levearterenol or phenylephrine as vasoconstrictors are sometimes suitable; the effects of epinephrine may be reversed in the presence of compounds with adrenergic blocking activity. If other analeptics seem indicated, 20 to 40 mg. of metamphetamine may be used intravenously. Another complication of the hypotension, which is fortunately quite rare, may be coronary thrombosis. Electrocardiographic changes may occur and some reservations about the use of phenothiazines and imipramine in cardiac conditions have been expressed.[48] (3) *Liver damage:* a small percentage of the patients on chlorpromazine develop an obstructive jaundice. If this occurs, it is generally seen early in therapy, within the first three months; its occurrence, probably based on a sensitivity reaction, is independent of amount or duration of dosage. Pre-existing liver disease apparently does not predispose to this complication. Among the phenothiazines, jaundice occurs most frequently with chlorpromazine and, perhaps, cannot be said truly to be a characteristic complication with the newer derivatives. Withdrawal of the drug and expectant therapy are generally sufficient measures. The incidence is estimated at one per cent. (4) *Blood dyscrasias and agranulocytosis* are rare but, of course, quite dangerous and have occurred early (within the first ten weeks) in therapy with most phenothiazines. The usual anticipatory routines of periodic blood tests are warranted but (since onset is often sudden) not necessarily practical. Attention should be paid to physical complaints and symptoms such as sore throat. (5) *Miscellaneous effects:* a light-sensitive dermatitis occurs with chlorpromazine (based possibly on an affinity of phenothiazines for melanin), a complication that is quite difficult to treat. Generalized melaninlike deposits throughout the body and in the lens or cornea were reported as a complication of sustained high dosage (over 1200 mg.) over years (ten) in some females, and further reports of this phenomenon should be forthcoming and be carefully considered. Even slight impairment of vision, however, is quite rare; nevertheless, if quantity of drug is a factor, this would argue for the more potent compounds in long-term treatment. With thioridazine in dosages over 1000 mg. daily, a few instances of retinopathy have been reported; and a harmless but strange side effect, orgasm without ejaculation, has been observed with this and other phenothiazines. When required, meprobamate, chloral hydrate or barbiturate sedatives can be given for sleep, but insomnia in the presence of an adequate dosage of phenothiazines might represent a variant of akathisia treatable with anti-Parkinson drugs. Whereas the drug is used successfully along with anticonvulsants, compounds of this class may occasionally evoke a pre-existing seizure disorder, especially with high dosage. Myasthenia gravis may be exaggerated because of neuromuscular blocking properties of the drugs. Overdose leads to extrapyramidal symptoms and collapse, but successful suicides have not been reported. Although usual doses are not contraindicated in pregnant and lactating women, a general rule would be for quite conservative pharmacotherapy in these states if drugs are to be given at all. To a degree, the drugs potentiate alcohol and sedatives, although this is not commonly a critical problem.

CHLORPROMAZINE DOSAGE The minimal dose of chlorpromazine generally employed for adults is 25 mg. three or four times a day; a commonly encountered dosage in compensated psychotic patients ranges from 300–800 mg. daily, and the maximal daily dose is 1500 mg. If somewhat larger doses are given at nighttime than during the day, an undesired drowsiness may be diminished; there is no good evidence that a periodic dosage during the day is necessary for effects in a large number of patients, but divided doses two to four times daily will meet most patient needs. In children, half a milligram per kilogram may be given. In uncooperative patients and in emergency situations, 25–50 mg. chlorpromazine may be given intramuscularly, slowly, and deep into the outer quadrant of the buttock; parenterally administered chlorpromazine is three times as potent as oral dosage.[49] Parenteral administration of some phenothiazines, although not defined as unsafe, is nevertheless best avoided when possible. In general, it is recommended to begin with small doses, preferably by mouth, and increase doses gradually for one or two days to effective levels, watching for desired effects and complications; if a dose level of 600–800 mg. daily is desired for psychotic patients, this can, if necessary, be easily achieved, usually within twelve hours. We use 300–600 mg. daily for psychotic patients who are not particularly agitated and 200–400 mg. of chlorpromazine to maintain patients who become relatively asymptomatic. The drugs may safely be abruptly withheld.

Other Phenothiazines

The newer phenothiazines probably vary critically in side effects; akathisia-inducing potential is greater than with chlorpromazine or thioridizine. The array of phenothiazines does provide flexibility in prescribing drugs since individual differences in response are encountered. Daniel X. Freedman and Jacob DeJong[32] were able to show that differences in individual sensitivity of the patient as well as in molecular configuration of the drug are responsible for the akathisia syndrome; surveys of extrapyramidal effects in large populations show that the piperazine group and the fluorinated group have a very high incidence of such effects.[6] Akathisia can be easily managed either by adjusting dosage, or with Benadryl or some of the atropinelike drugs used in the treatment of Parkinsonism, for example, Artane, Kemadrin, or Cogentin.

The drugs commonly used at present have received some objective trials and have been extensively observed in clinical practice. Some of these are perphenazine (Trilafon, minimum dose 6 mg., average dose 16 mg., maximum dose 75 mg. daily); prochlorperazine (Compazine, used also for antiemetic effects, 15–100 mg. daily); fluphenazine (Prolixin, 3–30 mg. daily); trifluoperazine (Stelazine, 6–32 mg. daily); and thioridazine (Mellaril, 150–800 mg. daily). One-fifth or less of the maximum dose is commonly used for maintenance. Drowsiness may occur initially with all phenothiazines, but patients usually adapt. Whereas these "alerting" compounds are used because of a lower (though not inconsiderable) incidence of drowsiness, and whereas they differ from chlorpromazine in motor and neural effects on animals, there is as yet no solid objective evidence that they have characteristic therapeutic effects radically different from chlorpromazine. Often therapists experiment until they hit on the right drug for their patient. There is a large number of other major tranquilizers (such as chlorprothixine, a thioxanthine derivative analogous to chlorpromazine) and also chemically unrelated drugs, such as haloperidol, which Jean Delay *et al.* used.

Rauwolfia Alkaloids

The other class of major tranquilizers (now no longer used extensively) are the rauwolfia alkaloids first used in psychoses by G. Sen and K. C. Bose and by J. C. Gupta in 1937. Reserpine, (see Figure 11–2) isolated from the alkaloid (and first used by R. A. Hakim in India; by E. Weber in Switzerland; and by Nathan S. Kline in the United States about fifteen years after the introduction of the alkaloid), has a marked calming effect in man and animals.

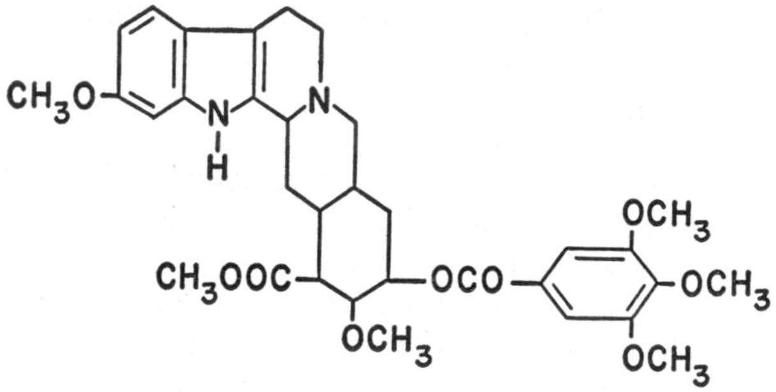

CH_3O — N–H — N — CH_3OOC — OCO — OCH_3 — OCH_3 — OCH_3 — OCH_3

Figure 11–2.

It has been assumed that the effect is brought about by a liberation of serotonin and catecholamines from storage sites; in any event, the use of reserpine as a basic tool to investigate the neurochemical basis of tranquilization or as a possible biochemical model for depression is still important. Its effect on the ascending reticular systems (apparently stimulated) is not entirely clear; a central parasympathetic activation occurs, and the drug peripherally produces a chemical sympathectomy. The drug (or its effects) has also a potentiating effect on LSD-25.[4,30,31] All these findings make it clear that mechanisms governing response to excitation operate through different pathways than in the case of phenothiazines. For this reason, and because we have observed a few patients over a period of time who do well only with reserpine, we think the drug should be reserved for a trial in patients who have not received it. J. A. Barsa and N. Kline[7] and others described three stages in the course of treatment of schizophrenia with reserpine: (1) the sedative stage of about three to ten days; (2) the turbulent stage, in which the patient becomes excited, complains about increased hallucinations and delusions, particularly nightmares, which lasts about three weeks (this may possibly be related to extrapyramidal effects and treated accordingly); (3) the integrative stage, in which the patient improves. Indications are very similar to those of the phenothiazines; needs for immediate sedation are better met by other drugs, but for a therapeutic course it may be used in both acute and chronic patients with or without phenothiazines. The drug is not recommended in the treatment of neuroses, depressions, and delirious syndromes. It also has been ineffective in organic psychoses such as Huntington's Chorea, but it has been useful in some very agitated, hostile, institutionalized senile or hypertensive patients who were unmanageable.

SIDE EFFECTS AND COMPLICATIONS Reserpine causes somnolence and fatigue as well as an uncomfortable nasal congestion and headaches. Acute initial large doses produce signs of parasympathetic stimulation, including vomiting and diarrhea (to which tolerance develops), but some miosis and slight bradycardia are characteristic throughout therapy, and some autonomic and serotonin effects persist weeks beyond drug withdrawal.[31] Hypotension is generally minimal; the pre-existing hypertension in hypertensive disease is, of course, affected, and these individuals may occasionally become seriously depressed with the drug. Depression in nonhypertensives is perhaps not as commonly seen but may occur. A few patients develop edema of the lower extremities. A Parkinsonian and dystonic syndrome occurs in about 5 per cent of the patients treated. Activation of peptic ulcers, melena, and hematemesis have been reported. The recommended dosage of reserpine for adults varies between 1 mg. and 5 mg. per day (the usual starting dose) and 20 mg. per day for very excited patients. It may be given orally or intramuscularly and combined with phenothiazines.

Minor Tranquilizers

These drugs have a calming effect in animals and man but do not in usual dosages produce the neuroleptic syndrome as do the drugs of the phenothiazine and rauwolfia groups. The most important of this group is Meprobamate. Other drugs are diphenylmethane derivatives such as hydroxyzine (Atarax, Vistaril) and benactyzine (Suavitil). Meprobamate is 2-methyl-n-propyl-1, 3 propanedial dicarbamate (see Figure 11–3).

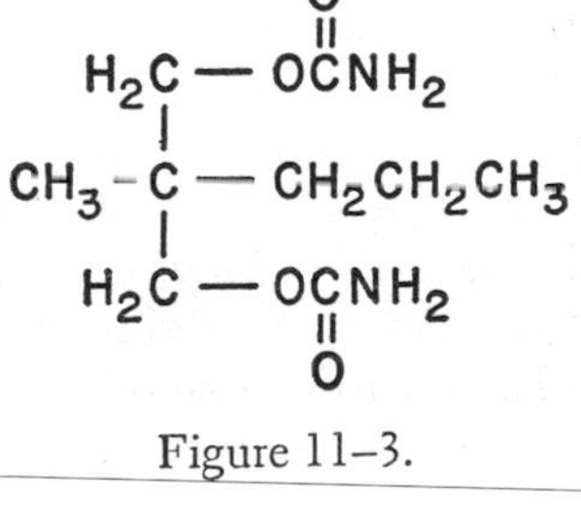

```
              O
              ‖
     H2C — OCNH2
      |
CH3 - C — CH2CH2CH3
      |
     H2C — OCNH2
              ‖
              O
```

Figure 11–3.

In animal experiments, Meprobamate has definite muscle-relaxant, anticonvulsant, and sedating properties. In human beings, it has a slight calming effect; the dose of Meprobamate for adults is 800 to 1600 mg. per day. It is used primarily in treating neurotics to relieve anxiety. Some patients are allergic to the drug. More serious is the possibility of habituation, with withdrawal symptoms similar to those produced by barbiturates; this has been observed with higher dosage levels than those advocated. Because the clinical effects of the drug are slight, and because addictive liability exists (or at least a liability for habituation), Meprobamate should be used sparingly (see Chapter 22). Benactyzine, an anticholinergic propanediol derivative, produces relaxation, but thought-blocking and depersonalization have occasionally been observed. In combination with Meprobamate (Deprol), it is used in tense and neurotically depressed persons, but one must be careful in dispensing the combination.

Another drug in this group is methaminochlordiazepoxide (7-chloro-2-methylamino-5-phenyl-3N-1, 4 benzodiazepineroxide hydrochloride [Librium]). (See Figure 11–4.)

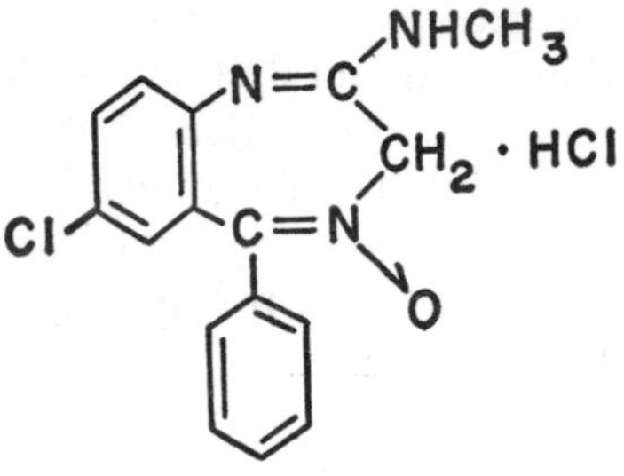

Figure 11–4.

The usual daily dose is 20 to 150 mg.; it acts rapidly and reduces anxiety in some patients. It is used for neurotic patients and for acute anxiety attacks and situational apprehension of any kind. In general, there are few autonomic effects, and there is a wide gap between the taming and the ataxic and hypnotic effects in animals. It is said not to produce somnolence and not to interfere critically with cognitive function in therapeutic doses. It may, however, produce ataxia and mild symptoms resembling alcohol intoxication. If it is withdrawn abruptly after sustained and very high dosages, convulsions may supervene within several days (see Chapter 20). Decreased visual acuity, phorias, and altered depth perception have been noted, and a study of a group of sixty patients on sustained dosage showed a significantly increased incidence of traffic accidents. Unlike Meprobamate, which has been used successfully for suicide, toxic doses of Librium have not been lethal. The basic neuropharmacology has yet to be extensively studied, but the array of effects already documented show undoubted activity. There may be a stimulant effect upon appetite. The drug has anticonvulsant properties and has been used in epilepsy. In alcoholism, it is perhaps most efficacious, but habituation to the drug may occur. The testimony of alcoholic patients who use it as a substitute warrants careful examination of the compound's effect in facilitating their avoidance of contact with the realities of their environment. In delirium tremens, doses of 100–200 mg. daily are quite effective, and an intravenous dose of 100 mg. will quite dramatically calm the hallucinating alcoholic, who immediately comes into improved contact. The drug is not particularly effective in the psychoses.

Antidepressant Compounds

The use of drugs in depression, although important for the development of newer compounds and research into neurochemical mechanisms, has still not replaced electroconvulsive therapy. When rapid relief of psychotic depression is required (for example, in a case of suicidal risk), electroconvulsive treatment is probably the most efficacious organic therapy we have. Nevertheless, many depressions can be treated without convulsive therapy (and its attendant confusion) in the proper therapeutic surroundings, and the drugs are of proven importance. The major antidepressants are:

(1) Inhibitors of monoamineoxidase
- (a) hydrazine derivatives:
  - iproniazid (Marsalid)
  - isocarboxazid (Marplan)
  - phenelzine (Nardil)
  - nialamid (Niamid)
- (b) a bimodal type with some amphetaminelike activity:
  - tranylcypromine (Parnate)
  - pargyline (Eutonyl)

(2) Dibenzazepines and isosteres
- imipramine (Tofranil)
- desmethylimipramine (Pertofrane)
- amitriptyline (Elavil)
- desmethylamitriptyline (Nortriptyline)
- chlorprothixene (Taractan)

(3) Minor antidepressants: amphetamine, metamphetamine, and piperidine derivatives:
- methylphenidate (Ritalin)
- pipradol (Meretran)
- deanol (dimethylaminoethanol, Deaner)
- chlordiazepoxide (Librium)

Hydrazides of isonicotinic acid such as iproniazid (Marsilid) were introduced in 1951 for the chemotherapy of tuberculosis, but hyperactivity, euphoria, and occasionally toxic psychoses led to its discontinuance. Later,

Marsilid (see Figure 11–5), perhaps therapeutically most effective of the MAO inhibitors in depression, was withdrawn because of liver toxicity.

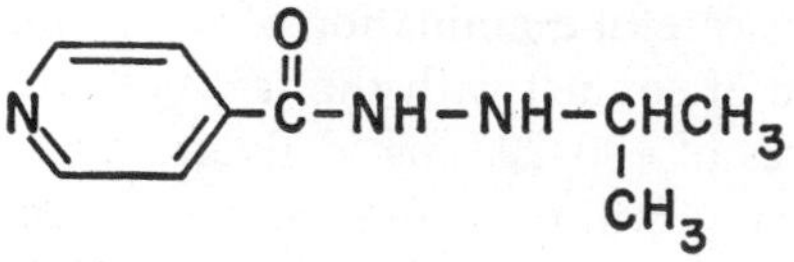

Figure 11–5.

Since 1957, a number of these compounds have been developed. We view this class of compounds as interesting but at present not necessary in the treatment of depression because of the availability of relatively safer effective compounds. As with all drugs, their availability provides a wider array of treatments and possibilities for trial in individual therapeutic problems. Whereas monoamine oxidase is inhibited and amines such as serotonin and norepinephrine are elevated in the human brain, their mechanisms of action must be based on the more general principle that these drugs interfere with a number of interrelated mechanisms governing the amines. These antidepressants can produce orthostatic and postural hypotension, which are generally mild. Occasional peripheral neuropathies, restlessness, and insomnia may be encountered, especially with higher dosages, and a mild hypoglycemia may intervene after prolonged treatment, leading perhaps to an increased appetite and weight gain. The serious concern, aside from the dangerous potentiation of a variety of drugs, as well as dietary amino acids (with associated hypertensive crises), is liver toxicity, which (unlike the reversible cholestatic jaundice induced by chlorpromazine) stems from hepatocellular degeneration and necrosis. It should be emphasized that each of these compounds differs possibly in effects on the "life cycle" of amines and clearly in liability to toxic and side effects. The major compounds in current use are Marplan or isocarboxazid (10–30 mg. daily), which has been reported to be potent and with only occasional instances of liver damage. The onset of action is slow and, as with all MAO inhibitors, effects continue (perhaps correlated with the recovery of MAO activity) for several weeks after withdrawal. Seizures have been precipitated by isocarboxazid, and it should not be used in epilepsy. Nialamid (Niamid, 50–200 mg. daily) is considered to have a lower potency but greater safety, while phenelzine (Nardil, 40–100 mg. daily) was reportedly well tolerated and useful in this series of compounds. Tranylcypromine (Parnate, 10–60 mg. daily) has both amphetaminelike action and monoamine oxidase inhibition. Clinically, it appears to be quite potent and safe with respect to liver and blood disorders but dangerous with respect to potentiation.

Imipramine, synthesized as an isostere of the phenothiazines, is closely related to their action in basic studies but shows specific differences. (See Figure 11–6.) R. Kuhn developed the drug in Switzerland in 1957 as an antidepressant.

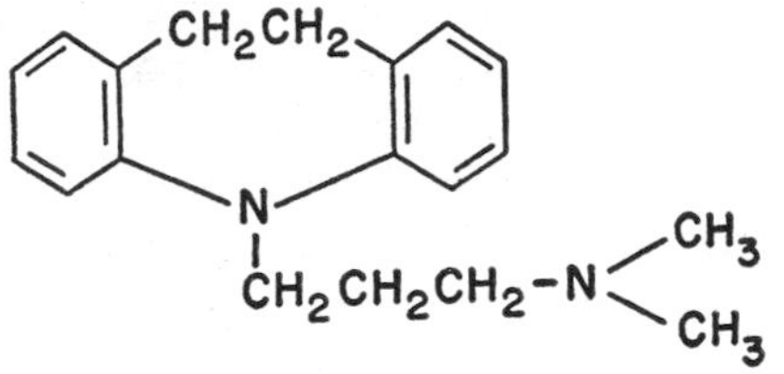

$$\text{(two benzene rings joined by } CH_2CH_2 \text{ and } N\text{; } N-CH_2CH_2CH_2-N(CH_3)_2)$$

Figure 11–6.

In normal subjects, it produces a sense of alertness and well-being, perhaps by stimulating motor activity, but is followed by sedation and psychomotor retardation, an aftereffect not seen in depressed patients. As with chlorpromazine, cholestatic jaundice has been encountered as well as pseudo-Parkinsonism; as with chlorpromazine, it is thought occasionally to activate seizures if anti-convulsive medication is not concurrent. Atropinelike side effects are characteristic and generally not troublesome (constipation, blurred vision, and dry mouth), but this would contraindicate use of the drug in glaucoma or high myopia and iritis. Pylorospasm may occur, and in elderly males a rectal examination should precede drug treatment since cholinolytic urinary retention can occur; in fact, in high dosage the drug has been effective in enuresis. Granulocytopenia is a small but nevertheless definite hazard, as is the use of the drug in cardiovascular disease. Dosage may range from 75–200 mg. daily, and the onset of effects generally may not be evident until five to ten days of treatment. The in vivo metabolite of imipramine, desmethylimipramine, has an antidepressant activity in animals (that is, given animals who are then administered reserpine) but it has yet to be established as superior in endogenous depressions. Amitryptyline (Elavil), 75–150 mg. daily, has frequently been used in patients unresponsive to imipramine, and it is claimed that its onset of action is faster. Chlordiazepoxide or a phenothiazine may be combined with these drugs if anxiety and tension are troublesome as the depression recedes. Chlorprothixine (Taractan), 200–600 mg. daily, as the previous compounds, shows effects on various components of amine metabolism but differs in its strong antagonism to the effects of serotonin and strong antiemetic effects. It has apparently both tranquilizing and alerting effects and produces extrapyramidal symptoms. As we move away from the more established compound imipramine, various mixed effects may be observed; and with all these drugs, especially those which have strong atropinelike effects, occasional exacerbations of hallucinations may be encountered. Not infrequently, depression which shifts to mania has been observed as well as psychotic symptomatology, especially in paranoid cases. For agitated depressions, combinations of imipramine and a phenothiazine are indicated. One critical contraindication is the use of imipramine after an MAO inhibitor, since unexplained hypotensive deaths have been reported. A period of several weeks should intervene between the use of these two antidepressant groups of drugs. Imipramine and non-MAO groups of antidepressants are often employed on a "target symptom" basis to combat depression in schizophrenic or neurotic disorders just as Librium or phenothiazines are used in neuroses and depressions for anxiety; this is not injudicious, but the landmarks and guidelines for such therapeutic decisions are poorly worked out; at present the approach can on occasion be used, but with a conservative and investigative attitude.

For the severe disorders, the amphetamines and piperadine derivatives are not important. In view of the symptomatic psychoses that may occur with continued high dosages of amphetamines, especially in prepsychotic or sociopathic individuals, caution should be observed. Amphetamine psychoses are difficult to distinguish from paranoid schizophrenia, but their occurrence nonetheless has been well documented. These drugs are rarely prescribed in depressions at the present time, except occasionally together with a sedative or tranquilizer to counteract the undesirable somnolent effects. They are still used in states of fatigue and in extreme situations when wakefulness is necessary. The drugs are recommended in organic cases of narcolepsy. Dosage of the d-form is 2.5 mg. to 15 mg. at daytime. Chlordiazepoxide may be used in mild depression with marked anxiety. Finally, there has been some interest in the use simply of phenothiazines for depressive target symptoms.

Psychotomimetics, Model Psychoses, and Psychedelic Drugs

With drugs that not only modify but also can induce behavior disorder, conceptual models for the involved neurochemical processes and behavioral processes can be tested with a powerful array of laboratory techniques. For Freud, a dream was a model psychosis, because the processes and laws he saw operating in the dream were quite similar to the waking state of psychosis. The dream differs, according to Freud,[36] only in its duration and mode of onset and termination; it is terminated by an act of one's own "will." The onset, duration, and termination of mental effects of a class of drugs, which includes LSD-25, mescaline, and psilocybin, are related to their biochemical actions; they have been of investigative importance because they reliably compel a period of altered mental function in which interesting subjective changes occur.[69] Drugs such as mescaline were studied in the nineteenth century. A number of compounds, for example, alcohol, can induce the release of irrational behavior, and the laughing gas reactions which Humphry Davy investigated a hundred and fifty years ago may be seen as a kind of model psychosis. Behavioral changes produced by alcohol, morphine, hashish and cocaine are well known; N-allylnormorphine (the morphine antagonist) may produce hallucinations, as may Serynl.[64] There are numbers of anticholinergic and atropinelike compounds that quite consistently induce altered mental states, and steroids inconstantly produce mood disorders. Combinations of MAO inhibitors with amino acids (tryptophan, methionine) produce psychoticlike states and exacerbate schizophrenic symptoms. Toxic confusional states, quite different from the effects of potent psychotomimetic agents, may be induced by an enormous range of drugs, and in certain dosages some of these (quinacrine) may imitate paranoid psychoses.[62]

The biochemical interest of compounds such as mescaline, LSD, and psilocybin lies in their structural similarity to such endogenous substances as norepinephrine or serotonin.[40] (See Figure 11–7.)

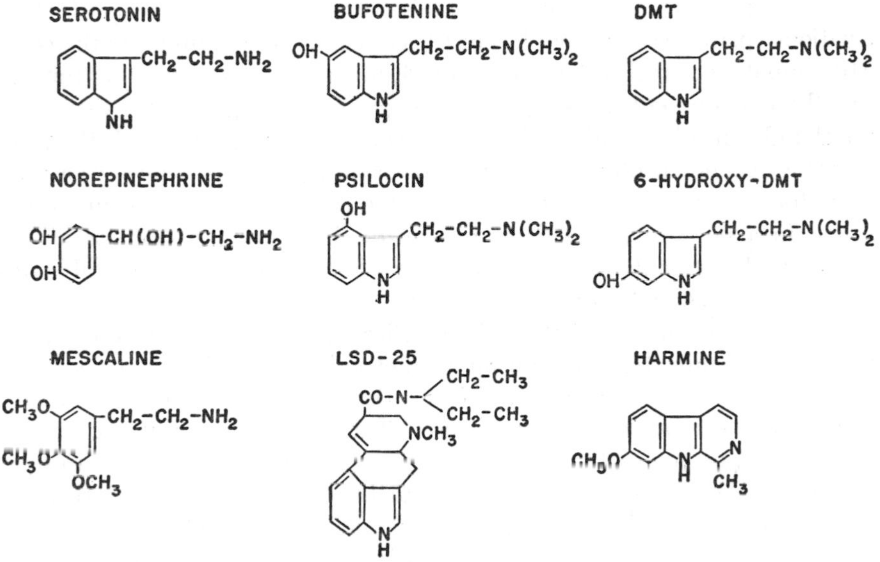

Figure 11–7.

Psychotoxic indolealkylamines, phenethylamines, or alkaloids (once called "telephathine") containing harmine and harmaline are widely distributed in plant life and consumed for ritual trance and altered subjective experiences; there has been a search for their occurrence in man. The mammal can N-methylate indole amines (producing the psychotoxic dimethyltryptamine as well as bufotenine); 5-hydroxylate indoles (which enhances their psychotoxicity); produce harmalinelike structures in the pineal; and O-methylate catecholamines such as norepinephrine (which is similar to mescaline).[40] The importance of these compounds is not necessarily that they are active agents in clinical disorder; rather, they offer a tangible way to see how a biochemical substance can act so as to produce a peculiar mental state.

Probably less than one half a millimicrogram of LSD per gram of brain is reliably sufficient to trigger a sequence of behavioral states for a period of ten hours. The drugs have the property of disengaging one's usual orientation to the everyday order of things, without clouded consciousness or marked physiological changes; some aspects of primary processes usually dormant or transient during wakefulness become "locked" into a persistent state.[14,24,84] The usual boundaries structuring perception and cognition become fluid. Awareness becomes vivid, and there is a diminished control over input. Momentary perceptions and feelings gain an independence from the normal corrections of logic; thoughts and perceptions which are usually suppressed come into awareness. In both animals and man, there is a failure to habituate to novel stimuli; the world appears new, and elements in it are unique and compel attention. The customary becomes illusory and portentous. Objects seen a moment ago may persevere in the mind's eye, giving rise to reports of hallucinations (perhaps since what has just been seen now contaminates the coexisting input from reality). Because the customary modes of viewing the self and the environment are shifted, and because the world seems somewhat novel and control is diminished, the drugs induce a state in which the individual is dependent on the environment, or on prior expectations, or a mystique for structure and support; at the same time, the person begins to see things in a new way. Psychiatry recognizes these primary changes as the background state out of which a number of secondary psychological states can ensue, depending on motive, capacity, and circumstance. The terminology that has grown around these drugs reflects this: if symptoms follow, the term psychotomimetic is used; if mystical experience, religious conversion, or therapeutic behavior change is the focus, then the term psychedelic (mind-manifesting) or psychoadjuvant is used. Socioculturally, these are "cultogenic" drugs or "utopiates," [10] and their use in religious ceremonies to bind groups together around a mystical state makes them of interest for therapy. Claims that a "psychedelic" experience occurs with a single trial of exceptionally high doses of LSD and that this leads to startling cures of alcoholism or neurosis require very careful investigation.[75, 76] It is obvious that these drugs can change the usual order of perceiving the world; they dehabituate and alter automatic modes of seeing, thinking, and defending. In smaller doses, they are used as adjuvants to therapy analogous to narcosynthesis. Such drug effects do not, however, guarantee reintegration, and this is of crucial importance if they are to be safely used in psychiatric therapy. Of itself, uncovering is not of particular interest in therapy (although it may satisfy the therapist's curiosity). What is required is a careful integration and synthesis on the part of the patient. There have been serious investigations in this country and in England and on the Continent concerning the therapeutic efficacy of these components.[1] At this juncture, the data are not sufficient to recommend the use of these drugs other than for investigative purposes, but their possible role in illuminating the genesis of psychopathological symptoms and their role in new learning and their mode of neuropharmacological action continues to be of great interest.

Hypnotics

Barbiturates, paraldehyde, chloral hydrate, and a few other drugs have been used for some time by psychiatrists to produce sleep and also for their sedating and anticonvulsant properties. Since the introduction of tranquilizers, these drugs are now primarily used as pure hypnotica and anticonvulsants. The potential danger in the use of barbiturates (and supposedly "safe" hypnotics) is discussed in chapters 18 and 22. Slowly injected, intravenous sodium amytal ranks perhaps next to electroconvulsive treatment as a powerful emergency sedative and is useful for narcoanalysis. *Continuous sleep therapy*, introduced by J. Klaesi, using a cocktail of hypnotics (and today also of tranquilizers), is a complicated and potentially dangerous technique. Patients are put into a light continuous sleep for a period of one to two weeks and are awakened only for food-intake and elimination. This technique requires very careful nursing to avoid the danger of pneumonia and has been given up in the United States but, with a number of modifications, is still practiced in some European institutions. There is some experimentation with electrically induced sleep treatments in the U.S.S.R.

Coma Therapies

In the early 1930s, Manfred Sakel introduced insulin coma therapy (ICT), and Ladislas J. Meduna independently developed a convulsive coma therapy, first using camphor and later metrazol to produce convulsions. A few years later, U. Bini and U. Cerletti introduced electrical convulsive therapy (ECT). Sakel first produced insulin coma in morphine addicts during the withdrawal period; later, with Otto Pötzl's blessing, at the Viennese Psychiatric Clinic, he extended his therapeutic attempts to schizophrenia. From the very beginning, there was strong disagreement at the Viennese Clinic about the effectiveness of insulin coma therapy. Karl Dussik, who worked closely with Sakel in the male division, was enthusiastic, and a recovery rate of 90 per cent was claimed; but Erwin Stengel, in the female division, remained skeptical and saw no successes beyond the expected spontaneous remissions. In the late thirties, insulin coma therapy and convulsive therapies were introduced into psychiatric hospitals all over the world. Today, after decades of these therapies and many conflicting evaluations,[50, 78] the techniques are now being used less frequently. ICT is still used in some European and South American hospitals but hardly at all in North America; and ECT has also been partly replaced by antidepressant drugs. Meduna's carbon-monoxide inhalation therapy is hardly used.[66] It would be a gross mistake, however, to view the introduction of coma therapies as a blind alley, without positive effect. These therapies actually revolutionized public mental hospitals; they have saved lives and have reduced time spent in hospitals, even if long-term results of large populations of patients are hardly better than those of control populations.[81] They created an atmosphere of optimism and stimulated medical and psychiatric research.

Meduna based his therapy on the erroneous assumption that schizophrenics only very rarely suffer from epilepsy. He felt, in a sense, that schizophrenia could be driven out by convulsions. Later, Meduna recognized with admirable candor that the coma therapies were crudely empirical and compared them to kicking a Swiss watch. There are no good general theories to explain the action of coma or, as they are often called, "shock" therapies. Sakel advanced some very complex hypotheses that could not be tested operationally. Some psychiatrists believed that the psychological shock itself was beneficial and referred to recoveries from catatonia following psychological trauma, such as fires, floods, and other severe illnesses and accidents (catatonic patients recovered temporarily when they fell into water). William Sargant felt that any severe emotional arousal or shock, whether it occurs through medical procedures, in psychotherapy, or in states of religious ecstasy, as through handling of venomous snakes in snake cults, can be "therapeutically" effective.[73] Some dynamic psychiatrists have also suggested that a punitive element often attributed to the success of shock treatment helps the guilt-ridden patient. It goes without saying that no punitive approach of any kind has any place in therapy.

Another explanation of the effect of coma therapy assumes that the nursing and mothering care that patients receive when they awake from coma is helpful; but this fails to explain why some patients improve and others do not.[53] A theory based on the selective amnesia after electric convulsive therapy postulates that the blotting out of specific painful memories enables the patient to overcome his depression, guilt, and anxiety and to learn new and more realistic responses.

INSULIN COMA THERAPY The aim of ICT is to produce reversible hyperglycemic coma by administration of high doses of insulin.[71] The technique is cumbersome and requires well-trained medical and nursing personnel. Some clinicians claim that in certain cases when drugs and psychotherapy fail, it is helpful. We will describe ICT only very briefly, because it has lost much of its practical importance. Patients receive an initial dose of 15 units insulin, with daily increases until coma is reached, usually after three hours. Routinely, patients are awakened after one to two hours from coma, which must not be too deep, by tubefeeding them with sugar solution and only in exceptional cases by intravenous injection of dextrose. When schizophrenic patients awake from coma, they are generally much more accessible than otherwise. Patients receive from thirty to fifty such treatments. There are complications, some of them quite dangerous; some patients fail to awake from coma and develop acute and lasting symptoms of cerebral and cardiovascular damage. Administration of glucagon, which promotes the mobilization of glucose, has decreased the danger of prolonged coma. Mortality is one per cent. Convulsions are frequent and considered desirable. The therapy is indicated only in schizophrenia. Contraindications are severe acute and chronic infections, caudal, renal, hepatic, and metabolic diseases, and pregnancy. Reports of results always have been very conflicting and do not exceed improvement rates of other organic therapies.

ELECTRIC CONVULSIVE THERAPY *Technique:* A current of from 70 to 130 volts administered from 0.1 to 0.5 seconds, applied to the head, is usually sufficient to produce a convulsion. This permits 200 to 1,600 milliamperes to flow through the brain. Lothar B. Kalinowsky, an energetic and experienced proponent of the procedure, recommends 70 volts in the duration of 0.2 seconds as the initial dose, with increases in both time and voltage if no convulsion occurs.[54] Patients are placed in loose hospital garments on a hard mattress, either in slight flexion or with hyperextension of the spine supported by sandbags. When the typical convulsion begins, a mouth gag is inserted to avoid tongue-bite. Trunk and upper extremities are gently restrained during the seizure. The convulsion is of the *grand mal* type. The apnea can be rather prolonged and may require administration of oxygen. Patients usually have an amnesia for the procedure, but they may remember vaguely that the whole experience was extremely unpleasant. This can be avoided by combining electric convulsive therapy with the administration of a quick-acting anesthetic such as intravenous sodium pentothal. For the prevention of fractures, Abraham E. Bennett introduced curarization[9] which was later replaced by the administration of a reversible muscle relaxant such as succinyl choline in doses of 1.5 to 2 mg. Usually, succinyl choline is combined with an intravenous anesthetic, which requires the assistance of an anesthesiologist. Patients generally receive from ten to twenty treatments in a series; occasionally, a few shocks suffice to produce marked remissions. Shocks are normally administered three times a week. We are opposed to the administration of very frequent and massive shocks, except, for example, for emergency sedation in catatonic excitement.

Indications and results: The primary indications for ECT are depressions and particularly involutional depressions. There is no other treatment that is as promptly effective in agitated depressions as ECT. The depressive cycles of manic-depressive psychoses also respond well; the manic phases are much more refractory. In general, reactive and neurotic depressions should not be treated with electric convulsive therapy, but by psychotherapy and antidepressant drugs. Occasionally in refractory, severe cases, ECT combined with psychotherapy has been helpful. ECT has been used in certain agitated symptomatic psychoses to produce rapid sedation. In schizophrenias, it is now quite evident that this facilitates remissions in those patients who would also remit under a less drastic therapeutic regime. The consensus today among the better therapists is that ECT should not be used in the treatment of schizophrenia, with the exception of some catatonic excitements for which the treatment may shorten the course substantially. Generally, neurotics should not be treated with electric convulsive therapy. Whether ambulatory patients should receive ECT is an open question.

Many investigators have reported that the percentage of remissions is consistently high in manic-depressive psychoses and in psychotic depressions; between two-thirds and three-fourths of the cases are reported to recover or improve markedly. It is less satisfactory in involutional paranoids; among these patients, half or less improve. In schizophrenia, the higher recovery rates reported by Meduna and other investigators shortly after the method was introduced stand in sharp contrast to the modest results reported in later work.[42] However, even Meduna, who, after all, is entitled to the bias of a pioneer, doubts that true schizophrenics recover after electric convulsive therapy.

Contraindications and complications: Severe cardiovascular and pulmonary disease, bone diseases producing a predilection to fractures, brain tumors, epilepsy, and progressive cerebral atrophies are contraindications. Electric convulsive therapy does not endanger life to a significant degree. Franklin G. Ebaugh reported two fatal cases in a large series of cases.[23] Hans Hoff pointed to a series of fifteen thousand shocks without fatality.[47] Perforations of an aortic aneurysm or of an intestinal ulcer in a diverticulum have occurred but are extremely rare. The most frequent complications are fractures of the mid-dorsal vertebrae, femur, acetabulum, and scapula. Tearing of ligaments and dislocation of joints, particularly of the mandible, are not rare. To avoid fractures in electric convulsive therapy, relatively weak currents with a slow increment are used usually in conjunction with curarelike drugs. Some psychiatrists are opposed to such a procedure because the paralyzing agent and anesthesia obviously increase the risk of electric convulsive therapy. However, muscle relaxants make it possible to treat patients with fractures, although in our opinion fractures are an indication for interruption of treatment. Facilities for endotracheal intubation with positive pressure respiration as well as for defibrillation should constitute standard precautions when anesthetics are used. Atropine may be used routinely to reduce secretions during the convulsion.

The most disturbing side effects are psychological deficit states: severe intellectual impairment; sweeping defects of memory and retention;[53] affective incontinence; and marked confusion. In most patients, fortunately, with the exception of patients with progressive brain disease, even severe defects improve within a relatively short time. Some cases have been reported in which subarachnoid hemorrhage developed.

Psychosurgery

Trephine holes have been discovered in a number of prehistoric skulls, and trephination is still practiced in primitive cultures as a form of magic medicine. The modern method was described by Egas Moniz of Portugal in 1936[67] and earned him the Nobel Prize. The observations of John Fulton[38] on chimpanzees with experimental frontal lobe lesions added to the scientific respectability of the procedure. Walter Freeman[35] became the outstanding advocate of the method in the United States and contributed much to a temporary burst of enthusiasm for the procedure in many countries.[11] There were serious objections to it from the outset. It is of some interest that the procedure has lost its popularity, although the results, though controversial, were not unfavorable.[44] We believe that the medical and popular climate of opinion was created mostly by ethical objections from such different quarters as the Roman Catholic Church, the Ministry of Health in Soviet Russia, and most psychoanalysts.

Neurosurgeons devised a number of procedures ranging from radical lobectomies to the transorbital lobotomy, which, according to Freeman, was so simple that a psychiatrist could do it.[35] The essence of most lobotomies is the cutting of tracts between cortex, subcortex, and basal ganglia. If cortical tissue is removed, the word lobotomy is in order; if only white fibers are severed, one speaks of a leucotomy. The standard operation by Freeman and James W. Watts,[35] a modification of Moniz's original prefrontal leucotomy, consists of cutting prefrontal thalamic fibers through burr holes. New technical refinements have enabled neurosurgeons to carry out very minute and precise ablations, chemical injections and stimulations in human beings. It is not impossible that such procedures, which Sem Jacobson advocates, will become more important in the future.

After the standard operation, the patient shows profound confusion. Most patients have a rather severe organic deficit state with disturbances of orientation, memory, initiative, and abstract thinking, which are of relatively short duration. During the immediate postoperative period, they are usually incontinent, a symptom which H. Houston Merritt called "Don't-give-a-damn incontinence." At this time, patients show such signs of cerebral lesions as unequal pupils and a positive Babinski sign, but even at this early stage, many patients show a lessening of preoperative tension and often euphoria. Within a few weeks, the massive signs of organic confusion disappear, and the patients' behavior becomes more normal. They are no longer incontinent; yet peculiarities in their toilet habits, such as endless sitting on the toilet, remain. This is probably just one of the expressions of a lack of initiative typical of this stage; it has also been considered an expression of aggressive infantile behavior.

In most reports, it is characteristically stressed that the lobotomized patient: (1) becomes less tense and anxious; (2) shows decreased incentive; (3) becomes cruder and less socially sensitive; and (4) does not deteriorate in gross fashion, but nonetheless shows some subtle evidence of a disturbance in his ability to think at abstract levels.[37] The clinical improvement of agitated, extremely anxious, deluded, and severely obsessive-compulsive patients is probably caused by a reduction of anxiety and replacement of very pathological defense mechanisms by more acceptable and normal defenses.

Freeman and Watts and a number of British psychiatrists at one time pleaded for early referrals of schizophrenic patients for the operation, but today no one advocates early lobotomy of schizophrenics.[63] We seriously question the use of lobotomies in any psychiatric syndrome except for desperate cases for whom all other interventions have failed. We oppose the use of lobotomy in the vast majority of depressive and neurotic patients. The method is also unsuitable for the treatment of sociopaths. An important indication for lobotomy, outside of the field of psychiatry, is the relief of otherwise intractable organic pain.

Lobotomy is far from a harmless procedure. There is a fatality rate of from 2 to 4 per cent; and postoperative complications such as cerebral hemorrhage and convulsive seizures are not infrequent. It is even more important to weigh the patient's relief from psychotic symptoms against the danger of the occurrence of such sequelae as tactlessness, insensitivity, crudeness, sloppiness, irresponsibility, and a rather general disregard for more refined social relations.[80] Even if slight, these traits can be very annoying to relatives and friends, although the patient typically is unaware of them. One husband said of his lobotomized wife: "She's not driven by all the devils of hell any more, but she has become so sloppy and smelly!" Fortunately, more severe ethical aberrations in lobotomized patients are rare. In any case, it is important to involve lobotomized patients in a program of psychotherapy and rehabilitation, which gives some degree of assurance that some of the undesirable consequences are minimized.

Other Somatic Therapies

For purposes of completeness, we should mention the utility of continuous tubs and hydrotherapies for relaxation. Indeed, "taking the waters" is still used in Europe for relaxation and "tonic" effects and exclusive resorts in the United States provide regimens of exercise, swimming, massage, and other adult and infantile pleasures. The psychological impact of spas and shrines is undeniable. We do not use the wetpack (see Chapter 2) which occasionally is still employed for manic and overly excited persons. Except for a few metabolic and nutritional diseases with deficiency syndromes, there is no indication in psychiatry to use therapeutic diets or prescribe vitamins.

In concluding this survey of organic therapies, we should recall that good "patient management" is required with any therapy. The physician must be alert to his patient's comfort and his practical difficulties, which range from symptomatic problems to everyday issues of "arrangements": getting to and from appointments; having money to procure his prescription; and so forth. The technicalities of either the organic or the psychotherapies do not require a suspension of empathy and courteous concern, and the course of treatment is always advanced when the physician can be informed (but not distracted) by what his patient might observe or feel.

NOTES

1. Harold A. Abramson, "The Use of LSD in Psychotherapy," *Transactions of a Conference on d-Lysergic Acid Diethylamide (LSD-25)* (New York: Josiah Macy, Jr., Foundation, 1960).
2. George K. Aghajanian, "The Effect of Chlorpromazine on Respiration of Brain Mitochondria as a Function of Metabolic State," *Biochemical Pharmacology*, 12 (1963), 7.
3. James B. Appel, "Analysis of Aversively Motivated Behavior," *Archives of General Psychiatry*, 10 (1964), 71.
4. James B. Appel and Daniel X. Freedman, "Chemically-Induced Alterations in the Behavioral Effects of LSD-25," *Biochemical Pharmacology*, 13 (1964), 861.
5. Julius Axelrod, "The Uptake and Release of Catecholamines and the Effect of Drugs," in Harold E. Himwich and Williamina A. Himwich, eds., *Progress in Brain Research*, Vol. 9 (Amsterdam: Elsevier, 1964).
6. Frank J. Ayd, Jr., "A Survey of Drug-Induced Extrapyramidal Reactions," *Journal of the American Medical Association*, 175 (1961), 1054.
7. Joseph A. Barsa and Nathan S. Kline, "Treatment of 200 Disturbed Psychotics with Reserpine," *Journal of the American Medical Association*, 158 (1955), 110.
8. Henry K. Beecher, "The Powerful Placebo," *Journal of the American Medical Association*, 159 (1955), 1602.
9. Abram E. Bennett, "Preventing Traumatic Complications in Convulsive Shock Therapy by Curare," *Journal of the American Medical Association*, 114 (1940), 322.
10. Richard Blum *et al., Utopiates* (New York: Atherton Press, 1964).
11. Board of Control, *Results in 1,000 Lobotomies* (England and Wales; London: H. M. Statistics Office, 1947).
12. R. Bozzi, A. Bruno, and A. Allegranza, "Urinary Metabolites of Some Monoamines and Clinical Effects under Reserpine and Chlorpromazine," *British Journal of Psychiatry*, 111 (1965), 176.
13. Bernard B. Brodie, F. Sulser, and E. Costa, "Theories on Mechanism of Action of Psychotherapeutic Drugs," *Revue Canadienne de Biologie*, 20 (1961), 279.
14. Sidney Cohen, *The Beyond Within* (New York: Atheneum Press, 1964).
15. Jonathan O. Cole, "Evaluation of Drug Treatments in Psychiatry," *Psychopharmacology Service Center Bulletin*, 2 (1962), 28.
16. Jonathan O. Cole, "Therapeutic Efficacy of Antidepressant Drugs," *Journal of the American Medical Association*, 190 (1964), 448.

17. Jonathan O. Cole *et al.*, "Phenothiazine Treatment in Acute Schizophrenia: Effectiveness," *Archives of General Psychiatry* (NIMH Psychopharmacology Service Center Collaborative Study Group), 10 (1964), 246.
18. John M. Davis, "Efficacy of Tranquilizing and Antidepressant Drugs," *Archives of General Psychiatry*, 13 (1965), 552.
19. Jean Delay, P. Deniker, A. Green, and M. Mordret, "Le Syndrome Excito-moteur Provoqué par les Médicaments Neuroleptiques," *La Presse Médicale*, 65 (1957), 1771.
20. José M. R. Delgado, "Pharmacological Modification of Social Behavior," in W. D. M. Paton, ed., *Pharmacological Analysis of Central Nervous Action* (Oxford: Pergamon Press, 1963).
21. Thomas P. Detre, "Countertransference Problems Arising from the Use of Drugs in the Psychotherapeutic Management of Psychotic Patients," in Gerald J. Sarwer-Foner, ed., *The Dynamics of Psychiatric Drug Therapy* (Springfield, Ill.: Charles C Thomas, 1960).
22. John Donnelly and W. Zeller, "Clinical Research on Chlorpromazine and Reserpine in State and Private Psychiatric Hospitals," *Journal of Clinical and Experimental Psychopathology*, 17 (1956), 180.
23. Franklin G. Ebaugh, C. H. Barnacle, and K. T. Neubuerger, "Fatalities Following Electric Convulsive Therapy," *Archives of Neurology and Psychiatry*, 49 (1943), 107.
24. Joel Elkes, "Effect of Psychotomimetic Drugs in Animals and in Man," in Harold A. Abramson, ed., *Neuropharmacology, Transactions of Third Conference* (New York: Josiah Macy, Jr. Foundation, 1957).
25. Joel Elkes, "Psychopharmacology: The Need for Some Points of Reference," in Robert M. Featherstone and Alexander Simon, eds., *A Pharmacologic Approach to the Study of the Mind* (Springfield, Ill.: Charles C Thomas, 1959).
26. Joel Elkes, "Psychotropic Drugs. Observations on Current Views and Future Problems," in Henry W. Brosin, ed., *Lectures on Experimental Psychiatry* (Pittsburgh: University of Pittsburgh Press, 1961).
27. David M. Engelhardt, N. Freedman, B. Rosen, D. Mann, and R. Margolis, "Phenothiazines in Prevention of Psychiatric Hospitalization. III. Delay or Prevention of Hospitalization," *Archives of General Psychiatry*, 11 (1964), 162.
28. Edward V. Evarts, "A Discussion of the Relevance of Effects of Drugs on Animal Behavior to the Possible Effects of Drugs on Psychopathological Processes in Man," in Jonathan O. Cole and Ralph W. Gerard, eds., *Psychopharmacology: Problems in Evaluation*, (National Academy of Sciences, National Research Council Publication No. 583 [Washington, D. C., 1959]).
29. John M. von Felsinger, Louis Lasagna, and Henry K. Beecher, "Drug-Induced Mood Changes in Man. 2. Personality and Reactions to Drugs," *Journal of the American Medical Association*, 157 (1955), 1113.
30. Daniel X. Freedman, "Psychotomimetic Drugs and Brain Biogenic Amines," *American Journal of Psychiatry*, 119 (1963), 843.

31. Daniel X. Freedman and Arnold J. Benton, "Persisting Effects of Reserpine in Man," *New England Journal of Medicine*, 264 (1961), 529.

32. Daniel X. Freedman and Jacob DeJong, "Factors that Determine Drug-Induced Akathisia," *Diseases of the Nervous System*, 22 (1961), Suppl. 2.

33. Daniel X. Freedman and Nicholas J. Giarman, "Apomorphine Test for Tranquilizing Drugs: Effect of Dibenamine," *Science*, 124 (1956), 264.

34. Daniel X. Freedman and Nicholas J. Giarman, "Brain Amines, Electrical Activity, and Behavior," in Gilbert H. Glaser, ed., *EEG and Behavior* (New York: Basic Books, Inc., 1963).

35. Walter Freeman and James W. Watts, *Psychosurgery* (Springfield, Ill.: Charles C Thomas, 1950).

36. Sigmund Freud, "An Outline of Psycho-Analysis" [1938], *Standard Edition* (London: Hogarth Press, 1949), 23.

37. Rudolf Freudenberg and J. P. S. Robertson, "Investigation into Intellectual Changes Following Prefrontal Leucotomy," *Journal of Mental Science*," 95 (1949), 826.

38. John Fulton, *Frontal Lobotomy and Affective Behavior, a Neurophysiological Analysis* (New York: Norton, 1951).

39. Silvio Garattini and V. Ghetti, eds., *Psychotropic Drugs* (Proceedings of the International Symposium on Psychotropic Drugs, Amsterdam: Elsevier, 1957).

40. Nicholas J. Giarman and Daniel X. Freedman, "Biochemical Aspects of the Actions of Psychotomimetic Drugs," *Pharmacological Reviews*, 17 (1965), 1.

41. Nicholas J. Giarman and G. Pepeu, "The Influence of Centrally Acting Cholinolytic Drugs on Brain Acetylcholine Levels," *British Journal of Pharmacology and Chemotherapy*, 23 (1964), 123.

42. Jacques S. Gottlieb and P. E. Huston, "Treatment of Schizophrenia," *Journal of Nervous and Mental Diseases*, 113 (1951), 237.

43. Milton K. Greenblatt, George H. Grosser, and H. Wechsler, "Differential Response of Hospitalized Depressed Patients to Somatic Therapy," *American Journal of Psychiatry*, 120 (1964), 935.

44. Milton K. Greenblatt and Harry C. Solomon, eds., *Frontal Lobes and Schizophrenia* (New York: Springer, 1953).

45. Roy R. Grinker and John P. Spiegel, *Men under Stress* (Philadelphia: Blakiston, 1945).

46. Harris Hill, C. H. Kornetsky, H. G. Flanary, and Abraham Wikler, "Effects of Anxiety and Morphine on Discrimination of Intensities of Painful Stimuli," *Journal of Clinical Investigation*, 31 (1952), 473.

47. Hans Hoff, "Indications for Electro-Shock, Tofrānil, and Psychotherapy in the Treatment of Depressions," *Canadian Psychiatric Association Journal*, 4 (1959), S55.

48. Leo E. Hollister, "Complications from Psychotherapeutic Drugs—1964," *Clinical Pharmacology and Therapeutics*, 5 (1964), 322.

49. Leo E. Hollister, S. L. Kanter, and A. Wright, "Comparison of Intramuscular

and Oral Administration of Chlorpromazine and Thioridazine," *Archives Internationales de Pharmacodynamie et de Thérapie*, 144 (1963), 571.

50. Gunnar Holmberg, "Biological Aspects of Electroconvulsive Therapy," *International Review of Neurobiology*, 5 (1963), 389.
51. Gilbert Honigfeld, "The Placebo Effect," Report No. 55, Cooperative Studies in Psychiatry (Veterans Administration, November 1963).
52. Samuel Irwin, "Drug Screening and Evaluative Procedures," *Science*, 136 (1962), 123.
53. Irving L. Janis, "Memory Loss Following Electric Convulsive Treatments," *Journal of Personality*, 17 (1948), 29.
54. Lothar B. Kalinowsky and Paul H. Hoch, *Somatic Treatments in Psychiatry* (New York: Grune & Stratton, 1961).
55. Eva K. Killam, "Drug Action on the Brain-Stem Reticular Formation," *Pharmacological Reviews*, 14 (1962), 175.
56. Gerald L. Klerman, Alberto DiMascio, Milton K. Greenblatt, and Max Rinkel, "The Influence of Specific Personality Patterns on the Reactions to Phrenotropic Agents," in Jules H. Masserman, ed., *Biological Psychiatry* (New York: Grune & Stratton, 1959).
57. Irwin J. Kopin, J. E. Fischer, J. Musacchio, and W. D. Horst, "Evidence for a False Neurochemical Transmitter as a Mechanism for the Hypotensive Effect of Monoamine Oxidase Inhibitors," *Proceedings of the National Academy of Sciences*, 52 (1964), 716.
58. Conan Kornetsky, "Alterations in Psychomotor Functions and Individual Differences in Responses Produced by Psychoactive Drugs," in Leonard M. Uhr and James G. Miller, eds., *Drugs and Behavior* (New York: John Wiley, 1960).
59. Else B. Kris, "Prevention of Rehospitalization through Relapse Control in a Day Hospital," in Milton K. Greenblatt, D. J. Levinson, and Gerald L. Klerman, eds., *Mental Patients in Transition* (Springfield, Ill.: Charles C Thomas, 1961).
60. Louis Lasagna, Frederick Mosteller, John M. von Felsinger, and Henry K. Beecher, "A Study of the Placebo Response," *American Journal of Medicine*, 16 (1954), 770.
61. Julian Lasky, C. J. Klett, E. M. Caffey, J. L. Bennett, M. P. Rosenblum, and L. E. Hollister, "Drug Treatment of Schizophrenic Patients: A Comparative Evaluation of Chlorpromazine, Chlorprothixene, Fluphenazine, Reserpine, Thioridazine and Triflupromazine," *Diseases of the Nervous System*, 23 (1962), 698.
62. David J. Lewis and R. B. Sloane, "Therapy with Lysergic Acid Diethylamide," *Journal of Clinical and Experimental Psychopathology*, 19 (1958), 19.
63. J. J. López-Ibor, "Limited Indications for the Use of Leucotomy," *Acta Luso-esp. Neurol.*, 4 (1948), 307.
64. Elliot D. Luby, J. S. Gottlieb, B. D. Cohen, G. Rosenbaum, and E. F. Domino, "Model Psychoses and Schizophrenia," *American Journal of Psychiatry*, 119 (1962), 61.

65. John Marks, "Predrug Behavior as a Predictor of Response to Phenothiazines among Schizophrenics," *Journal of Nervous and Mental Disease,* 137 (1963), 597.

66. Ladislas J. Meduna, *Carbon Dioxide Therapy* (Springfield, Ill.: Charles C Thomas, 1950).

67. Egas Moniz, *Tentatives operatiores dans le traitement de certaines psychoses* (Paris: Masson, 1936).

68. Gordon W. Olson and Donald P. Peterson, "Intermittent Chemotherapy for Chronic Psychiatric Inpatients," *Journal of Nervous and Mental Disease,* 134 (1962), 145.

69. Fredrick C. Redlich, L. J. Ravitz, and G. H. Dession, "Narcoanalysis and Truth," *American Journal of Psychiatry,* 107 (1951), 586.

70. Karl Rickels, "Psychopharmacologic Agents: A Clinical Psychiatrist's Individualistic Point of View: Patient and Doctor Variables," *Journal of Nervous and Mental Disease,* 136 (1963), 540.

71. Manfred Sakel, *The Pharmacological Shock Treatment of Schizophrenia,* ("Nervous and Mental Diseases Monograph Series," No. 62; New York: Nervous and Mental Disease Publishing Company, 1938).

72. Santo Salvatore and R. W. Hyde, "Progression of Effects of Lysergic Acid Diethylamide (LSD)," *Archives of Neurology and Psychiatry,* 76 (1956), 50.

73. William Sargant, *Battle for the Mind* (Garden City, N. Y.: Doubleday, 1957).

74. Gerald J. Sarwer-Foner, "Discussion," in Gerald J. Sarwer-Foner, ed., *The Dynamics of Psychiatry Drug Therapy* (Springfield, Ill.: Charles C Thomas, 1960).

75. Charles Savage, W. Harman, E. Savage, and J. Fadiman, "LSD: Therapeutic Effects of the Psychedelic Experience," *Psychological Reports,* 14 (1964), 111.

76. Charles Savage, J. Terrill, and D. Jackson, "LSD, Transcendence and the New Beginning," *Journal of Nervous and Mental Disease,* 135 (1962), 425.

77. Michael H. Sheard, "The Influence of Doctor's Attitude on the Patient's Response to Antidepressant Medication," *Journal of Nervous and Mental Disease,* 136 (1963), 555.

78. Virginia M. Staudt and Joseph A. Zubin, "A Biometric Evaluation of the Somato-therapies in Schizophrenia," *Psychological Bulletin,* 54 (1957), 171.

79. Hannah Steinberg *et al.*, "Animal Behaviour and Drug Action," *Ciba Foundation Symposium* (Boston: Little, Brown, 1964).

80. Ernst Stengel, "Follow-up Investigation of 330 Cases Treated by Prefrontal Leucotomy," *Journal of Mental Science,* 96 (1950), 633.

81. Ian P. Stevenson, "The Challenge of Results in Psychotherapy," *American Journal of Psychiatry,* 116 (1959), 120.

82. Fridolin Sulser, M. H. Bickel, and B. B. Brodie, "The Action of Desmethylimipramine in Counteracting Sedation and Cholinergic Effects of Reserpine-

like Drugs," *Journal of Pharmacology and Experimental Therapeutics,* 144 (1964), 321.

83. Leonard M. Uhr and James G. Miller, eds., *Drugs and Behavior* (New York: John Wiley, 1960).
84. Sanford M. Unger, "Mescaline, LSD, Psilocybin, and Personality Change: A Review," *Psychiatry,* 26 (1963), 111.
85. Abraham Wikler, *The Relation of Psychiatry to Pharmacology* (Baltimore: Williams and Wilkins, 1957).
86. Nathan W. Winkleman, Jr., "Chlorpromazine and Prochlorperazine during Psychoanalytic Psychotherapy," in Gerald J. Sarwer-Foner, ed., *The Dynamics of Psychiatric Drug Therapy* (Springfield, Ill.: Charles C Thomas, 1960).
87. Stewart Wolf and Harold G. Wolff, *Human Gastric Function: An Experimental Study of a Man and His Stomach* (New York: Oxford University Press, 1947).

CHAPTER TWELVE

Neurotic Behavior

◆ The term neurosis, introduced into the medical literature at the end of the eighteenth century by William Cullen, has become a household word,[15] but to define it precisely is difficult. Rather than a definition, we offer a brief preliminary description of neurotic behavior as consisting of acts that can be characterized as inappropriate, inadequate, unadaptive, and infantile, resulting in a subjective and objective discrepancy between psychological potential and actual performance. For psychoanalysis, "neurosis" refers to core conflicts around which symptoms are built. Metaphorically useful, the concept often implies a discrete entity and becomes reified rather than referring to sequences of observable behavior. For laymen the term seems to retain the connotation of "broken down" nerves. Eugen Kahn tried and failed to eradicate it by indorsing the comprehensive term "psychopathic personality" to refer both to symptoms and antisocial traits.[45] Rather than neurosis, we prefer to speak of "neurotic behavior" or, as L. S. Kubie[52] does, of neurotic acts; yet—as in the old question: how many trees make a forest?—one might ask how many neurotic acts make a neurosis? We succumb then, as do psychiatrists of varying persuasions, to the purely linguistic convenience of having a noun, neurosis, as well as an adjective available to discuss this range of behaviors.

To speak of a neurotic behavior disorder as a minor disorder is a euphemism, although compared with lasting psychotic disintegration, neurotic behavior is, in most cases, less crippling and catastrophic. Neurotic behavior is a variant of a normal personality development; its clear differentiation from normality is problematic. Most psychiatrists emphasize the importance of psychological events in the etiology of neurotic behavior. They are convinced that psychotherapy is the primary treatment and assume that neurotic behavior is largely learned and can also be unlearned. The variety of neurotic symptoms and character traits is extraordinarily large. For reasons that will become clearer later, no rigid differentiation is made between the subclasses of symptom neurosis, character neurosis, sociopathic disorder, and acute and chronic traumatic neuroses; we will consider all these behavior disorders in this chapter.

Incidence and Prevalence of Neurotic Behavior

Since neurotic behavior has not been clearly distinguished either from normal or psychotic behavior, we cannot say how widespread it is. Everybody commits a neurotic act at times. The severe and lasting forms of neurotic behavior occur only in a certain percentage of the population. Estimates of the prevalence of neuroses in medical practice range between 10 and 75 per cent and obviously are without much value. Such estimates are guesswork based on widely varying criteria of why neurotics seek help and on unrepresentative samples. Leo Srole *et al.*, found that 36 per cent of their metropolitan population had mild, 22 per cent moderately severe, disturbances;[70] but whether this segment of the population in the Midtown Study corresponds roughly to the neurotic group is not established. Neurotic behavior, contrary to popular opinion, is not limited to urban populations but is found wherever individuals in any society have been studied with sufficient care and intensity. From findings by August B. Hollingshead and Fredrick C. Redlich,[42] and also by Srole,[70] we can assume with some confidence that neuroses in the different social classes have different characteristics, but specific types are by no means limited to one social class. In patients under treatment, character neuroses are more frequent in the upper classes; symptomatic neuroses and psychosomatic diseases occur more often in the lower middle class; and most of the sociopathic disorders are found in the lower classes. Epidemiological data do not support the thesis that upward mobile persons are particularly neurotic. Downward mobility is correlated with sociopathy. Ethnicity is seemingly a factor, but correlations are purely impressionistic; various observers were impressed with the dominance of hysterical behavior in Latin groups; obsessive reactions in Anglo-Saxon, German, Scandinavian, and Japanese populations; and overt anxiety in Chinese and Indian peoples. The impact of religion on incidence is unknown. Jews have a tendency to assess themselves more easily as neurotic, which is not explained by their religion as such, but by their problems as a minority group. It is quite possible that fundamentalist religions, with their inflexibly imperative positions about taboo thoughts and conduct, aggravate neurotic conflicts; but fixed belief systems, by polarizing values, can also have stabilizing effects. Social factors may differentially influence not only definitions, but susceptibility, severity, prognosis, and rehabilitation.

Neurotic behavior occurs at all ages. Today, we are convinced that adult neuroses have roots that can be traced back to childhood neuroses.[53] Yet, in most cases we cannot state definitely when neurotic behavior begins. There is no evidence that neurotic behavior occurs more frequently in one sex than the other; only the conflicts differ.

General Characteristics of Neurotic Behavior

Neurotic persons act inappropriately. Their social, sexual, and occupational performance in general terms is below the level of their potential, and they suffer and/or impose misery on others. When John Dollard and Neal E. Miller called neurotics "stupid," they did not want to add to the vocabulary of abuse of such persons, but to draw attention to the fact that they do not learn from their mistakes.[16] The inappropriate behavior of neurotic persons is rigid and repetitive. They have not lost their hold on reality, but in certain segments of their organization of reality, neurotics show immaturity, egocentricity, and distortion, each of which is related to their neurotic acts. According to Lawrence S. Kubie, symbolic distortions and misinterpretations are cardinal features of the neurotic process.[52]

Neurotics misjudge their inner world more than their outer world. Either they are ignorant of their infantile wishes, or, suspending judgment, they attempt to satisfy them by inadequate or forbidden means. Neurotics do not clearly distinguish between wish and act; they feel guilty over fantasies and even unconscious wishes and invoke punishment for acts they did not commit. The over-all result is frustration, shame, despair, and fear of punishment. When they are loved they don't know it, and they seem to be incapable of loving in a mature way. They feel inferior over their incompetence, or they lose sight of their limitations and invite ridicule or abuse, which further lowers self-esteem and enhances isolation. Still, neurotics derive gains from their behavior; their symptoms provide outlets for impulse expression and relief, enabling them to benefit from the sick role and to gratify dependency needs. Neurotic behavior is usually a bad bargain but it has an economy and, from a clinical and dynamic standpoint, a necessary one.

A catalogue of neurotic behavior appears like a collage of nasty childishnesses. Obviously, there are appealing aspects to neurotics; a pretty, naïve woman, who is neurotically compelled to fail, charms her husband who needs to be a hero, although burned toast and weak coffee every morning, after every loveless or tormenting night, casts a pall on the bargain. The infantile sexual needs or inhibitions of neurotics; their inappropriate aggression; and their insatiable demands for care excite the attention and provoke the despair and retaliation of those close to them. Whether or not neurotics can be said to "want punishment" to atone for their forbidden impulses, its consequences are valuable to them. Punishment can be equivalent to blind attachment or may not be distinguished from it. They tend to want the familiar, to avoid unsought novelty, and to fear new solutions; punishment also enables them actually to check their impulses. The vicious circle of punishing and being punished and of destruction and self-destruction is one of the cardinal and most troublesome facets of neurotic behavior.

Symptom Neuroses, Character Neuroses, and Sociopathies

As long as neuroses are viewed by experts and the public as diseases, patients will complain about "symptoms" and psychiatrists will seek and find them. For a long time it did not occur to psychiatrists that they were studying a genuine behavior disorder manifested by innumerable symptoms and inhibitions; most of these are acts, habits, and traits that impress both therapist and patient by their resemblance to disease, and they earn the "patient" the sick role (see Chapter 7). Attention has only gradually shifted from "neurotic disease" with remarkable symptoms to "neurotic personality." Alfred Adler[3] and Sigmund Freud[34] recognized the existence of neurotic character traits early and Wilhelm Reich used the term explicitly and with imagination.[63] Today, we generally appreciate that symptoms coexist with character traits that are equally inappropriate expressions of behavior. Often it is impossible to state clearly whether we are dealing with symptoms or habits. Is a patient's excessive and lifelong anxiety a symptom or a habit?

Neurotic character traits or habits, such as aggressive or passive behavior patterns, are experienced as integral parts of one's personality, that is, as "ego syntonic." In contrast, the patient experiences symptoms as a foreign body, as "ego alien." At times, of course, anyone may experience vague displeasure with his characteristic traits and "disown them." The usual notion is that a man is not responsible for his diseases or his neurotic symptoms, yet he is held responsible for his character even though neither symptoms nor deeply ingrained traits can be changed at will. It often is very difficult or impossible to distinguish between symptoms and character traits. Should one speak of symptom or pathological trait in the case of a man who, constantly and against his better knowledge and judgment, becomes unrealistically passive and appeasing in the face of attack or, wishing to be understood, invariably loses his audience in detailed irrelevancies? How easily can an obsessive character change into a flexible, free person? Are not symptoms as well as inappropriate character traits best understood as responses to stresses and as solutions of conflicts? Thus, the borderline between symptom neurosis and character neurosis is rather obscure.

The differentiation of character neurosis and sociopathy, one of our sacred cows, is also open to question. It is ordinarily assumed that in sociopathies aggressive and primitive sexual impulses are more severe than in character neuroses. Still, how hostile and destructive does a person have to be to merit being called a sociopath instead of a character disorder? The sociopath supposedly does not suffer but makes only others suffer; he is not bothered by fear, guilt, and shame. Does he repress and avoid such affects, or does he lack the capacity to generate them? In general, he shows an intolerance for guilt, a faulty and primitive conscience rather than none at all, and in some cases there appears to be a fault in bond formation, a problem in identification and internalized response. The effect is that he does not learn through reward and punishment. In other words, sociopathic behavior, whatever its cause, is just as rigid, "stupid," compelled, and usually as inappropriate as neurotic behavior; further, any close analysis of neurotic behavior reveals its essential "antisocial" meaning, the masked struggle with rules, restrictions, and taboos, the revolt against becoming or being a responsible grownup.

Fundamentally, we would maintain that there is a continuity among the different symptom neuroses, character neuroses, and sociopathies. All types of neurotic behavior are variants of normal personalities, and all are characterized by inappropriate behavior. Whether subgroups of sociopathic disorders can be biologically distinguished is not as yet clear; when better tests become available to measure neurotic anxiety and anxiety-proneness, it may well become possible. Response to epinephrine and fine localized tremors on special tests have been reported to differentiate some groups of sociopaths.[66] There are undoubtedly many paths leading to diminished impulse control, and in psychiatry, the task of sorting out subgroups is far from complete. Yet the division of sociopathic from neurotic behavior has, as a matter of historical fact, derived from the value judgments and attitudes of society; the difference between neurotic symptoms and neurotic character traits cannot as readily be located in their psychopathology as in the differential assignment of the sick role. In most civilized countries, the sick role is assigned quite freely to persons with symptom neuroses; the arena in which their psychopathology is "acted out" is overtly internal and only covertly in interpersonal relationships. To persons with character neuroses and sociopathy we assign the sick role at best grudgingly or not at all; their dysfunction is expressed more directly in interpersonal transactions. There are clearer differentiations when sociopathic behavior becomes more inappropriate and uncontrolled, such as repeated fire-setting by a pyromaniac in contrast to the burning of a neighbor's house in vengeance. As experts learn more about the roots of the range of neurotic behaviors and as the public becomes more educated, a more reasonable assignment of the sick role hopefully will occur.

Theories of Neurotic Behavior

Freud considered neurotic behavior the result of unconscious conflict; this was the key to his formulations. Motivational conflict has also been emphasized by Pavlovian scientists and by learning theorists. To recapitulate, Freud explained that neurotic symptoms are constructed by the ego.[33] Symptoms emerge as a result of conflicts between forbidden, unconscious impulses of the id and strivings of the ego as the psychological representative of reality; the primitive superego can side with one or the other. Such conflicts generate anxiety and threaten stability. When conflicts cannot be solved, they are repressed by the ego or, as Robert Waelder put it, are "swept under the rug." [74] Such a repression may result in a simple inhibition of a function, such as paralysis of a limb, impotence, and so forth. If repression is inefficient, and in most cases it is, the conflicting needs and distress are not truly eliminated but split off and may return from the unconscious in a disguised form. They are then integrated as inhibitions, symptoms, and pathological personality traits. Aside from repression, the whole gamut of defenses is encountered in neurotic behavior.

In all neurotic behavior, Freud observed a regression to infantile patterns, which coexist with quite highly developed patterns. Regression in neurosis is selective and reversible in contrast to regression in the psychoses: a neurotic wife takes criticism of a meal to mean she is totally worthless, but recovers quickly. In Freud's genetic proposition, regression proceeds to points of fixation or previous neurotic conflict; the adult neurosis is a repetition of the "childhood neurosis." When the patient tells of a period in his childhood when he was afraid to go to school, or recalls a struggle with bed-wetting, or some specific phobia or recurrent dream, he is unwittingly pointing to the childhood neurosis—to some temporary, or more severe, problem that represents (usually in masked ways) his early stresses and struggles and may well color his present problems. Screen memories refer to shorthand capsule memories, a construction often concocted of fragments which express the sense of forgotten childhood problems and solutions. An effeminate man, too inhibited for any adult sexual activity, remembered the outside of a Victorian house, which later proved to contain memories of a stiffly unapproachable aunt, to whom he reacted by complying and imitating in order to please. The childhood struggles for attention and pleasure, the rebellions and atonements are, perhaps mercifully, forgotten; but the term, childhood neurosis, refers to the symptoms, strategies, and solutions developed in the everyday drama of childhood life.

Freud did not think that the *nature* of the conflict alone explains why normal or abnormal reactions occur. All human beings are subject to certain universal conflicts such as the Oedipal conflict; the Oedipal conflict is the occasion—it supplies the text—but it is not necessarily the cause for neurotic outcomes. Freud felt that it is the intensity of the conflict, or the quantities of psychic energies involved, that determine the neurotic outcome. If this view is correct, it is obvious that many variations in response to apparently similar familial configurations are possible. Freud also assumed that there was a contributory factor; that is, simply to maintain neurotic defenses requires the reallocation of available psychic energy. The maintenance of such "countercathexis" results in psychological impoverishment. Clinically, such patients seem under strain, less effective, and less able to employ alternatives. Freud did not propose a unified theory of neurotic behavior; he assumed that different neuroses exist, which require different explanations. He differentiated the so-called actual neuroses (neurasthenia, hypochondriasis, and anxiety neuroses), which he assumed to be caused by toxic substances that accumulate as the result of faulty and frustrating sexual habits; the transference neuroses (phobias, hysteria, and obsessive neuroses) caused by unconscious psychological conflict;[30] and the narcissistic neuroses (schizophrenias and manic-depressive disorders) where withdrawal of object libido (psychosexual interest and investment in others) is a crucial phenomenon. Traumatic neuroses are the result of an overwhelming stress that renders the individual helpless and forcefully reminds him of his helplessness. To a lesser degree, such narcissistic mortification[18] is characteristic for all types of neurotic behavior, and Adler's theory was based on the significance of inferiority feelings and attempts to overcome them in childhood and thereafter.[2]

Kubie distinguishes between the *neurotic potential*, the *neurotic process*, and the *neurotic state*.[52] The neurotic potential is man's unique ability to use, and also to distort, symbols. Symbols are seen as the chief vehicles, or tools, by which we represent ourselves to ourselves and to others, including representations of our body and the environment. By symbolic *activity*, Kubie refers essentially to *any* of the complex operations by which meaning is conveyed; false meanings are therefore compounded by symbolic distortions or misrepresentations, involving affect, cognition, and response. Man's relative independence from immediate stimuli produces both the power to think abstractly and the vulnerability to error (that is, the "neurotic potential"). In the "neurotic process," under the impact of stress, anxieties are generated, which induce repression of symbols.[39] Once this has happened, symbols are apt to be distorted, because they are no longer subject to conscious checking and learning. An entire "code" for a segment of reality is false but continues to be used. The resulting sequences of acts—the "neurotic state"—is nonadaptive, rigid, and repetitive; it is governed by inapparent and "secret" rules and goals. Kubie views as neurotic any type of rigid and repetitive behavior characterized by an unconscious distortion of symbols, regardless of the social or personal values that are the consequences of the act. According to Kubie, a very kindly and generous, but rigid, act which is not subject to conscious control is as neurotic as a senseless compulsive symptom.

Today, classical psychoanalysts, as well as neoanalysts, stress the role of the ego in controlling sexual and aggressive wishes and reaching acceptable compromises in the interest of adequate interpersonal relations and the maintenance of a personal equilibrium. Such emphasis had a definite impact on psychoanalytic theories of neuroses. Existentialists have added some subtle and some obscure descriptions of neurotic being, but no coherent theory. The experimental contributions by Pavlov and by some American experimental psychologists will be considered later in this chapter.

We come to the general view, then, that neurotic behaviors are faulty unconscious ways of coping with present and past stresses; their symptomatic expression utilizes mechanisms and processes that are present in each of us who must cope with sets of internal as well as external rules and inputs acquired at different stages of development. The process is characterized by a tendency to regress to, or remain fixated at, an infantile level of organization, rather than by the capacity for flexible regression and growth. The appearance of this neurotic state may be fleeting or persistent, mild or severe. From a communication standpoint neurotic "messages" are obscure, indirect, and relatively ineffective; however, they come across, because they are, compared with psychotic messages, less distorted.[65] Other aspects of the tenuous differences between neurotic and psychotic behavior were discussed in Chapter 9.

Etiology

Mechanisms and Functions of Neurotic Acts

To a certain extent, we can make sense out of the formation of neurotic behavior. With some notion of the equipment with which man copes, we have a glimpse of what can go wrong, of inherent strains in the system, for example, the long period of childhood dependence, and the capacity for internal structures to provide controls and autonomy, but also to distort input. We are a long way, however, from an understanding at the level of quantitative differences in disposition, and we know little about the basic laws governing the conscious and unconscious learning of neurotic behavior. The simple clinical example that follows elucidates, to a certain extent, the emergence of a neurotic act, and more specifically of a hysterical symptom.

> A young World War II soldier developed a complete anesthesia and paralysis of his right arm after marching to an outpost carrying a mortar piece on his shoulder. In a field hospital the diagnosis of brachial plexus paralysis was made; only in the general hospital to which he was evacuated were the symptoms recognized as a hysterical reaction. Some of the experiences at the time of the incident were reconstructed in hypnotherapy and the symptoms disappeared after treatment. He was afraid of being killed, and also to kill, but he was barely aware of these feelings. As a matter of fact, he considered himself courageous and was convinced that a good soldier must fight and not let his buddies down. When he began to hear heavy gunfire, he felt strange but not afraid; he experienced numbness of his arm and could not move it. Thus, the patient was torn by conflict between urges to run away from a very dangerous situation where the choice was to kill or be killed, and a desire to maintain his self-esteem and be a good soldier; when the conflicts and anxiety became too intense, they were repressed, and the patient regressed to the sick role or rather to the role of a child who had to be taken care of. He was unaware of his conflict, his emotions, of the repression and regression. We assume further that once the conflict became unconscious, it did not cease but was partially solved by a primitive type of unconscious reasoning: if I can't use my arm then I can't fight, and I will be evacuated; but I am still a good soldier.

We distinguish four steps in the emergence of a neurotic act. First, the single and multiple stresses, although possibly objectively minimal, are perceived in the light of predisposing past experiences as intense. Second, unmastered stress induces a state of being overwhelmed, helpless, and conflicted, and engenders overanticipation, fright, terror, guilt, shame, despair, and rage. The relatively ungoverned affects and the reduced range and efficiency of coping devices are not entirely novel but are a part of persisting or reactivated childhood experiences. Third, when stress is intense and coping seems impossible, defense mechanisms, primarily repression and sustained regression, are employed to eliminate awareness of conflict and demand. Fourth, defense mechanisms are inadequate, and conflicting needs return in the form of troublesome symptomatic acts or traits, which are integrated either apart from or into the general personality. Obviously, this sequence is laden with conjectures. It is not easy to identify the stresses, to discover the clashing needs and defenses, and to disentangle their hierarchical arrangements. The intermediate steps, such as the elimination of certain experiences from consciousness, the splitting of consciousness and the unconscious organization for their return to consciousness in a symbolic disguise and in the language of childhood, are extremely difficult to discern, even for experienced observers.

The neurotic act fulfills multiple functions more succinctly than normal behavior.[73] It attempts to reduce an individual's discomforts, anxieties, guilt, shame, and the like; to gratify repressed needs; and to reconcile the demands of reality and ethics with a mask of cogency and a degree of punishment. The function of neurotic behavior is to restore a psychological equilibrium that permits the neurotic person to regain or retain a precarious control over certain impulses while engaging in relatively stable interactions with others. Ineffective and troublesome as this compromise is, it nonetheless wards off something worse for the individual; if one could clearly understand just what the person is spared by the neurotic behavior—what he needs to overcome it—one would possess a truly rational key to treatment.

Predisposing Psychological Factors of Adult Neurosis

Our grasp of precipitating stresses and conflicts is more secure than our knowledge of predisposing causes. Excepting the traumatic neuroses, precipitating and predisposing stresses are usually closely linked, which makes an assessment of their relative significance difficult. More important than absolute strength of the noxious stimuli is how patients interpret them, and such interpretation usually depends on past experience. We have stated the basic assumption that neurotic behavior is learned. Precisely how neurotic behavior is reinforced, and just as important, how it is extinguished is largely unknown. Even after the thorough reconstructive efforts of psychoanalytic therapy and direct observations of children, our knowledge of predisposing causes—of why neurotic behavior takes hold, and in whom—remains unhappily scant. Freud's astute hunches about the major stresses comprise the crucial landmarks of development, but these are universal occurrences, and the extent to which they produce behavior disorders is said to depend on the magnitude of the stress and the resilience of the individual. Our present knowlege barely permits us to assess either. We assume that both learning and constitutional factors play a role. The fact is that some persons whose upbringing was exceedingly traumatic remain relatively healthy; others whose life was protected become neurotic. Margaret Sommers tells of a man who watched his mother carry on her trade as a prostitute from his infancy to his adolescence; yet he remained relatively healthy, presumably because his mother and some of her customers provided some emotional warmth and affection for him. In any event, it is clear that conflict, rapid changes of living conditions, and situations that impose vacillation and double binds make learning difficult and, through a confluence of well and poorly comprehended factors, an arrest of emotional development or fixation may occur. For reasons that similarly are obscure, all neurotics regress under stress. The notion that the inherent stress in each psychosexual stage gives rise to a specific type of neurosis has had a tenacious life, but empirical proof is largely lacking. However, empirical observation makes us certain that stress for the developing child is interpreted in the characteristic terms of his developmental stage and according to his needs and capacities.

The behavioral outcomes of the life crises were reviewed in Chapter 4; in this section, we add only some relevant clinical points. Neurotic behavior is infantile, and a developmental view enhances one's ability to isolate the pattern of infantilism in the adult. It should be clear that a review of fixations tells us *what* is going on; occasionally, *how* it came to be; and rarely, if ever, *why*. The discovery of a childhood neurosis does *not* mean we must automatically try to eradicate it; whether or not the patient must recall or redo all these developments in order to improve is quite open to question. All that is clear is that *internal* rearrangements and relearning must occur at some level for the patient to operate more efficiently in the present. As a rule, such "internal" change requires some act or activity on the patient's part, some experience in which he participates and works.

It has been assumed that early deprivations of food and love are related to neurotic depression.[9] The impact of early mother–child relationships may also result in an adult who is chronically prepared for "automatic" feelings of rejection, for example, by a mother, frightened and doubting herself, using rigid schedules to avoid easy reciprocal contact with the infant. Separation, experienced in infancy as emptiness and panic, could occur with simply an abrupt change in the way the mother attends to the child; some adults react this way with any change of supporting conditions. When infants use muscles and teeth aggressively and with affect, a new type of anxiety may occur, which is largely preverbal but related to recognized persons and losses. Ingrained, unrationalizable distrust and excessive insecurity over threats and excessive aggression have been related to predisposing experiences of this period. In the adult, a clenched jaw accompanying a silent bad mood may signify inner rage and tension—the frustration of the fourteen-month-old; if adults are asked what sensation they feel, they sometimes can note their tightened oral muscles and recognize a compelling, nameless tense mood that "automatically" accompanies it. Such a mood is one way of remembering and retaining an infantile bond; such early experiences cannot be easily represented in words and images, but rather there is "memory" through retained reactions. Excessive aggression and anxieties in toilet training can be generated by excessively policed demands for conformity. The child can say "no," but he can barely enforce his command, save through resistive and dirty means; instead of doing what he should in making a bowel movement, he waits, "forcing" the adult to "make me do it." And, instead of doing what he should when he should, he panics, has an "accident," and thus manipulates the adult. We see this behavior in every form of adult social life, for example, passive resistance, and the "dirty trick" of leaving someone else "holding the bag." Obsessive traits, atonement, and rebellion; ritualized rather than flexible controls; reaction formations (for example, in which the child masks his badness to "be good"); and manipulative power struggles are characteristic outcomes.

Some neurotic developments in adults are rather clearly related to the "second weaning," the resolution of intense attachments of the Oedipal period. If the child continues to seek exciting and comforting erotic pleasure, primarily through the parent; or if, because of parental ties, he overinhibits close attachments to peers and mild erotic pleasures; or if he spitefully "acts out" because of a fancied rejection, he will have trouble with sexual and other intimacies as an adult. Affection will always be charged with danger and temptation; the young adult will want more than others can give and behave in accordance with the rules of the past rather than the opportunities of the present. For such people, something is always missing in their adult satisfactions. One rather impulsive hysterical woman had a satisfactory premarital affair, but from her wedding night until her divorce, was frigid and furious with her puzzled husband and former lover; rebellion and "playing around" were permissible, but marriage and a *husband* were too uncomfortably close to her "forgotten" childhood romance, and she was "afraid" to grow up. The hysterical development of the phallic phase is related to forbidden excitement; imagined threats of punishment for "bad" sexual wishes are inhibiting to the child, who may then covertly cling to his fantasies and ties without "overtly" claiming them, that is, excite and seduce, but not gratify. What is permissibly erotic and exciting for a child is incest when the child reaches the age of sexual consequences. Latency experiences may have an as yet unappreciated role in reinforcing Oedipal solutions or in adding problems; reaction formations are common. Adolescence is the time when many clear-cut childhood neuroses appear to be reactivated.

Loss of the self, of a part of the self, of the parent or the parent's love and esteem, and later of his own self-esteem represent a genetic sequence of fears to which the child is vulnerable. In general, however, and in spite of an abundance of psychoanalytic data and speculations, we still have little solid evidence about predisposing causes of neuroses. Outside of being appreciative of the range of natural feelings, fantasies, problems and modes of coping of the child and the limits that parents require for sane living, we also cannot map out a general program for prevention of childhood neuroses.

A word about our language: When we speak of "abandonments" and "trauma" in a young child's life, we need not picture a child put out in the snow, never to darken his home again. If a man traces the history of any long friendship, he will find times when he has been disappointed or even betrayed and these occasions are strongly felt and reacted to. "Infantile" in psychiatric jargon might well be translated as "childish," since defensive maneuvers are already clear in children of three or four. Most of us can find memories relating to some part of this era in which our coherent biography begins, but preverbal experience—although crucially important—seems as distant from the inner world of the three-year-old as it does from the adult; neither child nor adult has words for it. It is clear that psychological time is somewhat deceptive. Further, our protective memory (which begins to operate quite early) gives to both the child and adult a false perspective about the distance of former infantilisms from the present era of—no doubt—adequate adjustment. A six-year-old has only a few years of experience in using the bathroom properly; a sixteen-year-old has had only two or three years to know his new sex characteristics and body; a twenty-one-year-old has usually had only a few years, if that, of sustained heterosexual gratifications and perhaps no experience at all in earning the position to support these aims responsibly. All this points to the relative closeness of the young adult to previous developmental eras, in spite of the distance provided at each stage by a protective amnesia for what has just transpired. To "catch on" to these facts and consequences of development as one reads psychiatric formulations and in any attempt to describe and formulate them, one must cope with one's own protective barriers; these impede finding an experiential root for the necessary abstractions. In our observation, experts continually try to perfect this uneasy marriage of intuitive, observational, and conceptual skills.

SOCIAL AND CULTURAL FACTORS Although neurotic behavior is found everywhere, only in Western cultures during the last few decades—and in those cultures influenced by Western thought—have the neuroses been explicitly recognized as behavior disorders. It seems that some mobile individuals are apt to suffer from a lack of identity and develop neurotic traits.[76] Very relaxed and even marginally deprived but stable societies have relatively few neurotic problems unless such a society begins rapidly to change and disintegrate.[6] It is thought that, within a given culture, persons and groups in marginal positions, such as persecuted minority groups and persons exposed to culture conflict, are more apt to develop neuroses than others. Lacking a realistic sense of security, such groups must rely on individual and group defenses such as withdrawal or overestimation of their own importance. Although specific recognition of neurotic behavior is quite characteristic of modern American society, tolerance of deviant behavior is greater in many other societies.

Group processes—from the family to the larger community—are clearly the means by which meaning, role definition, divergent, and congruent codes of conduct are conveyed and reinforced. Peer groups help children to emerge from the intensity of family involvement and childhood egocentricity; neurotic children are more likely to remain trapped or break all ties. Every child learns a special intrafamilial code, which is why family myths—as lovers' secrets—are difficult for outsiders to comprehend and enjoy. Why some children are limited by these small group instructions and others can freely—and at times all too freely—move to the code of the neighborhood, or subgroups of the society, is not completely known. Since family and milieu therapy has become of current interest, an understanding of the patient's communications is given real dimension and depth with explicit attention to the detailed and "loaded" signals of small group interactions.

CONSTITUTIONAL FACTORS Although most inquiries in the last fifty years have led to the assumption that neurotic behavior is learned, the role of genetic constitutional mechanisms and a constitutional disposition to neurotic behavior cannot be excluded. Freud's views of a complementary series of determinants, innate and learned mechanisms, in neuroses, have been cited.[32] Freud's "toxins" and other neuroendocrine theories of brain and behavior may well receive attention again in the growing field of neurobehavioral research. Biologists point to the universality of behaviors related to fear throughout the animal kingdom; the capacity for phobias is (or was) adaptive for man and perhaps the potential for overarousal to insufficient or confusing input, or to novelty or to sudden change cannot be easily extinguished and may vary in individuals. John Paul Scott and John L. Fuller have spoken of the link between distress and care-soliciting behavior with social behavior; this is clear in canines, where experiment can demonstrate that breed differences notably influence subsequent normal and abnormal behavioral patterns. There is, however, a sparsity of convincing attempts to link constitutional and bodily processes to human neurotic behavior. The pertinent contributions of Hans J. Eysenck, Daniel H. Funkenstein, Franz J. Kallmann, John Lacey, Robert B. Malmo, William H. Sheldon, and others have been reviewed in earlier chapters. In general, viewing the rapid developments of psychobiological methods and approaches, we have no doubt that the biological roots of neurotic behavior will become more relevant to clinical psychiatry than has been generally anticipated.

Experimental Neurosis

Pavlov's work became the basis for the production of disturbed behavior in animals that we call experimental neurosis. Essentially, such behavior disorder is produced by motivational conflict or by frustrations through external obstacles; internal handicaps; a tax on ability to discriminate cues; or a change of reinforcing conditions. Motivational conflicts in men and animals have been classified according to experimental psychologists into approach-approach conflicts, avoidance-avoidance conflicts, and approach-avoidance conflicts. Whereas it is easy enough so to label the laboratory procedures with which animals are studied, it is cumbersome (and at least unfamiliar) for psychiatrists to identify human conflicts in these paradigms. An example of an approach-approach conflict was told us by an officer who returned from overseas duty during World War II and saw, in the same instant he stepped off the ship, his wife and a milk bar; for a moment, he did not know where to turn. An avoidance-avoidance conflict is the dilemma of the taxpayer who does not want to pay his taxes, but also does not want to get into trouble. An approach-avoidance conflict might be the conflict of the young couple who are sexually attracted to each other but are deterred from pleasurable sexual activities by their rearing. Differences in the gradients of approach-avoidance or the capacity to tolerate high- or low-intensity objects (the degree of "arousal" represented by cues) may underlie "constitutional" variations in human learning.

In animal experiments, it is relatively easy to produce conflict that can be studied objectively and quantitatively. An important method involves responses to stimuli that become increasingly difficult to discriminate, as Pavlov's dog responding to a circle with a conditioned alimentary approach. As the circle and the ellipse are made increasingly similar, conflict ensues and so-called neurotic behavior can be observed. Other techniques involve randomly alternating reward and punishment after a certain set of responses is established, or delaying rewards, a technique Pavlov also used. Some experiments resemble natural situations; for example, the Russian experimental observations on an adult male chimpanzee who helplessly views his sexual partner copulating with another chimpanzee in an adjoining cage. Modern operant conditioning methods, neurophysiological techniques and computers have made possible very involved and refined techniques, which are designed to teach us not only about behavior in experimental neuroses, but also about the concomitant cerebral processes.

Kubie has aptly advised psychiatrists to keep in mind that the anxious, angry, and disorganized behavior of animals has only a superficial resemblance to human neurosis, because the conflicts are not unconscious and do not produce the symbolic distortions that are characteristic in humans.[51] Yet, this caveat overlooks what is systematically similar; symbolic thinking, far more complex than processing of signals, is not unrelated to the latter. The animal who shows fear or stops performing during a signal that precedes unavoidable shock is "interpreting" signals—or misinterpreting them. It is probably not correct to think that the signals that represent reality to the animal are perceived without error and distortion; indeed, Skinner and his students demonstrated "superstitious" behavior with a bird which pecked a key for food but "believed" it must also hop on one foot—a response accidentally associated with reward and unnecessary, in fact, to obtain it. The bulk of analytic theory, in fact, is built upon the idiosyncratic errors and the limitations of childhood learning that must be corrected with the advent of higher levels of organization. Nor is it correct to imply that human symbolic distortion cannot be as lawfully related to input-output contingencies as pigeons' errors. The admittedly consequential differences are those of complexity, level of organization, and method of study, not of principle. Although we gather data about neurotic behavior in terms of subjective experience and describe neurotic mechanisms by observing patterns of such experience, the fundamental operative mechanisms may yet be defined by objective studies.[54]

Diagnosis of Neurotic Behavior

There is a growing recognition, reflected in the literature, that the essence of neurosis is a chronically and consistently disordered life, not a discrete disturbance. On the basis of the preceding sections, we may now attempt a more precise diagnostic delineation of neurotic behavior, and offer the following criteria: (1) Neurotic acts are rigid, repetitive, and inappropriate. This inappropriateness is not accompanied by the disturbances of thinking and feeling that are characteristic for schizophrenias and behavior disorders associated with brain diseases. (2) Profound mood changes without any demonstrable cause are viewed as affective behavior disorders; if the mood changes are moderate and can be explained by antecedent behavioral events, they are customarily called neurotic. (3) Neurotic symptoms can be understood and explained as consequences of behavioral stresses and conflicts. (4) Neurotic symptoms and acts are not the result of demonstrable organ pathology. (5) They are more readily accessible to psychotherapy, the primary method of treatment, than any other behavior disorder.

When the term neurosis was used to refer only to symptom neurosis, the delineation of normal and neurotic behavior was not difficult: it was simply assumed that normal persons do not suffer from neurotic symptoms. As the umbrella concept of neurosis is extended to character neuroses and even to sociopathies, the problem of diagnostic boundaries becomes more troublesome. Inappropriate behavior occurs, at least at times, in all people. How often does it have to occur and how severe must it be? It would seem wise to restrict this label to rather severe forms of inappropriate behavior and not to use it lightly; psychiatrists' time might thereby be saved for severe dysfunctions. The fact that the processes that eventuate in a neurosis are universal should not be confused with the consequential result—the state we recognize as clinically significant.

In principle, the differential diagnosis of neurotic from organic signs or symptoms is simple: if demonstrable organ pathology is absent and significant behavioral antecedents can explain signs and symptoms, neurosis is diagnosed. In reality, the differential diagnosis between "functional" (which is bad jargon) and organic conditions may be exceedingly difficult. Since the advent of psychosomatic and comprehensive medicine, the dividing lines have become even more blurred. All diseases are influenced by psychological factors; many view the so-called psychosomatic illnesses as neuroses with somatic manifestations. Physicians' offices, clinics, and hospitals are crowded with neurotics who suffer from bona fide medical and surgical illnesses. Many of these patients exaggerate the symptoms and signs of their illness; we have no term to characterize this important group. Others deny their illness.[75] Although it is customary to attempt to reach a unitary diagnosis, it might be better in such cases, and perhaps in all cases, to make both a medical diagnosis and a psychosocial diagnosis; if they can be holistically unified, so much the better. The differential diagnosis of neurotic and schizophrenic behavior will be discussed in Chapter 14 and that of the different depressions, in Chapter 15.

Course and Prognosis

Chronicity and repetitiveness are essential characteristics of neurotic behavior except for the short-lasting disintegration of some traumatic neuroses. We disagree with the M. Shepherd and E. M. Gruenberg statement that neurotic behavior has a duration of one to two years, and it is our clinical impression that untreated neurosis persists throughout life.[69] It is our clinical impression that the majority get worse during the great crises of life: puberty, involution, and old age. Neurotics without benefit of therapy usually can be expected to learn little, although some undoubtedly do change and improve "spontaneously." [71] We occasionally see self-cures after a change of milieu and circumstances, through a fortunate decision, serious endeavor, or, rarely, the proper choice of mate or job. Erik H. Erikson stated that Freud, in his middle age, effected such a self-cure through his work.[21]

From a clinical point of view, we are more interested in those cases which get worse. Who are the neurotic patients who become disorganized? What happened to them? These questions focus on the great riddles in our field. In general, it is felt that severe disturbances are more apt to occur in those who have never approached maturity and always retained marked infantile and archaic mechanisms. This, of course, is highly relevant to an assessment of the chances for therapy, a problem that will be taken up in the next section.

Rapid and radical disintegration is seen if some important situational props ceased to function or if the only asset that permitted the patient to function adequately is lost. The authors have observed such a breakdown of relatively compensated neurosis in an athlete who developed poliomyelitis, in a widow who lost her only son, and in a refugee who had to leave his fortune behind.

General Remarks on Therapy of Neurotic Behavior

Since we look at neurotic behavior as acquired or learned, the logical therapy is psychotherapy, geared to an attempt to "unlearn" neurotic behavior and acquire adaptive behavior patterns. All psychotherapies, whether analytic or directive, whether based on Freudian or Pavlovian theories or merely pragmatic techniques, attempt to do this and all known methods have been reported successful, although reliable comparative evaluations are lacking.

In our opinion, the most suitable among the treatments for neurosis are the various forms of psychoanalytic therapy of individuals and groups. We are far from understanding what really helps the neurotic patient, but it is reasonably clear that corrective experiences can occur in a basically trusting and highly charged but regulated emotional relationship between therapist and patient. Both doctor and patient can get the current life situation into focus and, to a greater or lesser extent, most patients can appreciate that they, to some degree, are involved in their own symptoms and that symptoms have a past. With such support, patients can tackle some problems of current living previously beyond their abilities. Insight into unknown motivations and conflicts will free some patients to learn and see alternatives; recognizing the "child" within themselves, they may then be able to find the adult answers. With all neurotic patients, it is useful to talk about what transpires between therapist and patient, to identify within the hour the characteristic problem the patient brings and, in fact, "demonstrates." As therapy proceeds, the psychiatrist will assess the extent to which the patient can confront his dependency maneuvers and defenses and the wishes that motivate them. For a more detailed discussion of technique, we refer the reader to Chapter 10.

In general, the more infantile and immature the patient, the more difficult the treatment. Psychological sensitivity, intelligence, and what is vaguely referred to as ego strength—and "motivation"—are what therapists hope for in their patients; what to do when such qualities are lacking is a difficult and serious problem. We have no pat answer because we are just beginning to study the problem. It is important to differentiate between conscious and unconscious motivation of neurotic patients. Conscious verbal statements of either cooperation or antagonism to treatment may be quite irrelevant. It is also evident that the therapist can block the course of therapy, creating fear and estrangement by not hearing the patient, by being too intrusive and active or too impervious, too inviting and seductive, or too coldly ritualistic.

To create a favorable atmosphere for therapy, to reinforce and recognize the patient's wishes to work and get well, is not to be confused with "creating motivations" by phony role-playing and manipulations.

If a neurotic patient is not suffering, this is an unfavorable condition for therapy; after all, suffering that somehow touches and reaches a person is the greatest motivation to seek relief and even risk change through therapy and to cooperate with the therapist. It is said that, for this reason, sexual deviations and addictions are difficult to treat; although many of these patients undoubtedly suffer greatly, they are not able to overcome either the fear or the seductions that oppose a commitment to change. Masochistic traits, in particular, lead the patient to cling to symptoms. We have not learned well how to deal with antisocial persons; and we also have our troubles with infantile and self-indulging patients because, to a certain extent, even therapists may envy and hate such people and share the resentful jealousy society expresses toward them.

One of the important decisions a therapist must make is whether a given neurotic problem needs brief or prolonged and intensive therapy, provided the latter is available. The student should be cautioned against the assumption that the longest and most intensive therapy is always necessarily the best. Some patients have been helped by very brief therapy, even one session; but years of psychoanalysis have been a waste or even harmful to other patients. Psychoanalysis, the most thorough and ambitious treatment, is the recommended therapy for the intelligent neurotic patient who is not too "sick" and who is able and willing to enter into the serious commitment implicit in this process. It is available to a very few. Only exceptional and very severe cases require hospitalization.

Organic therapies such as lobotomy and electric convulsive therapy have no place in the treatment of most neuroses. Amytal interviews or hypnosis are occasionally useful in severe or in traumatic problems, but we see little general use—and many difficulties—for forced uncovering techniques. Psychotomimetics used for uncovering or transcendental experience have yet to be evaluated as a generally effective treatment. Carefully and discriminatingly used, the minor tranquilizers and antidepressants (replacing bromides and barbiturates) may be of modest help; the major value of major tranquilizers, of course, is in the psychoses and not in the neuroses. When the physician is not prescribing drugs to dull his own response to the tranquilized patient, but employs them as adjuncts of therapy, he may find occasions in treatment when they are useful; they may help to dampen intense anxieties sufficiently to permit psychological therapy to proceed or an equilibrium to be established. Some psychotherapists find the antidepressants such as amitriptyline or imipramine are useful in working with neurotic symptoms (phobia and anxiety), which they feel are sometimes secondary to depression, but such work with drugs is too new to be evaluated definitively. No matter how drugs are used, it is clear that neurotic problems, at present at least, cannot be dissolved or resolved chemically.

We have indicated how limited our knowledge is for generalized statements about prevention of neuroses. Even when we can identify causes in specific settings, we are usually unable to change parents, educators, and situations. Nor have we been able, except in a very limited way, to apply mental health principles to prevent neuroses in educational, industrial, and military organizations. The hope for such preventive measures exists; we are, after all, only at the beginning of a more rational approach to the conduct of human affairs. In the meantime, it is progress if we recognize and treat neurotic problems early, before they are too deeply ingrained or too overwhelming. To motivate neurotics to seek early treatment—provided such therapy is available—is an important task of mental health education.

Finally, it is well to remember that the following are common "good" outcomes of treatment: the patient may be "restored to function" without insight but with renewed strength after a brief crisis; he may explore alternatives, learn new attitudes, or be less perturbed and, hence, less reactive to existing traits and problems—and at any of these points he may be ready to stop treatment. Or, he may "uncover" many character problems, discovering their current activity and their origins and integrate his findings into new approaches. The psychiatrist may have learned little on which to base his hunches, but in these instances the patient, for the moment, may be relatively satisfied. What we can explain and what the patient needs for comfort are often different. Less satisfactory outcomes are not uncommon, and whatever the patient's momentary evaulation of outcome, it takes time before "effects" of therapy can be fairly evaluated by both patient and therapist.

Clinical Types

Current classification of neuroses, such as the one by the American Psychiatric Association, are satisfactory neither for the epidemiologist nor the research and clinical psychiatrist. Neurosis can rarely be characterized by one symptom; a patient labeled as an anxiety neurosis is often hysterical, phobic, or passive, and may have psychosomatic symptoms as well. Many symptoms and personality traits coexist in the same person, or different traits may occur in a person with the same diagnosis; a sexual deviant may be very anxious; an aggressive person may be hysterical or depressed. Why, then, refer to them by such a diagnostic label? The subcategories, moreover, do not constitute classes, but types. Hence, there are many patients who exhibit neurotic behavior that cannot be pigeonholed. Another objection, relating to the strict division into symptom neuroses, character neuroses, and sociopathies, has already been discussed. It is most important to keep in mind that these boundaries do not exist in the lives of human beings who become our patients, but in our minds. In psychiatry, there are cyclic periods of interest and revolution against "typing." Today, with a tendency to treat all neuroses by one method of psychotherapy, diagnostic distinctions are abhorred as intruding upon the encounter of one human with another. We do not share this phobia. Rather, we feel contemporary psychiatry requires a developed sense of descriptive diagnosis derived, in part, from evidence gathered from therapeutic interactions. An investigative attitude will sharpen our discriminations of neurotic and other forms of disturbed behavior; this precedes typing, which should emerge from advancing clinical and biological research. Divisions must be put on a better basis than exists at present.

For these reasons, the traditional subclasses of neurotic behavior will not be discussed here. Rather, we shall consider types of behavior with fluid boundaries, often occurring simultaneously in one patient or changing over a period of time. Drug addiction and alcoholism are discussed in chapters 22 and 23. Schizoid and paranoid personalities are taken up in Chapter 14 and depressive behavior in neurotics in Chapter 15. Certain syndromes with primarily somatic symptoms, such as impotence and frigidity (no less neurotic than hysterical reactions and phobias), are quite arbitrarily included in the chapter on psychosomatic medicine (Chapter 13).

Anxiety Reactions and Phobias

We usually stipulate that for a diagnosis of anxiety neurosis, frights, anxieties, and fears must reach a high level of intensity and occur in frequent attacks or as enduring states and in the absence of other gross psychopathology. Anxiety, of course, appears as a marked transient component in a variety of behavior disorders and was the only symptom occurring indiscriminately in all socioeconomic groups of the Manhattan Study.[70] It is well known that certain ethnic groups—for example, English, Scandinavians, Germans, and Japanese—do not permit the expression of anxiety to the degree that is tolerated by the Mediterranean peoples or Latin Americans. Neurotic anxiety states occur in attacks of varying degrees of intensity, from a vague, constant or intermittent feeling of unpleasantness and preoccupation to extreme panic, and also as a constant state of tension; both types occur in combination. By observing exactly how the patient avoids, interprets and escapes his dangers or endures them, the clinician can not only learn how daily living is concretely affected but also get clues about the underlying motives for the suffering. Fusions of anxiety with sadness, anger, and guilt are frequent. Many patients, unaware of their anxieties, experience only such effects as tachycardia, palpitations, breathlessness, urgency to urinate and defecate, headache, fatigue, insomnia, various aches, and impotence or frigidity. Whereas restlessness, agitation, muscle tension or tremors are symptoms, an anxious patient may feel tired, listless, and frozen. Chronic fatigue combined with mild depression, anxiety, and irritability is described as a separate syndrome, *neurasthenia*. Little is said today about this syndrome, and its independent existence is doubted.

Phobias are anticipatory, highly unrealistic fears and avoidance reactions to certain objects and situations. Certain phobias, such as fear of darkness, deep water, storms, lightning, wild animals, and strangers are widespread during the adult years and practically universal in childhood. Leland E. Hinsie and Robert J. Campbell list two hundred phobic reactions in their dictionary. Phobias that occupy the attention of psychiatrists may be crippling handicaps in a patient's everyday life or relatively harmless avoidance reactions. The most frequent phobias are agoraphobia, or a fearful avoidance of open spaces; claustrophobia, or the fear of closed, shut-in spaces; altophobias, fear of heights; the many zoophobias; and (naturally in a technological age) the fears of driving and flying. Paul Errera and Jules V. Coleman found that many of their phobic patients suffered from organic illnesses.[22]

In modern European practice the syndrome has emerged again under the frequently used label *vegetative dystonia.*

Although the riddle of anxiety is far from being solved, modern dynamic psychiatry can trace manifestations and rather specific meaningful causes. It takes much painstaking work to discover why a patient misinterprets stimuli and responds with fear, especially when the threats seem universal or specific causes are denied. General explanations are hazardous and list rather monotonously the themes of fear of injury, punishment, and temptation as causes. In well-studied adults, it is possible to disentangle the puzzle partially and trace many phobic reactions to infantile fears.

It is now widely accepted that adult phobias are modified repetitions of those of infancy, often reinforced by parental phobias. Phobias, of course, are a prime demonstration of the mechanisms of spreading displacement so that the original fear attaches to ever more remote and implausible substitutes. In a famous study of a phobic five-year-old boy, Freud demonstrated that little Hans wanted to have the undivided affection of his mother and eliminate his father, whom he feared, as a rival.[31] This wish created intensely uncomfortable feelings, which in turn were partly dissipated by development of an agoraphobia, permitting him to stay close to his mother, and a fear of horses, which, as demonstrated in the boy's conversation, was quite clearly a displacement to an animal of his fear and aggression concerning the father; the displaced fear of horses permitted the boy not only to stay indoors, but also at least to tolerate and cope with the father in the house. Some agoraphobias, particularly in women, ward off fear of abandoning sexual restraints, frequently with prostitution fantasies and fears that "If I let go, I won't stop." Many such fears spring from infantile loneliness, from a demand for love or a passive wish to give oneself up to anyone to be loved. Others involve aggressive wishes to be free, as the woman enviously assumes a man to be, or to destroy through "aggressive abandon." Anger and jealousy in many phobias are apparent if only in the cost to families who mistakenly support or exploit the patients' bizarre avoidances.

Altophobia has been explained as not only an infantile fear of injury by powerful and hostile persons but also a displacement of dangerous and dreaded masochistic wishes and impulses to let go and "come what may."

Behind claustrophobias lurks the infantile dread of being abandoned. The fears of driving and flying are related to fears of injuring others and the punishment for taboo wishes by being killed. Such a set of phobias seems to underlie the driving phobia in the following case.

DRIVING PHOBIA

The patient, a wan, beautiful, and self-effacing professional woman of thirty-two, referred herself for marital problems in which she masochistically endured much from her irresponsible, flamboyant, but passive husband. In her own selfless, quietly efficient way, she was quite domineering, did her work and managed the children, finances, and so forth. In marked contrast to her efficiency, her only apparent "weakness" was a striking and (for suburban life) curiously inconvenient fear of driving a car, a function she equated with power and masculinity. She felt the sports car she urged upon her husband was too bold an auto for her and (although solidly sensible about most matters) she irately asserted that without a mechanic's knowledge of mechanics, she or anyone would be an unsafe driver, endangering herself and her children. She accordingly avoided learning to drive (other than through exasperated, sporadic, and complicated demonstrations from her spouse) and, since she never asked for favors, she either walked or occasionally was offered rides by friends or her husband.

She really thought little of herself as a woman and of women generally and yet, in this one area, exaggerated "womanly helplessness" and in addition ridiculously overestimated the consequences of assertiveness; in this, her spoiled husband was only too willing to encourage her by calling reasonable requests "bossiness." Her phobia appeared to be an attempt to protect herself from complaints that she was aggressive and bossy (that is, in the driver's seat), and it expressed her need to be dependent, which she equated with weakness. As she ventilated guilt about dependency wishes and aggressive strivings and as she began to distinguish between competence and masculinity, the phobia lessened, and with firm encouragement from the therapist she undertook lessons.

Her background revealed a phobic mother and alcoholic father whose occupational status declined as she grew. Competence carried the danger of obviously criticizing both parents. She learned to appear self-effacing, to deny ambition while she quietly achieved. She hoped to run her father's life to make him happy (he wanted a son) but also feared loss of her mother's support. Her envy of the male was never directly stated, but she did recognize that she felt unreasonable awe at her husband's prerogatives and an inexplicable guilt if she too obviously encroached on them. The twice-weekly therapy over a year and a half focused mainly on her marital relationships as a springboard for disentangling her approach and feelings. The genetic sources of her problems (her penis envy, her masculine and feminine identifications, and her intense, furious disappointment with her body and her parents) were not discussed other than the few noted memories she occasionally touched upon and related to her present problems. As she made more sensible discriminations between legitimate wishes and fears of encroachment and as the husband's baiting became less successful, he became more attentive. She can now drive her *own* car or even comfortably ask her husband to run an errand but, even when the situation requires it, she still becomes quite anxious and avoids driving the husband's car!

Psychiatrists have attempted to treat anxiety, fear, and phobias by any means at their command. Supportive, suppressive, deconditioning and insight therapies in various forms are used. We encountered an example of suppressive "therapy" by an old but vigorous, benign tyrant, a widowed Italian farmer we visited, who kept three of his grown daughters on the farm to care for him; when one daughter remarked to us of her "panic" in church—she had to run out—the old man thundered at her, "Keep your eyes on the priest—not the young men!" The success of reassurance (that anxieties will pass) depends on the intensity and chronicity of the fear, the maturity of the patient, and the therapist's position as a trusted healer. More frequently than not, however, anxieties reappear soon after they are relieved. All psychiatrists rely in varying degree on a supportive, reassuring approach. It is often useful to the patient's self-esteem, so that he tries to reassert his own controls rather than exploit his phobia, even though insight into motivating fears is minimal. With insight-oriented therapy, the patient must learn the source of his fears and to apply such insight in real life. This matter is particularly important for phobias; sooner or later the patient must expose himself to the situation he dreads, and even analysts, at some juncture, will substitute for interpretive approaches a firm insistence on such confrontation, if therapy is to continue. Although the patient "deconditions" himself by stepwise exposure, we do not at this point see particular merit in the combined suggestive-reassuring deconditioning therapies, especially if they happen to lack appreciation of interpersonal and dynamic factors required in any treatment. No drugs have had a selective effect on fears and anxieties. Barbiturates are potentially dangerous; phenothiazines and reserpine are now considered useless for most anxiety neuroses by judicious therapists; and the more suitable Meprobamate and chlordiazepoxide may be habituating. We use the latter for temporary situational panic and anxiety, but this depends on the meaning of the symptom to the patient. A severely phobic man who had intermittent panic with tachycardia became more upset after reserpine, which abolished the rapid pulse: "Doctor, I have my panic but I don't feel it," he protested. For him, there was reassurance in the physical concomitants of anxiety.

Hysterical Behavior

We distinguish hysterical symptoms and hysterical character traits. Symptoms are divided into (1) conversion symptoms; (2) dysmnesic symptoms; and (3) dissociative symptoms. Conversion symptoms refer to the variety of bodily symptoms that can be produced by suggestion and autosuggestion. In general, these are disturbances of muscular functions and the sense organs;

autonomic functions may also be involved and division of hysterical from other mechanisms on the grounds of anatomy (or philosophy; for example, "voluntary and involuntary" nervous systems) cannot be justified. Some functions pertaining to body orifices, such as psychogenic vomiting, cannot normally be produced at will, but "gifted" hysterics are able to produce this and even more dramatic conversion symptoms, such as petechial subcutaneous hemorrhages. As we know, if only from reports about achievements of yogas, control over the body may be extended to an amazing degree. Conversion symptoms superficially resemble signs and symptoms of organic illness, and this is reflected in our tendency to perpetuate Latin and Greek names for the symptoms. All these signs, of course, occur without any organic pathology. Hysterical symptoms are, in most cases, easily differentiated from organic defects. A hysterically blind person has normal pupillary reactions to light. The patient with hysterical anesthesia has normal psychogalvanic skin reflexes, and the distribution of his anesthesia does not follow the anatomical distribution of skin innervation; for example, a hemianesthesia that abruptly cuts off in the midline. The hysterically paralyzed person has normal reflexes and electrical excitability of his muscles, although he may develop a disuse atrophy. The common conversion symptoms are: monoplegias and hemiplegias; hemianesthesias; and glove-and-stocking anesthesias; hysterical blindness; tubular vision; and deafness; complete anosmia and loss of taste; various attacks of pain without objective findings; attacks of choking and dyspnea; pseudoanginapectoris; fainting; certain types of anorexia and overeating; vomiting; diarrhea; constipation; and enuresis; and various types of impotence and frigidity.

Some hysterical patients exhibit the so-called hysterical stigmata, such as the "*clavus*" (literally nail) pressure over the vortex; *globus hystericus*, or a sensation of a choking ball in the pharynx; *ovarie*, or a painful sensation on slight pressure over the ovaries. Pseudocyesis, or false pregnancy, is a particularly dramatic hysterical syndrome. Most hysterical syndromes have an all-or-none character. The most striking hysterical attack is the hysterical fit, which resembles an epileptic seizure but can be distinguished readily from epileptic seizures in most cases. Hysterical patients rarely lose consciousness; they are not incontinent and do not injure themselves; there is no aura. The *arc de cercle*, which Charcot described, is reminiscent of an exaggerated imitation of a violent coital act and is not seen in epilepsy.[11]

The hysterical patient is convinced of the organic character of his illness. Characteristic is his *belle indifference*, an affective blandness in which the symptom speaks for itself. Many such patients, although dramatic, are oddly content, innocent, and "not curious" about their particular ailments. Their theatrical flair, when displayed, is quite recognizable. A raised skirt or a provocative gesture are similarly "innocent," and such common exhibitionistic and seductive traits are frequently encountered in life and in the clinic. Some patients come to recognize that they are enamored with drama, but then they simply ignore its display. In contrast to the *malingerer,* the hysterical patient makes no conscious efforts to produce the symptoms. However, differences between malingerers and hysterics are not absolute, and we often find many hysterical traits in malingerers and some near-conscious dramatic play-acting in the hysterical patient.

The most striking dysmnesic symptom is total amnesia, when persons temporarily forget their own identity; they cannot remember their names, ages, where they live, or what they do. This usually follows some relatively minor misdemeanor, which the patient is unable to remember, but which can be reproduced by special uncovering techniques, such as hypnosis or an interview under a light sodium amytal or pentothal anesthesia. The patient is bland and appears to be helpful in attempts to recover his lost identifying data but seems unable to do so. Minor dysmnesias, wherein the patients repress painful and highly charged experiences, are more frequent than total amnesias. The most common partial dysmnesic experience is the forgetting of names, events, and other data related to emotional conflict. Such events—the psychopathology of everyday life—are, of course, not limited to hysterical patients but are particularly frequent among them.

Related to the dysmnesic symptoms are the dissociative symptoms, in which certain experiences seem to be ego-alien, split-off, as it were. Dissociation is a basic mechanism operating in other and very different disturbances, for instance, in schizophrenia. In *depersonalization,* patients report a subjective feeling of strange and peculiar experiences.[43] The world looks different and unfamiliar; visual perceptions have changed, everything looks gray, colorless, cold; sounds and odors have also changed, and even tactile sensations are not the same; everything seems to be inert and dead; but most crucially, the experience of the self has changed. *Double personalities* are hysterical enactments of antagonistic roles in the patient. In a *déjà vu* experience, the patient feels that he has had the same experience before. He feels that he has met previously a person who obviously is a complete stranger or has seen or heard before some message that is really new.[5] Such experiences are usually found to be unrealistic attempts to master the unfamiliar; in any event, the motive (which generally is a search for some wished-for security) can only be specifically revealed by study in each case. In *somnambulism,* the sleeping patient gets up from his bed, walks about, and carries on complex acts, which he either cannot recall, or which he remembers vaguely as a dreamlike experience.[58] When interrupted in these activities, the patients react with surprise, irritation, or anger, as a person who has been awakened from sleep. A patient who had such attacks at the age of seven would be found roaming the house by her parents; she then would explain she had lessons to do (which she had in fact done); this worried, overscrupulous girl confessed a sin she did not commit out of need for parental assurance. Further analysis revealed the focus of some of her concern, masturbatory activity and an interest in what her parents were doing when she was supposed to be asleep.

There are other forms of hysterical attacks, such as the extraordinary behavior first described by Sigbert Joseph Maria Ganser.[37] The *Ganser syndrome,* often observed in prisoners under stress, consists of pseudodemented behavior during which the patient gives silly answers to obvious questions: grass is white; snow is green; two and two make five. *Fugue states* will be considered in Chapter 18.

Most patients with hysterical symptoms also display hysterical traits, but some hysterical personalities do not suffer from symptoms. Hysterical character traits are a flair for dramatic, exhibitionistic behavior; a certain infantile egocentricity; lability of mood; and, most of all, a high degree of suggestibility and gullibility, in the sense that such persons readily transform what is told them into their own imaginative and romantic schemes—an aspect of their reactivity and egocentricity. They hear what is said by "trying it out," much as a child who repeats what he has been told in order to make himself understand a parental order. The hysterical patient may be considered a compelled actor (not a dissembler), a person who dramatizes his unconscious conflicts by conversion, dysmnesic symptoms, and certain character traits.

Freud speculated on a predisposing factor, "somatic compliance," that is, a readiness for bodily organs to express mental conflict, as underlying the capacity for conversion.[32] Far more important than this speculation were investigations by Josef Breuer and Freud,[10] who demonstrated that not just suggestion but intolerable fear and guilt over sexual wishes motivated hysterical symptoms, and the denial and repression won the patient relief (or suspension of guilty worry, and hence the indifference). The meaning and message of the hysterical symptoms, traits, and conflicts can usually be discerned in thorough analytic investigation. At times, a relatively superficial inspection of the characteristic sex life of such patients may furnish important cues. Conflict over sexual and aggressive wishes and avoidance of external danger and temptations may lead to hysterical symptoms; the predisposing fixations will be fears over loss of love and the threats of injury and castration dating from early childhood. Paul Schilder maintained that concern over sickness in the families of hysterical patients is important.[67] Hysterical persons are not only apt repressors but also skillful identifiers. Their tendency to imitate is mostly unconscious. The hysterical patient, particularly in the face of threats and temptation (and in order to contain the anxiety), identifies with the person who provokes or seduces him. Oral mechanisms of incorporation can be discerned in such identification. L. Rangell has stated that such hysterical manifestations may occur at pre-Oedipal levels of development,[61] and some speculate that some of Freud's famous hysterical patients were possibly schizophrenic. They were certainly "sick," and it would be well to anticipate hysterical symptomatology occurring along a continuum of states, from mildly impaired persons to patients with little hold on reality. Indeed, this is true for any neurotic mechanism.

There has been some speculation whether the incidence of conversion reactions has decreased as a function of growing psychiatric sophistication at large. Two considerations are relevant to this speculation. One is that we see hysterical behavior without dramatic conversion and may thus miss a "modern hysteric." Some of these patients are startlingly naïve about what they do; as children, they succeed in being "innocent" about their seductive behavior and foolishly romantic and unrealistic about their attachments. Their pseudosophistication, often of the beatnik variety, merely expresses their irresponsible fascination with play, rather than achievement of gratification in a mature role. Diagnostically, they impress contemporary workers with their identity diffusion and borderline qualities; nevertheless, these cases often contain the mechanisms and history associated with hysterical disorders. A second important consideration is that psychiatrists may not see the bulk of hysterical disorders. It seems that this population still crowds the offices of neurologists, other medical specialists, and general practitioners, and such a patient is not referred unless the temporary problem becomes too persistent or troublesome to be dealt with by these specialists.

Psychotherapy of hysterical patients is erroneously considered a simple matter. The reason for such false optimism is the high suggestibility of these patients, who react easily and promptly to waking suggestion; unfortunately, they revert to the original or a different symptom after only a short time. Persuasive hypnosis, which has been recommended strongly since Jean Martin Charcot's time, may produce dramatic but not lasting results. The treatment of hysterical character disorders is particularly difficult. Even psychoanalysis, which developed its characteristic methods through adapting to the "needs" of hysterical patients to reproduce and reminisce or to resist such procedures, does not always succeed in getting to the bottom of a hysterical behavior in the sense of achieving lasting freedom from symptoms and a radical change of character structure.

Hypochondriacal Behavior

Hypochondriacal behavior refers to a habitual overconcern with health and unrealistic assumptions of being ill. The literature of this important syndrome, which is often lumped together with neurasthenia, is sparse.[12] It is manifested by a fear of illness; for those who like Greek names, we suggest the term "nosophobia." The most important type is cancerphobia. Syphilophobia has become less important since the development of antibiotic therapy, but fear of any infection is still quite prevalent. These patients are apt to exaggerate and misinterpret harmless and meaningless signs and symptoms; a headache indicates the existence of a brain tumor; a slight chest pain leads to the homemade diagnosis of a coronary thrombosis. Knowledge is not a sufficient protection against such behavior: physicians and medical students are notorious hypochondriacs. Many patients not only misinterpret but also actively search for signs and symptoms of illness. The severity of the hypochondriacal symptom or trait can be gauged by the inability of the patient to convince himself and thus be convinced of the falseness of his assumption. One of the most puzzling and aggravating problems in medical practice is created by patients who assert that they suffer from pain for which no "organic" cause can be found. The psychosocial and physiological determinants of such behavior are quite obscure.[72]

Hypochondriacal complaints are often seen as "entrance tickets" for persons who feel neglected to win attention from a physician or to relate to a hospital or clinic setting. Many observers of chronic clinic patients have noted their use of the waiting room, regular appointments, and the like as important social instruments to lighten their lonely or deprived lives. So-called iatrogenic illnesses, that is, illness produced by misleading statements or unwarranted procedures by physicians, are encountered. Often "thorough" examinations, designed to reassure the patient, actually reinforce his assumption of illness. These patients readily imagine themselves to be ill but are easily convinced that they are not, as illustrated in the following case.

> A depressed fifty-eight-year-old woman was convinced that modern medicine should relieve her of absolutely anything that hurt her. She had a few aches and pains, which she assumed were the basis for all the extensive tests she annually underwent in medical clinics. Each work-up meant that the doctors were further baffled and concealing from her the awful truth. She lost weight from worry and poor appetite. She was truly relieved of her conviction that she was "terminally failing" when told that her annual thorough examination was a search for dangerous diseases that doctors could help or cure, whereas modern medicine tended to be baffled but unworried about the everyday miseries she suffered. Astounded, she adjusted by turning her attention to her social life and grandchildren and putting aside her deadly romance with medicine.

The severe hypochondriac is not influenced that easily; neither persuasion nor suggestion nor insight into psychological causes produces changes. The psychotic hypochondriac has fantastic delusions of illness. He is convinced that he has no stomach, no brain, or that the vital organs have been eaten away by cancer. Such hypochondriacal delusions occur in depressions, in schizophrenia, and in organic reaction types. A reticent, laconic draftee in the United States Army from a backwoods farm was passed through several specialty clinics, including psychiatric examinations, in the search for causes of a mysterious gastric ailment; a bright intern, noting the patient's morning sickness, jestingly asked if he were pregnant and was amazed to find, with one "yes," that this was exactly a part of the taciturn man's (extensive) delusions. Usually, hypochondriacal symptoms occur together with anxiety and hysterical and obsessive symptoms. Hypochondriacal patients provoke anger, and many appendices and even more useful organs probably have been removed by an exasperated surgeon who acted in unconscious retaliation to the patient's relentless demands. In clinical practice, exaggeration of symptoms and a combination of hysterical and organic symptoms, which we so often see in medically ill patients, is much more important than pure "hysteria" or "hypochondriasis." The opposite reaction to hypochondriasis is a denial of illness, which is also of great practical significance. A person may take illness lightly, neglecting prevention as well as therapy; severe denial is seen in such syndromes as denial of blindness and anosogosia, a term used by Joseph Babinski to describe denial of hemiplegia. Its causes range from cerebral effects to pure psychogenic denial (see Chapter 16).

The more superficial causes of hypochondriacal reactions are lay ignorance of medical facts and possibly a cultural overconcern with health and illness: witness the ever-present phenomena of medical faddism and cultism. Freud had surprisingly little to say about hypochondriacs; he himself complained about minor ailments quite readily but stoically endured his long and severe illness. Freud rather casually considered hypochondriasis an "actual neurosis." The psychoanalytic literature speaks of an unconscious displacement of energy or interest from the sex organs to the hypochondriacally involved organ, in our opinion an unsatisfactory explanation. Prepsychotic hypochondriasis is seen as representing a shift in ego boundaries in an attempt to stabilize the fragmenting self-image. The self-punitive and punitive aspects of the behavior of hypochondriacal patients toward family and medical personnel, and their attempts to control their environment, are quite obvious. Understandably, psychotherapy of hypochondriacal behavior is very difficult. Often, the symptoms are rigid and deeply ingrained. Not infrequently physicians react to the provocative quality of hypochondriacal patients by rejecting or punishing them. Suggestive reassuring methods have little chance of success, and the results of psychoanalytic therapy are not remarkable. Analytic group therapy may turn out to be the best method for working with hypochondriacs.

Obsessive Behavior

Sandor Rado uses the term *obsessive behavior* rather than the customary tautological designation of obsessive-compulsive neurosis.[60] Obsessive behavior may be separated into obsessive symptoms and obsessive character traits. Symptoms are divided into obsessive thoughts, feelings, and acts. All obsessive symptoms have an ego-alien character; the patient considers them as strange, disturbing, and not compatible with his conscious thinking, feeling, and striving. In their more harmless forms, they occur frequently as the urge to reopen a letter already sealed or the superstitious reluctance to light more than two cigarettes on one match. The obsession may be superficially harmless, such as a preoccupation with insoluble or not very relevant problems or riddles, an obsessive concern over how many items justify the use of the word *much* (or what is an obsessive neurosis). Yet, obsessive behavior may also be so severe as to negate the old saw that neuroses are minor disturbances. Some of them are absolutely crippling: one patient with a washing compulsion could not tolerate furniture in his room because it was "unclean"; he lived for years in an absolutely empty room and slept on the floor.

Obsessive thoughts, feelings, and urges force themselves on the patient, giving him a feeling of apprehension and embarrassment. One of the most common obsessions is the urge to profane what is sacred, to use obscene language at ceremonial and solemn occasions in church, at funerals, or at public meetings. The aggressive and anal character of such speech is unmistakable. Some patients become worried lest they attack and kill a beloved person, child, or relative. Often, such a thought is related to phobic ideas, such as a fear of sharp objects or knives. Some obsessive patients become extremely upset unless certain acts are ritualistically carried out in a definite way or order. Again, there are many gradations of such behavior. Most persons prefer to have the table set in a certain fashion: deviation from such custom is noted and may even cause slight discomfort. The obsessive, however, becomes extremely upset if, say, a knife is pointed differently, and he fears that one of the persons at the table will die. One patient had to return to a certain spot on the road twelve times to check on whether the cherry stone he spat out had caused someone to break a leg. In most cases, obsessive patients cannot tell us what the magic meaning of their ritual is; their thoughts, words, and actions appear strange and ego-alien to them and others. Obsessive acts may produce a strange, stilted, ritualistic quality in these patients; they have to walk, sleep, eat, and talk in a certain way. If they do anything differently, they feel disturbed or fear they will upset the course of events; they avoid alterations of behavior at almost any cost. This avoidance behavior relates obsessive to phobic symptoms and to magical thinking and also highlights their defensive character.

All patients with obsessive symptoms show an obsessive character structure. Freud was impressed with a certain constellation of traits, the anal character. The obsessive character is obstinate, orderly, perfectionistic, and overly punctual and meticulous; he is usually parsimonious and frugal.[29] His thinking is characterized by an accent on form, by hair-splitting argumentation. He is inclined to intellectualism, and this often makes for a serious therapeutic problem because the patient verbalizes without feeling and engages in endless speculations and generalizations. Intellectually, these patients are steeped in overcomplexities and gnawing doubts that cannot be dissolved; feelings and actions tend to be indecisive and lack directness. One of the outstanding traits of the obsessive character complex is the patient's ambivalence: the normal tendency to see two or more sides of a controversy is enormously exaggerated. The obsessive person cannot help but have opposite feelings about everything; love and hate, positive and negative approval and action may coexist or alternate. They do and undo with rituals, or in social behavior, for example, they offer one a compliment and then a few insults. They may dress meticulously but cling to dirty underwear for several weeks.

Freud related obsessiveness to rebellious reactions centered around the period of bowel training. As such rebellion is dangerous and anxiety-producing, it becomes repressed. This repressed rage, according to Rado, is the key emotion in obsessions;[60] the "battle of the chamberpot," as he puts it, becomes embodied in the character structure. The housewife who cleans in a frenzy and is frenzied by others trespassing on her cleanliness demonstrates how close her behavior really is to a view of "dirty" childhood habits and their control, which she constantly caricatures. Repressed rage is then counteracted by defense mechanisms of undoing, reaction-formation, and innumerable rituals. Reaction-formation may produce a superficial, oily sweetness; sooner or later, however, the true aggressions break through. The obsessive vacillates between rage and attempts to undo by atonement. Atonement is symbolically achieved by rituals often of a rigid, magical, superstititious, or religious character. The megalomanic overestimation of mental products—magic of thought and wish—reflects the wish for autonomy; Erikson cites this as a developmental crisis of the two- to three-year-old when the problem of who and what makes things happen—such as bowel movements, for one—and the issue of power is important.[20] The obsessive defense may become more troublesome than the original impulse, and Rado speaks of the obsessive person as an overreactor.[60] Yet we really cannot assert that the root of obsessive behavior is in every instance referable to an actual battle of the chamberpot. It is more likely that the three-year-old's adaptations, his vulnerability to respond to the upset of his autonomy or ritualized order by overreacting, are of fundamental importance. This mode of reacting and thinking colors many experiences, including the experience of instinctual mastery, without toilet training necessarily becoming the provoking cause. Rather, the child may represent a range of experiences and adjustments in terms of the more familiar bodily concerns and magical theories centered about the experience of the making, elimination, and retention of feces and the periodicity of these functions. It is this displacement that may lead to the "anality" in obsessive characters, who have not ceased to appear since the admonitions of the Freudians and Dr. Benjamin Spock.

Treatment of obsessive behavior is difficult. The milder obsessive neuroses usually do reasonably well in analytic therapies. The resistances of all obsessive neurotics, through the defenses of intellectualization and isolation, are formidable and require much patience until a meaningful and positive emotional relationship is established.

Aggressive Behavior

The word aggression has many meanings; it denotes destructive or hostile behavior, a disposition to anger, but also, simply, a very active and vital personality who is more prone to approach, attack, and pursue than to avoid, retreat, and defend. The importance of aggression and passivity in our patients cannot be overestimated. To be meaningful in diagnosis and psychopathology, the term must be defined more specifically, and in psychiatric usage we limit it to hostile and destructive behavior. A related aspect, sadism, or a fusion of pathological sexual and aggressive behavior, will be taken up later. It is also important to differentiate between normal and neurotic aggressive behavior; the latter, generally speaking, is inappropriate and maladaptive. Habitual severe aggression in our culture is usually maladaptive, and we think of excessive nonadaptive aggression when we speak of neurotic aggression or of aggressive character disorders.

A distinction should be made between overt and unconscious aggression. In the former, the patient is aware of his manifest hostile and destructive behavior; in the latter, he is unaware of such behavior and intentions. We often encounter patients who are hostile to persons they are expected to love: to one or both parents, siblings, spouse, or children. This hostility may generalize to specific social and ethnic groups and, in some misanthropic persons, to all mankind. It may be accompanied and manifested by overt signs of anger, which, like anxiety, may be extraordinarily varied. Symptoms of acute anger produce muscular tension, gastric and vasomotor symptoms; and chronic rage, more difficult to detect by its somatic signs, is often associated with headaches, insomnia, fatigue, and muscular pains. Aggressive behavior is not always accompanied by overt anger; it may be deliberately suppressed, as in a cold rage, or it may actually be repressed and appear only in the form of unconscious derivatives. There is an endless variety of destructive behavior, ranging from insidious lovelessness to violence and murder. Much of the subtle diagnostic work of the dynamic psychiatrist consists of tracking down the behavioral derivatives of repressed anger and anxiety and detecting their true nature, meaning, target, and origin.

It is most probable that constitutional elements play a role in the etiology of aggressive behavior, a heritage from our primate ancestors.[56] Striking differences have been seen between demanding, aggressive infants and passive babies, although such temperament has not been proved to persist. On the whole, modern psychiatrists are inclined to assume that behavioral patterns of aggression and anxiety are learned and are developments of an inherent potential. We assume that severe aggression is reactive and develops from frustration and mishandling of defiant behavior in childhood and infancy. Just how this happens is unclear, but there is tentative evidence that aggressive behavior is likely to develop when it is harshly and severely punished or when it is endured without restraints. The tolerated amounts and patterns of aggressive behavior vary greatly, of course, in different social and ethnic groups.

In treating aggressive character disorders, therapists have the task of demonstrating the maladaptive nature of the aggressive behavior. Whether it is manifested in headaches or habits and traits that are not readily recognized as aggression (for example, a tremendous drive, arrogance, and coldness; or an inclination to manipulate), the true nature of these behavioral deviations must be uncovered first. After this is done, therapists may attempt to show their patients that their persistent aggressive behavior is an expression of an archaic rebellion, hatred or reaction to frustration; we induce them to wonder whether old interpretations of reality need apply in their adult world. Some aggressive behavior is motivated by anxiety, guilt, and need for punishment. Sustained virulence or envy often masks yearning for love and attention. It is necessary in therapy to uncover gradually, without injury to the patient's self-esteem, the fact that aggressive behavior often stems from weakness and not from strength; the child's weaknesses are his rightful limitations, not a permanent inferiority, and if the child was not helped to realize this, the adult, with the guidance of therapy, hopefully can. A basic principle is to break the vicious circle of provocation and punishment, in other words, to refrain from hitting back, as most persons in everyday life do; at times, it is indicated that the therapist turn the other cheek. The therapist can provide firmness and structure; if he really knows what he is about, this will be transmitted consistently in his behavior, without self-conscious attempts to "be firm." A therapist who recognizes his own limits will not be trapped into retaliating against a patient who has "exposed" the therapist's frailty; if he does get provoked, he has not "lost points" but rather can examine with the patient what is so provocative. Such self-knowledge on the therapist's part also means that he has learned that in saying "no," for example, his own omnipotence is not at stake. It may be important for the patient's welfare for the therapist to refuse a request; this responsibility does not entitle the physician to overestimate his importance. In general, it is difficult for therapists to distinguish between authoritativeness and authoritarianism, a distinction the aggressive patient requires.

Self-Destructive Behavior

Self-destructive behavior, occurring in its most severe forms in psychotic depressions and schizophrenias, is also a prominent aspect of many neurotic disorders. A certain pattern of self-destructive living has been called a neurosis of fate. Such patients seem to be pursued by bad luck. Whatever they attempt to do fails; they are victims of accident and misfortune. On closer study, it becomes apparent that this misery is not a matter of an impersonal fate; accidents and failure are provoked and carefully arranged, though not by conscious design. Unconscious motives often act in the following way: rational steps that would avoid failure or signal danger are left out of consideration, repressed, or "forgotten," and the result appears to be "fate." Freud was struck with the importance of this behavior and considered it an expression of the death instinct;[27] only some psychoanalysts accepted this formulation. Some persons respond to attack and threat with passive and self-abasing attitudes, which can provoke further hurt and lowering of self-esteem. One of the ways of self-limitation but also of "disarming" an opponent is clowning behavior, which may develop as a response in order to mollify rage and attack.

Freud introduced the concepts of feminine masochism and moral masochism.[28] Feminine masochism refers to an attitude of normal women to be passive, to endure, and to accommodate, with some pleasure and some pain (more precisely, to enjoy yielding) in sexual and maternal activities. Moral masochism is a trait encountered in persons with self-punitive behavior. It would be better to speak of moral sado-masochism. Such patients suffer for principles but also punish others through their "nobility"; a rational disagreement with these people leads one to feel guilty rather than correct. Whereas such behavior can be understood on the public scene in the service of great moral causes, the average moral masochist invites (and dispenses) punishment at home, in petty details of marriage or the office. The intransigence of a person who values work, prudence, saving for higher education, and who therefore refuses to take his family on a single holiday on these moral grounds, may merely mask his anger at giving anything to anyone and his revenge for not being given something he wanted but would not openly request. In brief, much infantile behavior can lurk behind morality, and morality can be used as a weapon for sado-masochistic needs. In analytic terms, the unconscious need for self-punishment is linked with the existence of an abnormally severe superego, which originates with the incorporation of an image of severely punitive parents. Such parents are, in some cases, objectively severe and punitive; in other cases, it is a fantasized image of a severe or unloving parent that becomes incorporated. Usually, such self-punitive, deeply entrenched attitudes are concomitant with depressive behavior and permeate the character and prevent enjoyment.

The essence of treatment lies in working through manifestations and origins of self-defeating and self-punitive behavior of the patient and in demonstrating to him over and over not only that he does not act in his own interest but also that some deprivation, fear, or hurt may sustain this. For example, one patient discovered that in enduring all kinds of defeat, he was still concerned with a forgotten battle; defeat meant he really wasn't a bad, obstreperous, demanding boy, and he recalled his parents forgiving him if he admitted he was wrong, even when he was, in fact, not wrong. The self-destructive habits of such patients also reveal themselves in therapy, by their attempts to defeat the efforts of the therapist to help them. In their profound need to hurt themselves, they manage to alienate and frustrate anyone who wants to help. They gain insights but are unable to apply them. Freud referred to this phenomenon as negative therapeutic reaction.[35] Punishment becomes a secondary reward; it seems that, for some persons, suffering, as long as it is under their semiconscious control, as long as it is familiar, is preferable to the exposure and courage required to change habits and views. This behavior becomes a formidable problem in life and also in treatment because the ordinary incentives for learning and improving seem to be perverted.

Passive Behavior

Passivity, as the term is used in psychiatry, refers (like its counterpart, aggression) to a number of rather different phenomena: psychological inactivity, inertia, indolence, laziness; but also a lack of responsiveness; a yielding to aggression and hostility; or to a need for support, guidance, and domination. We have distinguished receptivity from pathological passivity. Many passive persons create much mischief through their passivity and provoke strong aggressive responses from their fellow human beings. Often, there is a combination of passive with aggressive traits, for which we use the awkward term "passive-aggressive." In studying such patients, we learn that their provocations are not meaningless by-products but that there are unconscious wishes to be hurt and mistreated; such patients feel justified and "confirmed" in their avoidance by mistreatment. Some experience vicarious pleasure and secret pride at the exasperation or "wasted" energy of others. In some, passivity is a reaction-formation to an underlying aggression, and the opposite also occurs. Clinically, the most important aspect is a need to depend, be cared for and be dominated, needs that, in turn, create considerable anxiety and, more importantly, decrease in self-esteem. Freud spoke of an unconscious fear of the wish to be in a passive feminine role as the most difficult psychological problem in the treatment of any male.[35] One characteristic of infantile passivity (and magic) is found in the majority of neurotics: they expect their thoughts and wishes to be known without making them public and explicit and accordingly feel they are not understood and are easily slighted. They depend on others for what efficiently they could only do for themselves and overreact by distrust and withdrawal. They strike secret "bargains" expecting that what they themselves do without stint earns them the right to demand (of course, without asking) a favor in return. If a patient cannot say no and refuse a request, one should be alert to the fact that he probably cannot permit others to refuse his stated or unstated requests. If he does "permit" refusal, he exaggerates and courts rejection, nurturing either grudges or disappointments as the excuse for personal failures.

Just as with aggression, psychiatrists assume that genetic and constitutional determinants probably exist without being able to specify them. One striking feature of the persisting passive and masochistic behavior is that there is reward in not changing such patterns; losing these requires enormous trust and appetite for change. When the patient can "disown" these patterns and rebel more openly against them, some therapeutic gain may be made.

Passive patients are difficult to treat. They manipulate the therapist into a position of an authoritative parent, leader, and manager and avoid responsibilities and decisions when they can. Only a great deal of patience in working through the patient's problems can alter such attitudes.

Inadequate and Infantile Behavior

By the generic term, inadequate behavior, is meant behavior by persons who are unable, and often seemingly unwilling, to solve the ordinary tasks of life which are posed to adult members of a society because of personality factors. There are cases of arrest in development, apparently because of an impoverished sociocultural background, in which there is a reduced capacity to cope with personal relationships of any complexity. These people are seen by psychiatrists because they are in trouble: sometimes depressed, sometimes simply displaced from their accustomed environment, as in military service. Other variants are character disorders, such as the "schlemiel," the inveterate bungler. Such character types, people who play characteristic roles in a group, have been identified from time immemorial in folklore. The man who is always spilling soup, or the "poor soul" who invariably gets soup spilled on him, are recognized in psychiatric jargon as inadequate personalities. A quite subordinate role in a group may be the refuge for the truly borderline mentally retarded; similarly, many neurotics in these roles are assumed, erroneously, to be dull.

Inadequate persons behave as children; hence, the traits inadequate and infantile are intimately linked; infantile personalities, however, are not necessarily neurotic.[64] Neurotics usually feel dissatisfied and inadequate; they feel that they have not fulfilled their potential and want to be different. The infantile person may be at ease with himself; he does not want to change, nor does he complain that he has not actualized himself. Characteristic infantile traits are emotionality and inability to delay, resist, and control impulses. Infantile persons have explosive outbursts of anger, childlike temper tantrums, and they express their sexual and erotic needs, which are often quite primitive, without restraint; at times, they are described as flagrantly egocentric and narcissistic. Lack of control over aggressive infantile sexual drives makes some infantile personalities markedly antisocial or asocial. Some, however, are conformists; others are creative and useful nonconformists.

Freud used the term narcissism to describe the attachment of libidinal energy to the ego.[27] In complicated speculations, he distinguished primary narcissism from secondary narcissism; in the former, psychosexual energy is invested in the body and the ego; in the latter, libido is withdrawn from objects to the ego; this Freud assumed to be the case in schizophrenia, and also in depression, which he called narcissistic neuroses. Today, the term narcissistic behavior is generally used descriptively to designate a high degree of self-love, beyond what is required for healthy self-regard. Narcissism means more than egocentricity. Like Narcissus, who fell in love with his reflected image, narcissistic personalities are characterized by an unusual degree of vanity, and absorption with self (self-image, bodily appearance, achievements), overevaluation of their own interests, and loose ties with other persons except when they seek immediate gratification. As such clusters of traits are frequent in infantile character neuroses, and also in schizoid and some antisocial personalities, the term has descriptive value. Blatant narcissistic behavior is disapproved in Western society; most people, including therapists, react to it with the annoyance and resentment that they display toward aggressive provocation. Some infantile narcissists powerfully attract persons who need to nurture such traits and to partake vicariously in the egoism they cannot directly express.

Treatment of infantile personalities involves an educational approach. Long-term intensive psychotherapy used by analytic psychiatrists is such an educational approach. Many infantile personalities, with their inability to control behavior and to delay impulses, require considerable modification of the analytic method. Such modifications are in the direction of more structuring. The therapist guides and provides opportunities to establish relationships and identifications with a reliable adult person. For some patients, this kind of emotional re-education is best done in an open institutional setting.

Impulsive Behavior

Impulsive behavior disorders are manifested by irresistible acts, which are incompatible with overt social and ethical standards and do not serve a useful purpose. In the older literature, there was considerable discussion about the difference between compulsive and impulsive neuroses. According to Otto Fenichel, compulsive neurotics are ego dystonic; impulsive neurotics are ego syntonic.[23] The differentiation is doubtful because the impulse-driven individual cannot explain or justify his behavior any more than the compulsive. Compulsives, however, are more ritualistic and more clearly defensive, in impulsive neurotic behavior the naked, antisocial instinct is more discernible. Yet, impulsive behavior has a defensive function as well, because, as in addictions and perversions, it supposedly protects against discharge of even more dangerous impulses, which would produce anxiety and depression. Usually included in the category of impulsive behavior are kleptomania, or impulsive stealing; poriomania, or impulsive running away (closely related to fugue states and considered in Chapter 16); pyromania, or impulsive fire-setting; and impulsive gambling. Some patients with impulsive behavior suffer from cerebral syndromes, such as postencephalitic states; some are epileptic; and some are mentally deficient. In children, an important syndrome, the hyperkinetic child, has been described. This syndrome is characterized by problems of an often good-natured child with poor impulse control; hyperactivity; short attention span; problems of maintaining and shifting a mental set; and difficulty in fine sensorimotor control. These disorders generally dissipate by adulthood. In general, and in view of the relationship of "organicity" to impulse control, the most strategic investigative attitude is to recognize the possibility of brain dysfunction in some groups of impulse disorders. Eugen Kahn and Louis H. Cohen recognized such complex and largely unexplored relationships when they described the syndrome of organic drivenness.[46]

The kleptomaniac, in contrast to ordinary thieves, steals objects often of little value. The difference between *kleptomania* and thievery is not always clear-cut because impulsive traits are also found in certain habitual thieves who act against their own interests. Usually, the stealing in the kleptomaniac is a symbolic act of restitution of a real or imaginary tort that the patient suffered.[36] A calm, intelligent schoolteacher compulsively stole change from a roommate's purse; generally she had forgotten to cash a check or was a bit short of funds. She finally brought herself to pay attention to her thoughts when doing this. She found herself saying, "It's my right to take it if I need it." Surprised at this childlike assertion, in therapy she recalled for the first time her childhood tempers, a flood of notions that her mother owed her what she wanted, attention from her father being the dominant wish. Put simply, then, "I want what I want when I want it," is quite seriously the emblem for those adults who still battle for the rights of infancy. Theft of vehicles by adolescents is typically a rebellious act against an authority figure. Impulsive acts such as inexplicable cruelty to pets, or compulsive braid-cutting, usually occur in patients who are psychotic or mentally retarded. These acts can be understood without much difficulty as unconscious retaliation for injury, with displacement to a less feared object; as all impulsive acts, they produce a reduction in unconscious anxiety. In all these cases, including those of *pyromania*, a gratification of primitive sadistic needs is also present. Another behavior disorder in this category is *impulsive gambling*. There are many normal persons who gamble and probably fulfill needs very similar to those of impulse neurotics: to conquer fate, to prove omnipotence in a childlike, playful fashion without effort, or to exhort fate (personified by parents) for a beneficence that is overdue. The normal gambler is able to stop. The impulsive gambler cannot; he must gamble to protect himself against deep unconscious anxieties and threats and to try to prove his worth to a parental figure, or himself, by being smiled on by "lady luck."[7] As in all impulsive neuroses, addictions, and perversions, there are strong self-destructive and destructive tendencies involved. In the professional gambler, as in many sociopaths, behavior is determined by group influences from the underworld in which he lives. The treatment of impulsive neurotics by insight-oriented therapy is a difficult but not unrewarding task.

Deviant Sexual Behavior

Sexual deviations of adults, also called perversions, are patterns of sexual behavior that predominantly and habitually satisfy other sexual needs than those gratified by normal coitus. Sexual deviations are impulsive and inflexible acts; the individual feels he is under pressure to commit the act and does not have the ordinary capacity to resist or to change his behavior. Becoming aroused by the sight, touch, or smell of a female garment as an optional prelude to coitus is a normal characteristic of male sexual behavior, but a fetishist who achieves orgasm *only* if he sees, touches, or smells a woman's underwear is sexually deviant. Sexual deviations are widespread; prevalence data on some specific deviations, mostly from the work of Alfred C. Kinsey and his co-workers, are given in the next sections.[49, 50]

Cultural attitudes toward adult sexual deviations undoubtedly influence their incidence. There seems to be, however, no direct relation between the degree of permissiveness of the culture and the frequency of deviation. Attitudes toward sexual behavior that are displayed in child-rearing are very likely more decisive factors in deviant behavior than attitudes toward adult sexuality. The relationship of sexual deviations to normal sexual habits was first pointed out by Freud in his fundamental work, *Three Essays on the Theory of Sexuality*.[26] Freud demonstrated that everybody in his infancy and childhood is polymorphously perverse and that such infantile behavior under certain not completely unspecified conditions persists in the adult sexual deviant. In the normal adult, strivings for genital satisfactions gain primacy over infantile strivings; in the sexual deviant, infantile strivings remain dominant. Because neurosis was considered the "mirror image" of perversion (that is, defended against it), it was thought that no anxiety attended perversion; this is not so, and now we recognize that the perversion is maintained against many threats—heterosexual anxiety, incestuous, or more regressive needs.

It is characteristic for normal adults that sexual needs are fused with erotic and social needs that permit instinctual gratification along with love, care, and appreciation of another. In many deviations, this is not the case; instead, sexual deviates behave not only in an infantile but also in an asocial or antisocial manner. At times, there is severe aggression compounded in deviant sexual behavior, for example, seduction of children, or overtly destructive behavior. However, this is usually not the case, and most sexual deviates are people who damage mostly themselves. To a certain extent, the antisocial behavior of sexual deviants is a consequence of the strongly disapproving and punitive attitude of society. It is particularly marked in the case of male homosexuality in Western society. On the whole, disapproval of deviant sexual behavior is less severe in many non-Western cultures. Fortunately, in our own culture, certain changes in sexual mores are becoming noticeable. Under the impact of such changes and of modern psychiatric findings, persons committing deviant sex practices, if not damaging to others or public nuisances, are nowadays less likely to be punished if apprehended; afflicted persons are increasingly advised or ordered to obtain therapy. It is obvious that even in those cases in which harm is done, mere punitive measures such as incarceration are not helpful. Generally speaking, to help severe sexual deviates is a very difficult matter; only intensive insight-oriented psychotherapy offers modest promise. Yet, surely every sexual deviant with reasonable motivation deserves a chance for treatment. Very often a prognosis cannot be made before therapy is undertaken, and not infrequently a perversion may be found to represent a fairly isolated and treatable manifestation of immaturity.

Homosexuality

Homosexual behavior is sexual behavior directed at a person of the same sex. In addition to the 5 per cent of the general population who are exclusively homosexual, there is a much greater number, possibly one-third to one-half of the male population, who have at least some homosexual experiences, and 10 to 20 per cent who have engaged in sexual behavior with both sexes regularly.[49] Homosexual behavior is seen in children, adolescents, adults, and in many species of animals. Occasional homosexual behavior in children and adolescents cannot be considered abnormal. The variety of homosexual behavior is as great as the variety of heterosexual behavior. Sexual intercourse often is not the dominant mode of sexual experience but is substituted in both sexes by pregenital modes of gratification (fondling, kissing), by genital-to-mouth contact or, somewhat less frequently in male homosexuals, by genital-to-anus contact (often called sodomy, which also refers to relationships with animals). There is often a rather aggressive element in homosexual practice; hostile fantasies play a large role in homosexual relationships; and it is also noteworthy that, in contrast to normal heterosexual relationships, aggression may not be dissipated by homosexual behavior. Parenthetically, some psychotic homosexuals have become involved in murder or other violent crimes. Sexual behavior in which children are objects is clearly destructive; perpetrators, if not defective or psychotic, are found to fear adult contacts or to act out, concretely, a childhood wish or seduction in which they were traumatized or seduced.

When homosexual needs are repressed, psychoanalysts speak of latent homosexuality, a term that is often used loosely. Such repressed homosexuality is always infantile homosexuality and is usually revealed only in such derivative character traits as passivity and an interest in feminine occupations and hobbies in the male; and a certain aggressive interest in male occupations and recreations in the female. Latent homosexuality refers to a repressed nucleus of the dormant psychology of the opposite sex; for example, the basic attitudes of a little girl toward her body and her father—her wish for a penis or power from him—are repeated in some form in the boy. These repressed attitudes are critically important both as a basis for one sex understanding the other as well as in trait- and symptom-formation. Not all male homosexuals are permissive or effeminate; nor are all female homosexuals masculine, aggressive, and assertive. It cannot even be stated, as was once popular among so-called sexologists, whether a homosexual is active or passive; homosexuals often change roles in these relationships. Another form of sexual misidentification, different from but closely related to homosexuality, is transvestitism, in which individuals have the urge to wear the clothes and in general to assume typical habits of the other sex. Transvestites invariably are very disturbed persons; many of them are schizophrenics, but the symptom does occur in neurotic character disorders.

In all likelihood, homosexuality occurs in all cultures, but the attitudes of societies differ markedly; in large parts of Africa and Asia, the attitude toward homosexual behavior is not so severe and condemning as it is in contemporary Western society. Social attitudes toward male and female homosexuals differ; discrimination is less pronounced against female homosexuals. Female homosexuals also are less noticed than males, and not infrequently two homosexual women manage to have a fairly peaceful, untroubled relationship, which is more difficult and rare in male homosexuals. A fair number of male and female homosexuals "cruise" promiscuously and move compulsively from conquest to conquest. Some patients describe the need for this adolescent level of relationship as like an addiction and speak fearfully of growing old and unattractive. In big cities, homosexuals form their own "society" with its own rules, roles, and lingo. In these societies, homosexuals also try to justify their neurotic sexual choice and to protect themselves against what they consider unfair, discriminatory, and punitive practices by the heterosexual population. With an inverted pride, many homosexuals cite (and exaggerate) the number of gifted artists, writers, and actors among them. This does, however, point to the problem of identity, the psychic mobility and exaggerated self-assertion that can be involved in homosexual life as well as in exhibitionistic and creative life. Although the great majority of homosexuals are unhappy but harmless and decent people, there is a definite connection between these homosexual societies and such underworld activities as crime and prostitution; pimps play an important role, and some homosexuals are prone to become involved in illegal activities. This may be largely because homosexuals are driven through our laws into an underground existence. The dynamic reason for "getting caught," however, is their strong need for self-punishment.

Much has been written about the causes of overt homosexual behavior, but there is no consensus, and opinions differ widely. One group points to the importance of an innate constitution and the presence of "bisexual" disposition that exists in all people and, depending on the relative strength of heterosexual or homosexual factors, may lead to one or the other or to mixed forms of sexual behavior. Kinsey,[49] and Clellan S. Ford and Frank A. Beach[24] adhere to a bisexual theory. The latter refer to the well-established fact that both sexes produce male and female sex hormones. Contrary to some expectations, however, there are no biochemical data to support a constitutional abnormality in homosexuals.[47] The constitutionalists refer, among other data, to Kallmann's findings of a very high incidence (80 per cent) among siblings of identical homosexual twins. Identification in identical twins is clearly important in the establishment of the sex role, however; thus, such observations do not settle the question of etiology conclusively. There has been an abundance of publications on the psychogenesis of homosexuality, particularly in the psychoanalytic literature. The typical focus has been a sexual identification with the parent of the opposite sex, presumably because of a high castration anxiety. The male homosexual is horrified by the penisless female, and the female homosexual feels threatened by the male penis; she may need to be a boy to please the father or to appease her inferiority feelings. As these factors are also made accountable for many other sex deviations and neuroses, this does not solve the problem. In some cases, homosexual behavior represents a neurotic retreat from desired but feared heterosexual relationships; rather than firmly fixed homoerotic choice, these people seem ready for heterosexual choice if they can overcome their specific fear or inhibition. Freud cited a mechanism that is frequently encountered in narcissistic characters; a little boy, overindulged and petted, suddenly ceases to be the object of affection.[26] He then searches for his lost image in other boys, whom he can treat as he was treated. Others seek for mothering from the father; still others attempt through female wiles to attract a father or to mother him. Recently, Irving Bieber and his co-workers, on the basis of psychoanalytic studies of male homosexuals, pointed to some provocative parental constellations.[8] A possessive mother and a cold, detached father make it difficult for the growing boy to develop a heterosexual orientation. In general, we are inclined to think that further detailed, controlled studies into the life history of homosexuals will reveal a number of different constellations that contribute to different patterns of overt homosexuality.

Therapy of the overt homosexual yields results that are far from encouraging. Even psychoanalytic treatment cannot boast of great success, and superficial methods are of no use whatsoever. Homosexuals can be treated only if they sincerely and strongly want treatment. A real change of sexual orientation in the overt and exclusive homosexual is not common. Often, the patient and therapist have to be satisfied with a better general adjustment of the patient, a lessening of the self-destructive neurotic tendencies. The well-adjusted homosexual who has accepted his deviant sex role is in fact virtually untreatable; he may seek help for his anxieties or depressions, but not his sexual choice. He may also seek help with his heterosexual attachments without wishing to give up his homosexual practices. Somewhat paradoxically, our results with very neurotic homosexuals, provided they desire treatment, are somewhat better.

MALE HOMOSEXUAL WITH SELF-PUNITIVE TENDENCIES

A twenty-four-year-old landscape architect, an active homosexual, asked for therapy. The patient, a masculine and intelligent man, elegant in dress and manner, said that he was deeply disgusted with his homosexual practices, considering them unnatural and sinful; he wanted to be married. His first homosexual relationship occurred in college with a classmate. With the exception of one homosexual affair with a social equal, which lasted almost a year, his contacts were usually short, with socially inferior persons whom he met in parks, taverns, and public toilets. He usually had the partner perform fellatio, although he had reached orgasm in all kinds of practices. He also masturbated regularly, usually with homosexual fantasies. Very rarely, he had vague heterosexual fantasies, for example, dreams in which he had sexual intercourse with a woman whom he beat, hurt, and who tortured and threatened him. He had twice been arrested for homosexual behavior and escaped sentence only with the aid of skillful lawyers. He had also been discharged from the Air Force for his homosexual behavior. He had seen two psychiatrists previously, whom he felt could not help him, and whom he antagonized by his flagrant, self-punitive homosexual escapades. The patient always had one or more girl friends whom he dated. He engaged in pleasurable kissing and embracing with them, but was horrified by the possibility of genital contact. He never had an erection during such contacts, but was sexually potent with homosexual partners. His parents learned about his difficulties following one of his arrests, after which his mother tried to force him into marriage.

In psychoanalytic therapy, an attempt was first made to stop his practice of frequenting bars and other public places to meet homosexual partners. This behavior usually followed scenes with one of his girl friends, or with his mother. These women made demands, which he could not clearly describe, but which made him guilty and anxious. The patient was able to reduce these dangerous homosexual contacts at least to the point that his social existence was no longer threatened. During therapy, a good deal of material about his background was uncovered, although he was only superficially cooperative in such explorations because they provoked much anxiety. In the transference to the therapist, he tried to maintain a distant but pleasant and overtly compliant relationship, reflecting his passive, compliant orientation to his father. He said he liked the therapist, felt he did his duty by coming to the hours and paying his bills, and felt generally protected by the therapeutic contacts.

The patient comes from a socially ambitious Italian Catholic family who are not devout. He tends to deny his background, preferring to associate with upper-class Anglo-Saxons or with skid row bums. The father, a tree surgeon, always remained a distant, overdemanding, aloof authority figure whom the patient could neither trust nor like; he never protected the patient against the seductive, domineering, and very unstable mother, who was given to irrational emotional outbursts against her husband and the other family members. There was much arguing in the household. An older sister much resembled the mother. Undoubtedly, the patient was afraid of these "dangerous" females. He was unable usefully to identify with the distant but weak father; instead, he superficially complied with demands while unconsciously parodying the father's weakness through his own symptoms. Why he seemingly identified so strongly with the aggressive, man-hating mother and sister whom he feared was not clear to him nor to the therapist. His strongest asset was his intelligence, and he did well in college. His father wanted him to become a scientist but, surprisingly, he failed the prerequisite courses and (the son of a tree surgeon) he turned instead to landscape architecture, a profession that he dislikes.

After two years of therapy, both therapist and patient felt that some improvement had occurred. He had become more independent, had established his own household, and socially and professionally had a more satisfactory existence. He continued with his homosexual relations, but endangered himself less. He felt that he and the therapist had come close to understanding his key conflicts but did not consider them solved by any means. As the patient was not satisfied with a "more normal" homosexual life and wanted a "cure," he was referred by mutual agreement to another analyst for more extensive treatment.

The psychoanalytic treatment of intense anxiety over "latent" homosexuality is a very different matter; in such cases, psychoanalytic therapy may do a great deal. It should also be stressed that psychoanalytic therapy may contribute to the management of many homosexuals who get into legal difficulties by working through their aggressive, defiant, and self-punitive needs. It is important to distinguish the worry and identity confusion of the young adult from lasting homosexual fixations. It is very common for neurotic young people to question their virility and attractiveness and to react to homosexual impulses with the conviction that they are different. Often, *any* difference is perceived as "queer" by the adolescent, who is not confident that there are different ways to be a man other than the stereotypes, and ways unrelated to sexual perversion. The psychiatrist always attempts to find out precisely what the patient who feels he is odd really means by such statements.

Other Sexual Deviations

Next to homosexuality, the most frequent perversion is sexual intercourse with domestic animals, referred to by the loaded words, sodomy and bestiality. The habit is less harmful than popular disapproval would indicate. In *fetishism*, persons can be sexually aroused only by certain objects or specific conditions that are incidental or unrelated to copulation.[55] One patient could be aroused only if prostitutes with whom he had sexual intercourse smoked cigars. The habit changed eventually; after he discovered his unconscious homosexual attachment to his father, who was a cigar smoker, he was satisfied when the prostitutes smoked cigarettes. This patient later married a nonsmoker!

In *exhibitionism*, individuals achieve sexual gratification by exposing their genitalia in public.[13] Pathological exhibitionism is usually limited to males; in Western culture, females are granted some display of their legs and the upper part of their torso, strictly regulated by the culture and the setting in which it occurs. The exhibitionist, as has been found in psychoanalytic therapy, suffers from very high castration anxiety and identification with a female; he asserts his masculinity in an infantile fashion by showing his genitalia, usually to minors; he may behave "counterphobically" and try to shock women to avoid his own concerns about the women's penisless genitalia. The ordinary punitive approach to exhibitionism is highly inappropriate from a psychiatric point of view. It is relatively easy to treat exhibitionists, unless they are homosexual or psychotic. Exhibitionistic behavior vis-à-vis minors may be damaging to the child; this, however, is the kind of impulsive behavior that, in most cases, can be dealt with effectively by an understanding psychotherapy.

Scotophiliacs achieve sexual pleasure and orgasm only by looking at primary or secondary sex organs or by witnessing sexual activities.[1] To a degree, scotophilic behavior is part of the normal preparation for the sex act, and it is usually more pronounced in males; derivatives, such as nosiness and gossip, occur in both sexes. Scotophilic individuals are infantile or adolescent nuisances surely, but certainly not dangerous. Many are more or less gratified by "legitimate" channels of stimulation, for example, by certain types of magazine "art," striptease, and burlesque.

There are many forms of sexual behavior, including such kinds of heterosexual stimulation as cunnilingus, fellatio, anal intercourse, and the numerous variations of the *ars amandi*, which should be considered perversions only if they become the exclusive modes of sexual gratification.

Sexual Sadism and Masochism

The word *sadism* immortalizes the writings of the Marquis de Sade on sexual activities that gratify by inflicting pain. The opposite is sexual *masochism*, in which gratification is obtained by suffering and enduring pain. Often, both are combined, and we speak of sado-masochism. A certain sadistic component is certainly a part of normal male sexual behavior, just as a certain masochistic element is characteristic for the normal female. In extreme forms, the love object may be destroyed, for example, in sexual murder or in the cannibalistic behavior of certain psychotic individuals, in whom otherwise universally repressed oral sadistic impulses have invaded conscious behavior. The etiology of sexual masochism remains obscure in spite of our insights into self-punitive and atoning tendencies. It seems much easier to understand why individuals are driven to destroy others than why they will destroy themselves or enjoy pain; the fact that they do, however, is indisputable.

Certain forms of hypersexuality are seen as expressions of infantile sexual behavior and are much akin to perversions. Both the "Don Juan" with a need for sexual intercourse with countless women and an inability to enter into a deeper relationship, and his counterpart, the nymphomanic woman, have profound character neuroses.[62] Usually, seduction in childhood and pathological attachments to frustrating or permissive parental figures are found in the life histories of such patients; paradoxically, the promiscuous "save themselves" for an unobtainable "true love." Nymphomanic women are usually frigid; prostitutes also rarely enjoy intercourse with paying partners. Impotence and frigidity are discussed in Chapter 13.

Masturbation

Masturbation is autoerotic; it is sexual gratification without a partner and is an almost universal practice before sexual maturity is reached. According to Kinsey, over 90 per cent of men report masturbatory experiences in their adolescence.[49] In women, the reported percentage is lower, but women may be less inclined to admit masturbation or may not even be clearly aware of it.[50] Persistent or occasional masturbation in a large percentage of the population continues into the adult years, especially if other forms of gratification are unavailable or difficult to attain. In most cases, men masturbate the penis and women the clitoris by hand; more rarely, women perform vaginal masturbation manually or with suitable objects. Psychologically, the accompanying fantasies are of particular interest: through such fantasies, the gratification of infantile and forbidden impulses is possible, and to some degree masturbation thus may have a socially protective function. Developmentally, it may permit the growth of sexual interest in the opposite sex, freeing the individual from infantile fixations or from generalizing the incest taboo; fantasies may serve as a transition to mutual sexual activity. Such fantasies, however, can also have the opposite effect. Until recently, masturbation was considered a very harmful practice, leading to impotence, frigidity, neurasthenia, and even psychosis. Today, we are convinced that the "harmful" effects of masturbation are due to the intense anxiety, guilt, and shame that may consciously or unconsciously accompany the practice. As compulsive masturbation is the usual sexual outlet of psychotic and deviant "derelicts," one can readily see why such a symptom was taken to be the cause of the disorder.

"Normal" masturbation in teen-agers certainly does not require profound therapy. Instructions about its nature and an attempt to provide opportunities for healthy sexual and social living is all we can and should do. In our own society, however, this is often easier said than done, and at times we are powerless to do more than relieve some of the shame and guilt. If masturbation is recognized as a symptom of profound neurotic or psychotic behavior, therapy must be directed toward such disorder.

Sociopathic Behavior

In the older literature, the term *psychopathic personality* was used for what we now prefer to call *sociopathic behavior*. Nowadays, we are disinclined to assume that sociopaths are born as such and tend to believe that they have acquired their behavior in a social setting. Nevertheless, an adequate classification based on biological as well as social-psychological research of the number of different disorders grouped into the category of sociopathic personality does not exist yet and is greatly to be desired.

Asocial and antisocial behavior varies from relatively mild cases, with unreliable and irresponsible interpersonal relationships, to very severe destructive and dangerous cases. It must be remembered that value orientation influences diagnostic and therapeutic endeavors with the sociopathic group. A behavioristic diagnosis—a list of facts—that does not include the psychosocial context in which they occurred is of little use. Western societies in general disapprove of slackers, drifters, hobos, gamblers, beggars, prostitutes, persons with poor work records, and pathological liars. In such cultures, this disapproval is quite casual; in others, it is severe and reinforced by legal sanctions. The attitudes of society toward severe forms of deviant aggressive, sexual, and acquisitive behavior are punitive and codified by criminal laws. Crime is a legal, not a psychiatric term, referring to behavior that violates the penal code. From the psychiatric point of view, there is a difference only in degree between legally defined criminal groups and other classifications. The function of value judgments is particularly evident when an "antisocial" member of one culture or social class is evaluated by a member of a culture with different mores. A young, lower-class Okinawan woman may see nothing wrong with prostitution that permits her to support herself and her family, although the chaplain of the American Army post on that island condemns her behavior and calls her antisocial. We do not, however, clearly know in terms of psychological makeup, whether such a woman differs from her Western colleagues. Social class undoubtedly influences our classifications and descriptions. The range of impulse disorders from the neurotic to the sociopathic is wide; pathological liars, given to childish senseless and fantastic lies, often have marked hysterical traits. The "instinctual" roots of the lies are unmistakable. Many persons well situated in stable social roles and professional groups show in their character problems a large "component" of sociopathic disregard for bonds and feelings; their behavior, although legal, is hardly covertly social.

Although clear demarcation from what is ordinarily called neurotic and psychotic behavior is often not possible, we note certain more or less typical traits of asocial personalities. Such individuals are immature; they cannot postpone or inhibit their impulsive behavior. Although they may be intelligent, they have not learned to consider the consequences of their acts. Their relationships with other persons are typically shallow, and they do not enter into lasting associations. They are disinclined to assume responsibility, or assuming it, are irresponsible in conduct. Their acts are provocative and either very aggressive or extremely passive; their sexual behavior is infantile and often "polymorphous-perverse." Seemingly, they do not learn; neither ordinary rewards nor punishments affect them. In working intensively with sociopaths, one often is impressed that they unconsciously seek punishment and are stimulated by punishment. In some cases, such punishment is incarceration and is sought because it protects them. Hervey M. Cleckley,[14] and others have pointed out the proximity of this sociopathic group to psychotics. Unlike psychotics, the asocial personalities retain contact with reality, yet their hold on reality may be quite tenuous. We have observed that families may have both psychotic and sociopathic members; though as yet we do not clearly appreciate how and when these links occur, our impression is that, for some persons, sociopathic and "action" traits "ward off" hallucinatory and delusional symptomatology. In the group of pathological liars, for instance, it is clear that, at times, their lies serve opportunistic and fraudulent purposes; at other times, their lies are utterly fantastic and express only preconscious strivings and conflicts. It has often been said that this group makes others suffer while they themselves, in contrast to neurotics, do not suffer. The confidence man, and indeed many charming scoundrels with an ability to overlook inhibitions and normal reticence, and an inability to feel real bonds, irresponsibly stirring the passions and bypassing the inhibitions of others, leave havoc in their wake. Every psychiatric hospital administrator knows he must watch the balance of diagnostic entities on a ward, for one or two sociopaths too many leads to chaos. Therapeutic communities composed of sociopaths, however, may be successful.

Habitual criminals fall into the group of sociopaths. Since the pioneering work of August Aichorn,[4] and William Healy and Augusta F. Bronner,[41] psychiatrists, together with psychologists and sociologists, have concerned themselves with the psychological and social causes of crime and have made contributions to the understanding of the complex and extremely varied behavior of adult and juvenile delinquents. Obeying the existing demands of courts of law, psychiatrists have, until recently, considered only whether or not criminals suffer from major psychiatric disorders. Many crimes undoubtedly are committed by schizophrenics, epileptics, and patients with organic disorders, but most criminal offenders do not fall into these diagnostic categories. We know, today, that many habitual delinquents are arrested in their development and that most varieties of delinquent behavior are specifically learned in unfavorable psychosocial settings. Seduction, pronounced inconsistency in upbringing, harsh punishment alternating with overindulgence, a real or imaginary tort, and incessant attempts to remedy this tort are elements that recur in the histories of delinquents.[19] Studies of the motivations and psychosocial backgrounds of different types of criminals, such as aggressive, sexual and possessive offenders, are just beginning to appear.[25] Erik H. Erikson developed the useful concept of a malignant identity diffusion,[21] in speaking of youngsters without proper models for constructive identification, who are pushed to identify with models that they find in disapproved subcultures. However, since juveniles as well as adult sociopaths undoubtedly constitute various distinct subgroups, our current psychodynamic formulations should not be overgeneralized.

Psychiatrists have been only dimly aware of the social conditions that facilitate, but do not solely determine, the genesis of criminal behavior. They are more inclined to search for the specific experiences that produce sociopathic behavior. The work of Sheldon and Eleanor Glueck and of other experts highlights the importance of the social environment, where a different set of rules of conduct is established and where delinquent behavior is learned and rewarded.[38] Sociologists have also stressed that deviant behavior is the result of expectations that are not matched by opportunities. Sociologists, following Émile Durkheim's theory, emphasized that crime is related to normlessness or *anomie*, a very broad concept concerning psychosocial isolation, which has been used to explain many forms of abnormal behavior.[17] The majority of criminals in all societies is found in the lowest social class, where opportunities for normal and orderly development are scarce. In the New Haven studies, the highest concentration of sociopaths (defined, of course, by upper-class psychiatrists) was found in the lowest social status positions.

Older theories, for example, that sociopathic behavior was solely constitutionally determined and that sociopaths have definite somatic stigmata, have not been verified. The study of patients with such specific diseases as epilepsy, hypoglycemic states, and organic and functional behavior disorders who have committed crimes teaches us relatively little about the fundamental nature of crime. It is difficult for experts on behavior to free themselves from the values of their culture and dispassionately investigate these problems, which lack the conventional signs of "illness."

Aichorn has shown that the very heterogeneous group of juvenile sociopaths can be approached therapeutically and that gifted and persistent therapists can help even some of the very difficult cases.[4] To underestimate the difficulties, provocations, and disappointments of such an endeavor would be foolish. The initial step is to gain the confidence of a patient who has never trusted anybody and may be unbelievably cynical. Later, it may be possible to demonstrate to the patient the self-defeating nature of his behavior and induce him slowly and patiently to accept new models and identities and to replace impulsive acting out with more considered actions and thoughts. Such therapy has been carried out successfully, particularly with groups in prisons and in special institutions and schools for juvenile offenders.[45] With such sociopaths, particularly those confined to reform schools and prisons, group therapy is probably the most effective approach a psychiatrist can employ. Lawyers, criminologists, and penologists are gradually becoming cognizant of such interventions.

Sociopathic Personality

In this patient's first contact with a psychiatrist he complained of "compulsive gambling," which, he said, became a problem when he married fifteen years earlier and was now ruining his life. His wife was about to leave him; his parents and brothers were "furious"; and he "wanted to get straightened out once and for all."

He was a cheerful, ruddy, fat little man of thirty-six whose charm immediately made him well liked by both patients and staff. He had a gift for caricature and mimicry and often disrupted therapy by gently lampooning a fellow patient or his therapist.

His Italian parents had immigrated to this country before the birth of their six children. The oldest, a girl, married when the patient was eight. The five boys grew up together, and the patient, who was the youngest, saw himself as the clown: "No matter how bad things got, I could always get a laugh." His father got up at three o'clock every morning to open the family grocery stand. The boys would work at the fruit stalls until time for school. The patient early began to steal from the store or from his father's clothes and, at the age of eight, was playing "craps" in the alley behind their home with stolen money.

He had always felt that he was his mother's favorite, but he resented her "because she always treats me like a little kid." He remembered his mother's awe at the large sums of money exchanged by gamblers in the neighborhood bookie parlor. He saw his father as stable and stupid, "a working stiff" who never had enough money for his wife or anything else. The father did beat him occasionally for stealing, but he felt that his father "never had the guts" to discipline him as he deserved. No matter how angry his father got, his mother could always bring him around. On several occasions, the patient ran away from home, but was always welcomed back and forgiven.

He was one of the youngest members of several loose gangs and neighborhood ball teams, but he formed no consistent alliances. An exceptionally good baseball player, he was restored to the parish team as often as he was dismissed for "clowning." Similarly, he was repeatedly readmitted to school in spite of chronic delinquency (fights, thefts, fire-setting) because he was charming and quick-witted. He said that he never needed to do any homework in order to "snow" his teachers, and he maintained better-than-average grades. All his brothers finished high school and the oldest became a dentist. The patient wanted to "make lots of money" and did enough desultory schoolwork to get through two years of college.

In the fall of his junior year, he awoke one morning late for class and decided that marriage would give him the stability he needed. He packed and left college to marry a girl for whom he felt sorry because she was a patient in a tuberculosis sanitarium—where she remained for the first fourteen months of their marriage. He worked sporadically, but gambled constantly and was again bailed out of difficulty by his family. He referred to gambling as "The Fantastic" and "Ecstasy." He said that he felt transformed when at the race track: "Nothing else matters as long as I'm out there."

After three years of marriage, his wife had a complicated delivery and he "nearly cracked up." He felt that he had almost killed her and that this proved that their life together was hopelessly jinxed. When she became pregnant for the second time, he rapidly amassed several thousand dollars of gambling debts and fled to Cleveland, hiding there during the next nine months. He attempted to promote popular records and had some spectacular flops; on one occasion, he hired a full bill of nationally known entertainers, rented a fourteen thousand-seat auditorium, and then was able to sell only two hundred tickets.

His wife found him one year later, but they have been repeatedly and turbulently separated since that time. They have four children, debts of "more than $50,000," and "more enemies than the Pope." All of his relatives and in-laws had paid off threatening bookies, or lent the patient "a last stake" and gradually abandoned him; the father would not allow his name to be mentioned in the home. Nonetheless, at the time of the patient's hospitalization, the father reopened his fruit stand, although he was seventy years old and retired, to pay off the bad checks and "save the family name."

The first hospitalization lasted less than a week because the police located and arrested him for forging checks. Within a few days he reappeared, having persuaded the court that he wanted to reform. He had been given a suspended sentence of four months after his father had promised to make good the checks.

There were many instances of misbehavior: he forged checks and went on alcoholic binges. During his wife's visits he twice disappeared from the ward and had intercourse with girl friends in a car on the hospital lot. With the expiration of his suspended sentence, his misdemeanors seemed to taper off. He frankly discussed his relationship with his therapist and spent long periods talking about his efforts to get other people interested in him. He spoke of himself as "a 205-pound prick" and saw most of his behavior as exhibitionistic efforts to impress people. As he began to work on this material in therapy, he became increasingly depressed.

Early in treatment, it was noted that his superstitions had been extreme, but he always seemed bemused and embarrassed at his own gambler's mythology. Gradually, he began to talk of God's influence or his wife's jinx with increasing anxiety; he complained of constant "crazy thoughts" and began to suspect the staff of eavesdropping on his therapy hours. The jokes and superstitions of his earlier badinage became delusions. As he continued to examine his immediate behavior, he talked of Abraham and Isaac and villains from Italian opera in a loose context, and began to think of murder and suicide as "the solution."

During one hour, he rather frantically confessed that he had once robbed a blind man and raped a cripple; he insisted that he was trying to be "perfectly honest" and yet was continually tormented by wild thoughts. He said he was sure that his therapist hated him and that there was no hope. He then became highly agitated and had to be transferred to a locked ward. Following this episode, he rapidly regained his poise. His wife agreed to take him back and with some hazy plans for moving to a new town and starting over, he was, though moderately depressed, discharged from the hospital, ending his therapy.

During the two years following, he was twice briefly committed to another hospital for depressive episodes but rapidly recovered and returned to his wife. We last saw him when he had collected court summonses for forgery in five counties and was, somewhat cheerfully, expecting to go to jail "for a long, long time."

Traumatic Neuroses

The term, traumatic neuroses, refers to acute and chronic maladaptive behavior following psychological trauma that produces intense anxiety in a previously well-functioning person. The traumatic incident may involve physical injury, but this is not a necessary condition for the development of traumatic neurosis. However, injury to the traumatized person or to others, illness, or extreme exhaustion may substantially increase the impact of the trauma. Whether the inability to escape is an additional factor in the genesis of a traumatic neurosis is not certain. Roy R. Grinker and John P. Spiegel, who studied and treated intensively soldiers with traumatic reactions after combat, so-called combat exhaustion, feel that the reactions in war and in civilian life are essentially the same.[40] There are wide individual differences in the ability to withstand stress, but everyone has his breaking point. One may distinguish an acute phase, a subacute phase, and a chronic phase.[48] Military physicians and combat psychiatrists also learned to recognize prodromal symptoms preceding combat exhaustion: poor appetite, insomnia, headaches, unusual fatigue, restlessness and apathy, and a careless, inadequate performance. In the *acute phase*, the person reacts with intense anxiety. The anxiety may be consciously experienced and manifest itself by its usual physical concomitants; it is often accompanied by impotent rage, which probably is an important causal element in the chain of reactions leading to a traumatic neurosis. The most frequent manifestation, when escape is impossible, is a stuporous reaction, a freezing of the organism, almost like sham death; random and disorganized attempts to struggle against the threat may also occur. In general, overt reactions of rage and anxiety seem more adaptive, and the prognosis for recovery is better when the traumatized person has been able to fight or "blow off steam." In the *subacute phase*, the patient seemingly is trying to master the overwhelming event; to this end, a variety of available defenses, for example, repression, denial, projection, are observed. The universal phenomenon during this time, while awake and asleep, is a repetitive attempt to master the trauma by re-experiencing it in frightening dreams and in vivid flashes. In the *chronic phase*, the patient who has not been successful in mastering the stressful experience slips, as Abram Kardiner pointed out, into a parasite existence.[48] Rado interpreted the anxiety and hysterical symptoms of this phase as attempts to elicit pity.[59] When secondary advantages, such as pension or insurance payments, are in the foreground, we speak of *compensation neuroses*; when the reactions follow illness, we speak of *invalidism*. During the chronic phase, the patient is dependent and helpless. If dependency was a marked trait before the trauma, the chances for the development of chronic reactions are greatly heightened. If the patient's dependent and narcissistic needs are not gratified, he may develop a characteristic clinging and clawing hostility. These reactions are not conscious; pure malingering or conscious exaggerations are rare. Karl A. Menninger and others have drawn attention to an aggressive and self-destructive type of personality that is accident-prone.[57]

In dealing with traumatic neuroses, the goal of treatment is to prevent the patient from reaching the chronic stage. The essence of the technique used by the military is not to reward the patient for withdrawal from activity by discharging him or reassigning him to the noncombat duty, but to keep him in his natural environment and help him to master his tasks and not to escape into invalidism. The important implications of such an orientation for military psychiatry will be considered in Chapter 25. The recurrent, repetitive nature of the traumatic neurosis is interpreted as a recurrent attempt to master overwhelming input (flooding of the "stimulus barriers") and failure to master provokes ever new attempts to do so; prompt treatment tends to provide a way to "put the trauma in its place." The persistence of a wide variety of neurotic symptoms in adults may, according to some analysts, derive from the traumatic quality of infantile neuroses, leaving areas of function which the patient repetitively attempts to master—but with the inefficient techniques of the young child. The old saw about an ounce of prevention applies well to traumatic neuroses. In spite of the new discoveries of dynamic psychiatry, many patients with traumatic neuroses have become the chronic "beneficiaries" of insurance agencies, of welfare and medical institutions and particularly of veterans' hospitals. The task of understanding and treating traumatic neurotic behavior as well as neurotic behavior in general is still far from being solved.

NOTES

1. Karl Abraham, "Restrictions and Transformation of Scoptophobia in Neuroses," in *Selected Papers* (London: Hogarth Press, 1926).
2. Alfred A. Adler, *Study of Organ Inferiority and its Psychical Compensation* (New York: Nervous and Mental Disease Publishing Co., 1917).
3. Alfred A. Adler, *Über den nervösen Charakter* (München: J. F. Bergmann, 1928).
4. August Aichorn, *Wayward Youth* (New York: Viking Press, 1935).
5. Jacob A. Arlow, "The Structure of the *Déjà Vu* Experience," *Journal of the American Psychoanalytic Association,* 7 (1960), 611.
6. Gregory Bateson and Margaret Mead, *Balinese Character* (New York: New York Academy of Sciences, 1942).
7. Edmund Bergler, "The Gambler, a Misunderstood Neurotic," *Journal of Criminal Psychopathology,* 4 (1943), 379.
8. Irving Bieber, *Homosexuality* (New York: Basic Books, 1962).
9. John Bowlby, *Maternal Care and Mental Health* ("W.H.O. Monograph Series, No. 2," [Geneva: World Health Organization, 1951]).
10. Josef Breuer and Sigmund Freud, *Studies on Hysteria* (New York: Basic Books, 1957).
11. Jean Martin Charcot, *Leçons du Mardi à la Salpétrière* (Paris: La Bataille, 1892).
12. Gerard Chrzanowski, "Neurasthenia and Hypochondriasis," in S. Arieti, ed., *American Handbook of Psychiatry* (New York: Basic Books, 1959), Vol. I, pp. 258–271.

13. H. Christoffel, "Male Genital Exhibitionism," in Sandor Lorand and Michael Balint, eds., *Perversions Psychodynamics and Therapy* (New York: Random House, 1956).
14. Hervey M. Cleckley, *The Mask of Sanity* (St. Louis: Mosby, 1955).
15. William Cullen, *First Lines of the Practice of the Physic* (3rd ed.; Edinburgh: Wm. Creech, 1781).
16. John Dollard and Neal E. Miller, *Personality and Psychotherapy* (New York: McGraw-Hill, 1950).
17. Émile Durkheim, *Suicide: A Study in Sociology,* translated by John A. Spaulding and George Simpson (Glencoe, Ill.: The Free Press, 1960).
18. Ludwig Eidelberg, "An Introduction to the Study of Narcissistic Mortification," *Psychiatric Quarterly,* 31 (1957), 657.
19. Kurt R. Eissler, ed., *Searchlights on Delinquency* (New York: International Universities Press, 1949).
20. Erik H. Erikson, "Identity and the Life Cycle: Selected Papers," *Psychological Issues,* Vol. I, No. 1 (New York: International Universities Press, 1959).
21. Erik H. Erikson, "The First Psychoanalyst," *Yale Review,* 46 (1962), 40.
22. Paul Errera and Jules V. Coleman, "A Long-Term Follow-Up Study of Neurotic Phobic Patients in a Psychiatric Clinic," *Journal of Nervous and Mental Disease,* 136 (1963), 267.
23. Otto Fenichel, *The Psychoanalytic Theory of Neuroses* (New York: Norton, 1945).
24. Clellan S. Ford and Frank A. Beach, *Patterns of Sexual Behavior* (New York: Harper, 1951).
25. Lawrence Z. Freedman, "Sexual, Aggressive and Acquisitive Deviates," *Journal of Nervous and Mental Disease,* 132 (1961), 44.
26. Sigmund Freud, *Three Essays on the Theory of Sexuality* [1905] in *Standard Edition,* Vol. 7 (London: Hogarth Press, 1956).
27. Sigmund Freud, "On Narcissism: An Introduction" [1914], in *Standard Edition,* Vol. 14 (London: Hogarth Press, 1957).
28. Sigmund Freud, "The Economic Principle of Masochism" [1924], in *Standard Edition,* Vol. 19 (London: Hogarth Press, 1961).
29. Sigmund Freud, "Character and Anal Eroticism" [1908], in *Standard Edition,* Vol. 9 (London: Hogarth Press, 1959).
30. Sigmund Freud, "Notes upon a Case of Obsessional Neurosis" [1909], in *Standard Edition,* Vol. 10 (London: Hogarth Press, 1955).
31. Sigmund Freud, "The Analysis of a Phobia in a Five-Year-Old Boy" [1909], in *Standard Edition,* Vol. 10 (London: Hogarth Press, 1955).
32. Sigmund Freud, "A General Introduction to Psychoanalysis" [1916–1917], in *Standard Edition* (London: Hogarth Press, 1955), 15–16.
33. Sigmund Freud, "The Ego and the Id" [1923], in *Standard Edition* (London: Hogarth Press, 1961), 19.
34. Sigmund Freud, "Inhibitions, Symptoms and Anxiety" [1926], in *Standard Edition* (London: Hogarth Press, 1959), 20.

35. Sigmund Freud, "Psychoanalysis Terminable and Interminable" [1937], in *Standard Edition* (London: Hogarth Press, 1961), 23.
36. M. Friedman "Cleptomania: The Analytic and Forensic Aspects," *Psychoanalytic Review*, 17 (1930), 452.
37. Sigbert Joseph Maria Ganser, "Über einen eigenartigen hysterischen Dämmerzustand," *Arch. Psychiat.*, 30 (1898), 633.
38. Sheldon Glueck and Eleanor Glueck, *Unraveling Juvenile Delinquency* (New York: Commonwealth Fund, 1950).
39. Roy R. Grinker, S. H. Korchin, H. Basowitz, R. A. Hamburg, Melvin Sabshin, H. Persky, J. A. Chevalier, and F. A. Board, "A Theoretical and Exploratory Approach to Problems of Anxiety," in Jules H. Masserman and Jacob L. Moreno, eds., *Progress in Psychotherapy* (New York: Grune and Stratton, 1957).
40. Roy R. Grinker and John P. Spiegel, *Men under Stress* (New York: Blakiston, 1945).
41. William Healy and Augusta F. Bonner, *New Light on Delinquency and Its Treatment* (New Haven: Yale University Press, 1936).
42. August B. Hollingshead and Fredrick C. Redlich, *Social Class and Mental Illness* (New York: John Wiley, 1958).
43. Edith Jacobson, "Depersonalization," *Journal of the American Psychoanalytic Association*, 7 (1959), 581.
44. Maxwell S. Jones *et al.*, *The Therapeutic Community: A New Treatment Method in Psychiatry* (New York: Basic Books, 1953).
45. Eugen Kahn, *Psychopathic Personalities* (New Haven: Yale University Press, 1931).
46. Eugen Kahn and L. H. Cohen, "Organic Drivenness, a Brain-stem Syndrome and an Experience" *New England Journal of Medicine*, 210 (1934), 748.
47. Franz J. Kallmann, *Heredity in Health and Mental Disorder* (New York: Norton, 1953).
48. Abram Kardiner, *The Traumatic Neuroses of War* (Menasha, Wisc.: G. Bonta Publishing Co., 1941).
49. Alfred C. Kinsey, Wardell B. Pomeroy, and Clyde E. Martin, *Sexual Behavior in the Human Male* (Philadelphia: Saunders, 1948).
50. Alfred C. Kinsey, Wardell B. Pomeroy, Clyde E. Martin, and Paul H. Gebhard, *Sexual Behavior in the Human Female* (Philadelphia: Saunders, 1953).
51. Lawrence S. Kubie, "The Experimental Induction of Neurotic Reactions in Man," *Yale Journal of Biology and Medicine*, 11 (1939), 541.
52. Lawrence S. Kubie, "The Neurotic Potential, the Neurotic Process and the Neurotic State," *U. S. Armed Forces Medical Journal*, 2 (1951), 1.
53. Seymour Levine, "The Effects of Infantile Experience on Adult Behavior," in Arthur J. Bachrach, ed., *Experimental Foundations of Clinical Psychology* (New York: Basic Books, 1962).
54. Frank A. Logan, *Incentive: How the Conditions of Reinforcement Affect the Performance of Rats* (New Haven: Yale University Press, 1960).

55. Sandor Lorand, "Fetischismus in Statu Nascendi," *Internationale Zeitschrift für Psychoanalyse*, 16 (1930), 87.

56. Konrad Lorenz, *Über die Natur des Bösen* (Wien: Borota Verlag, 1963).

57. Karl A. Menninger, "Purposive Accidents as an Expression of Self-Destructive Tendencies," *International Journal of Psycho-Analysis*, 17 (1936), 6.

58. Chester M. Pierce and Harry H. Lipcon, "Somnambulism," *U. S. Armed Forces Medical Journal*, 7 (1956), 1143.

59. Sandor Rado, "Pathodynamics and Treatment of Traumatic War Neurosis," *Psychosomatic Medicine*, 4 (1942), 362.

60. Sandor Rado, "Obsessive Behavior," in Silvano Arieti, ed., *American Handbook of Psychiatry*, Vol. I (New York: Basic Books, 1959).

61. Leo Rangell, "The Nature of Conversion," *Journal of the American Psychoanalytic Association*, 7 (1960), 632.

62. Otto Rank, "Die Don Juan-Gestalt," *Imago*, 8 (1922), 142.

63. Wilhelm Reich, *Character Analysis* (New York: Noonday Press, 1949).

64. Jurgen Ruesch, "The Infantile Personality," *Psychosomatic Medicine*, 10 (1948), 134.

65. Jurgen Ruesch, *Disturbed Communication* (New York: Norton, 1957).

66. Stanley Schachter, "The Interaction of Cognitive and Physiological Determinants of Emotional State," in Leonard Berkowitz, ed., *Advances in Experimental and Social Psychology*, Vol. I, p. 89 (New York: Academic Press, 1964).

67. Paul Schilder, "Concept of Hysteria," *American Journal of Psychiatry*, 95 (1939), 1389.

68. John Paul Scott and John L. Fuller, *Genetics and the Social Behavior of the Dog* (Chicago: University of Chicago Press, 1965).

69. Michael Shepherd and E. M. Gruenberg, "Neurosis," *Milbank Memorial Fund Quarterly*, 35, No. 3 (July, 1957), 258.

70. Leo Srole, Thomas S. Langner, Stanley T. Michael, Marvin K. Opler, and Thomas A. C. Rennie, *Mental Health in the Metropolis* (New York: McGraw-Hill, 1962), 1.

71. Ian P Stevenson, "Processes of 'Spontaneous Recovery' from the Psychoneuroses," *American Journal of Psychiatry*, 117 (1961), 1057.

72. Thomas S. Szasz, "Language and Pain," in Silvano Arieti, ed., *American Handbook of Psychiatry* (New York: Basic Books, 1959), Vol. I, 982–999.

73. Robert Waelder, "The Principle of Multiple Function," *Psychoanalytic Quarterly*, 5 (1936), 45.

74. Robert Waelder, *Basic Theory of Psychoanalysis* (New York: International Universities Press, 1960).

75. Edwin A. Weinstein and Robert L. Kahn, *Denial of Illness* (Springfield, Ill.: Charles C Thomas, 1955).

76. Allen Wheelis, *The Quest for Identity* (New York: Norton, 1958).

CHAPTER THIRTEEN

The Psychosomatic Diseases

General Reflections

The term psychosomatic has many, perhaps too many, meanings. Psychosomatic diseases may be loosely referred to as a group of somatic diseases of unknown etiology in which psychological factors play a variably important role and one that is supposed to be greater than in diseases in general. Often chronic and relapsing, disorders such as asthma, hypertension, peptic ulcer, and ulcerative colitis are related to stress and to personality organization in complex ways. Frequently, emotions are correlated with exacerbation of symptoms and occasionally with relief; but clear-cut etiological relationships between behavior and disease have not been demonstrated, nor do all individuals with these diseases show significant behavioral disturbances. Yet, an impressive number do, and recent work has indicated that, within limits, the degree of personality disorganization in persons with asthma or ulcerative colitis is correlated with the severity of somatic pathology.[35, 74] Not only tissue change, but changes in heart rate, blood pressure, and other physiologic concomitants of stressful emotional states are frequently thought of when the term psychosomatic is used. Nevertheless, such conditions as enduring impotence, tics, or stuttering are also "psychosomatic" reactions; such dysfunctions may involve psychodynamic mechanisms encountered in neurotic symptom-formation. For convenience, all these dysfunctions may be discussed under the rubric of psychosomatic disorders. The related term, "comprehensive medicine," emphasizes the fact that emotional and social factors are of importance in diagnostic and therapeutic decision-making in all aspects of medical and surgical practice. The principles involved are taken up in Chapter 25.

Pioneers in psychosomatic medicine were such European clinicians as Felix Deutsch, Victor von Weizsäcker, and Erich Wittkower, but psychosomatic medicine's foremost development occurred in the United States. However, there are notable workers in other countries, such as the late K. M. Bykov and his student E. S. Airepetianc in the Soviet Union, J. L. Halladay in Great Britain, and Arthur Jores, Alexander Mitscherlich, and Thure Uexküll in Germany.

Psychosomatic medicine, then, may best be viewed simply as an approach in which the focus is on the exploration of the relationship between emotional and bodily symptoms. This relationship should not be thought of as implying psychogenesis of somatic disease nor be viewed in a static or unidirectional sense. Chronic diseases, for example, have emotional consequences, which may in turn influence the course of these diseases; if one has a passion for labels, one could speak of "somatopsychic" sequences. Theodore Lidz cautioned that the term "psychosomatic" should not be used as a euphemism to obscure the presence of clear-cut neurotic conflicts;[86] nor need it connote a soul mysteriously acting upon matter. Yet, even those who are offended by a dualistic concept must accept Alexander Mitscherlich's teaching that the therapies of severe psychosomatic diseases invariably are dualistic.

Three trends that account for the present thinking and directions of psychosomatic medicine can be identified. Some time ago, internists began to realize that psychological factors could be looked at systematically. Second, research tools were developed both for physiologic and for behavioral processes, internists and psychiatrists began to exchange ideas. Third, psychoanalytically oriented psychiatrists were stimulated by ego psychology, which provided a framework in which regulatory mechanisms and adaptation were of central importance. These lines, converging in the founding of the American Psychosomatic Society in 1939, were described by Bernard Bandler[7] as the "beachhead" that dynamic psychiatry established in general medicine. It was important that clinical investigators would begin to conceive of the organism as coordinating numerous regulations *both* of psychologic and physiologic functioning. A response to stress could discoordinate normal regulations, upsetting the balance among subsystems, and this would become evident either in mental symptoms or disordered bodily function, or both.

Basic Considerations: Neurobehavioral Mechanisms

Pavlov's demonstration that visceral responses can be conditioned and that viscera may be selectively responsive to discrete stimuli provides the fundamental demonstration of a link between bodily and behavioral events.[27] This supports the broad view that organs respond to environmental input and to memories, images, and wishes. The crucial puzzles about details and mechanisms remain;[118] how are specific organ systems conditioned, and how do they "escape" from "inhibitory" control? Direct conscious control of most autonomically innervated organs is not possible. For example, localized brain "centers" for *discrete* regulation of the bronchiolar lumen (analagous to discrete flexion and extension of somatic muscles) are not demonstrable. How, then, do such organs become integrated into complex behavioral transactions? How does the yogi "learn" to control his heart rate? How does hypnotic suggestion produce blisters? Apart from local and peripheral neurohumoral regulations, how, and to what extent, do central processes govern (or cease to govern) autonomically innervated organs? If focal centers for discrete and direct (rather than generalized) visceral control are largely lacking, then some central integrative activity of the various component systems must be required. Are functional brain "centers" patterned and acquired through a cycle of peripheral and central reactions? If so, a stress acting centrally could eventually directly activate a sensitized segment of the vasculature or bowel. Does excitement affect such central control? Are constitutional and genetic factors involved, so that one rather than another organ represents the "weak link," perhaps acting as a predisposed focus to be triggered by the general effects of a future stress? We do know that functional differentiations involving subcortical systems occur throughout development; for example, the gastrocolic reflex present at birth soon differentiates so that the infant can eat at one time and defecate at another. Thus, learning and differentiation of visceral adjustments occur early in development;[121] preferential response systems are developed on the basis of experience, hormonal patterns, and neuroendocrine interactions, as well as "constitution." The group at Fels Institute, for example, studied longitudinal and developmental aspects of individual patterns of psychophysiological response,[80] and other workers focused on longitudinal studies of specific endocrine patterns in the individual. Yet, how are such patterns linked to disturbed behavior? Do the early patterns of autonomic function really emerge with psychological regression (in the same sense that more primitive neuromuscular patterns emerge following brain injury)? Finally, what are the *specific* component systems (biochemical, endocrine, neuronal, and so forth) involved in any one psychophysiological sequence of events? These and other problems explicitly or implicitly underlie viewpoints advanced in the area of psychosomatic disease. We have no firm answers to these questions, which are crucial for a basic biological understanding of clinical sequences. Much of our recent attention has been focused on discovering basic neural and humoral regulations rather than on the study of their significance for behavior and disease.

Brain and Viscera

One way to ask questions about these links is to focus on brain-visceral functions. A. G. Langley, around 1900, connected the "autonomous" peripheral autonomic system to the spinal cord. The later work of Philip Bard, Walter B. Cannon, and others extended this link to the cortex and hypothalamus and to behavioral and physical regulations, which now include among others, complex neural-pituitary-adrenal or gonadal-neural feedback sequences. It was Cannon's[28] description of emergency behaviors of fight and flight that demonstrated that sympathetic systems were integrated into the defensive and coping behavior of the organism. Yet, in view of newer detailed knowledge of the families of bioactive amines, their selective distribution in brain and their neuromuscular and metabolic feedbacks, broad generalizations about the behavioral significance of the various neurohumoral and autonomic systems are precarious. Current research has been occupied with detailed sequences, which undoubtedly will provide the basis for future links of neurochemical systems with significant behavior patterns. There is, of course, no question that anatomically and chemically differentiated central nuclei and neural systems (from the medulla to the hypothalamus and the surrounding limbic system) *could* be critically involved in psychosomatic diseases. Stimulation and ablation of components of these systems have produced: gastric ulcerations (not identical with the clinical variety); specific changes in nitrogen balance and endocrine output;[101] the induction of hepatic enzyme systems;[77] spasms of the gastrointestinal and other smooth muscle; pulmonary edema[97] and cardiac arhythmia;[14] and changes in blood volume and renal excretory patterns.

Speculation on the role of brain mechanisms in psychosomatic disorders centers on the function not only of hypothalamic nuclei but that of activating systems and the limbic system. The latter is thought to regulate patterned visceral and neuroendocrine response, to mediate perception of crude feeling as well as an array of viscerally linked behavioral patterns including oral behaviors (mouthing, biting, eating) and sexual, aggressive, and avoidance behaviors. Paul D. MacLean[93] broadly relates these sets of behaviors to preservation of the species and the self. Links between the highly differentiated nuclei of the hypothalamus and the amygdala have been of special interest, and the function of the phylogenetically old limbic cortex may be to integrate the component sequences controlled by these specialized nuclei. MacLean on many grounds (including cytoarchitecture) speculates that the limbic structures analyze inputs in terms of their visceral and affective significance for primitive action. Immediate and sensory qualities as well as intensities of input, rather than sequentially ordered adaptations in space and time, are subserved; smell, for example, may differentially guide the behaviors of lower animals.

Vulnerability to confusion between internal input (or visceral "feelings") and external input is built into the nervous system at this and at lower levels.[51] MacLean notes that inputs from the environment are registered in the responses *both* of the limbic system and the neocortex; environmental events can thus either be cognized or be "interpreted" and felt and responded to as if they were "gut" processes. There are many clinical examples of such confusion; George L. Engel and Franz Reichsman,[48] for example, observed that in an infant with a gastric fistula, the stomach reacted to the appearance of the child's favorite doctor as if he were food. Patients often refer to worries or persons as being inside them and eating them up; they "chew over" a problem and "swallow pride." At some levels, these metaphors may have concrete meaning and vividness for the patient, and this may be based on the arrangement of underlying neural systems. For example, lesions of the amygdala may produce stupidly fearless animals that indiscriminately mouth the environment (bolts, feces), or stimulation may produce components of attack or sexual behavior. In man, stimulation may be followed by visceral hallucinations and compulsive sexual thoughts and feelings as well as physiological responses; in psychomotor epilepsy, the automatisms and illusions are referred to lesions in deep temporal lobe structures. The notion is that in some disorders dissociations between the old and new brain could occur; activation of visceral systems could then persist without check or restraint and thus be linked to disease states.

Limbic systems organize some component sequences of primitive bodily functions; they are brought into play by activating systems that are influenced by a confluence of internally and externally directed processes. Autonomic input and autonomic "centers" of the brain are anatomically and functionally linked not only with motor mechanisms but with the electrical, physiological, and behavioral activating systems of the brain (which facts should temper overly artificial divisions of behavior into "autonomic" and "voluntary"). These activating systems are involved with intensity in behavior, both in the sense of "triggering" response and modifying the magnitude of response. They provide a link between alertness and the psychophysiological implements of awareness, such as muscle tone and reactivity. Physiological concomitants of activation are the psychogalvanic response, palmar conductance, change in local blood volume and various sets of muscle potentials, shifts in alpha amplitude and frequencies recorded from scalp electrodes; and shifts of pulse rate. Of course, a single peripheral measure alone does not indicate the presence of stress; a low heart rate may be observed with inactivity or with hyperactivation. Activation is not an undifferentiated dimension of behavior; a variety of responses occur; for example, pulse rate differs according to whether one actively attends to mental or to environmental input. In psychophysiological measurements, the *law of initial values* applies so that the pre-existing levels of activity set the range over which subsequent responses can fluctuate.[145]

For different peripheral autonomic responses, there appears to be an optimal range of "activation" in which flexible adaptations can occur. For example, experimental asthma in guinea pigs is critically affected either by general excitation (overarousal) or by dampening of central activation (underarousal); animals who were deeply or very lightly anesthetized died with anaphylaxis, whereas animals in the midrange (or those with midbrain lesions) survived.[51] Thus, the general state or level of excitation, acting through complex component mechanisms, can determine whether wheezing is a passing episode or an epitaph. If peripheral disorders (a heart attack) lead to central overactivation, a number of uncontrolled regulations and secondary symptoms could ensue.

In summary, many observations suggest that activating systems can affect the regulation of bodily states. Control over the intricate neural subsystems, which, in sum, constitute the general arousal mechanism of the brain, evolves with development and requires integrated neocortical and subcortical interactions; a developmental vulnerability to maladaptive regulation and organ dysfunction could occur. In the most general sense, whatever the exact neuroendocrine and neurobehavioral mechanisms turn out to be, psychosomatic diseases appear to involve maladaptive dissociations of functions, subsystems operating without brakes and to the detriment of the total integrated activity of the organism. Responsive to local metabolic, peripheral vascular and chemical, as well as neural inputs, activating systems may provide a mechanism through which emotional intensities lead to unregulated activity of peripheral organs.

Behavior and Viscera

Measurement of the effects of stress on steroids, amines, and autonomically innervated organs require exquisite experimental control of behavior as well as sophisticated biochemical measures as indicated in the studies of the Walter Reed research group led by D. McK. Rioch, J. V. Brady, and J. W. Mason. For example, in studies of stress-induced ulcer, it was clear that stress consists of more than electric shock. An "executive" monkey who could work to avoid shock got the ulcer; his companion, who could do nothing about the schedule of shocks, did not.[21] Stress, therefore, must be defined in behavioral terms, but the link between stress and somatic reactions is complex. For example, the periodicity of shock-avoidance performance is critical to the production of ulcers; long continuous periods of shock-avoidance (eighteen hours on; six off) may not produce ulcers. In this case, an interaction of behavioral and biochemical regulations, each with its own periodicity leading to enhancement or inhibition of stress-induced changes, is suggested. Measurements of biochemical "rebound" phenomena showed quite different periods of elevated plasma pepsinogen levels and rates of gastric secretion occurring after cessation of shock;[117] this depended upon the duration and periodicity of stress as well as genetic or individual differences. It is, in fact, common to observe "after reactions" when a period of stress and coping is terminated; it is as if visceral subsystems do not "know" when to stop their hyper- or hypofunction.

Howard S. Liddell, in experiments with infant goats, showed not only that temporal parameters of shock differentially affected autonomic response but that the availability of "objects" (the mother goat) greatly modified stress.[84] Even more critical is the fact that the physiology of stress is not limited to the pituitary-adrenal system. As Cannon[28] noted, many experimentally induced stressful situations (producing fear and extreme inhibition) seem to involve an overactivation not only of peripheral sympathetic but also of parasympathetic discharge. Carl P. Richter produced an apparently vagus-mediated shock and death in wild rats by simply clipping their whiskers, which are critical for activation and orientation; such rats put into a tank do not exert effort and thereby drown.[122] The experimental syndrome of "giving-up" remains to be further investigated.

We are impressed not only with the role of conditioning but with temporal factors in stress and the organism's task of coordinating a gamut of regulations of component systems which can operate unchecked. The general role of arousal states of high intensity in the regulations of adaptive response is striking. Behavioral dyscontrol is also important; in some diseases (experimental ulcer and asthma), misdirected instrumental efforts to compensate for stress appear to be more damaging at the physiological level than the actual absence of effort. An animal in bronchospasm, who locates the source of air deprivation as external, aggravates the condition by useless attempts to remove the obstruction (and to no more avail than the overdependent human who denies his inner wishes by excessive activity). In view of the difficulty experimentalists have in specifically and precisely regulating and dampening visceral-motor responses, and in view of the integration of such responses into the totality of behaving, the search for mechanisms that protect or regulate bodily dysfunction would logically range from structuring activities at the psychological level to a more precise understanding of the neural and chemical controls of physiological regulations.

Basic Considerations: Clinical Observation and Theory

When psychosomatic disease and severe behavior disorder coexist, the disease is likely to have a poor prognosis and to be more refractory to treatment. The behavior disorder may have preceded, followed, or been concomitant with the onset of disease; occasionally, remarkable periodic alternations of a psychosis and symptoms of disease are observed. Most clinicians are impressed with the striking infantile attributes of many patients with psychosomatic disease. Marked dependency wishes, however, may be "encapsulated" or masked by an overcompensatory style of life adjustment; such patients may or may not show psychological regression under stress but are generally thought to express their persisting warded-off needs in organ dysfunction. When such regressive needs are built into the personality, they may at some point seriously restrict flexible adaptation. For example, an intense, disturbing attachment of a woman for her mother may not be evident until overt or covert abandonment occurs; this psychological trauma or conflict may then be followed by a thyroid crisis.[85] Many such clinical examples convince investigators that diseases are often manifestations of adaptational failure. In order to explain such phenomena, a number of theories of dubious biological validity and psychological reliability were elaborated and often generalized with an appalling lack (or unmanageable surplus) of supporting data; nevertheless, certain of these approaches deserve notice because they represent serious attempts to formulate relationships among a very complex range of phenomena.

Psychoanalytic Views

A general thesis underlying many points of view in American psychosomatic medicine obviously derives from Sigmund Freud. In Freud's theories, somatic events, through a hierarchy of restructuring processes, were translated into affects, ideas, and actions; energies could, by "conversion," be channeled back to "compliant" body systems—the "mysterious leap from mind to body" as Deutsch termed it.[38] Conversion symptoms are usually confined to processes which have, or can have, ideational content; a conflict has to be perceived to some extent, then repressed and later symbolically expressed in symptoms. For example, vomiting in a woman conflicted about wishes to perform fellatio is a dramatic symptom symbolically communicating an unconscious problem that can be made conscious by appropriate techniques. Vomiting may also be the concomitant of anxiety and tension; the organic expression of such tension in itself has no psychological meaning although it might tax the total economy of the organism. Both types of vomiting, according to Franz Alexander, would be manifestations of a "vegetative neurosis," [3] which may be the precursor of a psychosomatic disease.

How can an organ system become overresponsive? Some workers envisage a sequence of psychological events. Thus: persons with marked dependency needs regress; the wish for love unconsciously becomes a wish to be fed, and (since severe ego impairments presumably do not permit either direct adult satisfaction or neurotic symptom-formation) this persisting need becomes a chronic stimulus for gastric hyperactivity, which in itself accomplishes nothing for the patient. Other regressive chains of events could lead to particular unconscious wishes that activate their appropriate automatic "visceral concomitants." This view led Jurgen Ruesch and others to discern the general role of regressive wishes in psychosomatic disorders.[125, 126] Some workers speculated about physiological as well as psychological regression. What was sought were explanations of how intense regressive yearnings could lead to actual organ damage. Sidney Margolin argued that regression induced wide fluctuations in visceral activity and hence organ damage.[98] Thomas S. Szasz postulated that some individuals might have parasympathetic hyperactivity as a concomitant of regression; these individuals would be liable to asthma, peptic ulcer, and ulcerative colitis. For others the concomitant regression might be sympathetic hyperactivity, thus disposing them to hypertension or arthritis.[139] It should be noted that attempts to classify the range of symptoms by autonomic criteria are inherently difficult, since autonomic and somatic response are, in the central nervous system, intrinsically interlocked. "Autonomic" symptoms such as blushing or fainting may be hysterical, and symptoms such as coughing or vomiting involve an array of chemical, vestibular or vagal initiating "triggers" and, primarily, are a response of the somatic musculature of the upper trunk.

Other Approaches

Notable approaches to psychosomatic research have involved experimental or clinical exploration of objectively defined psychophysiological response to stress in humans. Stress has to be meaningful to individuals. It becomes meaningful in terms of inherited disposition, early conditioning, later life experiences, cultural stresses, and current life situation. Harold G. Wolff and his co-workers clearly demonstrated the interaction of these different factors. In some cases, they noted a summation effect of psychological and somatic causes; in allergic disorders, the effect of pollen was experimentally enhanced by the specific emotions of anger, fear, and resentment.[153] Characteristic affects, conflicts, and modes of solution were discerned in various disorders. Wolff was criticized by psychoanalytic investigators who felt that he did not sufficiently emphasize unconscious factors in the meaning of stress, but his work was usually clinically relevant and methodologically sound. We still need to know what basic behavioral patterns are linked to characteristic sets of bodily response. At what level of description can one sort out those "attitudes" which are linked with bodily adjustments? Are there fairly simple neurobehavioral "sets" or attitudes by which the organism copes and which are the true correlates of organ dysfunction? Basic coping attempts—riddance, avoidance, approach, hunger, aggression, trying or making an effort—are "sets" or attitudes with which (consciously or not) the organism engages the environment; frustration or enhancement of these attitudes is often evident with organ dysfunction. It is not at all apparent that the fine details of mental mechanisms will be as useful in understanding bodily and behavioral responses as are the simpler but specific over-all attitudes Wolff discerned.

The Problem of Specificity

In Alexander's view, the specific target-organ in a psychosomatic disease would depend upon specific regressive psychological needs and their appropriate biological expression. For example, in asthma, a psychological conflict about separation from the mother would activate the respiratory system rather than, for example, the gastric system.[3] (Alexander also reasoned that, since respiration represents the first separation and the first step toward independence, and, since crying represents a wish for reunion, the separation conflict of asthmatics was biologically expressed in a compromise in wheezing as a "suppressed cry.") In general, it was thought that if a persisting emotion were not contained through neurotic symptom-formation it could be linked to an "appropriate" organ system that would be overactivated and become diseased. As early as 1912, Alfred Adler had pointed to organ inferiority as a basis for the occurrence of a specific symptom.[2] Flanders Dunbar drew up profiles from her psychoanalytic interviews and assigned specific clusters of traits to each disease.[41] On the other hand, George L. Engel and co-workers proposed that unresolved loss and separation manifested by the affects of helplessness and hopelessness are the powerful and universal emotions that precede the onset of a wide variety of somatic reactions.[43, 44, 45, 46]

Some psychoanalysts refer to all psychosomatic conditions as "pregenital neuroses" because the pertinent psychological conflicts and solutions in such patients are apparently rooted in adaptations prior to the genital phase. Whereas these psychological theories about specific or general conflicts and disease may offer valuable clues to the clinician, I. A. Mirsky warned of the glib application of concepts such as regression to somatic symptoms.[108] It is questionable, for instance, whether the symptoms of ulcerative colitis may be considered an anal or oral condition, or whether such thinking helps to explain anything. Mirsky also challenged traditional medical models for the etiology of ulcers, pointing out that gastric hypersecretion occurs before, during, and after the healing of duodenal ulcers.[109] Similarly, one should be wary of the too facile translation of bodily symptoms into "organ language," colitis meaning, for example, a wish to defecate on one's enemies. Engel, in fact, showed that vascular and mucosal changes occur prior either to constipation or diarrhea.[45] Meticulous study of pathophysiological (as well as psychopathological) sequences is required before the expressive and communicative aspect of the symptom is given primary etiological significance. The end result of any disease—the way it is valued by patients and family—will inevitably have symbolic and psychological meaning and influence what ensues; but this must not be confounded with prior sequential processes, which may be quite differently determined. Deep regressions and a profoundly disturbed personality are, in fact, often observed in severe psychosomatic illness. Yet, this does not establish a prime cause; rather, it reflects the total psychophysiological maladaptation involved in the disease. Why it is that pregenital fixations should lead, in some cases, to schizophrenia or to affective behavior disorders; in others, to obsessive neuroses; and in still others, to psychosomatic diseases cannot be stated. The hard facts to back up such etiological assumptions are not known, the concrete clinical details elude crisp summary, and the proposed theoretical models are too broad to suggest the truly critical differentiating mechanisms.

Of course, any theory linking emotions with specific organs is limited since we do not know why, nor under what conditions, the vegetative symptoms of excessive or deficient autonomic function could be transformed into the more lasting structural changes of a psychosomatic disease. In fact, the presumed precursors to organic pathology, hyperemia of the gastric mucosa or labile hypertension, have *never* been directly observed to shift into organ pathology.[114] We must conclude that sustained or transient abuse of autonomically innervated organs is connected to structural somatic lesions more by empathy than by evidence. Correlations of altered brain or somatic function with symptoms can perhaps only be made with certain *components* of pathophysiological processes and not directly with the tissue change, organ dysfunction, or the clinical expression of symptoms.[52]

Simultaneous occurrence of several diseases in one patient militates also against the specificity theory; similarly, the clusters of psychological mechanisms by which specificity is defined constitute a monotonous repetition of similar problems (repressed rage, dependency) that are not convincingly specific. The simple assertion that the patient shows a passive-dependent attitude does not predict his patterns of problem-solving, relationships to specific persons, or coping mechanisms in specific crises. Yet it is still possible that specific patterns of impulses, coping mechanisms, and personality organization associated with psychosomatic disease will emerge. An approach that studies conditioning of interoceptive processes, which is linked to psychodynamic and developmental theories, and which is tested with modern descriptive and neurobehavioral techniques, appears promising. The task, one that clinical research always entails, is to move from broad views to tactics appropriate for research in order to rescue useful clinical observations from premature oblivion. After all, for centuries physicians and astute observers have noted that the way a person experiences and feels about his life and the way he is "built," or copes with his situations and feelings, influences the course of, or occasion for, medical illness. With modern concepts and skills, we should begin to clarify how and when such constitutional, developmental, behavioral, and adaptational factors play a specific or general role in organ dysfunction.

An important contribution to the problem of specificity has been made by Mirsky *et al.*, who found that pepsinogen and uropepsinin levels in patients with peptic ulcers are significantly higher than in control populations.[110, 111] These levels are higher from an early age in certain persons and their families, and Mirsky assumes that under critical psychosocial conditions ulcers will then develop in such persons and not in others.[109] He could, for example, fairly successfully predict ulcers in a population of army recruits. A predisposition, possibly genetic, is therefore one factor determining specific organ choice. Presumably, similar somatic predispositions will be found in other psychosomatic conditions; Mirsky mentions such possibilities for pernicious anemia, not strictly a psychosomatic disease, and hyperthyroidism.

Etiology

We assume that in each case there is a varying balance of causative factors. It is important to determine necessary and essential causes and the relative weight of the different factors that could account for differences in course, severity, and resistance. Thus, with a high genetic predisposition, less severe psychological impairments would be required for a disorder to occur. Different sets of psychological or organic factors would be relevant for the study of predisposition, reparative processes, and resistance. In gastric ulcer and essential hypertension, there is a heavy weighting of the genetic factor in the dimension of predisposition; in a "somatic" disease, such as tuberculosis, sociocultural and economic factors play a significant role both in resistance and exposure.[65] It has, for example, been suggested that the rising rate of tuberculosis among Negroes and the diminishing rate among Irish reflect the role of changing living patterns.

In thinking about etiological factors, we must envision sequences through time where various different processes become, at one juncture or another, of special interest. Schematically, one might search for predisposing factors, "sensitized pathways" determined by an interaction of genetic, physiological, and experiential factors. Psychological factors can influence the readiness for such pathways to be activated since they condition much of what is and is not exciting in a person's daily experience. Once such cycles of excitement are under way, some individuals, for psychological or physical reasons, can contain it and cope with it; others give way to further excitement and panic. The availability of alternative pathways for coping with excitement are strongly conditioned by psychological mechanisms. Presumably, a defect in the organization of drives, defenses, and coping devices can render a physiologically predisposed individual vulnerable to activation of organ systems and subsequently less protected against further stress.

When symptoms do develop, they have different consequences according to the personality and "strength" of the patient. Many highly capable individuals cope adequately according to social and occupational criteria but demonstrate some "cost" or weakness in their somatic symptoms. It is not easy for such successful persons to find those readjustments that might concomitantly diminish organic dysfunction. The successful scientist may ignore his needs to be cared for and refuse to modify his productive pace of work and interest, leaving his ulcer to "speak for" his tension and need. On the other hand, the alternation of psychoses with organic dysfunction indicates the crucial position that the symptomatology can occasionally hold in the total organization of personality. And finally, a developed psychosomatic symptom, as any symptom, can reinforce regression; the symptom can absorb the attention of the patient and come to replace many discriminations and efforts to achieve differentiated modes of coping. This schematic view of etiological factors, which considers predisposing and precipitating factors and conceives of major or minor weaknesses in the psychophysiological links comprising adaptive behavior, is not a satisfactory explanation of any specific case; rather, it represents an orientation that is open to data from many levels whenever this should be forthcoming from basic and clinical research and observation.

Treatment

The methods psychiatrists have used in the treatment of psychosomatic diseases vary from classical psychoanalysis to supportive and conditioning therapy. If psychiatrists treat psychosomatic illness, they should assume responsibility for the total treatment—for which they are rarely equipped—or they must cooperate closely with a medical specialist. One often reads that psychotherapy of psychosomatic patients needs to be modified from those methods used in treating neurotics; but usually no precise statement, either about the treatment of neurotics or the proposed modification, can be found. We also do not know in detail what the results of such therapies are. One over-all estimate of results was made by Wolff, who felt that over a period of years, two in three patients were helped by psychotherapy and two in five benefited greatly.[153] George E. Daniels *et al.*[35] felt that, in ulcerative colitis, psychotherapy was beneficial in terms of both psychological adjustment and somatic manifestations when the treated patients were compared to an untreated group. Regardless of its therapeutic effectiveness in psychosomatic disease, it should be kept in mind that psychoanalytic treatment has furnished us with important new data about the meaning and motives of behavior and valuable hunches about psychophysiological reactions.

In studies of ulcerative colitis, Erich Lindemann and others were impressed with the intense dependency needs of such patients[89] and devised a method of supportive therapy (involving gratification of needs), which Sidney Margolin once described under the name of anaclitic therapy.[99] The generally unsatisfied dependency needs of most patients with psychosomatic conditions may respond to treatment by paternalistic, warmly authoritative, and interested practitioners. It must be kept in mind, however, that the dependency needs may be activated by severe illness. We believe that, for practical reasons, treatment of most psychosomatic diseases must be in the hands of nonpsychiatrists. This requires, of course, a different training of these practitioners than has been customary until now. To understand the commitment demanded in working with these disorders, the student is urged to read Engel's paper on the management of ulcerative colitis.[47]

The student may not be familiar with the difference psychotherapists make between their understanding of the connectedness of things (as derived from the coherence of the patient's fantasies, current conflicts, and their genetic roots) and the decision of what to focus upon with the patient in therapy. The psychotherapist can track clusters of themes that begin to spell out a coherent story about basic instinctual strivings and attempts to solve them; in fact, we are better able to predict the sequence of symbolic and fantasy material, to link it with the patient's overt behavior, than we are to control behavior with this knowledge. Whatever psychiatrists may think about such connections, in their therapeutic work—from psychotherapy to psychoanalysis—they look for detailed and explicit behavior, in order to get a concrete picture of the patient's view of life, his current life situation, and his way of coping. Predisposition is a difficult dimension to investigate, but every physician can be curious about the patient's current life situation and be supportive in doing this; this may be far more important than any depth exploration of personality. The following case report shows that brief psychotherapy, in a patient with psychosomatic symptoms, can be effective, especially when the approach is based on interest in the patient rather than a crusade against the disease.

Brief Psychotherapy in a Patient with Mucous Colitis

The patient was referred because of severe bouts of mucous colitis of one year's duration, which was unresponsive to medical treatments. A thirty-six-year-old woman of Irish extraction, a highly intelligent mother, housewife, and leader in church and community affairs, the patient had had two brief prior episodes at the time of leaving home for college, and college for work. In addition to her colitis, she had developed a severe allergic response to insect bites, which meant that she had to curtail the extensive gardening she enjoyed with her family. She restricted her activities, was depressed and irritable, over-involved and oversensitive to the boyish depredations and "mess" of her sons, and was depreciative of her husband's frantic efforts to cheer her up. She felt guilty about her situation, was angry at the inability of doctors to help her, and insisted that her only difficulty was her colitis. At the time of onset of symptoms, her mother had visited (which she remembered as mildly irritating) and, ultimately of more relevance, her husband was then considering a change of job, which, in view of her sensitivity to change and loss of control, was probably a major stress.

In the initial therapeutic hours she tried to control therapy by flattering the therapist's undoubted intellectual prowess; she demanded guarantees of cure and pressed for "theories" to link her colitis to her mental function. Denied these, she finally threatened to stop treatment and after a vituperative explosion returned the following week, now having "decided" on her own that the therapist was not being stubborn but was really trying to help. She was told that there might or might not be connections between her feelings and her symptoms. If they were discovered, fine. If not, she was more important than her colitis and had problems; and for these, both the doctor and she could, perhaps, try to find some solutions. The therapist admired her capacity to manage, sympathized with her distress (sanctioning her need for care) and, recognizing her daily concerns, focused on the details of her problems with her boys and her husband. Although part of perhaps one or two hours was given to discussion of her background, there was no genetic focus to the interaction. She had risen above a shabby background, rife with domestic discord, superstition, and prejudice and had a disparaging attitude toward her mother while defending her not very successful father. In all, she thought of her parents' home as a "mess" and felt superior. Her fear of her own anger and a capacity to control, and her difficulty in seeking and using support was countered by a need to believe in "some" power upon which she could depend, a power greater than she could manage or destroy. Highly idealistic, she held to a private belief in her own version of God.

After sixteen once-a-week sessions, she had resumed her work, and the colitis was slowly disappearing. For the past ten years, she has written occasionally, speaking about her family and social projects, which she again manages. The intensity of her allergic response had diminished the summer following therapy so that she could again engage in outdoor life. Perhaps, just as she had "permitted" the therapist to do what he could do, she also decided to support her husband in the job change and, resuming control of herself and her situation, no longer had the loss of control, possibly symbolically represented by her symptom.

Schematically, one could trace her concern with messiness; her need for order; her managerial strivings and ability, which deteriorated into domestic tyranny; her magical sense of her own power; and her denial of any wish to be cared for. These constitute a cluster of traits that quite clearly refer to behavioral modes of the anal period and to regression from the probably phallic identification with which she had benignly and successfully coped. We can speculate about how this occurred in her childhood setting, but the strategy of therapy was simple, supportive, and concretely focused on current real problems with her family, and her view of herself and the therapist.

From what has been said about the general principles of etiology, diagnosis and treatment of the so-called psychosomatic diseases, it is obvious that we feel it is not a well-defined field. Just what diseases should be called psychosomatic is an open question. From the point of view of therapy, this should encourage any physician to approach his patient pragmatically and sympathetically without avoiding or becoming confused by the fact that there may be a strong psychological component, a severe social conflict, or a temporary life crisis (the occasion for, or memory of which, the patient may be unable, at first approach, to define). On the following pages, some of the diseases, which, according to current knowledge, are significantly influenced by psychological factors, are discussed.

Respiratory Psychosomatic Diseases

Respiration is a sensitive index of emotions. Emotional expressions such as laughing, yawning, and crying are modifications of respiratory movements. In fear, anger, and depression, changes of respiratory rhythms (holding one's breath, deep breathing, sighing) are well known. Changes in the "driving" or pacing of respiration are closely linked (perhaps through connections to the activating systems) to changes of mood and states of consciousness. Anesthesiologists who "bag breathe" for the patient, thereby controlling each respiratory cycle, report that this alone is sufficient to induce amnesia and muscular relaxation. Deliberate overbreathing can induce attacks of wheezing, which have been found to replace sad mood and depression in asthmatic subjects.[90]

Bronchial Asthma

Psychological events play a role as precipitating and probably also as predisposing causes in many but by no means in all cases of this complex disease.[92] Peter H. Knapp *et al.* felt psychological factors were significant in more than half of their patients.[75, 76] These investigators have been carrying on sustained clinical and experimental studies of the problem of asthma, attempting predictions of the course of the disorder from psychological data. Marvin Stein and his co-workers are systematically studying the pathophysiology of the disorder, as well as the psychodynamics, and we can expect increasingly focused and explicit data from such full-time psychiatric research efforts.[130, 135]

Although all that wheezes is not asthma, Jules H. Masserman and C. Pechtal with monkeys;[102] W. Horsely Gantt with dogs;[56] and R. Schiavi, M. Stein, and B. B. Sethi[130] with guinea pigs have all produced wheezing by psychological stress and conflict. E. Dekker[37] believes that "wheezing" can occur (but probably there is no bronchiolar involvement) and that normal controls can be "taught" to wheeze. Ian Stevenson and Harold G. Wolff assumed mechanisms in bronchial asthma to be similar to those in vasomotor rhinitis:[136] the patient wants to get rid of a person or a relationship but feels conflicted over such wishes. Thomas N. French and Franz Alexander not only related asthma to a suppressed cry in a dependency-independency conflict but observed the frequency of water symbolism in the dreams of asthmatic patients.[53] The relationship of the patients to their mothers was found to be disturbed. The patients were overdependent and demanding as children; their mothers were inadequate, inconsistent, and ambivalent in their care, expecting premature independence of the child, but at times they were also overprotective. The fear of closeness and the fear of the threat of a loss and separation seem to be important experiences in patients with bronchial asthma.

Knapp cites, among other factors, the role of excitement in the pathophysiology. Anger, anxiety, frustrations, and temptation can be identified in many asthmatic attacks. In chronic cases, however, the patients generally also develop depressive, hopeless attitudes and become completely absorbed by their physical illness. Such observations, of course, are not specific and are encountered in other psychosomatic illnesses and also other types of asthma. Erich D. Wittkower found that the problems of children with cardiac asthma were very similar to those of children with bronchial asthma.[147] Stein and P. Ottenberg found that certain odors can precipitate asthma,[135] and Joseph G. Kepecs and co-workers pointed to the interesting fact that asthmatics are oversensitive to odors.[71] D. Funkenstein found a group of asthmatics who alternated between episodes of psychosis without asthma, and asthma without psychosis.[55] When these patients were psychotic, even mecholyl (a parasympathetic agent that provokes wheezing) could not induce asthma. Whether this resistance depends on a heightened sympathetic tone in smooth muscle during the psychosis is not known. Although numerous observers note the role of excitement in inducing or terminating wheezing, notions that crying or sobbing are specifically relieving are not tenable, since vomiting may be equally efficacious in terminating an attack. In any event, it is clear that a number of regulatory mechanisms and thresholds may be shifted in asthma.

Treatment of asthma consists of somatic methods and a psychologically sensitive approach. Few physicians are available for such sophisticated treatment of asthma. Experienced clinicians, such as Alvin L. Barach, combine somatic and psychotherapeutic methods according to the specific needs of the patient.[8] To treat asthmatics by individual or group psychotherapy alone is not indicated.

Hyperventilation

This is a frequent disorder, which often causes fainting, grayouts, and blackouts. Patients are usually aware of it but are unable to stop breathing deeply and rapidly; this leads to a fall of blood CO_2, dizziness, anxiety, faintness, syncope, and, in some cases, to tetanic spasms of hands and feet. Often, such patients have hysterical personality structures and hysterical symptoms. Attacks can be frequently ameliorated by identifying for the patient that he is in fact overbreathing and by exploring the usually obvious provoking factors in his present life situation. In cases of acapnia, CO_2 inspiration will often stop the attack. The capacity for respiratory processes to be under conscious control is counterbalanced by the numerous signals controlling respiration, which are unconscious, and by the close and "built in" neurobehavioral association of panic and hyperventilation. Thus, when physiological cues initiate overbreathing, it is difficult to assert conscious control, and when hyperventilation is initiated consciously, "escape" from control readily occurs. Another troublesome form of faulty inspiration leads to swallowing of air (*aerophagia*), distention of stomach, ructus, and vomiting. Coughing and throat-clearing are also commonly encountered, often as "nervous habits." One of our patients, too proud to cry, but sensitive and yearning for attention, would cough paroxysmally with deafening loudness when injured and resentful. (Unable to "rid" herself of conflict she evoked anguish and pain in her household.)

Common Cold

From clinical impression, it seems likely that certain psychological stresses lower the resistance of the organism to colds. Friedrich Nietzsche once wrote: "Contentment preserves one even from catching cold. Has a woman who knew that she was well dressed ever caught cold? No, not even when she had scarcely a rag to her back." It is a common clinical observation that the common cold follows slights, humiliations, and disappointments in love. Wolff and his co-workers consider the symptoms of vasomotor rhinitis and related disturbances of the entire respiratory tract as attempts at ridding the organism of noxious stimuli, such as dusts or gases, but also of undesirable psychological stimuli. Repressed resentment, rather than diffuse fury or irritable anger, is the outstanding emotion encountered in such patients.[64] Stress-induced changes of the oropharyngeal flora are reported.[67]

Cardiovascular Psychosomatic Diseases

It is well known that emotions influence cardiovascular function to produce tachycardia or bradycardia, a rise or fall in blood pressure, vasoconstriction, or vasodilation. Rage produces reddening of the face or pallor, increase in blood pressure, and tachycardia. It is less well known that, in careful observations, Wolff, Stewart Wolf, and others demonstrated that anger and anxiety also produce changes in stroke volume, circulating blood volume, peripheral resistance, and oxygen consumption.[149, 150] Albert F. Ax reported different patterns of polygraphic measures (including cardiovascular measures) with fear or anger.[5] Non-esterified free fatty acids may be elevated with stress,[20] and it is possible that a differential binding and release of the various catecholamines in vascular tissue is preferentially related to different affects. It is, however, not clear that such physiological alterations play a major role in the pathogenesis of heart disease.

Essential Hypertension

The pathogenesis is complex and largely unknown; renal, neural, humoral, and emotional factors play a role. Experimentally, centrogenic hypertension has been produced in dogs. The disease may be symptomatic for years, and its course is followed mostly in terms of its complications, of which cerebrovascular accidents are the most important ones. It is to be differentiated from a malignant hypertension in which there is a rapid and often lethal progression of cardio-renal and retinal symptoms. In some groups of hypertensives, there is apparently a strong predisposing factor. When the gamut of psychophysiological responses to stress, including pulse and blood pressure, were recorded, Lacey found a group who showed consistent patterns of response;[79] another group that varied in the response systems that most reflect stress; and yet a third group of random and erratic responders.

At one time, it was hoped that the hypertensive reaction could be predicted, since lability of blood pressure may precede clinical hypertension. About 25 per cent of soldiers of various nations showed higher elevations of blood pressure the closer they were to the front; following the disaster of the Texas City[127] explosion, a large percentage of survivors showed a temporary persistence of quite elevated blood pressures. Experimental stress can also create a population of temporary hypertensives. Yet, in all of these instances, pressures returned to normal, and progression to hypertension has not in fact been documented. In one study, hypertensives were found to be persons with strong ambivalence and conflicts over hostility and dependency.[119] Such patients restrained overt hostile behavior, but vascular mechanisms appeared to express the covert anger. A precipitating factor cited by Carl A. L. Binger was the sudden loss of security with respect to authority figures—among them physicians—on whom the patients depended.[13] Stewart Wolf *et al.* stated that such patients suffer from conflicts between aggressive drives and approval gained by maintaining peace,[150] but certainly such conflicts occur in large populations and are not specific. A. M. Ostfeld and B. Z. Lebovits tested one group with essential hypertension and one with renal hypertension, using the Rorschach test and personality inventories; they found no difference between the groups.[115] Many of the symptoms usually attributed to hypertension, for example, fatigue, dizziness, palpitation, insomnia, headaches, and weakness, are quite unspecific and in all likelihood are related to anxiety, anger, and various psychological conflicts over aggressive and dependent needs.

Angina Pectoris and Myocardial Infarction

Hans Selye proposed that stress and myocardial damage precede occlusion.[132] It is popularly assumed that psychological factors play a significant role in the etiology of coronary heart disease. The available data, however, are even more obscure in the coronary diseases than in hypertension. Some have commented that angina pectoris attacks are correlated, at times, with upsetting fantasies of aggressive, sexual, or dependent content and feel that anxiety and anger in such patients may contribute greatly to their misery. In view of the general psychology of pain, in which anticipation has been shown to be a major factor, this would not be surprising. Evidence that emotional upset produces coronary thrombosis is largely speculative. Edward Weiss and O. Spurgeon English point to so-called anniversary reactions when a coronary attack occurs on the anniversary of previously upsetting events.[142] Harry H. W. Miles and Stanley Cobb, in their catamnestic study, failed to confirm this impression,[105] although V. R. Hilgard and M. F. Newman have established the general significance of anniversary reactions.[62] Vascular diseases, with their threat to life and social and economic security, will produce realistic and unrealistic fear and thus bring into play powerful defense mechanisms, particularly denial of serious illness, which are manifest in disregard of medical regimen, confusion, and uncooperative attitudes. Unwise medical management may induce invalidism. Morton F. Reiser and Herman Bakst rightly stress that we know more about the somatopsychic side of cardiovascular diseases than about the psychosomatic aspects.[120]

Other Cardiovascular Psychosomatic Syndromes

Much has been written about so-called *neurocirculatory asthenia.* The symptoms grouped by Sir Thomas Lewis under the label *effort syndrome*[83] —some call it vegetative dystonia—are breathlessness, palpitation, tachycardia, chest pain, faintness, fatigability, and anxiety. Miles and Cobb feel that such patients may be divided into two groups, ranging from pure anxiety neuroses to patients with organic cardiac pathology, presumably on a constitutional basis.[105] Most of these patients are minimally disabled and respond well to psychotherapy. The syndrome is important in military medicine because it provides obvious secondary gains for the sick soldier. Two other neurovascular diseases in which psychological factors probably play an important role are *Reynaud's disease*[106] and *causalgia.*[88] *Stress polycythemia*[81] has been documented and, since red cell mass is normal, phlebotomy and therapy with radioactive phosphorus would be contra-indicated. Experimental studies from Cannon to the recent past indicate a definite link of anxiety and blood viscosity.[82]

Studies of surgical cardiac patients show that such patients frequently exhibit severe anxiety and regressive defense mechanisms.[17] The sudden loss of a chronic ailment calls for a major readjustment. Occasionally physicians, delighted with their progress in the war against disease, can overlook the concerns and the difficulties involved for their postoperative patients who must find new adjustments.

Gastrointestinal Psychosomatic Diseases

Some of the most important work on the influence of emotions on somatic functions has been done in patients with gastrointestinal disorders. A relationship between G.I. functions and feeling states has long been postulated on the basis of clinical experience. Anger and anxiety may decrease appetite; depression may result in loss of appetite or overeating. Anxious anticipation and sustained tension may produce diarrhea or constipation. Vomiting occasionally accompanies general anxiety and is a specific concomitant of disgust. Such symptoms are even more pronounced in children than in adults. We all know the pervasive readiness with which we view the world through our mouths, stomachs, bowels, and anus; the way to a man's heart, how armies travel, what a good fighter has, and a number of other personality attributes, are commonly appraised in a vernacular which runs the gamut of the gastrointestinal system. Indeed, as Theodore Lidz and Robert Rubenstein put it, pleasure and displeasure during the first few years of life are largely centered in the gastrointestinal tract.[87] Feelings of gratification, of love, trust, and security are experienced after being fed, whereas hunger produces intense displeasure. Defecation is accompanied by both tension and release, or variants of these affects. If one seriously considers the amount of time and activity and effort centered around gastrointestinal functions through every day of life—and this is even more true for the starving than for the well-fed population of the world—it is hardly surprising that such activities and the affects surrounding them are prepotent in organizing early experience. Early experience forms the model for fantasies and thoughts about a wide range of modally related activities involving gain and loss, care and protection, pleasure and frustration. Having acknowledged this, we can only assert that we know of no evidence that, for example, can firmly link patterns of early feeding to the occurrence of subsequent disease. Infants with gastric fistula or a history of severe organic problems involving the gastrointestinal tract have not, to date, been demonstrated to produce significant pathology in adult life. In any event, speculation concerning etiology is probably useful only in pointing out areas that will require finely detailed investigation.

Peptic Ulcer

Many somatic and psychosocial factors seem to play a role in the etiology of peptic ulcers, but no definitive etiology has been established so far. In addition to clinical observations, considerable experimental work on gastric motility and secretion has provided the groundwork for current psychosomatic theories in peptic ulcer. The first to demonstrate a relationship between gastric secretion and the emotions was an American Army surgeon, William Beaumont, in his observations of Alexis St. Martin, who suffered from gastric fistula after a gunshot wound.[11] Very elaborate observations of such correlations were made by Wolf and Wolff on their patient, Tom;[151] by Margolin with particular attention to unconscious affect and gastric function,[99] and most recently by Engel, F. Reichsman, and H. L. Segal, on Monica, an infant with a gastric fistula.[49] Monica responded to the approach of her trusted doctor or nurse with increased gastric secretion; when depressed or approached by strangers, however, there was a marked hypoactivity. Gastric secretion did not discriminate between joy or anger; rather, there was an increase with arousal of any intense affect and a decrease with an apparent inhibition of affect. A brief episode of fear can lead to suppression of gastric secretion; George F. Mahl found that chronic, rather than acute, fear in animals produced hyperacidity, but that neither condition led to ulcers.[95] A combination of hunger and electric shock to the feet led to gastric lesion in rats.[129] Work with the executive monkey and Mirsky's important studies of pepsinogen, the role of hormones, as well as central lesions producing gastric erosions, have been discussed.[103, 110]

Many experienced clinicians have been impressed with the correlation of emotional components in ulcer. One of the most discussed questions in psychosomatic medicine was whether specific conflicts and personality patterns, or simply fear in general are involved. It has been postulated by quite a number of investigators that the ulcer patient has a specific conflict centering around his unconscious unfulfilled needs for food and love. Deprivation of such needs in infancy and repeated in adult life were thought to result in increased demand for food and love with concomitant hypersecretion which, under certain circumstances, would lead to an ulcer.

One of our patients with an ulcer is a highly competent woman who would love to retreat from the world and be cared for. However, she feels she must constantly be alert, manage, take care of her husband and children, and forestall any imminent disaster since she can, in her opinion, rely on no one else. As a child, she was a good girl who was a little adult, looking after her rambunctious sister, who made a lot of noise and got all of the parental attention. We could not find an infantile deprivation in this woman, but certainly there was deprivation by the age of four or five, when these character traits described above had begun to crystallize. In any event, we have described a covertly demanding, controlling, and hyperactive personality type whereas, in contrast, Frederic T. Knapp, M. Rosenbaum, and J. Romano described the occurrence of peptic ulcer in shy, passive persons with prominent, latent homosexual conflicts.[68] The problem with such summary descriptions is exemplified by the fact that our hyperactive patient showed prominent, latent homosexual conflicts (she had a man's role in her family). Socially, she was notably shy and retiring, patiently waiting for others to discover her virtues and strength; she would not overtly demand help or attention, but she expended much energy in expecting it. As in all descriptions of the psychological and personality organization of patients, it is quite difficult to pin down discriminating features. S. I. Cohen and A. J. Silverman, in a controlled study, found compliant attitudes and features (somewhat similar to "anger in" types) in patients with ulcer but not with gastric carcinoma; a significantly low basal level of urinary norepinephrine was correlated with the ulcer personality.[32]

Psychogenic Vomiting and Dysphagia

Psychogenic vomiting is a very frequent symptom both in children and adults. Some, particularly hysterical and anxious persons, react to a wide variety of psychological stresses with nausea, vomiting, and also with chronic disturbances of appetite, epigastric pain, and discomfort. Psychogenic vomiting is usually a harmless neurotic symptom and is quite amenable to a wide variety of suggestive and insight-producing therapies; in many cases, these may uncover more specific fantasies and experiences that induce the patient to express sexual and aggressive conflicts of incorporation and ejection by vomiting. In some patients, however, psychogenic vomiting and its equivalent, psychogenic hiccoughs, are refractory to simple treatment. Hypnosis may be used to stop an acute attack, but more extensive psychotherapy may also be required.

In a number of patients with cardiospasm, apart from purely organic cases of achalasia, emotional factors, which contribute to the understanding of the main symptoms, have been found. Usually, the patients are anxious, excitable persons with hysterical traits; they like to eat and have a great need for love and succoring but also have difficulties in entering into a dependent relationship. Typically, they have a history of feeding and eating difficulties in infancy and childhood. The characteristic hysterical difficulty of swallowing, with a feeling of obstruction in the pharynx, the globus hystericus, should be differentiated from the more severe and complex cases. In most cases, the treatment of cardiospasm is a taxing problem that is best approached with the combined efforts of gastroenterologists and psychiatrists.[94]

Ulcerative Colitis

The etiology of this disease, characterized by remissions and relapses and often by fatal outcome, is unknown; infection, allergic diathesis, disturbances of enzyme metabolism, and psychological factors may all contribute. Melitta Sperling found unconscious rage reactions in her patients,[133] which, of course, have also been incriminated in many other psychosomatic diseases. The role of families should be studied in this disorder; such studies will enhance our picture of the psychological development of these patients. They may not yield differentiating factors; but they could empirically reveal the profound disorders in the environment that foster or inhibit growth and development, and this could be clinically useful. Engel and his co-workers studied a large patient population, and found in all their patients a striking immaturity and marked dependency needs which had not been fulfilled by a pathological mother; this produced helplessness and despair in the patients. These authors maintain that the pathology of the bowel is an unspecific response to the grief of separation anxiety.[43,44,45,46] Engel has also noted an interesting shift in symptoms; symptoms of colitis, which are associated with helplessness ("I cannot help myself") and hopelessness ("neither I nor anyone else can help me"), are often replaced by symptoms of headache when the patient has achieved a more active psychological position, expresses more aggressive fantasies, and seems to be in a period of decision-making ("I am going to try to help myself"). Occasionally, psychosis has been reported to "replace" colitis or to coexist with it. Wolff assumed that a variety of emotions may cause hypermotility and hypersecretion of the colonic mucosa, leading ultimately to ulceration.[153] Recently, there have been theories that autoimmunity is etiologically significant. One could conjecture that pathogenic emotions alter the immunity of the patient; data for such hypotheses do not exist yet.

Most psychiatrists who have had experience with the treatment of ulcerative colitis stress the importance of a supportive approach.[89] Even more than in peptic ulcers, the dependency needs of the patient must be recognized and gratified. Psychodynamic, psychogenic, and psychotherapeutic assumptions similar to those about ulcerative colitis have also been made concerning different intestinal diseases of unknown etiology, such as mucous colitis, regional ileitis, and the irritable bowel.[134]

Psychosomatic Disease of the Skin

Emotional states are accompanied by changes in the skin. Blushing occurs in shame; enraged persons turn red or pale; and fear can produce blanching, gooseflesh, and sweating. It is conceivable, though not proven, that enduring emotions lead to increased vascularization, changes in moisture of the skin, and consequently to skin disease, or at least to the facilitation of skin disease.[148] Joseph G. Kepecs produced blisters with an irritant and observed exudate into the blisters after the evocation of sad mood with crying; when crying was suppressed, there was first a lag and then the exudate.[70] The hypnotic induction of blistering also indicates that some element in the skin is responsive to neural or neurohumoral control. P. F. D. Seitz demonstrated that an underlying neurotic conflict can persist and be expressed in various multiple symptoms; hypnotic suggestion could cause the disappearance of the skin disorder only to be "replaced" by another symptom.[131]

Some outstanding dermatologists admit the possibility of multiple psychological and somatic causation for diseases of the skin; others express skepticism and believe that neurotic traits are not the cause but the consequence of itching and disfiguring skin disease. Some conservative dermatologists believe there is only one skin affliction, in which psychogenesis is undisputed, *self-inflicted excoriations.* Persons who scratch their skins, often ferociously, are angry, self-punitive, and masochistic persons who can best be treated by a psychotherapeutic approach. Anger and self-destructive tendencies have also been considered to be important contributory factors in *chronic eczema or neurodermatitis.* Another fairly general observation is the striking exhibitionism of some patients with chronic and particularly with disfiguring skin disease. They often are unusually aggressive, flirtatious, and even promiscuous; probably such behavior is often at least compensatory in patients who feel unattractive and crave affection and bodily contact. Wittkower and B. Russell comment on the fact that patients with *seborrhea* and those with acne vulgaris suffer from social isolation.[148] It is a common observation that psychological stress aggravates any number of skin diseases, particularly *psoriasis.* However, there are times when exacerbations cannot be related to stress, even by a considerable stretch of imagination.

Patients with *pruritis ani and vulvae* are often sexually immature and suffer from disturbances of potency or from frigidity. In men with anal pruritis and eczema, latent homosexual tendencies are typically prominent; scratching of the anus often provides sexual excitation and may be considered a form of masturbation. In some cases of pruritis ani, we find excessive concern over dirt and cleanliness. *Common warts,* in some persons but not in others, can be removed by hypnosis, suggestion, and placebo therapy.[141] Other puzzling dermatoses are *general alopecia* and *alopecia areata,* in which the sudden loss of hair is related, among other factors, to nonspecific emotional upset.

Psychological Factors in Allergic Diseases

In this group of diseases, we might distinguish two populations, with a high allergic and low psychological factor at one end of the continuum, and the opposite weighting of factors at the other. The effect of psychological factors on the immune response or sensitivity is harder to establish than effects on reactivity to an existing sensitivity.[18] Apart from the diseases such as seasonal and perennial rhinitis and conjunctivitis, bronchal asthma, urticaria, and various skin diseases, migraine and various gastrointestinal syndromes have been thought to occur at times on an allergic basis. In many of these disorders, psychological factors complicate the course of illness and can be predisposing and precipitating. Allergic patients strike some observers as even more labile, depressive, oversensitive, and resentful than other chronic patients with diseases of comparative severity. The affects and conflicts described in the discussion of vasomotor rhinitis and bronchial asthma play a comparable role in the allergies. Irritation, resentment, and anger have been identified particularly in urticaria. P. Marty assumes that allergic patients suffer from lack of identity, and overidentity with whomever they interact, anxiously fulfilling unconscious expectations of their environment without any real gratification of their own needs.[100] When no interaction is possible, they feel empty and deserted without any inner resources. Leon J. Saul has also stressed the allergic patient's dependency needs and fear of isolation.[128]

A summation of psychological and physical effects can be readily observed; for example, repressed anger during the ragweed season at a relatively low pollen count will often produce a violent sneezing attack. Occasionally, the nature of the allergen may be psychologically significant and linked to aggressive and sexual conflicts; in other patients, for instance, in the majority of hay fever cases, it seems to have no psychological meaning. Yet even in such obviously organic cases, a general reduction of anxiety and hostile conflicts may result in improvement of the allergic condition. Drugs such as antihistamines, which act locally on the nasal mucosa, also act on brain stem activating systems and on the reticulum surrounding the sensory nucleus of the vagus; change in the background tone of smooth muscle could conceivably alter response to allergens. Harold A. Abramson, an allergist and psychotherapist with a comprehensive orientation, finds that exploration and treatment of psychological conflict is of importance in the majority of allergic cases.[1]

Psychosomatic Aspects of Endocrine and Metabolic Diseases

Our knowledge of stress and endocrine functions is more advanced than our knowledge of specific psychosomatic aspects of endocrine diseases.[19] Behavior disorders associated with internal diseases may be divided into three groups: the psychosomatic, the somatopsychic, and the behavior disorders, which are primarily the result of brain pathology associated with such diseases. In the case of behavior disorders of endocrine and metabolic diseases, this division seems particularly relevant; in some cases all three types of reactions may coincide in the same patient. In Chapter 6, some of the organic and toxic psychoses and organic deficit states that occur in endocrine and metabolic diseases are discussed and the question of whether certain abnormal personality traits are the result of endocrine dysfunction are considered. It is also obvious that certain endocrine and metabolic diseases produce severe psychosocial stresses; to be an endocrine or metabolic cripple—a dwarf, a hermaphrodite, a severe diabetic—calls for an extraordinary adjustment. In this chapter, we will consider only whether certain psychological stresses contribute significantly to the etiology of endocrine diseases. A. Conrad pointed to interpersonal difficulties that preceded manifest hyperthyroidism[34] and noted that female patients are afraid of losing maternal affection. Lidz found, in his intensively studied cases, an overattachment of patients to their mothers and also to their own children, and an inability to relinquish such relationships.[85] George C. Ham, Alexander, and Hugh T. Carmichael assume that an extreme fear of not surviving can be demonstrated in such patients and maintain that this plays a contributory if not a specific role in the etiology of the disease.[61] Ruesch and others found that about one-third of their female hyperthyroid patients were essentially normal personalities and that the other two-thirds were highly anxious and hysterical types.[126] Wittkower and his co-workers also cautioned against the assumption of a generic psychogenic theory.[40] Whether psychogenic factors play an important etiological role in other endocrine diseases, such as in Addison's disease and Cushing's syndrome, remains to be seen.

Obesity

Obesity is defined by marked increase over the ideal weight. This is not an altogether satisfactory criterion because it does not consider constitutional variations in fat deposits. However, there is little doubt about the diagnosis of more extreme forms of obesity. Hypothalamic lesions produce hyperphagic (and often ferocious) animals; in some instances, it is clear that the defect is an inability to stop eating rather than an enormous appetite motivating the animal to work for food. Such start-and-stop mechanisms may be relevant to more complex human disorders since the sequence of feedback signals, which comprise the component parts of the complex act of eating, appear to be fractionable by discrete chemical, surgical, and electrical manipulations of the brain; for example, the role of perception of satiety in overeating has been under study in humans.[137, 138] Although hypogonadism and hypothyroidism, diseases of the pituitary and of the hypothalamus, may be associated with obesity or contribute to it, the most apparent cause of obesity is overeating.[22] In our opulent culture, obesity is common in civilized countries. It is particularly frequent in the lower classes. Thirty per cent of lower-class women and 4 per cent of lower-class men were judged obese in a recent survey of a U.S. sample.[112] Digestion, absorption, and metabolism in most obese persons are not disturbed, although there is some direct evidence that due to inactivity, caloric output is reduced in many obese people. Obese persons have faulty eating habits; they eat too often and too much, particularly too many carbohydrates and fats. An old Zen proverb recommends that a man should eat when he is hungry and drink when he is thirsty, and obese persons often do not follow this rule. Their eating excess is not caused by hunger for food but by a compulsion to eat, possibly as a magical means to gain love and affection; their faulty eating habits usually have psychological causes. A. Stunkard found that some of his obese patients ate in an orgiastic fashion and at irregular intervals, often at night; yet they failed to perceive stomach contractions when they were hungry and overtly denied their hunger.[137] Hilde Bruch, who has intensely studied the psychopathology of obese adolescents, points to the dominant mothers of such patients, who push their children emotionally or withhold love and food.[25] It should be remarked that dominant mothers have been credited with an etiological role in bronchial asthma, the allergies, peptic ulcer, and also in schizophrenias and depressions; what their distinct contributions are still remains to be seen. Stunkard and his co-workers warn of coming to easy conclusions about the problem of obesity. They specifically disproved the thesis of the dominant mother, the weak father, the femininity of obese men, and the high anxiety of obese patients.[146] However, the striving of obese patients for independence is usually thwarted; their self-esteem remains low; tolerance of loss and frustration is typically poor. Particularly, in obese girls there is also a rejection of sexual role that precedes the onset of obesity. To be sure, there are secondary gains: obese patients get special attention, although the attention is not sufficient to prevent their depressive moods. Mild cyclic mood-swings are frequent in older persons. During the depressive phase, which is often precipitated by psychological events such as rejection or temptation, obese patients eat excessively and gain weight; they then become remorseful and ashamed and start to diet rigorously. Bruch draws attention to the fact that the basic personality of an obese person, after diet and weight-loss, remains unchanged, and the cycle will be repeated unless a more profound psychological attack can be made on the problem.

Treatment, consisting of a combination of dietary and if necessary pharmacological measures combined with psychotherapy, is far from an easy task. By definition, patients with psychogenic obesity are addicts to food, and psychotherapy of confirmed addicts is notoriously difficult. Trangressions in eating and relapses in most cases have to be expected, although over-all results in the hands of patient and skillful therapists are fair.

Anorexia Nervosa

Although psychogenic underweight is symptomatically the opposite of psychogenic obesity, the causes of both conditions are more similar than dissimilar. There are, in fact, cases that fluctuate between overweight and underweight. Lack of appetite in children, often combined with finickiness and true or pseudo food-allergies, is usually a symptom of defiance and protest.

An extreme form of underweight is anorexia nervosa,[16,140] properly considered a syndrome rather than a unitary disease. The syndrome occurs mostly in young girls but has been observed in both sexes and all age groups. Anorexia nervosa is accompanied by pronounced distaste for food and often by nausea, psychogenic vomiting, and constipation. It is frequently followed or preceded by amenorrhea; the latter is probably caused by general physiological tension and not by primary endocrine dysfunction: follicle stimulating hormone (FSH) secretion in some cases is low. Patients are withdrawn and shy and often are mistaken for schizophrenics. Borderline cases, such as Ludwig Binswanger's famous patient Ellen West, are difficult to classify, but usually differentiation from schizophrenia and depression is possible. Helmut Thomä and others in thorough studies drew attention to the secret snatching of food, raiding of the icebox and the cooky-jar, kleptomanic behavior, and marked guilt feelings over such actions. These patients suffer a severe puberty crisis and are unable to assume the adult sexual role.[140] J. E. Meyer called attention to the mild cases that are frequent;[104] and these girls reject their sexual role and express this by changing their body by food fads and starvation. Food intake seems to be highly sexualized, but the notion that adolescent girls with anorexia always have unconscious fantasies of incestuous oral relations and oral impregnation has not been demonstrated.[16] They may, however, suffer from near delusional ideas of poisoning. In the literature, there has been confusion between anorexia nervosa and *Simmonds' cachexia:* the latter is a serious pituitary illness; its diagnosis rests on evidence of severe hypofunction and radiological evidence of destruction of the pituitary gland. In an interesting paper, Cannon drew parallels between anorexia nervosa and voodoo death in terms of adrenal malfunction.[29] He considers both disorders expressions of self-destructive tendencies, in which adrenal mechanisms play a role. Anorexia nervosa can be a serious therapeutic problem; although one-third of the patients recover spontaneously, some die unless they are expertly treated. They are accessible to psychotherapy, and recovery of severe cases under intensive psychotherapy and proper hospital management may be dramatic and rewarding.

Young Woman with Anorexia Nervosa

A twenty-one-year-old white girl of average height was transferred from the medical service for treatment of severe cachexia. Her weight, never exceeding 87 pounds, was usually maintained by a variety of food and health fads. Some months prior to admission, the patient began to lose interest in eating; this was reported by the family as a gradual, almost imperceptible process. Always a dawdling eater, she spent even more time than usual over her meals. The patient's menstrual periods ceased; and, in addition to not eating, she frequently became nauseated. At that time, her father, who recently was hospitalized for a bleeding ulcer, became quite concerned both about the girl's eating habits and her passivity and seclusiveness (she had made no effort to obtain a job in the three years since she left high school). He thought that she perhaps needed a vacation, yet he was also worried about her growing disinterest in her appearance and her tendency to spend the day in pajamas and robe, lounging in bed. Both parents were distressed by the long nightly conversations between the patient and her twenty-six-year-old sister. These conversations stretched far into the early morning, depriving the girls of "much-needed rest." In fact, plans were being made to give up the parental bedroom to the patient and thus separate the daughters. In the presence of such turmoil and indecision, the girl's weight continued to drop. Her family physician administered thyroxine and vitamin shots, and the patient dutifully trudged off to the doctor each week, observed her rapidly diminishing weight being recorded, and returned home regularly reporting that all was well. The mother recalls that she had a suspicion that her daughter was losing weight but asserted that no urging would get the girl onto the bathroom scale: "So what could we do?" Finally, when she had lost one-third of her original weight, dropping from 87 to 64 pounds, she was admitted to the local hospital and following a medical and endocrine workup, she was referred to the psychiatric service.

History taken there revealed that the parents were in their late forties. The patient's father was successfully employed as a traveling salesman. All described the family as "close-knit" in which the members freely exchanged their thoughts and troubles(!). In the five years preceding hospitalization the parents were confronted with failures of each of the three children; the elder sister retreating to home following failure at a drama school, finally, settled after three years of indecision as a bank clerk. The patient's brother, absorbed in writing science fiction, failed his engineering course despite high abilities. The mother, a tiny, rather tired-looking woman maintained that she was the only person who understood her children, even while her daughter pointed out her failings in vain. The father, a ruddy-faced, stout man, seemed to view the world with a perennial, sad half-smile. The family denied any history of mental illness.

Concern over the patient's health dated virtually from the time of her birth when a loud nonsymptomatic heart murmur was detected; she was restricted in her physical activities thereafter. The father, in particular, was zealous in protecting her, a worry he related to the death of his own sister of rheumatic heart disease at age twenty-one. The mother also valued the daughter's ailment, claiming with some pride that when the girl needed a dental extraction, it had to be performed in a hospital with "three doctors" in attendance. The patient had few close friends and dated boys only twice in her life. It was accepted by the family that she would not seek work after completing high school, where she was a good but compulsive student. She took on the role of mother's assistant around the house.

On admission, the patient presented a bizarre appearance. She was dressed in a black shift, which accentuated her extreme gauntness. Her straight black hair fell in disarray to her waist, and she kept her features hidden behind layers of thick, pale makeup, which emphasized a vivid green eyeshadow and long false eyelashes. Silvery polish on dagger-like fingernails completed the picture. The first encounter with the family was almost as bizarre. The patient was lying across her mother's lap, screaming and crying, demanding to be taken home, since she had had no idea that she was being sent to a psychiatric ward. The father insisted that since all else had failed, she might die at home, and that she would not have to stay. To this the mother responded by slapping the father, telling him not to upset the child. The mother then began to pace, asking her son's opinion, since "he had a semester of psychology at college and got an A." The patient's sister was weeping and agreeing that the patient should go home if she wanted to. The patient then began to chant, between her sobs, "They won't make up their minds, they won't make up their minds." Finally, the mother grudgingly agreed to permit her daughter to stay "for a few days for a rest," but with the implication that she would be removed to die peacefully at home if treatment did not meet her approval. The patient promptly stopped crying and went to bed.

It was decided that no emphasis should be placed on eating and that attempts at psychotherapeutic intervention would be kept at a minimum. Weight would not be an issue, and like all other patients, she would be weighed once a week. However, the psychiatrists of the service were ready to start tube-feeding if she began to lose weight. This last measure was not to be discussed with the patient unless she did indeed begin to lose.

Her response was dramatic. She not only began to eat, but ate incessantly. She went everywhere (even to bed) clutching a box of dry cereal or popcorn, and munching continuously. As her weight increased to 85 pounds, she gradually discarded her more bizarre embellishments. She complained of a feeling of fullness in her stomach, but never vomited. A complication was the development of severe generalized edema, presumably related to rapid weight gain in a cachectic patient: this responded to salt restriction.

Family and individual therapy then became intensive. The patient verbalized remarkable insights into her problems but was discouraged about her family's inability to change. The mother threatened weekly to remove the girl, asserting steadfastly that there was nothing wrong with her mind. The father continued to smile sadly, even though it was dramatically disclosed that his heavy drinking had been a family issue for years. Attacking her mother more directly, the patient began talking of wanting to move out of the house to begin a life of her own. She also was able to express her affection, mixed with a certain contempt, for her father. After four weeks of improvement, the mother abruptly (and with but little resistance by the father) took the patient home against the physicians' advice. For two years, the patient has been able to attend school; her weight has remained steady since her discharge.

Diabetes Mellitus

There are few diseases that are better studied than diabetes; in this respect, the general definition of psychosomatic disease as an illness of unknown etiology, in which emotional factors play a decisive role, does not quite fit. The symptoms can be related to an inadequate production of insulin and an inability to metabolize carbohydrates. There is, however, considerable lack of clarity about the role of heredity and the factors that precipitate the illness or influence its fluctuating course. It is generally assumed that emotions have some impact on the physiological mechanisms underlying diabetes. Evidence cited are anecdotal tales such as those about the increase of diabetes after the Wall Street crash in 1929. More important, it is clear from experience in managing these patients that psychological conflicts aggravate the illness. In response to these conflicts, patients tend to mismanage their regimen, and this leads to metabolic crises.[124] In the psychosomatic literature, there have been some reports of specific personality profiles of diabetics, but controlled studies establishing this beyond doubt are lacking. William C. Menninger assumed that many diabetic patients are depressed and anxious and are essentially passive personalities who overtax themselves and suffer from chronic fatigue and frustration in not fulfilling their own expectations and those of their environment.[103] In observations of diabetic children, Bruch found that specific characteristics do not exist but noted that chronic and serious diseases such as diabetes reinforce dependency conflicts.[24] Mirsky was impressed with the severity and the regressive character of psychological disturbance in his patients.[107] In the psychoanalysis of a diabetic patient, George E. Daniels was struck by the strong fear of being overpowered, but he did not suggest that this is necessarily a typical pattern.[36] L. E. Hinkle, F. M. Evans and Stewart Wolf found that a variety of life and experimental stresses caused ketonuria in their patients.[63] They were impressed, as was Mirsky, with the tendencies of diabetic patients to respond to stress by overeating. In addition to well-established principles of dietary treatment and insulin therapy, it is clear that attention to psychological factors, and particularly to self-destructive, dependent, and hypochondriacal needs, is important.[124]

Spontaneous Hypoglycemia

This syndrome is characterized by a fall of blood sugar below 50 mg. per 100 ml. In the early stages, patients are hungry, feel weak, sweat profusely, and are quite anxious and tremulous. Many anxiety states have been taken for hypoglycemic states, and vice versa.[33] It is assumed that early symptoms are related to an increased epinephrine output and increased tissue utilization of glucose. The more severe symptoms consist of coma and general or focal seizures. This stage is rarely reached, but there are reports that patients have died from untreated spontaneous hypoglycemia. There are also reports of longer-lasting confusion; in one case, Joseph Wilder assumed that criminal behavior was the result of hypoglycemia.[144] In a number of cases, severe emotional disturbances of an unspecific nature have been found; in others, faulty eating habits are clearly present. Occasionally, mild hypoglycemic states account for temporary anxiety, irritability, and fatigue in normal and neurotic persons. Psychotherapy in severe and obstinate cases may be warranted.

Emotional Factors in Genital Dysfunctions

In this section, psychosomatic and somatopsychic dysfunctions involving the organs of reproduction are described. The most frequent of these dysfunctions are impotence and frigidity—essentially as we see them today, forms of neurotic behavior with disturbances in the ability to copulate effectively and pleasurably. The role of emotions in other dysfunctions, such as amenorrhea, dysmenorrhea, and infertility, is more complex and obscure. A number of genital somatopsychic syndromes, such as the different forms of hermaphroditism and Cushing's disease, will be described in Chapter 16. The psychosocial aspects of pregnancy and parturition are taken up in Chapter 25.

Impotence and Frigidity

Impotence is the partial or total inability of the male to perform and enjoy sexual intercourse. *Frigidity* is the corresponding disturbance in the female. Some cases are relatively simple inhibitions and others very complex characterological disturbances. The criteria for these symptoms are, in fact, elusive; we have no definite norm for potency or for a woman's capacity to perform and enjoy sexual relations. Frequency of sexual intercourse, duration of its length, and degree of enjoyment vary tremendously. According to Alfred C. Kinsey *et al.*, the number of performed sexual acts ranges from zero to 100,000 in a lifetime; the intensity of sex behavior decreases from puberty on. Twenty per cent of the male population retain capacity for intercourse beyond the age of 70.[72]

Total or partial impotence occurs if any of the steps in the normal sexual performance is impaired: desire for intercourse, erection, ejaculation, orgasm, and relaxation.[60] Only in severe cases is the desire completely absent, but the need for intercourse may vary greatly in the same individual, depending on the partner, circumstances, and other factors. The completely potent male who can copulate at any time, at any place, and with any woman, does not exist in reality: if he did, he would be a social monstrosity. At least for long-lasting relationships, we postulate a fusion of sexual and affectional needs. Lack of erection, disappearance of erection immediately before intercourse, or soft erection is characteristic of total impotence. *Premature ejaculation* is the most frequent form of "partial" impotence. As we cannot always know how long intercourse should last for a given couple, we cannot define premature emission categorically. In any case, emission before, or immediately after, introduction of the penis is a disturbed function for which patients frequently seek therapy. Female partners of the upper social classes in Western culture, who require a longer time for arousal and satisfaction, may complain about intercourse of short duration, although the sources of such complaints may be a displacement of guilt and envy. Most compatible couples can permit mutual pleasure and adapt themselves readily to achieve it. Disturbed orgasm or lack of orgasm, as in extreme cases of retarded ejaculation in the male, is relatively rare. Lack of relaxation after intercourse and postcoital depression are usually complex disturbances and must be considered within the context of the patient's general attitudes about sex. Although derision and contempt for the impotent male is marked, frigidity is likely to be condoned. The behavioral components of frigidity—for example, lack of desire, inability to be aroused, inability to achieve orgasm, and inability to relax after intercourse—are not as easily and readily distinguished as in the male. In most cases, frigidity is characterized by a lack of enjoyment of intercourse and an inability to achieve orgasm. In severe cases, there is pain in intercourse (dispareunia); an inability to admit the penis because of contractions of the pelvic floor muscles (vaginismus); or a complete absence of lubricating secretion in vagina and vulva. The most important complaints of the female are various degrees of aversion to sexual union, ranging from indifference to high anxiety and guilt. Transient shifts of satisfaction can occur, but anger, fatigue, indifference or disgust are dominant affects. Obviously, such emotions in both male and female interfere with adequate functioning during the sexual act.

The frigid woman may be afraid of "the masculine assault," and the impotent male may be concerned essentially with being castrated or humiliated by an aggressive female. Both sexes sometimes "go on strike" and punish the partner (or atone to their consciences) with diminished performance. Very few diseases, such as tumors of the spinal cord or tabes dorsalis, causing the destruction of neural mechanisms essential for erection and ejaculation will cause impotence. Some metabolic diseases, such as diabetes, are said to impair potency, but findings are by no means unequivocal, and in all likelihood psychological disturbances play a role in causing impotence in these diseases too. Certain phenothiazines (thioridazine) may rarely depress ejaculation without affecting orgastic gratification. Even in males who were castrated before puberty and in various forms of pseudohermaphroditism originating before and after puberty, relatively normal function has been observed; psychosexual identification—being a male or a female—depends as much on experience and attitude as equipment. Frigidity due to genitourinary disease, injury, or malformation is also exceedingly rare.

In human beings, emotions more than any other factors control sexual functions; desire, orgasm, and gratification are defined primarily by their psychological value and meaning, and variations in any one person in the experience of these components of sexual behavior are the rule. They are determined by a complex of attitudes and concurrent feelings, attachments to the loved person, and internal needs. The term "psychic impotence" merely reflects the absence of physical symptoms in what essentially is always an experientially significant behavioral function. Virtually all cases of impotence and frigidity are caused by anxiety, guilt, shame, and anger. These affects are in some cases the result of realistic danger, as in undesirable sexual intercourse, or the result of moral prohibitions. The inhibitions produced by these affects may be relatively slight, superficial, and temporary, or severe and enduring. A typical instance of a temporary disturbance is the sexual inhibition that frequently occurs on the honeymoon of the newlywed or in a situation of first sexual experience, when the necessary skills are not yet acquired, and anxiety, often with guilt and shame, is excessive. Although sexual inhibitions of cultural origin are not as pervasive as in the Victorian era, they are still sufficiently marked to produce at least temporary dysfunction in a great many persons. It is often forgotten that masturbation is the chief sexual experience prior to intercourse and that, although intercourse is "natural," it may take time even for the excitable young person to learn how to achieve the pleasures available. Normal individuals certainly vary in acquiring these skills. Often, we find specific experiences of punishment for sexual behavior in the history of impotent or frigid patients. The resulting anxiety may be overt or repressed; the resulting symptom may be part of a general anxiety state or hysterical reaction. The causes for more severe sexual inhibitions have deeper origins; such patients display a certain infantilism usually found to be related to childhood fantasies or ambitions and persisting attachment and taboos.[39] Obviously, a profound homosexual orientation is accompanied by heterosexual impotence. Some "bisexual" persons may be able to copulate satisfactorily with partners of both sexes, although in most of these cases there is some impairment of function.

From a therapeutic standpoint, it is very important to assess whether impotence or frigidity occurs temporarily or permanently, and whether it is manifest with a particular partner or under specific conditions. Obviously, impotence with a spouse is more serious than a "protective" failure with a prostitute or pickup. Difficulties that are largely due to transient situational stresses or to inexperience and to the ubiquitous but too severe guilt and anxiety over sex in our culture, are not as serious in therapy as the impotence or frigidity that is the result of severe previous sexual trauma (usually in childhood), the disturbances that accompany severe perversions, or disturbances based on fairly entrenched neurotic conflicts. In the first case, sexual instruction, general reassurance, and possibly prescription of a tranquilizing drug—or even a drink or two—may be effective; in the other cases, only psychotherapy will help. Psychiatrists and other medical practitioners should keep in mind that certain cases of mild frigidity may well be left alone if the partners are compatible and function well otherwise.

Character Neurosis and Impotence Treated by Analytic Psychotherapy

A twenty-seven-year-old lawyer begged the therapist on his knees(!) to take him into therapy. He suffered almost constantly from such severe anxiety that he could not work. Although he was brilliant, with a superior law school record, he was told that he would lose his position if he did not take serious steps to change. A small, wiry man who talked incessantly and at high speed with lively gestures, the patient was able to check his logorrhea only as treatment progressed.

Apart from his anxiety, associated with gastric pains and frequent bouts of diarrhea, he complained of impotence. In repeated attempts at intercourse with girls of his own social group, he always failed to have an erection. His desire was great, but he did not frequent prostitutes for fear of acquiring a venereal disease. Just before entering treatment, he fell in love with a young woman; it came to heavy necking and cunnilingus, but he was unable to have intercourse although his experienced partner tried to encourage it and be helpful. In general, he complained that women treated him like a little boy and made fun of him. He was usually interested in more than one woman and talked readily to them about his sexual problems. He masturbated excessively—as much as ten times a day. He freely admitted he would like to be a woman; there was, however, no history of overt homosexual activity except for mutual masturbation at puberty with a partner of the same age. A good part of this behavior proved to be a manifestation of fear and self-contempt. He provoked his colleagues by talking too much and at the wrong time and in a self-belittling way, thereby inviting their aggression and condescension.

The patient was the only son of a lower-middle class family. The father, a tense, anxious tailor, was dominated by his wife, the matriarch in the family, and a demanding, aggressive, and possessive person. To the patient, the father could be critical, harsh, and belittling. At one time, he gave him a good thrashing before other children because he did not want to fight with a bigger boy. From an early age on, the mother took the patient into her confidence, telling him details about her marriage—among other things, about her frigidity and also her disappointment in her incompetent husband. She was given to hysterical outbursts and incessantly complained about minor, imaginary, and major real illnesses including a bilateral mastectomy and a hysterectomy. After these operations, she became particularly seductive and exhibitionistic to the patient; this was extremely upsetting to him.

Appreciated by his teachers and colleagues for his intellect, the patient was nevertheless despised for his cringing and yet aggressive behavior. He obtained an excellent job but was unhappy in it because of his unsatisfactory personal relations. In particular, he provoked anti-Semitic comments and also felt deeply hurt by them. Never in robust health, he had many nervous symptoms, and his fingers were chronically infected from nailbiting.

The patient tended to confuse therapy by intellectualizing and punning; it took time before he felt compatible enough to communicate simply and directly rather than clown and demean himself in trying to make the therapist laugh. During therapy, he became emotionally involved with another patient of the therapist, a seductive, promiscuous woman, who soon treated him like a slave. When he discussed this, including his fantasies about the therapist's relationship to this female patient, much of his relationship to his father and mother became more comprehensible to him. Gradually, he became more openly aggressive to the therapist; he was relieved to find he was taken seriously and would not be belittled, and he finally stopped the masochistic relationship with the other patient. He slowly worked through his fantasies concerning "dangerous and castrating" women and as he became more assured he also felt less compelled to be in the foreground, talk, provoke, assert, or belittle himself. He masturbated less and felt physically more fit. There were still a few bouts of anxiety with diarrhea and vomiting, but in general, after some hundred hours of therapy, the patient felt much improved. He arranged to take another job where he would be taken more seriously. Two years after termination, it was learned that he was married and had a reasonably good emotional and sexual relationship with a warm and supporting wife.

Menarche and Menopause

Physicians are frequently consulted about behavioral and somatic difficulties connected with the onset and cessation of menses. The onset of menses, even without any somatic dysfunction, usually is an upsetting event, especially if no psychological preparation has taken place; it mobilizes earlier fantasies over the dangers and "dirty" nature of sexuality. Physicians can help girls (either directly or through their mothers) overcome such concerns and prepare them realistically for their sex role.

The great majority of women develop mild symptoms of discomfort during the menopause, but only a small fraction requires endocrine and psychological therapy. During the menopause, the ovaries produce a markedly diminished amount of estrogens, which results in a cessation of ovulation, cessation of the menstrual cycle, and a gradual but slight atrophy of inner and outer genitalia, and also of the breasts. Some authors believe that an oversecretion of gonadotropic hormone also plays a role in the genesis of the menopause syndrome. Vasomotor changes such as hot flushes, sweating, fatigue, sensation of coldness, dizziness, headaches, nausea, and dyspepsia are the common complaints during this period. Many women also become markedly depressed, anxious, and irritable. They feel that life has lost its purpose after the "change of life," and react with anxiety and depression to bodily changes. Feelings of having become barren and sexually unattractive are experienced as severe narcissistic injuries. In neurotic women, menopausal symptoms are apt to be more pronounced. William S. Kroger and S. C. Freed make the interesting observation that many women develop menopausal symptoms within a year after a simple hysterectomy.[78] They explain this phenomenon in women with normally functioning ovaries and with adequate blood supply, as a result of the patients' castration anxiety. The therapy of the menopausal syndrome usually relies on medication with estrogens or stilbesterol and, depending on the needs of the patient and the skill of the therapist, on supportive or brief psychotherapy. The psychological effects of hormones, especially in an era where they are used for birth control, require further research.

It should be mentioned that in a fair number of men, mild depressive symptoms occur in the fifth decade, perhaps related to the fact that these men have passed the peak of their careers and feel useless and unwanted. Physical symptoms such as headaches, dizziness, and hot flushes are noted but are relatively rare, and the pathophysiology of the "male climacterium" is quite obscure.

Amenorrhea

Endocrinologists distinguish between primary amenorrhea, when menses have never occurred, and secondary amenorrhea, when menses have ceased. The causes for primary amenorrhea are hormonal dysfunctions, associated with psychological infantilism. There are also otherwise healthy young girls, with normal hormonal assays ruling out endocrine deficiency, in whom physical and psychological signs and symptoms of immaturity are found. Many of these patients have a childlike or boyish appearance; they are shy, withdrawn, anxious, and often hysterical. On more thorough investigation, rejection of the feminine role and overt or covert conflicts with their mothers are often discovered; possibly such disturbances are contributing causes of the syndrome. Secondary amenorrhea, like primary amenorrhea, may be caused by organic conditions such as almost any serious illness or malnutrition, as well as by endocrine and gyneocological disorders. In a large number of patients with amenorrhea, however, no organic causes are found. In amenorrhea of "unknown origin," the women were psychosexually immature and could not accept adult sexuality.[69]

Amenorrhea may be the direct consequence of tension and anxiety; many women and girls with amenorrhea consider their menses dirty and disgusting. Delay or absence of menses after guilt-evoking intercourse is quite frequent and may be understood as an expression of fear of (or wish for) pregnancy. A well-known type of hysterical amenorrhea occurs in pseudocyesis or hysterical pregnancy. Such patients look and act like pregnant women; their abdomens are distended by meteorism; they report bizarre appetites like other gravida, and complain about nausea and vomiting. There may be enlargement of the breasts, lactorrhea, and even a softening of the cervix; everything is there except the baby! In women with pseudocyesis, strong unconscious wishes for impregnation are often found, usually with an incestuous tie to their fathers. Nongaseous abdominal bloating, or Alvarez syndrome, also a condition with many hysterical aspects, often occurs in middle-aged women without amenorrhea.[4] It is not difficult to deliver such patients from their dramatic symptoms by suggestive therapy, which may be followed by intensive psychotherapy directed at the central conflict. Most psychogenic amenorrheas are not treated as easily.

Dysmenorrhea

This syndrome consists of general discomfort, abdominal and pelvic cramps and pains, lassitude, headache, dysepepsia, nausea, irritability, and depression accompanying menses. It is caused by a number of medical and gyneocological diseases, but in many patients the symptoms are psychogenic. They often occur in anxious and hostile women who reject the feminine role.

Therese Benedek and Boris B. Rubinstein found that such women were particularly anxious and irritable during the premenstrual phase: in psychoanalysis, such patients expressed an unconscious fear of castration.[12] During the menstrual phase, fear and irritability change to depression; feelings of being dirty and worthless are interpreted as unconscious disappointment at not being pregnant.[6] In our opinion, the question whether such dysmenorrhea is the result of rejection of the feminine role, or a correlate of undefined hormonal processes has not been satisfactorily answered.

In the older literature, so-called menstrual psychoses were described. In some schizophrenic and epileptic patients, an aggravation of symptoms at the time of menses has been noted. The existence of severe episodic behavior disorders solely attributable to endocrine changes and behavioral stresses connected with the menstrual cycle is, however, not certain.

Other Gynecological Diseases

LEUKORRHEA This disease often stubbornly persists in spite of gynecological and general somatic therapy and is also considered a psychosomatic disturbance. In some patients with *menorrhagias* and *metrorrhagias*, somatic causes were excluded by careful gynecological examinations; psychological causes were therefore assumed to be of etiological significance. The underlying mechanism possibly consists of vascular congestion and hyperemia produced by intense emotions.[15] A sober scientist like Wolff also assumed that the development of tumors may be accelerated by psychogenic factors.[153] F. Wengraf reported that he had successfully treated fibromas by psychotherapy.[143] Kroger and Freed state that they have not been able to produce such effects.[78]

INFERTILITY The important problem of infertility is extraordinarily complex. Experts in the field explored thoroughly and systematically a variety of structural, physiological, and pathological causes for infertility in both partners.[26] In many cases, however, no organic factors to explain sterility can be found. It is, of course, possible that a low sperm count or dysfunction in ovulation may be accounted for by psychological causes, but evidence for such assumptions is usually lacking. Occasionally, couples simply do not have intercourse. In a number of cases, the problem may be solved by proper advice about sexual matters; precise determination of ovulation by temperature measurements will permit intercourse at the right time; proper position of the partners and avoidance of adverse practices, such as douches before or after intercourse, may help. Many infertile couples are fatigued and under stress when they have intercourse, and this may somehow have an untoward effect on fertility. At times, simple clarification may help to correct adverse habits and facilitate impregnation. In some cases, a more intensive psychotherapeutic effort may help to tackle the sexual difficulties or the unconscious motivation to avoid having children. Unfortunately, there are no controlled studies that demonstrate the role of psychogenic factors in sterility. Fertility after psychotherapy of husband and wife, or either one, has often been observed; whether this is the result of psychotherapy is difficult to establish. An interesting and not infrequent observation concerns previously infertile couples who had children of their own after adopting a child, which presumably produces a better attitude to parenthood.[113] Artificial insemination may create considerable anxiety and conflict in both partners and requires sensitive psychological handling. Proper advice about contraceptives always requires psychological sensitivity and knowledge.

HABITUAL ABORTION Some women who suffer from habitual abortion have conscious and unconscious wishes to get rid of the child and perhaps excessively miss a warm, paternal support and approval by the husband. On the other hand, there are innumerable women who, in spite of such wishes and unsatisfactory husbands, carry their pregnancies through to term. Criminal and therapeutic abortions are usually very stressful experiences for women who often, consciously or unconsciously, interpret them as infanticide. A program of sterilization was carried out on a psychiatric population in Sweden; the behavioral consequences ranged from minimal to very severe upsets[38] and seemed to be related to psychodynamic factors.[12] The question of indications for therapeutic abortion are discussed in Chapter 24.

Emotional Factors in Musculo-Skeletal and Neurological Syndromes

Low Back Pain

A frequent, troublesome, and often puzzling symptom is pain in the low lumbar, sacral, and sacroiliac regions of the back. It may be caused by a variety of diseases and injuries of bones and joints of the vertebral column or its adjoining structures, such as neoplasm of prostate, rectum, uterus, or retroperitoneal structures. The most frequent causes of low back pain are fibromuscular spasms and strains with and without *herniation of the intervertebral* discs of the lumbosacral spine; back strains and herniated discs are mercurial syndromes with obscure etiologies, even in cases with definite traumatic histories. A thorough orthopedic and neurological examination will permit detection of organic etiological factors of such back pain in a fair number of cases. In many instances of proven herniated discs and pain after trauma, psychological factors contribute to the symptom and complicate the picture. Besides such cases, there are many cases of back strain without any organic pathology or with inconsistent and bizarre signs; in such cases, one is particularly inclined to explain the syndrome psychologically.[23] Conversion reactions, especially after accidents with palpable secondary gains, and particularly when compensation is involved, are frequently observed. The majority of psychogenic backaches are found in anxious persons, perhaps with poor postural habits, and usually with muscular tension and unconscious motivation to escape from disagreeable tasks; in some of these instances, exploration of causes for tension and exploitation of secondary gains may be successful. It is understandable that backaches from bad posture are frequent in occupations where marching (soldiers), standing (waiters, sales personnel), and sitting (office workers, psychotherapists) are important.

Collagen-Vascular Diseases

A wide group of diseases, such as *lupus erythematosus, scleroderma, dermatomyositis,* and *periarteritis nodosa,* involve lesions of blood vessels and connective tissue. Some of these diseases affect the brain and are taken up in Chapter 16. Therapies with steroids are sometimes employed for inflammatory aspects of these often grave disorders. Emotional factors have not been well investigated, although emotional complications could be expected, not only on the basis of reaction to the disease, but perhaps also in the basis of central nervous system involvement. *Rheumatic diseases,* which are pathophysiologically related to the above diseases, are similarly little understood. Sero-inflammatory processes are known to be exacerbated during emotional stress, but the etiology of the whole group of rheumatic symptoms is essentially unknown; infection, or metabolic, autoimmune, and endocrine abnormalities may play a role.

The group of diseases referred to as *rheumatoid arthritis* is characterized by multiple afflictions of the joints and chronic inflammation of the periosteal and subcutaneous connective tissue. Since 1923, when Eli Jelliffe pointed to a number of relevant psychogenic factors, rheumatoid arthritis has been considered a psychosomatic disease.[66] Stanley Cobb, W. Bauer, and I. Whiting stated that, in thirty of fifty arthritic patients, upsetting life events had a relationship to the onset of exacerbation of symptoms.[31] Unconscious hostility, rebellion against authority, guilt, and preoccupations with morality problems probably play an important role in such patients. Alfred Ludwig stressed loss of security and dependency needs as etiological factors.[91]

Weiss and English feel that a psychotherapeutic approach, particularly in the patient with chronic rheumatoid arthritis, has much to offer.[142] They feel that excessive medication, too much physiotherapy, and prolonged bed rest may be harmful and only increase invalidism. However, few psychiatrists would try to deal with the complex and frustrating therapeutic problems of chronic rheumatoid arthritis by psychotherapy alone. Etiological and therapeutic statements similar to those made about chronic rheumatoid arthritis, which occurs mostly in the young-age range, have also been made about *osteoarthritis* in middle and old age.

Tics

Involuntary, sudden, repetitive, circumscribed muscular movements, or tics, have been considered an expression of neurotic behavior for a long time. The symptoms are twitching movements of face and neck and blinking. Grimacing and more complex mannerisms are not easily differentiated from tics. These motor symptoms occur in a wide variety of basal ganglia diseases, but many tics are expressions of affects, even if an eye disease or nerve injury originally triggered the behavior. They become quite automatic and, although modifiable, can recur under tension even in successfully treated cases. The simplest assumption, by no means totally satisfactory, is to regard them as an expression of tension. Tics have been considered as a playful attempt to express aggression and frighten others. They often occur in patients with obsessive personalities. In some rare cases, tics are associated with coprolalia, which is quite striking in the *maladie des tics*, or *Giles de la Tourette's syndrome*. In the psychoanalytic literature, there is considerable discussion of whether tics are primarily expressions of defenses or of pregenital and aggressive drives. Many therapies, including analytic psychotherapy, cathartic hypnosis, suggestive hypnosis, and other persuasive and conditioning therapies, as well as pharmacological treatment with neuroleptics and even, in severe cases, lobotomy have been recommended, but the results generally have been modest. Tics are, in fact, rarely cured, but they can be relieved by a variety of techniques.[57]

Stuttering

Stuttering is usually defined as a labored, difficult, hesitant, or explosive form of speech. Dominick A. Barbara distinguishes it from stammering for which articulation difficulties are characteristic.[9] In very severe cases, communication is highly disturbed, and often the patients are also troubled by tics and general motor discoordination. Severe defects usually appear in childhood. Even such severe defects fluctuate, and all stutterers speak normally at times. There is actually a short period between the ages of three and five in which very many children stutter for a short time. The etiology of stuttering is obscure; as is usually the case in such disorders, theories are rampant, with relatively little factual evidence. Some authors consider stuttering a cerebrally caused disorganization. It has been thought by some to be related to handedness, because a considerable number of stutterers are left-handed or ambidextrous. Others have focused on cross-lateral dominance (for example, left-handed and right-eye preference) as contributory. The factor of heredity in this disorder is controversial. There is a high concordance of stuttering in twins, and the disorder occurs frequently in several members of a given family. Emil Froeschels and Anton Jellinek who called stuttering a dissociative aphasia, believes that it is a learned disturbance.[54] A number of authors see in it essentially a failure in social communication as a result of neurotic development. Stuttering is a way of delaying communication, related to many tactics of speech whereby the speaker "buys time" and controls the pace of verbal communication. There is much to support a psychogenic point of view without denying the relevance of other etiological factors. Speech habits easily become automatized, and effective control may require special training if faulty patterns become established. Since speech is closely linked to imitation as well as to communication, in development, attitudes, identifications, and emotions will condition speech, and speech patterns will reflect aspects of object relationships and identifications. Anxiety and tension definitely have a disorganizing effect on speech that resembles mild stuttering, and emotional stress definitely aggravates stuttering.[96] It seems likely, though not conclusively proven, that stutterers have severe, demanding, and rejecting parents. They are often able but compulsive, vacillating and hesitating personalities, struggling with problems of aggressive assertion; sadomasochistic traits may be evident and these personal problems are reflected in the consequences of stuttering as a mode of communication. It is important to distinguish between primary and secondary characteristics of stuttering. Secondary characteristics are the reaction to an embarrassing and handicapping defect, which is apt to isolate the stutterers and make them hostile, bitter, and resentful.

Therapy of stuttering consists of speech therapy, based on the premise that stuttering is a learned form of speech, and perhaps also intensive psychotherapy aiming to improve the basic lack of security, trust, and self-esteem of the stuttering person as these are manifest in his current life situations. Therapies should start early, in childhood, soon after the defect is diagnosed, but not all children with the disorder require therapy. The decision should be made only after observation of the relative intransigence of the symptom. Close rapport with the parents, if necessary by individual or group therapy aiming at relaxing parental demands and attitudes, is often helpful.

Insomnia

This is a complexly determined symptom found in many neurotic-psychotic patients. From the fundamental work of Nathaniel Kleitman, we know that the need for sleep varies considerably[73] and that muscular fatigue and relaxation play a predominant role in the physiology of both sleep and in the rest that accompanies sleep (see Chapter 6). Apart from patients with encephalitis or postencephalitic states, in whom the sleep-regulating mechanism of the brain stem is damaged, insomnia can be caused by physical pain, a considerable variety of physical discomforts, and, most frequently, by psychological events that either prevent patients from falling asleep or interrupt their sleep. Sleep disturbances in schizophrenia are discussed in Chapter 14 and disturbances in depression in Chapter 15; the consequences both of sleep deprivation and of a loss of a customary behavioral pattern may be quite disorganizing for vulnerable persons (see Chapter 6). The most important emotions that disturb sleep are anxiety and anger. Lawrence S. Kubie told us that insomnia produced by anxiety is treatable by ordinary sedatives such as barbiturates but that inability to sleep caused by rage did not respond to such drug therapy. Patients are often unaware not only of the context of such emotions but even of their existence and complain simply of their effects. Night terrors and bad dreams are reported by some patients as sleep-disturbing events and often furnish clues about the nature of the disturbance. Patients vary in their attitudes toward sleep disturbances, and some find any disruption a psychological deprivation equivalent to being denied food or a basic right; others acknowledge discomfort but are less conscious about the deprivation. In any event, sleep is an episode integrated into the entirety of the patient's life, and the causes and treatment of disturbances cannot be isolated from links with waking life. Therapy of insomnia includes treatment with sedatives, general measures to produce fatigue and relaxation, and psychotherapy. One might also remember that appropriate sexual gratification is an excellent sedative and that persistent sexual excitement may prevent patients from falling asleep. Some psychiatrists, aware of physiological requirements, instruct their patients that sleep is not necessary as long as the patient is able to rest and relax in bed. Such advice is of little help because what troubles the patient and keeps him from sleeping is too much anger or too much anxiety. The most rational way to deal with insomnia is to treat the underlying disturbing affect. Such psychotherapy, however, is often a difficult and time-consuming task, and therapists often rely solely on sedatives with all the potential dangers of addiction and denial of the critical problems of daily living, which the patient may also prefer to avoid. Treatment of a really acute state in which re-establishment of a sleep pattern is required is facilitated by judicious and adequate sedation (even though therapists often chasten themselves with the worry that by giving a sedative they are reinforcing the patient's basic tendency to avoid reality). To the contrary, they actually may thereby help the patient to be in a position to cope more effectively.

Fatigue

One of the most common and most obscure symptoms encountered is the complaint of fatigue. We distinguish fatigue or general lassitude associated with mental and psychomotor energy from muscular weakness or asthenia contingent upon a loss of muscular power.[10] When patients complain of symptoms of asthenia, they usually also complain of fatigue. Thorough medical examination may locate causes of asthenia in a range of medical illnesses, particularly obscure infections, undetected neoplastic diseases, anemia, Addison's disease, and myasthenia gravis. In the last two diseases, psychological stress definitely aggravates them. According to a verbal communication by Eugene W. Meyer, psychological trauma can even precipitate myasthenia gravis. It is not uncommon to find neurotic patients who, as many so-called normal persons, have not learned to recognize their bodily needs in illness; they may overcompensate and deny a fatigue, which, for example, follows a viral infection. They do not recognize that their reserves are diminished and they overcompensate with the result of increasing depression, frustration, and inefficiency. When no physical causes of asthenia can be detected, existence of psychogenic causes is assumed and sometimes is clearly evident. It is believed that such patients suffer from unresolved unconscious anxiety, anger, and frustration, as in so many other diseases and syndromes.

Fainting

Syncope, or fainting, means sudden loss of consciousness with quick and complete recovery. It is usually differentiated from coma and subcoma in which loss of consciousness is less transient. Syncope, with the exception of hysterical fainting and loss of consciousness in the cerebral dysrhythmias, is in the last analysis due to a chemical, physical, or reflexive interference with cerebral oxygenation. Many clear-cut syndromes of syncope are referred to by their causes: bradycardia, tachycardia, carotid sinus reflex, orthostatic hypotension, hyperventilation, hypoglycemia, and the strictly psychogenic forms. Psychogenic factors usually play a role in orthostatic hypotension and in hypoglycemia; they are always present in hyperventilation.

The pure psychogenic forms of syncope are differentiated by Romano and Engel into an anxiety type and a hysterical type.[123] In the anxiety type, which may be associated with a hyperventilation syndrome, the individual at the onset of the syncope feels anxious, sweaty, dizzy, has blurred vision, ringing in the ears, and feels faint. In the hysterical type the above prodromata, which also occur in the predominantly "organic" types of syncope, are absent. Hysterical syncope comes on suddenly, and the patients are usually bland and surprised. It has symbolic meaning, usually signifying escape from an aggressive or sexual conflict. Cultural factors have reduced the incidence of social fainting, the prerogative of the supposedly delicate Victorian woman. In syncope caused by hysterical conflicts and anxiety, only a psychotherapeutic approach offers any promise if the disorder is repetitive and disabling.

Headache

Headache is surely the most common medical symptom. Yet the pathogenesis of most headaches, and particularly the psychogenic headache, is far from clear. According to Wolff, nine out of ten headaches are psychologically determined.[152] Psychiatrists should be familiar with the differential diagnosis of organic headache and should try to rule out the headaches that are not psychogenic. Intelligence and memory tests should be performed, and a thorough medical workup, including tests of visual acuity, X-ray of the skull, EEG, urinalysis serum, nonprotein nitrogen, and blood sugar, and, in some cases, lumbar punctures with examination of the spinal fluid, needs to be undertaken. Usually, these procedures will establish possible organic causes such as tumors; acute febrile infection; diseases of nose, ear, or paranasal sinuses; eye diseases (particularly glaucoma); increased intracranial pressure; head injury; vascular and renal diseases; and possibly diseases of the cranial and cervical sensory nerves.

The above methods of examination help to identify specific syndromes, of which the most important is *migraine*. This syndrome probably has a multifactorial etiology; heredity plays a role, but psychological stress often precipitates attacks; a rigid and perfectionistic character trait has been observed. The headache is characterized in typical cases by paroxysmal, circumscribed, usually one-sided pain; it occurs in attacks with prodromal signs such as scotoma, visceral symptoms, nausea and vomiting. It often responds specifically to therapy with vasoconstrictors. Pain is associated with dilation of the cranial vasculature. There may be local edema, which has been ascribed to neurohumoral factors and the release of polypeptides, serotonin, acetylcholine and histamines. Water and electrolyte retention may occur concomitantly with an attack, and aminoaciduria has been noted; these may be secondary to pain and muscle tension.[30, 74]

Other related syndromes are *histamine headache* and headaches caused by *spasm of the temporal artery*. In both, emotional factors may contribute to the precipitation of attacks. The responsible physical mechanisms of psychogenic headaches are muscular tension or vasomotor changes. It is particularly apt to occur when the patient is exhausted and helpless in his effort to cope with a difficult situation or an overpowering adversary. Organic headaches are usually intermittent; an experienced clinician such as H. Houston Merritt teaches that enduring headaches are always psychogenic. In many cases, psychotherapy will help to identify such emotional affects and permit better handling of the problem.

Vertigo

Vertigo refers to the unpleasant feeling of circular and falling movement, often connected with sensations of nausea and faintness. True vertigo should be distinguished from giddiness, in which unsteadiness but not the sense of turning is present. Disturbances of equilibrium such as ataxia in various neurological disorders also occur without vertigo. The physical causes of vertigo are otological, ophthalmic, neurological, and general illness involving the vestibular system. One of the most frequently encountered syndromes with an obscure etiology is Ménière's Disease, characterized by vertigo, tinnitus, and deafness. Psychological factors aggravate symptoms of Ménière's Disease and other forms of vertigo.[50] An important disturbance related to vertigo is motion sickness, induced by a complex of physically defined components of motion (pitch, yaw, angular velocities) acting on the inner ear. Psychological factors (for example, anxiety, often related specifically to a particular form or purpose of travel), fatigue, and general poor health are contributory factors. In all likelihood, there is also a constitutional vestibular oversensitivity present. Ninety-five per cent of experimental subjects adapt to the specific physical component of motion that induced sickness.[58]

In a large number of patients with subjective vertigo and giddiness, however, no organic pathology is found, and a search for psychological causes commonly reveals abnormal anxieties, anger, and dependency needs. At times, the psychotherapeutic exploration of anxieties and irritations over threats and conflicts brings relief; but in other cases, little tangible improvement has been produced. Results are difficult to evaluate, as vertigo and giddiness in some patients stop as mysteriously as they begin.

Enuresis

In adults, enuresis, or involuntary bed-wetting during sleep, is a troublesome and by no means infrequent symptom. During World War II, between two and three per cent of American soldiers suffered from nocturnal enuresis. Adult enuresis is practically always preceded by childhood enuresis. Enuresis must be distinguished from urinary incontinence, which is the result of a variety of somatic conditions. A thorough general medical, neurological, and urological examination should be carried out to establish the most important organic causes of incontinence, such as urological defects and irritations, spina bifida, localized damage to cerebral and spinal centers for micturition, or diffuse brain damage. It should also be kept in mind that emotional problems, invariably present in such patients, aggravate incontinence. Enuresis of adults occurs most frequently in deteriorated patients with chronic brain disease, and in epileptics, schizophrenics, and mental deficients. It is also a social symptom and occurs relatively frequently in institutional settings, such as prisons, barracks, and schools. The majority of patients reveal psychological tension and conflict by their enuresis. By his symptoms, the enuretic expresses his aggression and resentment of situations over which he feels he has no control and which he has to endure. He may respond to a sexual temptation by enuresis. Most enuretics are infantile personalities; mild-to-severe sexual infantilism, such as persistent masturbation, ejaculatio praecox, impotence, frigidity, and overt or near-overt homosexual behavior are not uncommonly correlated with enuresis. Treatment of enuresis in adults is not an easy matter. Common-sense procedures, for example, restriction of fluids and urination before retiring, are practically never sufficient. Advocates of a conditioning approach claim remarkable successes. The prevalent psychiatric approach in North America is to help the patient, through psychotherapy, to understand the nature of the symptoms and to induce him to relinquish his infantile needs and conflicts and assume responsibility for this elemental physiological function. Involuntary defecation (*encopresis*) in adults, apart from fecal incontinence caused by rectal or circumscribed neural lesions, is a severe symptom usually observed in deteriorated and very regressed patients.

Overview of Psychosomatic Medicine

Claims that psychological stresses produce anatomic and physiological alterations, or at least contribute to them, have been made in many "purely organic" diseases. Some of the outstanding examples are the claims by W. A. Greene, I. F. Young, and S. N. Swisher that loss of an object plays a role in the genesis of leukemia,[59] or statements that psychological conflicts and stresses contribute to the etiology of cancer.[116] In another chronic disease, tuberculosis, many clinical and literary observations, such as Thomas Mann's *The Magic Mountain,* point to the influence of behavior on the illness. Such propositions are easily misunderstood; if they are cited to give the impression that psychological trauma directly causes cancer, leukemia, or tuberculosis, they make no sense. On the other hand, it is theoretically and practically plausible to assume that psychological stress and loss—the attitudes of hopelessness or helplessness—may contribute to the etiology of many more illnesses than we customarily assume, but they do so through component physiological mechanisms related to stress. These require extensive neurobehavioral research. Psychiatrists have learned to match their methods to their needs and are beginning to avoid overdesigned and highly complex correlative studies when exploratory work is required. Similarly, focused studies are replacing anecdotal accounts and fiats based on no data. We can expect a more sharply refined behavioral description of traits and a better appreciation of the variable role of current motivations on the one hand, and of the role of developmentally and constitutionally determined predispositional factors on the other. The "conditioning" of various component systems, their mode of integration into organismic behavior, is a very real problem and requires more than psychodynamic explanation. There is, fortunately, a growing tendency in the field for a sustained series of discrete studies in which the intention is to tackle a sequence of processes and to weigh multiple factors, rather than to explain everything at once. A more critical but also wider application of psychotherapeutic medicine is also noticeable; this will be discussed further in Chapter 25.

NOTES

1. Harold A. Abramson, *Somatic and Psychiatric Treatment of Asthma* (Baltimore: Williams & Wilkins, 1951).
2. Alfred Adler, *The Neurotic Constitution* (New York: Moffat, Yard, 1921).
3. Franz Alexander, *Psychosomatic Medicine* (New York: W. W. Norton, 1950).
4. Walter C. Alvarez, "Ways in Which Emotion Can Affect the Digestive Tract," *Journal of the American Medical Association,* 92 (1929), 1231.

5. Albert F. Ax, "The Physiological Differentiation between Fear and Anger in Humans," *Psychosomatic Medicine*, 15 (1953), 433.

6. Michael Balint, "Contribution to the Psychology of Menstruation," *Psychoanalytic Quarterly*, 6 (1937), 346.

7. Bernard Bandler, "Some Conceptual Tendencies in the Psychosomatic Movement," *American Journal of Psychiatry*, 115 (1958), 36.

8. Alvan L. Barach, *Physiologic Therapy in Respiratory Diseases* (Philadelphia: Lippincott, 1948).

9. Dominick A. Barbara, "Stuttering," in Silvano Arieti, ed., *American Handbook of Psychiatry* (New York: Basic Books, 1959), Vol. I, pp. 950–963.

10. S. Howard Bartley, "Fatigue and Inadequacy," *Physiological Reviews*, 37 (1957), 301.

11. William Beaumont, *Experiments and Observations on the Gastric Juice and the Physiology of Digestion* (Plattsburgh: F. P. Allen, 1833).

12. Therese Benedek and Boris B. Rubenstein, *The Sexual Cycle in Women*, "Psychosomatic Medicine Monographs," 3, National Research Council (1942).

13. Carl A. L. Binger, Nathan W. Ackerman, A. E. Cohn, H. A. Schroeder, and J. H. Steele, *Personality in Arterial Hypertension*, "Psychosomatic Medicine Monographs," 8, American Society for Research in Psychosomatic Problems (New York, 1945).

14. Rudolf P. Bircher, T. Kanai, and S. C. Wang, "Mechanism of Cardiac Arrhythmias and Blood Pressure Changes Induced in Dogs by Pentylene Tetrazol, Picrotoxin, and Deslanoside," *Journal of Pharmacology and Experimental Therapeutics*, 141 (1963), 6.

15. J. B. Blaikley, "Menorrhagia of Emotional Origin," *Lancet*, 257 (1959), 691.

16. Eugene L. Bliss and C. H. H. Branch, *Anorexia Nervosa* (New York: Hoeber-Harper 1960).

17. Eugene L. Bliss, W. R. Rumel, and C. H. H. Branch, "Psychiatric Complications of Mitral Surgery," *Archives of Neurology and Psychiatry*, 74 (1955), 249.

18. Jeanne Block, H. Jennings, E. Harvey, and E. Simpson, "Interaction between Allergic Potential and Psychopathology in Childhood Asthma," *Psychosomatic Medicine*, 26 (1964), 307.

19. F. Board, H. Persky, and D. A. Hamburg, "Psychological Stress and Endocrine Functions," *Psychosomatic Medicine*, 18 (1956), 324.

20. Morton D. Bogdonoff and E. H. Estes, "Energy Dynamics and Acute States of Arousal in Man," *Psychosomatic Medicine*, 23 (1961), 23.

21. Joseph V. Brady, "Ulcers in 'Executive' Monkeys," *Scientific American*, 199, No. 4 (1958), 95.

22. John R. Brobeck, "Neural Regulation of Food Intake," *Annals of the New York Academy of Sciences*, 63 (1955), 44.

23. Thornton Brown, J. C. Nemiah, J. S. Barr, and H. Barry, "Psychologic Fac-

tors in Low-Back Pain," *New England Journal of Medicine,* 251 (1954), 123.

24. Hilde Bruch, "Physiologic and Psychologic Interrelationships in Diabetes in Children," *Psychosomatic Medicine,* 11 (1949), 200.
25. Hilde Bruch and G. Touraine, "Obesity in Childhood: V. The Family Frame of Obese Children," *Psychosomatic Medicine,* 2 (1940), 141.
26. Charles L. Buxton and Anna L. Southam, *Human Infertility* (New York: Hoeber-Harper, 1958).
27. Konstantin M. Bykov, *The Cerebal Cortex and Internal Organs,* (trans. and ed. by W. H. Gantt), (New York: Chemical Publishing Co., 1957).
28. Walter B. Cannon, *Bodily Changes in Pain, Hunger, Fear and Rage* (New York: Appleton, 1929).
29. Walter B. Cannon, "Voodoo Death," *American Anthropologist,* 44 (1942), 169.
30. Loring F. Chapman, A. O. Ramos, H. Goodell, G. Silverman, and H. G. Wolff, "A Humoral Agent Implicated in Vascular Headache of Migraine Type," *Archives of Neurology,* 3 (1960), 223.
31. Stanley Cobb, W. Bauer, and I. Whiting, "Environmental Factors in Rheumatoid Arthritis," *Journal of the American Medical Association,* 113 (1939), 668.
32. Sanford I. Cohen, A. J. Silverman, W. Waddell and G. D. Zvidema, Urinary Catechol Amine, Gastric Secretion and Specific Psychological Factors in Ulcer and Non-Ulcer Patients," *Journal of Psychosomatic Research,* 5 (1961), 90.
33. J. W. Conn and H. S. Seltzer, "Spontaneous Hypoglycemia," *American Journal of Medicine,* 19 (1955), 460.
34. Agnes Conrad, "The Psychiatric Study of Hyperthyroid Patients," *Journal of Nervous and Mental Disease,* 79 (1934), 505.
35. George E. Daniels, John F. O'Conner, Charles Flood, Aaron Karush, Leon Moses, and Lenore Stern, "An Evaluation of the Effectiveness of Psychotherapy in the Treatment of Ulcerative Colitis," *Annals of Internal Medicine,* 60 (1964), 587.
36. George E. Daniels, "Analysis of a Case of Neurosis with Diabetes Mellitus," *Psychoanalytic Quarterly,* 5 (1936), 513.
37. E. Dekker, E. Van Vollenhoven, and J. During, "Further Experiments on the Origin of Asthmatic Wheezing," in Arthur Jores, and Hellmuth Freyberger, eds., *Advances in Psychosomatic Medicine,* No. 1 (New York: Robert Brunner, 1960).
38. Felix Deutsch, ed., *On the Mysterious Leap from the Mind to the Body* (New York: International Universities Press, 1959).
39. Helene Deutsch, *The Psychology of Women* (New York: Grune & Stratton, 1945).
40. M. Dongier, F. D. Wittkower, L. Stephens-Newsham, and M. M. Hoffman, "Psychophysiological Studies in Thyroid Function," *Psychosomatic Medicine,* 18 (1956), 310.

41. Helen F. Dunbar, *Psychosomatic Diagnosis* (New York: Paul B. Hoeber, 1943).
42. Martin Ekblad, "Prognosis after Sterilization on Social Psychiatric Grounds," *Acta Psychiatrica et Neurologica Scandinavica*, 37 (1961), Suppl. 161.
43. George L. Engel, "Studies of Ulcerative Colitis," *Psychosomatic Medicine*, 16 (1954), 496.
44. George L. Engel, "Studies of Ulcerative Colitis, II," *American Journal of Medicine*, 16 (1954), 416.
45. George L. Engel, "Studies of Ulcerative Colitis, III," *American Journal of Medicine*, 19 (1955), 231.
46. George L. Engel, "Studies of Ulcerative Colitis, IV," *Psychosomatic Medicine*, 18 (1956), 334.
47. George L. Engel, "Studies of Ulcerative Colitis, V, Psychological Aspects and Their Implications for Treatment," *American Journal of Digestive Diseases*, 3 (1958), 315.
48. George L. Engel and F. Reichsman, "Spontaneous and Experimentally Induced Depressions in an Infant with a Gastric Fistula," *Journal of the American Psychoanalytic Association*, 4 (1956), 428.
49. George L. Engel, F. Reichsman, and H. L. Segal, "A Study of an Infant with a Gastric Fistula," *Psychosomatic Medicine*, 18 (1956), 374.
50. Edmund P. Fowler and A. Zeckel, "Psychophysiological Factors in Meniere's Disease," *Psychosomatic Medicine*, 15 (1953), 127.
51. Daniel X. Freedman and G. Fenichel, "Effect of Midbrain Lesion on Experimental Allergy," *Archives of Neurology and Psychiatry*, 79 (1958), 164.
52. Daniel X. Freedman, F. C. Redlich, and W. W. Ignersheimer, "Psychosis and Allergy: Experimental Approach," *American Journal of Psychiatry*, 112 (1956), 873.
53. Thomas M. French and Franz Alexander, *Psychogenic Factors in Bronchial Asthma*, "Psychosomatic Medicine Monographs," 4, G. Banta (Menasha, Wisc., 1941).
54. Emil Froeschels and Anton Jellinek, *Practice of Voice and Speech Therapy* (Boston: Expression Company, 1941).
55. Daniel H. Funkenstein, "The Relationship of Experimentally Produced Asthmatic Attacks to Certain Acute Life Stresses," *Journal of Allergy*, 24 (1953), 11.
56. W. A. Horsley Gantt, *Experimental Basis for Neurotic Behavior*, "Psychosomatic Medicine Monographs," American Society for Research in Psychosomatic Problems (New York, 1944).
57. Margaret W. Gerard, "The Psychogenic Tic in Ego Development," *The Psychoanalytic Study of the Child* (New York: International Universities Press, 1946), Vol. II, p. 133.
58. Leslie N. Gay and P. E. Carliner, "The Prevention and Treatment of Motion Sickness," *Bulletin of the Johns Hopkins Hospital*, 84 (1949), 470.

59. W. A. Greene, Jr., I. F. Young, and S. N. Swisher, "Psychological Factors and Reticuloendothelial Disease," I, *Psychosomatic Medicine,* 16 (1954), 220; II, *Psychosomatic Medicine,* 18 (1956), 284.

60. Emil A. Gutheil, "Sexual Dysfunctions in Men," in Silvano Arieti, ed., *American Handbook of Psychiatry* (New York: Basic Books, 1959), Vol. I, p. 708.

61. George C. Ham, Franz Alexander, and Hugh T. Carmichael, "Dynamic Aspects of the Personality Features and Reactions Characteristic of Patients with Graves's Disease," in Harold G. Wolff, ed., *Life Stress and Bodily Disease* (Baltimore: Williams & Wilkins, 1950), p. 451. In Research Publications of Association for Research in Nervous and Mental Diseases, Vol. 29, 1950.

62. Josephine R. Hilgard and M. F. Newman, "Anniversaries in Mental Illness," *Psychiatry,* 22 (1959), 113.

63. Lawrence E. Hinkle, F. M. Evans, and S. Wolf, "Studies in Diabetes Mellitus," *Psychosomatic Medicine,* 13 (1951), 184.

64. Thomas H. Holmes, T. F. Treuting, and H. G. Wolff, "Life Situations, Emotions, and Nasal Diseases," *Psychosomatic Medicine,* 13 (1951), 71.

65. Thomas H. Holmes, N. G. Hawkins, C. E. Bowerman, E. R. Clarke, and J. R. Joffe, "Psychosocial and Psychophysiologic Studies of Tuberculosis," *Psychosomatic Medicine,* 19 (1957), 134.

66. Smith Ely Jelliffe, "The Neuropathology of Bone Disease," *Transactions of the American Neurological Association* (1923), p. 419.

67. Stanley M. Kaplan, Louis A. Gottschalk, and D. E. Fleming, "Modifications of Oropharyngeal Bacteria with Changes in the Psychodynamic State," *Archives of Neurology and Psychiatry,* 78 (1957), 656.

68. Frederic T. Kapp, M. Rosenbaum, and J. Romano, "Psychological Factors in Men with Peptic Ulcers," *American Journal of Psychiatry,* 103 (1947), 700.

69. Kenneth Kelley, G. E. Daniels, J. Poe, R. Easser, and R. Monroe, "Psychological Correlations with Secondary Amenorrhea," *Psychosomatic Medicine,* 16 (1954), 129.

70. Joseph G. Kepecs, M. Robin, and M. J. Brunner, "Relationship between Certain Emotional States and Exudation into the Skin," *Psychosomatic Medicine,* 13 (1951), 10.

71. Joseph G. Kepecs, M. Robin, and C. Munro, "Responses to Sensory Stimulation in Certain Psychosomatic Disorders," *Psychosomatic Medicine,* 20 (1958), 351.

72. Alfred C. Kinsey, Wardell B. Pomeroy, and Clyde E. Martin, *Sexual Behavior in the Human Male* (Philadelphia: W. B. Saunders, 1948).

73. Nathaniel Kleitman, *Sleep and Wakefulness as Alternating Phases in the Cycle of Existence* (Chicago: University of Chicago Press, 1939).

74. Robert W. Kimball, "Studies on the Pathogenesis of Migraine," in Joseph Wortis, ed., *Recent Advances in Biological Psychiatry* (New York: Grune & Stratton, 1961), Vol. III, p. 200.

75. Peter H. Knapp and S. J. Nemetz, "Acute Bronchial Asthma, I," *Psychosomatic Medicine*, 22 (1960), 42.

76. Peter H. Knapp, "Acute Bronchial Asthma," II, *Psychosomatic Medicine*, 22 (1960), 88.

77. W. E. Knox, "The Adaptive Control of Tryptophan and Tyrosine Metabolism in Animals," *Transactions of the New York Academy of Sciences*, 25 (1963), 503.

78. William S. Kroger, *Psychosomatic Gynecology* (Philadelphia: W. B. Saunders, 1951).

79. John I. Lacey, D. E. Bateman, and R. VanLehn, "Autonomic Response Specificity. An Experimental Study," *Psychosomatic Medicine*, 15 (1953), 8.

80. John I. Lacey and B. C. Lacey, "The Law of Initial Value in the Longitudinal Study of Autonomic Constitution: Reproducibility of Autonomic Responses and Response Patterns over a Four-Year Interval," *Annals of the New York Academy of Sciences*, 98 (1962), 1257.

81. John H. Lawrence, "Polycythemia: Physiology, Diagnosis and Treatment, Based on 303 Cases," *Modern Medical Monograph* (New York: Grune & Stratton, 1956).

82. Jacob Levine, E. Luby, A. Rauch, R. Yesner, "Blood Viscosity of Psychotics and Nonpsychotics under Stress," *Psychosomatic Medicine*, 16 (1954), 398.

83. Sir Thomas Lewis, *The Soldier's Heart and the Effort Syndrome* (New York: Paul B. Hoeber, 1920).

84. Howard S. Liddell, *Emotional Hazards in Animals and Man* (Springfield: Charles C. Thomas, 1956).

85. Theodore Lidz, "Emotional Factors in the Etiology of Hyperthyroidism," *Psychosomatic Medicine*, 11 (1949), 2.

86. Theodore Lidz, "General Concepts of Psychosomatic Medicine," in Silvano Arieti, ed., *American Handbook of Psychiatry* (New York: Basic Books, 1959), Vol. I, pp. 647–658.

87. Theodore Lidz and Robert Rubenstein, "Psychology of Gastrointestinal Disorders," in Silvano Arieti, ed., *American Handbook of Psychiatry* (New York: Basic Books, 1959), Vol. I, pp. 678–689.

88. Theodore Lidz, "Causalgia," in Russell L. Cecil and Robert F. Loeb, eds., *Textbook of Medicine* (Philadelphia: W. B. Saunders, 1963).

89. Erich Lindemann, "Psychiatric Problems in Conservative Treatment of Ulcerative Colitis," *Archives of Neurology and Psychiatry*, 53 (1945), 322.

90. John W. Lovett-Doust and D. Leigh, "Studies on the Physiology of Awareness, The Interrelationships of Emotions. Life Situations, and Anoxemia in Patients with Bronchial Asthma," *Psychosomatic Medicine*, 15 (1953), 292.

91. Alfred Ludwig, "Psychogenic Factors in Rheumatoid Arthritis," *Bulletin on Rheumatic Diseases*, 2 (1952), 33.

92. Neil T. McDermott and S. Cobb, "A Psychiatric Survey of 50 Cases of Bronchial Asthma," *Psychosomatic Medicine*, 1 (1939), 203.

93. Paul D. MacLean, "Psychosomatic Disease and the 'Visceral Brain,'" *Psychosomatic Medicine,* 11 (1949), 338.
94. John M. McMahon, F. J. Braceland, and H. J. Moersch, "The Psychosomatic Aspects of Cardiospasm," *Annals of Internal Medicine,* 34 (1951), 609.
95. George F. Mahl, "Effect of Chronic Fear on the Gastric Secretion of HCI in Dogs," *Psychosomatic Medicine,* 11 (1949), 30.
96. George F. Mahl, "Some Observations about Research on Vocal Behavior. Disorders of Communication," *Research Publication A.R.N.M.D.,* 42 (1964), 466.
97. Frederick W. Maire and H. D. Patton, "Neural Structures Involved in the Genesis of 'Preoptic Pulmonary Edema,' Gastric Erosions and Behavior Changes," *American Journal of Physiology,* 184 (1956), 345.
98. Sydney Margolin, "The Behavior of the Stomach during Psychoanalysis," *Psychoanalytic Quarterly,* 20 (1951), 349.
99. Sydney Margolin, "On Some Principles of Therapy," *American Journal of Psychiatry,* 114 (1958), 1087.
100. P. Marty, "The Allergic Object Relationship," *International Journal of Psycho-Analysis,* 39 (1958), 98.
101. John W. Mason, "Plasma 17-Hydroxycorticosteroid Levels during Electrical Stimulation of the Amygdaloid Complex in Conscious Monkeys," *American Journal of Physiology,* 196 (1959), 44.
102. Jules H. Masserman and C. Pechtal, "Neurosis in Monkeys," *Annals of the New York Academy of Sciences,* 56 (1953), 253.
103. William C. Menninger, "Psychological Factors in the Etiology of Diabetes," *Journal of Nervous and Mental Disease,* 81 (1935), 1.
104. J. E. Meyer, "Diagnostische Einsellunger und Diagnosen in due Psychiatrie," in Hans W. Gruhle, R. Jung, W. Mayer-Gross, and M. Muller, eds., *Psychiatrie der Gegenwart* (Berlin: Springer, 1960).
105. Henry H. W. Miles and S. Cobb, "Neurocirculatory Asthenia, Anxiety and Neurosis," *New England Journal of Medicine,* 245 (1951), 711.
106. John A. P. Millet, H. Lief, and B. Mittelmann, "Raynaud's Disease: Psychogenic Factors and Psychotherapy," *Psychosomatic Medicine,* 15 (1953), 61.
107. I. Arthur Mirsky, "Emotional Factors in the Patient with Diabetes Mellitus," *Bulletin of the Menninger Clinic,* 12 (1948), 187.
108. I. Arthur Mirsky, "The Psychosomatic Approach to the Etiology of Clinical Disorders," *Psychosomatic Medicine,* 19 (1957), 424.
109. I. Arthur Mirsky, "Physiologic, Psychologic, and Social Determinants in the Etiology of Duodenal Ulcer," *American Journal of Digestive Diseases,* 3 (1958), 285.
110. I. Arthur Mirsky, P. Futterman, and S. Kaplan, "Blood Plasma Pepsinogen," II, *Journal of Laboratory and Clinical Medicine,* 40 (1952), 188.
111. I. Arthur Mirsky, Stanley Kaplan, and Robert H. Broh-Kahn, "Pepsinogen Excretion (Uropepsin) as an Index of the Influence of Various Life Situ-

ations on Gastric Secretion," *Association for Research in Nervous and Mental Disease Proceedings*, 29 (1950), 628.

112. Mary E. Moore, A. Stunkard, and L. Srole, "Obesity, Social Class, and Mental Illness," *Journal of the American Medical Association*, 181 (1962), 962.
113. Douglass W. Orr, "Pregnancy Following the Decision to Adopt," *Psychosomatic Medicine*, 3 (1941), 441.
114. Adrian M. Ostfeld, "Stress, Semantics, and the Vascular System," *Angiology*, 10 (1959), 406.
115. Adrian M. Ostfeld and B. Z. Lebovits, "Personality Factors and Pressor Mechanisms in Renal and Essential Hypertension," *Archives of Internal Medicine*, 104 (1959), 43.
116. G. M. Perrin and I. R. Pierce, "Psychosomatic Aspects of Cancer," *Psychosomatic Medicine*, 21 (1959), 397.
117. E. Polish, J. V. Brady, J. W. Mason, J. S. Thach, and W. Niemeck, "Gastric Contents and the Occurrence of Duodenal Lesions in the Rhesus Monkey during Avoidance Behavior," *Gastroenterology*, 43 (1962), 193.
118. Gregory Razran, "Conditioning and Perception," *Psychological Review*, 62 (1955), 83.
119. Morton F. Reiser, A. A. Brust, and E. B. Ferris, "Life Situations, Emotions and the Course of Patients with Arterial Hypertension," *Psychosomatic Medicine*, 13 (1951), 133.
120. Morton F. Reiser and Hyman Bakst, "Psychology of Cardiovascular Disorders," in Silvano Arieti, ed., *American Handbook of Psychiatry* (New York: Basic Books, 1959), Vol. I, p. 659.
121. Jules B. Richmond, E. L. Lipton, and L. Lustman, "Cardiac Rate and Skin Temperature Responses in Newborn Infants," *Psychosomatic Medicine*, 17 (1955), 475. (Abstract.)
122. Curt P. Richter, "On the Phenomenon of Sudden Death in Animals and Man," *Psychosomatic Medicine*, 19 (1957), 191.
123. John Romano and G. L. Engel, "Studies of Syncope, III, Differentiation between Vasodepression and Hysterical Fainting," *Psychosomatic Medicine*, 7 (1945), 3.
124. Harold Rosen and T. Lidz, "Emotional Factors in the Precipitation of Recurrent Diabetic Acidosis," *Psychosomatic Medicine*, 11 (1949), 211.
125. Jurgen Ruesch, *Chronic Disease and Psychosomatic Invalidism*, "Psychosomatic Medicine Monographs," 9 (1946).
126. Jurgen Ruesch, C. Christiansen, L. C. Patterson, S. Dewees, and A. Jacobson, "Psychological Invalidism in Thyroidectomized Patients," *Psychosomatic Medicine*, 9 (1947), 77.
127. Arthur Ruskin, O. W. Beard, and R. L. Schaffer, "Blast Hypertension: Elevated Arterial Pressures in the Victims of the Texas City Disaster," *American Journal of Medicine*, 4 (1948), 228.
128. Leon J. Saul, "The Relation to the Mother as Seen in Cases of Allergy," *Nervous Child*, 5 (1946), 332.

129. W. L. Sawrey, J. J. Conger, and E. S. Turrell, "An Experimental Investigation of the Role of Psychological Factors in the Production of Gastric Ulcers in Rats," *Journal of Comparative and Physiological Psychology*, 49 (1956), 457.

130. Rau Schiavi, M. Stein, and B. B. Sethi, "Respiratory Variables in Response to a Pain-Fear Stimulus and in Experimental Asthma," *Psychosomatic Medicine*, 23 (1961), 485.

131. Philip F. D. Seitz, "Symbolism and Organ Choice in Conversion Reactions," *Psychosomatic Medicine*, 13 (1951), 254.

132. Hans Selye, *The Stress of Life* (New York: McGraw-Hill, 1956).

133. Melitta Sperling, "Psychoanalytic Study of Ulcerative Colitis in Children," *Psychoanalytic Quarterly*, 15 (1946), 302.

134. H. M. Spiro and M. L. Pilot, "The Irritable Bowel," *Connecticut Medicine*, 23 (1959), 12.

135. Marvin Stein and P. Ottenberg, "Role of Odors in Asthma," *Psychosomatic Medicine*, 20 (1958), 60.

136. Ian P. Stevenson and H. G. Wolff, "Life Situations, Emotions and the Bronchial Mucus," *Psychosomatic Medicine*, 11 (1949), 223.

137. Albert Stunkard, "Obesity and the Denial of Hunger," *Psychosomatic Medicine*, 21 (1959), 281.

138. Albert Stunkard, "Hunger and Satiety," *American Journal of Psychiatry*, 118 (1961), 212.

139. Thomas S. Szasz, "Physiologic and Psychodynamic Mechanisms in Constipation and Diarrhea," *Psychosomatic Medicine*, 13 (1951), 112.

140. Helmut Thomä, *Anorexia Nervosa* (Stuttgart: Huber Klett, 1961).

141. Montague Ullman, "On the Psyche and Warts," *Psychosomatic Medicine*, 21 (1959), 473.

142. Edward Weiss and O. Spurgeon English, *Psychosomatic Medicine* (Philadelphia: W. B. Saunders, 1957).

143. Fritz Wengraf, *Psychosomatic Approach to Gynecology and Obstetrics* (Springfield: Charles C Thomas, 1953).

144. Joseph Wilder, "Psychological Problems in Hypoglycemia," *American Journal of Digestive Diseases*, 10 (1943), 428.

145. Joseph Wilder, "Modern Psychophysiology and the Law of Initial Value," *American Journal of Psychotherapy*, 12 (1958), 199.

146. Norris Weinberg, M. Mendelson, and A. Stunkard, "A Failure to Find Distinctive Personality Features in a Group of Obese Men," *American Journal of Psychiatry*, 117 (1961), 1035.

147. Erich D. Wittkower, "Studies of Influence of Emotions in the Functions of the Organs," *Journal of Mental Science*, 81 (1935), 533.

148. Erich D. Wittkower and B. Russell, *Emotional Factors in Skin Disease* (New York: Paul B. Hoeber, 1953).

148. George A. Wolf and H. G. Wolff, "Studies on the Nature of Certain

Symptoms Associated with Cardiovascular Disorders," *Psychosomatic Medicine,* 8 (1946), 293.

150. Stewart G. Wolf, Ph. V. Cardon, Jr., E. M. Shepard, and Harold G. Wolff, *Life Stress and Essential Hypertension* (Baltimore: Williams & Wilkins, 1955).

151. Stewart Wolf and Harold G. Wolff, *Human Gastric Function* (New York: Oxford Press, 1943).

152. Harold G. Wolff, *Headache and Other Head Pain* (New York: Oxford Press, 1948).

153. Harold G. Wolff, *Stress and Disease* (Springfield: Charles C Thomas, 1953).

CHAPTER FOURTEEN

The Schizophrenias of Adults

Basic Problems

There is no generally accepted definition of schizophrenia. Points of view vary widely, from the traditional consideration of schizophrenia as a severe disease characterized by specific disturbances in thinking and feeling, to Thomas S. Szasz's notion that schizophrenia is a pseudoproblem such as that of ether in yesterday's physics.[188] Notwithstanding, there are millions of people who are diagnosed as schizophrenics; they fill our mental hospitals. Patients and their families often suffer beyond description.

A tremendous amount has been written on the subject of schizophrenia. Leopold Bellak's second volume of references lists 4,000 articles and books published in the decade 1946–1956.[15] Yet, despite this full measure of dedicated work, the important questions of diagnosis, prognosis, etiology, and therapy are still unanswered and constitute psychiatry's greatest challenge. Can the behavioral processes and changes be described with any precision and order? Is schizophrenia a group of ill-defined syndromes, or is it a true nosological entity? Is it a disease? A maladjustment? A way of life? Is the irrationality of schizophrenia transmitted by genes or by interpersonal relations? What are the best methods of treatment?

Historical Remarks

The first reasonably good description of what today is called schizophrenia appeared in the French psychiatric literature in the late eighteenth century under the label *Vesania*, a word meaning total madness without fever. Esquirol described and differentiated acquired or accidental forms of idiocy from congenital idiocy.[55] In the middle of the last century, Morel coined the term *démence précoce* for a form of degenerative stupidity[141] (everything was "degenerative" in those days). Karl L. Kahlbaum described catatonia,[104] and Ewald Hecker, hebephrenia.[88] Emil Kraepelin built on such earlier work in his classical description of the symptoms, course, and prognosis of dementia praecox, which he viewed as a disease with many subtypes (many more than we remember today); early onset; and inevitable deterioration, attributable to some unknown metabolic disorder. Although Kraepelin was aware that there were cases of dementia praecox that did not deteriorate, he maintained his ideas and his diagnostic classification with considerable rigidity.[116] An excellent observer and systematizer, he described the rich symptomatology and natural history of schizophrenia in great detail and clarity. Eugen Bleuler, like Kraepelin, believed it was fundamentally an organic disease, although he described it in psychological terms. He pointed out that the disorder neither always starts early nor inevitably leads to deterioration.[22] He saw its essence—the primary symptoms—in a diminution and leveling of associative affinities. Primary symptoms often cannot be discerned directly; the familiar observable symptoms are secondary symptoms. They are either direct consequences of the primary symptoms or perhaps attempts at reintegration. Bleuler divided the secondary symptoms into fundamental symptoms, which only occur in schizophrenia, and accessory symptoms, which are incidental in schizophrenia and also occur in other mental diseases. Fundamental symptoms are the disturbances of thinking and feeling, such as splitting and blocking of thoughts and affects and the more complex disturbances of autism or withdrawal and detachment from reality and a deep ambivalence. Other secondary symptoms were hallucinations, delusions, illusions, and catatonic symptoms. In calling the illness schizophrenia, Bleuler stressed the lack of unity and coherence of the patient's personality. Although he admitted the possibility of psychological causes (and indeed stressed the fact that symptom *content* had to reflect life experience), and although he was interested in therapy, he felt the basic cause was organic and manifested in a weakened psychological structure. He used the analogy of osteomalacia predisposing to fractures, which occur with slight stress. In general, his views of schizophrenia were strikingly modern and have remained the basis for contemporary considerations. Adolf Meyer called schizophrenia parergasia and regarded it as a reaction, which could be explained in large part by the detailed study of the patient's life history.[137] Such a point of view was later elaborated in terms of the role of communications in interpersonal relations by Harry Stack Sullivan.[185] This led to a focus on psychotherapy in mental hospitals and to a sharp attention to mother–child relationships and to the developmental roots of schizophrenia. Jung, who seriously entertained a theory of a toxic factor operating at a certain phase in the illness, still looked at it fundamentally as a psychologically meaningful disorder.[103] He related the phenomena of schizophrenia to normal sleep, dream and awakening, and studied the role of the introvert personality type in the disease. Similar ideas about the wishfulfilling function both of dreams and hallucinations were expressed by Freud, whose chief clinical contribution to the problem of schizophrenia was an ingenious interpretation of the memoirs of Judge Daniel Paul Schreber, an intelligent paranoid schizophrenic.[71] Freud noted the narcissism in schizophrenia and spoke of an initial withdrawal of libido from objects to the self; delusions and hallucinations represented restitutive attempts in which the return path of libido to objects was inexplicably diverted and abnormal. Paul Federn was the first psychoanalyst to consider schizophrenia explicitly as a disorder characterized by weakness of the ego, a notion which, among other implications, extends the pathology to far more functions than thought and affect;[60] an altered experience of the internal and external world was implicated. Most contemporary approaches are based on these beginnings, some representing old observations in a new language, some extending earlier approaches in ways consequential to the study or treatment of schizophrenia.

Incidence and Prevalence

There are no reliable estimates of the incidence and prevalence of schizophrenia. This is not surprising for a disorder in which agreements on diagnosis are far from satisfactory. Statistics of hospitalized patients indicate that female schizophrenics are more frequently admitted than are males. Female schizophrenics also stay longer in mental hospitals than males. According to hospital statistics, most schizophrenics appear in psychiatric facilities for the first time in young adulthood; however, onset of adult schizophrenia as early as puberty and as late as the sixth and seventh decade has been reported. The onset of the disorder in women is reported to occur later than in males. Data from hospitalized patients, however, do not give any information about true prevalence and incidence in the total population. Reported prevalence in the total population is said to be roughly 0.3 per cent,[123] in the authors' opinion, a significant underestimation. In the New Haven prevalence studies of cases under treatment, schizophrenics comprised almost half of the total patient population.[95] About one-quarter of the first admissions to mental hospitals in the United States are schizophrenics, and up to half of the population of most mental hospitals is made up of schizophrenics. Thus, the disorder constitutes a formidable health and economic problem.

The Problem of a Cardinal Disturbance

A basic question is whether schizophrenia is a single disorder or disease or whether the term is a "catch-all diagnosis," a conglomeration of many different entities. Bleuler thought he would avoid this troublesome question by speaking of the group of schizophrenias,[22] but the question of what belongs to the group still remains. Most workers are committed to the assumption that the schizophrenias have some sort of common denominator regardless of far-reaching differences in overt symptomatology and course. This is the position taken by those who view schizophrenia as a disease, as well as by those who look at schizophrenia as a way of life characterized by unique modes of experiencing. For some investigators of somatic factors, however, the assumption of groups of different disorders (or different pathways to similar behavioral endpoints), or of a different physiology for different phases of the same disorder, has seemed the best approach.

Schizophrenia presents as disordered behavior; even proponents of the organic viewpoint describe the basic symptomatology in the language of psychology and behavior. Some have focused on listing symptoms without regard to the persons living with such symptoms or the mechanisms generating them; others have been concerned with the formal structure of thought, language, and defense mechanisms, either analyzing or simply describing these; others have stressed the meaning, function, and purpose of schizophrenic behavior—what the behavior is behaving for.

It is not easy to find one's way through the varied approaches to the disorder or the attempts to pinpoint what fundamentally is at fault. The student will find that descriptions and explanations are often intermixed. These various formulations have been undertaken sometimes to catch the "essence" of the disorder, sometimes mercifully to bring order into the intermittent chaos experienced by most observers of schizophrenia. Each new item that catches psychiatric interest (such as narcissism, symbiotic mother–child relationships, family dynamics, social roles, identity, logic and paleologic, the archipallium and the ARAS, mescaline, serotonin, twins, and so forth) has provided a text around which the "story of schizophrenia" can be written. Of itself, this should be testimony enough to certify that we are confronted with a dysfunction involving the organization of behavior at every level. Schizophrenia touches on many problems with which the behavioral sciences are concerned because it entails an impairment of mechanisms that organize and coordinate segments of behavior; the ultrastructure of behavior is thereby revealed, thus exposing much that we ordinarily do not see when the parts are working well.

Because it is a dysfunction that often extends over a lifetime, and because observers approach it at different phases and stages with different intentions in mind, the problem for contemporary students is to become acquainted with the major approaches and to question whether a given explanation provides both the necessary and sufficient details to account for the disorder. The power to work with and comprehend schizophrenic behavior has grown, but we have not yet penetrated and formulated those aspects of behavioral processes that most parsimoniously explain and differentiate the behavior. The search is for a comprehensive definition of the fundamental variables that would serve those interested in prediction, etiology, therapy, and prevention. In the meantime, we, along with other scientists engaged in complex psychosocial and biological work, have to rely on partial approaches.

For Bleuler, the disruption of associations constituted a hypothetical primary symptom, but one does not get the impression that he assumed the existence of *one* basic or cardinal behavioral dysfunction, as have some psychiatrists.[21] Bleuler described "simple" disturbances (thinking and feeling) and "compound" disturbances (such as autism or self-absorption and ambivalence). Obviously, there is a connection between the two. The reason one tends to describe a basic compound disturbance in schizophrenia throughout its course is our difficulty in consistently pinpointing distinct manifest disturbances of thinking and feeling in the very early stages of the disorder.[133]

From clinical experience and patients' own accounts,[29, 107] we are inclined to see the cardinal disturbance as a disorder in the organization of communications, resulting in a profound alteration of the patient's self-experience and his experience of the world. This, of course, implies a fundamental dysfunction in the psychobiological equipment by which information is coded and decoded. The essential communicative signals and operations by which the stability of the self is normally maintained function poorly. These sets of signals include personal and social bonds, memories, habitual activities, and stable but adaptable modes of perception of, and attention to, external and bodily cues.

The dissolution of essential communications involves a shift of attention and activity from an engagement with normal communications to an absorption in the self, to an occupation with simply maintaining stability and basic boundaries. There is a concomitant loss of focus and coherence and a profound shift in the meaning and value of social relationships and goal-directed behavior. This is evident in the inability realistically to implement future goals and present satisfactions; they are achieved magically, or through fantasy and delusion. Some of the "withdrawn" behavior, especially of the more advanced schizophrenics, appears to have the crude (though unsuccessful) function of differentiating the self from others; of keeping intensity (which is now difficult to control) at a minimum; and of coping with the threat of change. The altered world threatens to continue to dissolve. In short, there is a profound disturbance of identity. This is highlighted in a sequence of early changes described by Claus Konrad,[115] which emphasizes the patient's altered subjective world, whatever his overt behavior.

It seems that, at a very early stage, boundaries between the self and the world become unstable, fluid, and difficult to maintain. Clinically, this is evident in somatic delusions that involve a vanishing differentiation of the self and others, and of inside and outside. Communication may at first flow easily, but the contents of the heightened consciousness cannot be clearly and precisely allocated. Aspects of relationships not normally attended to are highlighted; schizophrenics focus on ordinarily disregarded details and attributes rather than usual goals and meanings.[22]

Behaviorally, one sees a sensitivity and an "insight" which are "too good," too clearly revealing of, and penetrating into, the fabric of feeling and too perceptive of attributes of situations and persons. It is as if all the implements by which the self is maintained—the operations normally occurring without consciousness or attention—are exposed for the patient's attention. Much of what *we* try to disentangle for scientific purposes seems all too clear to our patient. (No wonder he is confused!) Such knowledge is, on examination, useless; it is, for the moment, "helpless" insight without selective purpose and reality checks. A patient in this fluid state told us the world and everyone in it (whom he wished to "unite" in a special society) had a rhythm, and he was having trouble getting his rhythm to oscillate in time with ours; communication was, therefore, odd and difficult. It is striking how taxing it is for schizophrenics to hold to a level where they may have some degree of stability; the push toward disorganization is usually massive.

Following the weakening of ego boundaries, or concomitant with it, some schizophrenics experience themselves as being in the center of the universe. With a loss of moorings to reality, there is a loss of conventional perspectives, and the self becomes magically magnified; events in the world and around the patient acquire a new meaning. In this state, the unstable, fragmenting self can be only magically restored, so the world now revolves around the patient, and each and every event and personal interaction acquires a special magical and often uncanny significance. These interpretations are unshared and lead rapidly to enormous isolation or autism and to a profoundly unrealistic assessment of reality, or *dereism.* Harold F. Searles noted that schizophrenics, as children also do, identify easily with nonhuman or inanimate objects.[172] Human contact and relationships are too intense, as well as distorted, for the patient; weaknesses in his prepsychotic relationships become exposed. In any event, the structure of human relationships clearly shifts in its utility to the patient; the normal function of interpersonal activities as an object and a source of communications, satisfactions, and meaning is altered. As the patient becomes deficient (or different) in discriminating his outer and inner reality, primitive, infantile, sexual, aggressive, and passive wishes, as well as fantasies and drives, gain prominence, surface to consciousness, and often appear uncontrolled.

Some of the varied manifestations of this early disturbance in self-experience are remindful of sudden shifts of mental organization that can be seen in a few minutes following LSD-25. Yet, even with this experimental drug, it requires a passage of time for the various mental operations that are altered to be clearly manifest to subjects and observers. Thus, while the drug reaction "unfolds" through time, and a variety of behavioral strategies may be successively employed, the fundamental shift in the organization of experience is probably present instantaneously, affecting simple and compound functions. Many similarities to the disturbances of the identity experience and to the perceptual and cognitive confusions may be found as transient or permanent components of a variety of conditions. In the schizophrenic, these are far more profound, more lasting, and cannot be easily influenced. Not all the phenomena are constant; some may be manifest and recur only in specific interpersonal stresses when, instead of coping, the patient disorganizes. To avoid confusion, it should be clear that these deductions about perception and experience, although often clinically evident, are not necessarily descriptions of the overt behavior the psychiatrist or family initially may see;

a person experiencing in this way may be quiet or noisy, secretive, retentive, bemused, or self-absorbed and "odd," or highly intense and excited to the casual observer. Overt behavior depends on the interactions of a particular patient with his particular ongoing environment. Self-accounts, clinical probing, as well as direct observations of clear-cut manifestations of these cardinal changes, constitute the source for our assumptions. Thus, we offer no more than a tentative sketch of a cardinal disturbance in self-experience, which seems to exist in all phases and all types of certain partially organized (rather then integrated) states which, taken as a whole, we recognize as schizophrenia.

How the course of the disorder modifies and influences the basic disturbance is outlined in the following sections. We must be alerted to the clinical fact that some patients show changes within moments that may take years to develop in others. This, of course, makes the task of explaining schizophrenia more difficult. The processes observed in a person who has lived from the age of fifteen to forty-five years with clear evidence of schizophrenia may have quite a different consequence and significance than processes described in the height of a schizophrenic break occurring at age forty-five. The study of schizophrenia, if it teaches us anything, points to the necessity and value of defining the context in which the behavior occurs. Many workers vainly seek a shorthand, one-sentence definition of the disorder.

General Remarks about the Course of Schizophrenia

The great variety of schizophrenic symptoms, then, is related to differences in the course of the disorder. Some schizophrenias progress very rapidly; others slowly; some forms are almost static. In some cases, we observe a spread of symptoms to many behavioral activities—the whole personality seems to be affected and invaded—and other cases remain oligosymptomatic. Some present to the psychiatrist in acute breaks with reality; others, only when a crisis forces the patient and family to recognize a disorder of longer standing.

When schizophrenias change from incipient to advanced and easily recognized forms, they pass in a rather lawful fashion through certain more or less delineated phases:[57] (1) the early or initial phase; (2) the phase of disintegration or clear-cut schizophrenic dissociation; (3) the phase of deterioration. Schizophrenias may run the whole course to the bitter end, but many become arrested at an earlier stage. Under stress, symptoms can recur at any time. There are also reversals of the pathological processes—we speak of "remissions"—in which reparative actions gain the upper hand. At present we are, in spite of a few leads, unable to account for factors that determine a benign or malignant course.

Are the characteristic remissions and relapses expressions of endogenous processes, or are they responses to psychosocial variables, or both? Some patients recover, apparently completely; when such recovery occurs without treatment we speak of spontaneous remission. The term need not imply an independent endogenous process; it is just as likely that the spontaneous remission is a response to nondeliberate but nonetheless favorable psychosocial stimuli other than specific therapeutic activity. Many schizophrenics, of course, do not recover completely; they reveal some persisting defects, which, after an attack, may be very slight—a certain blunting of the personality; a slight withdrawal; a certain unpredictability; or a continuing hypersensitivity. Unfortunately, we have not undertaken full psychodynamic and biological studies of such "recovered" schizophrenics. Estimates of a tendency to remission vary between a conservative 6.6 per cent observed by Otto Kant[106] in public mental hospitals and a high of 24.5 per cent reported by Thomas A. C. Rennie.[157] The remission rate and the degree of change is understandably of great importance in any evaluation of therapy. If the rate of therapeutic successes is lower than the remission rate, one can hardly speak of therapeutic success. Some conservative psychiatrists believe that current methods of therapy have been able to induce or to increase the chance for remission only in certain benign types. They anticipate that as a rule two-thirds recover or improve, while one-third continues to regress or fails to improve; and they accurately note that the longer the disorder proceeds without change, the worse the prognosis.

Early Symptoms

In essence, the early symptoms of typical schizophrenias are those we have described as schizophrenic identity disturbances. Schizophrenias rarely start as full-blown syndromes; the beginning is more often insidious than abrupt. Even in the relatively rare patient with a seemingly dramatic onset, careful histories usually reveal either a gradual onset or prodromal warnings over long periods. Modern psychological investigators have concentrated on trying to understand how schizophrenic symptoms develop from the idiosyncratic and disordered communication pattern in certain families. There are cases that can be convincingly traced back to childhood; in most cases, however, we are unable to detect undisputed symptoms before puberty. If prodromal warnings and childhood defects are apparent, they usually are so *after* the fact, when we know we are dealing with schizophrenia. Although the history may reveal covert delusions or fragmented thinking, many prodromal symptoms and signs are not specific; accordingly, we usually cannot recognize that specific alteration which will lead to schizophrenia. It should be noted that this chapter is not concerned with the schizophrenias of childhood or with autistic children; these seem to be a different matter, and it is rather doubtful if even the diagnostic label of schizophrenia should be attached to such children.

Prodromal symptoms, then, are not distinctive, and most schizophrenics show a host of neurotic symptoms before the onset of the manifest disorder. They are hysterical or obsessive, quite frequently depressive and hypochondriacal, and may or may not have symptoms of neurotic depersonalization. Although older textbooks make the point that schizophrenics have no insight into their difficulties, many patients not only notice and report changes in their way of experiencing, but have periods of frantically heightened attempts to resolve problems of which they are too keenly aware. Alterations of body scheme and body experience are characteristic early changes. In a dramatic case, the body was experienced as flattened out like a canoe; in another, the penis shrank as in Koro, a behavior disorder reported to exist in Southern China. At the beginning, these feelings are vague, and the patient may try to correct the experiences himself. Hilde Bruch and Lawrence C. Kolb stress the importance of such alterations of the body image in their patients. Later, these altered bodily perceptions, which often present clinically as hypochondriasis, may develop into full-blown somatic hallucinations and delusions.[32, 114]

Many patients gradually or suddenly become anxious. Anxiety connected with overt or latent homosexual impulses seems particularly prevalent when they reach this stage of panic. It is quite conceivable that the frightening instability and alteration of the world, the inability to cope at some juncture, precipitates panic that (in young people especially) will reflect sexual identity problems more frequently than sustained (goal-directed) homosexual or incestuous desires. This does not mean that the patient's self-perception of incest-images, as with other images, is not vivid, concrete, and frightening.

Harry Stack Sullivan viewed anxiety in schizophrenics as a repetition of infantile, preverbal, "uncanny feelings," which were evoked when the child temporarily lost his security and sense of self.[185] People undergoing anesthesia, feeling themselves slip away, experience something far less overwhelming but related to such uncanny feelings. Security operations and defensive maneuvers may obscure the actual feelings; patients may then become withdrawn, indifferent, apathetic and, searching for the roots of their uncanny experience, they develop strangely exaggerated religious and philosophical ideas. We sometimes doubt whether the term anxiety should be used so freely in schizophrenia. If it is anxiety, one should remember the inability to focus and cope that accompanies it; one patient told us he did not know whether he was exhilarated, in pain, or imperiled and frightened: "I felt all of these and could not tell the difference." When we observe carefully, we always notice the crucial symptom—some difficulty in the patient's ability to communicate. Even at this early stage, the observer may be struck by a private language, a façade of blandness, emptiness, ambivalence, and autistic withdrawal; however, stormy, impulsive, aggressive, and destructive behavior, and sexual deviations are more characteristic. Sexual regression is often manifested by compulsive masturbation with infantile oral and anal fantasies or often without the report of any fantasies; orgasm may be experienced as painful.

The Phase of Disintegration or Schizophrenic Dissociation

The coexistence and intertwining of a dream world and adult experience of reality has become more manifest. Otto Pötzl astutely said in his lectures that schizophrenia is a disease in which a dream penetrates existence like a malignant tumor; healthy and pathological aspects coexist. Eugen Bleuler speaks of double bookkeeping, the compelling coexistence of private and public reality, as one striking aspect of the disunity and strangeness of patients in this phase. (It was such disharmony—or splits in experience—which in part induced him to coin the surprisingly durable term, schizophrenia.[22]) The distintegrative phase is clearly recognized by the phenomena that Bleuler described as fundamental and accessory symptoms. It is estimated that about half of all patients reach this stage under present methods of treatment.

Formal Aspects of Higher Mental Functions in Schizophrenic Behavior

Most authors still view the fragmentation of thinking as the most important schizophrenic symptom. It is admittedly a striking symptom, but more importantly, it is an aspect of the basic disorder that can be clearly described and discerned by the clinician (perhaps this is why Bleuler called it a "simple" function). Thinking becomes incoherent; its binding logical quality and certain over-all guiding concepts seem to be missing. Patients report that their thoughts break off and are withdrawn from them. Their thoughts become vocal and hallucinated. Others can hear them, and they can hear the thoughts of others; Kurt Schneider felt these are the most significant symptoms.[170] The schizophrenic thinking disorder has been studied by analysis of the schizophrenic's language.[108] Norman Cameron classified three types of thought and language disturbance: (1) Asyndesis, a deterioration of connecting links. (2) Metanymy, imprecise labeling, hitting at the periphery rather than the bull's-eye (for example, a patient has a "menu" rather than meals). (3) Interpenetration—or mixing—of ideas relating to fantasy and to reality.[36] As the disorder progresses, the language of schizophrenics ceases to convey accurate data about reality and presumably distorts inner experience as well.

The fragmentation or splintering of thoughts can reach extremes in which verbal productions become if not obtuse, stilted and beside the point or a conglomeration of *neologisms* and a *salad of words*. The formal aspects of these schizophrenic thought disorders have greatly impressed psychiatrists[198] and induced Henrious C. Rümke to say: "The secret of schizophrenia lies in its form." [165] We believe that the formal aspects of schizophrenic thought and language, and generally of schizophrenic behavior, including communications and object relations, deserve much more extensive research, even though certain features are already quite clear. What Sigmund Freud described as primary-process thinking, Heinz Werner as physiognomic thinking, Silvano Arieti as paleologic, and what Alfred Storch calls archaic behavior refers to the level at which the schizophrenic is operating. Max Levin points out that a child often cannot even *think* of the details of a story unless it is reread to him, whereupon he appears to know it word for word and objects to the slightest deviation from the text.[124] Hearing in order to think is one type of "concrete" or sensory thinking; similarly, the schizophrenic, in order to think, may "hear" something, whereupon he thinks other people can hear what he thinks. E. von Domarus,[49] and later Arieti,[6] pointed out that the logic in this concrete thinking is based on linking two things together on the basis of a few common aspects, not on the basis of distinct categories. In normal logic, "A" is always "A" and never "B"; but in paleologic thinking, "B" may be "A" if it has only a single aspect of "A." Categories thus lose their distinction. A patient with the delusion that she was the Virgin Mary followed the reasoning that, since she was, or wished to be, a virgin, she was, in fact, identical to the Virgin Mary. Arieti also gives the example of a paranoid schizophrenic who wanted her child to become an angel; since angels are nourished only by "spiritual food" she did not feed her child.[6] In this instance, the simile is lost and a wishful and concrete identification of the child and angel occurs. The identity of categories is blurred, and relational logic is replaced by primitive logic. If there is no distinctiveness in the categories of what can disturb someone, then passionate love and hate can be equated, simply because both perturb. With this defect in the ability to identify categories, words tend to lose their ability to identify classes and are used much more concretely and literally. I. Matte Blanco[129] expressed the conviction that the tool of symbolic logic will help us to disentangle schizophrenic thought disorder. David Shakow[175] remarked on the bewildering schizophrenic world: a patient refused to eat because the menu listed soup, which disgusted him since he read it as so-u-*p*. The proverb "A bird in the hand is worth two in the bush" may lead to a confused dissertation on horticulture. Frequently, when asked to sort different colored cardboard squares and circles, the patient cannot group them; he looks for different shades of color, notices irregularities in the cards, and the like. The proper boundaries of tasks or thoughts are lost. Thoughts acquire a perceptual intensity; for example, truth is gold and slightly lighter than water; synesthesias, in which, for example, sound has visual qualities, are observed.

The following are recorded fragments from an interview with a thirty-nine-year-old chronic schizophrenic, which illustrate severe disturbance of thinking.

Patient: Fundamentals of ideas, principles and, ways and means and this and that, I understand this business isn't a discussed too much, but aah personally speaking I believe that aah this has arisen in the facts that this situation is brought to my attention. The reason I say my attention because I thought anything like this discussion would be brought up into three parties. I believe in dancing or party or anything like that, the third part or something like that, or any parts that people discuss. I aah generally feel that the situation calls for aah, well you know I just don't, understand that aah this principle discussions.

Doctor: You don't understand why we get together.

Patient: I can see that now, I can understand that in more ways, then let's say aah, one, I say to myself, why not use what I can think I'm able to think about and personally speaking I say to myself, well why did you think of this idea. You take tomatoes, you take potatoes, a then you say well people have a bought things and discussed things, but principally speaking they said well why not accomplish an idea that this situation called for strategy, and I personally could not involve myself because I personally had to a, bring in this idea because I realized this person qualified for this certain job. . . .

Doctor: Why didn't you share your problems?

Patient: Well because this principle of the idea, people are always discussing different facts, of different ways, different terms and oh you know, you sort of kind of disgusted and burned up about this situation. . . . I personally didn't understand, kind of disgusted I says this got to stop, so, we reminisce and this and that, and seen the situation, there's people try to accomplish this and that, they picked up this idea that idea, they just couldn't move this ideas, well write it down or something, why not, says I haven't anything in my hand, why can't I use that?

Doctor: Was it that you didn't have confidence in anybody?

Patient: I said anybody? I think that's a very bad word. Ah, when you say anybody, I, my situation call for the strategy, baskets or something I don't know, people brought this, this principle of this idea, this situation, I couldn't understand why this situation always brought this attention and this realistic facts. So you can see that I kind of got, kind of pissed off at times. . . .

Disturbances of Communicative Behavior

The failure to distinguish categories and maintain goal-directed thinking affects the communicative and social functions of the patient. Consensus about the relationship of persons and events (which characterizes what is stable in any social system) becomes difficult or impossible. The names of things are known, but categories, roles, and functions are confused. A patient believes the doctors are his family since they take care of him. Descriptions of the theories of children and primitive peoples refer to this type of animistic thinking in which things are identified, not by what they are, but by an aspect of what they do or by incidental qualities they have. Children and primitives, however, use this logic and manner of thinking differently from schizophrenics; it does not play the central role in their relationships to persons and objects that it does in schizophrenia. Characteristics of primitive or primary process thinking such as displacement; condensation; symbolization; coexistence of opposites; disregard for time, space, logic, syntax, and causality are fitted into the scheme of living differently by the dreamer, the primitive and the child on the one hand, and the schizophrenic on the other. If one watches the child in his use of such logic, he is obviously experimenting and discovering the way things are and the way they can be linked in categories; if he calls people in the far distance "toy people" he is nevertheless also asking and ready to learn about perspective and to accept the proposition that in fact these are real people. The use of such thought is indeed a part of a creative learning and testing process. But this differs markedly from the way a schizophrenic functions, when the use of such thought represents either anergic or desperate attempts to keep a thought just the way he wishes it to be. Schizophrenic language and logic often is mistakenly compared to that of poets and seers. The fact that the schizophrenic will speak in metaphors or in seemingly profound or poetic language (rather than directly to the point and conventionally) often puts young psychiatrists in awe of them or, worse, makes them suspect a hidden schizophrenia in poetic talent. Needless to say, the patient is not an Eastern mystic and usually cannot sustain the life and discipline either of a poet or a seer (though there have been schizophrenic artists who continued to be creative). The patient's use of language reflects his isolation and lack of confident relationship to social realities; it is used out of necessity and not because he has a wide range of choice. For most of the schizophrenias, the thought disorder was not clearly manifest prior to the illness; the patient had been able to function at some level, utilizing conventional codes. Thus, unlike a child, the schizophrenic patient to some extent contaminates his already developed skills—a key fact differentiating the normal, creative, and integrative from the schizophrenic use of primitive thinking.

From investigations of the family history and current familial interactions there is evidence (which we will discuss in more detail later) that schizophrenic thinking is often the end result of a long coaching in the use of irrational modes of thinking. The fact that we sometimes can decode schizophrenic language, linking the content and mode of thinking with the patient's experience, and that we always see him as a person with a biography and motives convinces us that schizophrenic behavior is not meaningless; but the discovery of meaning is not necessarily identical to the discovery of cause. We have noted that the irrationality in schizophrenia is related but not equivalent to the behavior of primitive people, of children, and of neurotics. Similarly, his adjustment and situation in life is related to that of his family—but certainly not equivalent. If both the intact family and the impaired patient have a thought disorder, thought disorder alone is not a sufficient cause of schizophrenia. If we are not to lose the identity of the person and the category "patient" who lives a profoundly different life from his irrational relatives, such distinctions must be borne in mind. Why schizophrenic persons who live in a nightmare or think with dream logic can only with great difficulty shift from this primitive level of functioning is simply not known. If we can conclude from this that the schizophrenic, conditioned by familial ties, lives in a world that is altered, that this is real to him, that he lives with several simultaneous sets of meanings (which are bound to be confusing), that his links with reality are in some sense impaired, and that this is a compelled state (even though fluctuating), we are in a better position to understand schizophrenic behavior. We have not satisfactorily explained it, however, with any of these approaches.

To summarize: A primitive, illogical, and irrelevant way of thinking coexists with precise, factual thinking. We frequently observe such contamination when a patient uses normal speech but has a highly personalized meaning in mind so that, in fact, the formal qualities of thinking have lost their boundaries and utility. A schizophrenic frequently is not able to control his tendency to see aspects of things and to contaminate normal communications with his special twists. This characteristic feature of schizophrenia, an aspect of the multiple levels of functioning, is perhaps what is most baffling about the disorder.

Attention, Perception, and Learning

It has been generally agreed that certain psychological functions such as perception, attention, intelligence, memory, and consciousness are not fundamentally disturbed in schizophrenia. However, we are less sure about this today than we were a decade ago. For one thing, we are not dealing with "faculties" that are present or absent; we now want to know how mental processes are organized and function, at what rate, and under what circumstances. Even investigations of mental deficiencies have been enhanced by studying the conditions under which learning can take place, rather than focusing on an assumed absence of ability; if temporal and rate factors in the acquisition of information are controlled and properly reinforced, deficient children can learn some complex operations. We have yet much to learn from laboratory studies of optimal conditions for reinforcement in schizophrenia. In a disturbance in which motivation is so clearly altered, it is evident that attention cannot function normally. Consciousness in the ordinary sense is not disturbed except in some catatonic episodes and in oneirophrenic psychoses. Time sense, as measured by estimation of one second duration, was altered in a significant number of patients.[126] Shakow has summarized studies of psychological function undertaken with E. H. Rodnick, P. Huston and others (many of whom became leaders in the psychobiological study of schizophrenia and began their work in the 1930's at Worcester State Hospital).[175] According to Shakow, the schizophrenic fails to habituate or he perseverates: the patient responds when the stimulus is slight and underresponds when it is great. If the interval between stimulus and response in tests is too long, the patient is distracted by intervening stimuli; if it is too small, he cannot choose among alternatives. Thus, he may perform as well as normals but only if he is offered a very narrow and optimal range of time intervals. Patients, even cooperative ones, seem unable to maintain a set for any period of time, showing slower reaction times. Thus, good performance in the patient is dependent on highly specific circumstances. E. Callaway III, R. T. Jones, and R. S. Layne observed, in recording evoked potentials to two trivially dissimilar tones, that the patients continue to attend to both stimuli, whereas the normals will lose interest in the slight differences.[35] The patient apparently attends to too many inputs and, from the experimenters' viewpoint, unnecessarily assigns each input some value. The patient shows difficulty in sustaining attention to what we conventionally require of subjects because of his fragmented percepts and concepts; his "set" or strategy of attending is geared to multiple and minor categories. Changes in value assigned to inputs are also evident in Rodnick's studies, which show that personalized cues (a picture of a familiar person) will lead to response in patients when signals (lights) will not. In general, the performance of paranoids on these various tasks most closely approaches that of normals. Whether we should view the primary defect in schizophrenia as one of "intake"—altered perception of what is to be thought about (which is unlikely) —or as an altered experiencing of such perceptions and altered integration of them, or whether we should conceive of a true impairment of the equipment for logical thinking remains to be clearly resolved. Since a schizophrenic can at times think logically and even "observe" and remember the altered experience of the psychosis, it is likely that his basic defects are prior to the capacity for logical thought. On the other hand, any sustained experience of this kind will eventually be bound to be manifest in a predominance of illogic, of unintegrated use, and dilapidation of logical powers. Later in this chapter, when we discuss the phase of deterioration, we will consider issues related to the problem of intelligence in schizophrenia.

Affects and Drives

Grossly fragmented perception and thought, clearly inappropriate primitive affect, and gross ambivalence must be viewed together as fundamental symptoms during the second stage of schizophrenia. Bleuler emphasized the incongruity between feeling and thinking; the lack of unity; of a splitting of the mind; of ambivalence, or a coexistence of love and hate. Patients may speak of dreadful things with bland expressions or a smile. A woman tells of being raped and beaten with the expression she might use to speak about the beginning of a tender love affair. In point of fact, she may be referring to two things at once: to her love for her father (tenderness) and a primitive way to achieve it (rape); and her bizarre affect is not without meaning. *Incongruity of affect* may also be seen in emotional blunting, which coexists with extreme sensitivity and often appears to be protective. The schizophrenic German poet Friedrich Hölderlin speaks of his own feelings as a volcano covered by a cap of ice and snow. Again, this is more than a metaphor; it directly expresses the experience of being split; it indicates a self that is unable to focus, direct, and coherently feel its own energetic feelings. The infantile drives and impulses of the schizophrenic in this stage are closer to the surface of consciousness, less controlled, and in some cases quite dangerous. Some ghastly sexual and murderous crimes (such as cannibalistic murder) have been committed by schizophrenics, as well as some of the most dreadful suicides.

Usually, drives are not goal-directed in the actual environment; the schizophrenic tends to be unable energetically to focus wishes on the environment; he "dreams," experiences images, but lacks directedness. His drives are instead usually manifest in regressed oral or autoerotic behaviors, in florid thoughts and vivid beliefs, which seem to entail withdrawal from objects in the world in favor of fragmented or blunted autistic relationships. There may, however, be disorganized thrusts into the world of activity and attempts to transform it, manifest in bizarre—and occasionally dangerous—social behavior.

In the standard description of this group of disorders, *blunting of will power* is listed as an important symptom. Patients are described as inactive, unable to make decisions. Two considerations lie behind this observation. It is more correct to say that in many situations patients are not interested in making decisions, just as they are not interested in using their judgment; they are too preoccupied with themselves and their overwhelming experiences and fantasies. Their weakness of will is essentially a disengaged attitude in a situation where the nonschizophrenic believes will power or judgment should be exercised. Schizophrenics can be very active whenever they are really involved; their involvement, however, is unpredictable and not easily fathomed, even in well-studied patients. In a second sense, the effort required to focus on all that is necessary for decision-making is too great for them. The level of organization in which decisions are expected requires something more of the patient than magical solutions. Focus and involvement that is sustained and that can stand reversals and distractions are entailed; this is not easy for the patient to achieve, even when he is sufficiently aroused to try to do so.

Hallucinations, Delusions, and Illusions

Whereas Bleuler considered hallucinations, illusions, and delusions as usually *accessory symptoms*, others, such as Josef Berze and Hans W. Gruhle, viewed them as fundamental features of schizophrenia.[19] The manifold delusions, illusions, and hallucinations are consequences and representations of a primitive mental set in which the motivation or capacity to test reality is lacking. It is not clear whether these phenomena should be viewed as attempts to structure and order reality and the chaotic inner world, or whether they are primary manifestations with a secondary defensive function. Hallucinations are frequent; most often they are auditory, but visual, tactile, olfactory, and gustatory hallucinations also are observed. Hallucinations are very definite and realistic in some patients; in others, they are more dream-like—vague or fantastic. Auditory hallucinations in the form of voices are threatening, aggressive, and insulting; more rarely, they are neutral or seductive and even friendly. Some hallucinations are tactile, of a sexual nature, and some patients report more complex somesthetic hallucinations, such as being beaten or sexually abused. Illusions or misperceptions of reality are frequent. Patients report experiencing *déjà vu* and secret signs and revelations. Hallucinations and illusions are woven into the fabric of false and incorrigible beliefs. Delusions of being controlled, hypnotized, influenced, and manipulated are quite frequent, if not universal. These may develop from ideas of reference into elaborate systems, which direct thoughts and actions, such as the deluded schizophrenic's "influencing machine," studied by Victor Tausk.[190] The loss of autonomy, of balanced controls, provides the basic ground against which the simplistic explanatory power of delusional thinking can be appreciated. Schizophrenics equivalently "save" their fragmenting selves, their families, and the world through delusion. They attempt to abolish problems of war and peace at one fell swoop. Occasionally, they resort to action. Newspaper accounts of senseless crimes frequently stress the incongruous affect of the culprit who, on examination, may have slaughtered innocent bystanders in order to have peace or to quell the voices in his head. In all these descriptions, the human capacity for dissociation, for segments of organized behavior blandly to proceed without the checks, guidance, and steering of reality—which includes emotional comprehension and responsiveness—is apparent.

Catatonic Symptoms

Catatonic symptoms, another accessory symptom of Bleuler, are psychomotor acts frequently seen in schizophrenic patients and by no means limited to the so-called catatonic type. The two most extreme catatonic symptoms are *catatonic stupor* and *catatonic excitement*. In stuporous states, patients are mute and immobile; they are negativistic and will not eat or drink (or even, at times, defecate); they do not take care of their bodily needs, such as clothing themselves adequately, avoiding extreme temperatures, washing themselves, or using toilet facilities when required. They seem to be less bothered by fatigue than normal persons would be. From clinical observation, it appears that sleep is not disturbed. Some Indian yogas are probably stuporous catatonics. There is danger that stuporous patients will starve to death or die from exposure or infection unless they receive proper care. Most catatonic patients do not develop stupor; some seem to approach it without developing the full syndrome. W. Mayer-Gross *et al.* maintain that the stuporous patient does not experience anything whatsoever, but we disagree.[130] Those stuporous patients who can be induced to speak about their experiences give accounts of a strange dream-state, such as being bewitched. Frequently, the catatonic will relate his immobility to an excruciating paralysis of decision; he is poised between murder and suicide and believes that the slightest activity is momentous and will bring destruction. In fact, catatonic excitement may precede or follow stupor. We have known patients who, after long-lasting stupor, gave rather clear descriptions of experiences that could be verified; it may be embarrassing but instructive for the attending staff to hear about their behavior when they think they cannot be observed by a patient who is "out of contact." One patient, a Turk who spoke no German at the time of his admission to a provincial mental hospital near Vienna, learned to speak the Austrian dialect of the province during ten years of stupor. The striking thing about stupor is that the musculature is dissociated very much in the way that a patient can be "taught" in hypnosis that his will and his actions can be separated. In catatonic stupor, any action is deemed dangerous by the patient, and action sometimes may be inhibited even in situations of external danger, such as fire. Harry Stack Sullivan considered catatonic stupor an extreme form of withdrawal.[185]

Catatonic excitement is a severe state of agitation with sudden onset and indiscriminate violence. Some of the exotic forms of agitation, such as Amok, Latah, and Arctic hysteria, may well be states of catatonic excitement. Patients in such a condition must be considered dangerous to themselves and to others and treated accordingly. Catatonic symptoms include slight mannerisms and odd behavior and extend to marked stereotypy (identical phrases or gestures used for a wide range of meanings and situations). One sees grimacing; bizzare gestures and postures; the repetition of what has just been said (echolalia) or done (echopraxia); negativism; and, rarely, catalepsy, for which neurological explanations have been advanced. H. H. DeJong[43] has compared the waxy flexibility of the musculature and posture of catatonics to the effect of bulbocapaine acting on the midbrain. R. Gjessing's observations of a "periodic catatonia" with concomitant imbalance of nitrogen metabolism refer to a small but biochemically interesting subgroup of schizophrenics.[79] Lesions of the central gray substance and tumors impinging on the third ventricle will produce stupor, and in view of the links with the hypothalamus, metabolic shifts might be expected. Response to drugs indicates an altered central state, since some catatonics, with sodium amytal, "wake up" to speak about their thoughts and appear to sleep after intravenous metamphetamine. These findings of Joel Elkes would suggest that, whereas the musculature in the catatonic is protected from activation by internal and external input, some paradoxical central state maintaining this barrier is disturbed by drugs acting on brain stem systems.[53]

Schizophrenic Deterioration

In the phase of deterioration an extreme loss of efficiency in performing tasks occurs. One observes empty, silly, helpless, and unresponsive behavior, or even automatisms such as mouthing, sucking, plucking, and scratching movements. Arieti differentiates the "burned out" schizophrenic, who may be employable and rehabilitated, though quite impaired, from the preterminal progressive cases.[5] Dilapidation, stemming in part from long years of disuse, lack of practice in social conduct, work, and pleasure, represents an impairment that is observed to fluctuate and is to some degree reversible. It is evident that the phase and stage in schizophrenia must be clearly described if research on presumably homogeneous populations is to take place. A simple division of patients into acute and chronic groups is far from sufficient.

General deterioration in schizophrenia, whatever its predisposing cause, seems to be the result of living with a disorder in which there is an impairment of those functions that lead to sustained, integrated, and goal-directed behavior. Although there may or may not be a diminution of applied intelligence (social skills, the elementary skills required for group living and so forth), there is certainly no absolute loss of specific learned abilities or general intelligence in schizophrenia. The differentiation of schizophrenic and other deterioration, however, is far from solved. Whereas Kurt Goldstein emphasized [81] the similarity in the deterioration of schizophrenic and organic disorders, Kraepelin and others stressed differences, such as the wide fluctuations in performance, which are more characteristic for schizophrenic than organic patients.

> During the early days of World War II, an extremely regressed back-ward patient seemed utterly out of contact, grunting only an incomprehensible word from time to time. Periods of mutism were interrupted by outbursts of ferocious violence; for this reason he was kept in one of those bare cells which we call isolation rooms. He ate like an animal, masturbated without any concern for others who might observe him, urinated and defecated on the floor, and smeared himself with feces. But one day, he wrote on the wall with feces, the only writing material he possessed: "Buy War Bonds."

This capacity for unexpected performance clinically distinguishes schizophrenic deterioration from organic deterioration, in which the deficit is relatively constant and covers a much wider area of performance. Memory and recall, which are characteristically disturbed in organic disorders are—clinically—intact in deteriorated schizophrenics, although conditions for optimal function may be quite special. In schizophrenia there is accordingly considerably more scatter in various segments of standard intelligence tests than in organic dysfunctions. As noted, schizophrenics do have greater difficulties than normals in learning, especially when sustained efforts and social involvements are necessary. It is likely that there are subtle disturbances of concept-formation, manifested by impaired judgment in real life and also in certain tests, such as the Kohs Block Test. Nevertheless, the young schizophrenic who gradually or suddenly performs poorly in school and shows impairment on tests is incapacitated less by a loss of aptitude than by apathy, lack of interest, and withdrawal, which may be secondary to the primary perceptual and experiential problems. Some schizophrenics are, and remain, highly intelligent, particularly those paranoid patients who do not disintegrate; their maintenance of vigilant and reactive contact with, and activity in, the environment generally differentiates them from other subgroups. It seems that patients with high initial intelligence are less likely to deteriorate than patients with lesser endowment. Familial and social patterns that sustain an "intelligent attitude" rather than simply require intellectual achievements may be the critical differential factor. Many observers have been struck by the fact that some geniuses, such as Vincent Van Gogh and Robert Schumann, who became schizophrenic, continued to be productive and creative during their psychoses. Ernst Kris expressed to us the interesting idea that creativeness may be a defense against the destructive impulses of such schizophrenics.

Manfred Bleuler estimates that about one-fourth of all schizophrenics reach a state of deterioration or extreme deficit behavior.[24] This observation was confirmed by many other psychiatrists. Today the extremes of such deterioration are relatively rare, unless the patients are badly neglected. Such neglect is not infrequent; the deterioration of the unfortunate patients on the chronic wards is probably in part an indignant withdrawal from contact after extreme hurt and humiliation (both in the world of the hospital and the uninterested world outside). Nevertheless, it would be misleading solely to blame unsatisfactory social and hospital conditions. We cannot underestimate nor cease to investigate those intrinsic and interpersonal factors that reinforce the relative inability of the patient to transcend his impaired states. We may call this impairment an ego weakness, integrative weakness, "a regressive preponderance" (as Sullivan put it), or "a predominance of the unconscious forces" (in Carl G. Jung's terms);[103] but whatever we call it, we have not defined it. Whether differences in endowment, personality, interpersonal experience (for example, lack of reinforcement of goal-directed behavior at critical phases of development or of the illness), or all of these and more determine deterioration, is unknown. A few experiments have been undertaken in which dilapidated patients have been transferred to highly intensive treatment wards, and it still remains a mystery why some of these patients can be reached by treatment and others not.

Types of Schizophrenia

There is much confusion about the classification of schizophrenias. The criteria for such classification are crude descriptions of symptoms, which, as we well know, fluctuate and change during the course of the disorder. Reality only approximates the types that exist in our minds and in textbooks. The types most frequently are, to use the current American terminology, "undifferentiated" or mixed types. All too often, classification is based on hindsight. Like Kraepelin,[116] and more recently Henri Ey,[57] we propose to differentiate types primarily according to their courses. The most important task thus would be to differentiate the benign types, which are relatively stable, from the malignant types, which disintegrate and deteriorate. If we mention types in the following section, we do this more to acquaint the student with the kaleidoscopic richness of the syndromes without, for the moment, undue concern over rigid boundaries. We differentiate: (1) The classical types. (2) The border states, which obviously cannot be clearly allocated. (3) The diagnostically troublesome category of the paranoid syndromes.

Classical Types

Kraepelin, the great taxonomist, described many types of dementia praecox, all now forgotten except the basic types also mentioned by Eugen Bleuler. The *hebephrenic type* is characterized by early onset, massive disturbances of thinking and feeling, and a tendency to rapid deterioration of behavior that is clearly regressed, fragmented, and silly. A hebephrenic disorder "grafted" upon mental deficiency is referred to in the German literature as *Propfhebephrenie*. The *paranoid type* (dementia paranoides) suffers from hallucinations, persecutory and fantastic delusions, with a tendency to behavioral disintegration and pervasive disturbances in thinking and feeling. The *catatonic type* exhibits a variety of hyperkinetic and hypokinetic symptoms with the extremes of stupor or excitement. These three types are generally recognized because, on occasion, a pure type has been observed, but there has been considerable controversy about the fourth, *dementia praecox simplex*, first described by O. Diem.[48] Eugen Bleuler stated that dementia praecox simplex is characterized by the presence of the primary symptoms and the absence of secondary symptoms. Even the primary symptoms may not be very marked. An oddness that has always existed becomes more evident, and the patients gradually become asocial and their affect shallow, blunt, or indifferent. Over a period of time, a person with few symptoms other than occupational or social decline may show streaks of autistic or fantastic thinking, often surprising in view of a bland, well-maintained front. Followed over the years, these patients insidiously decline in functions and status. Many petty criminals, habitually unemployed hobos, and prostitutes belong to this category. The changing population of symptoms and subtypes requires careful investigation. K. A. Achte reported that there has been a decrease of catatonic, and an increase of hebephrenic, types.[1] More important than shifts in the incidence of particular symptoms or types, however, is the realization that since we possess better therapies fewer advanced and terminal states of classical schizophrenia are seen.

Border States

We distinguish four different border states: (1) The schizophreniform—in all likelihood atypical schizophrenias. (2) The oneirophrenias and related states, which are close to the symptomatic psychoses (a psychosis that is a symptom of another disease). (3) The "pseudoneurotic" states, which are, according to American usage, "borderline" states in the more narrow sense of the word. (4) The schizoaffective reactions, "hybrids" between the schizophrenias and the affective behavior disorders, which will be considered in Chapter 15.

Gabriel Langfeldt found, in catamnestic studies, that certain cases, which he called *schizophreniform psychoses*, exhibited the basic symptoms of schizophrenia but had a markedly better prognosis.[121] Somatic, reactive, and also psychogenic elements can be discerned, and onset is relatively acute. Langfeldt assumed that the schizophreniform psychoses respond well to the various organic therapies and that the true schizophrenias are therapeutically refractory. In American psychiatry, the schizophreniform psychoses are lumped with the acute schizophrenias. The rare syndrome of *oneirophrenia* was described by Ladislas J. Meduna and W. S. McCulloch.[136] The word oneiroid means dreamlike and was introduced by W. Mayer-Gross.[130] Typically, it is a syndrome characterized by disturbance of thinking and affect with clouding of the sensorium, ranging from mild confusion to delirium. Some patients have fever and leucocytosis. Meduna, F. J. Gerty, and V. G. Urse also reported metabolic disturbances in such cases.[135] In our opinion, many of these patients would be better described as behavior disorders associated with acute mild encephalopathies.

Two rare types of catatonia are of more theoretical than practical interest. One is *recurrent catatonia* with classical catatonic symptoms and spontaneous remissions with symptom-free intervals, in which R. Gjessing reported a retention of nitrogen (responsive to thyroid treatment) during the catatonic episode.[79] The other is R. Stauder's *lethal catatonia*, a fulminant disease with a characteristic severe psychomotor agitation, which changes into a hypokinetic phase, followed by clouding of the sensorium, exhaustion, coma, and death.[182] Pathological findings reveal submucosal hemorrhages, swelling of the brain, and hyperemia but no specific disturbances. Encephalitis and meningococcus septicemia must be considered carefully in the differential diagnosis. "Lethal catatonia" need not be lethal; early electric convulsive treatment usually is life-saving. We consider Stauder's lethal catatonia an acute brain syndrome and a symptomatic psychosis, an encephalopathy rather than a form of schizophrenia. Stauder's lethal catatonia should not be confused with the occurrence of "mysterious" sudden death in schizophrenia, which, of course, generally has a negative correlation with the level of medicine practiced in public mental hospitals and with the competence of their pathologists. Certain pregnancy psychoses probably fall into the border group between schizophrenia and severe behavior disorder associated with brain diseases.

More important than the rare types discussed are some young persons presenting in an acutely disturbed, almost toxic state of confusion and identity diffusion, who emerge from their psychoses with a relatively good sense of identity. We also see dangerous and exhausting catatonic excitements in young schizophrenics (without known organic disease), which are too extreme to be controlled by drugs but respond well to ECT, and these must for the moment be classified with the schizophrenias. During World War II, some soldiers, under conditions of extreme stress and isolation, developed short schizophrenia-like episodes from which they promptly recovered under more favorable conditions. Similar reactions were reported by Poul M. Faergeman as "psychogenic psychoses." [58]

Clinicians have been troubled over those border states, which appear to lie on a continuum between neurosis and schizophrenia.[31] Such patients have characterological ego-syntonic abnormalities and relatively few and mild schizophrenic symptoms; they do not disintegrate or deteriorate. The best-known grouping is the so-called *pseudoneurotic schizophrenia* described by Paul Hoch and Phillip Polatin.[93] These patients suffer from diffuse and severe anxiety, a panoply of neurotic symptoms and polymorphous perversions, and, to a slight but significant degree, basic schizophrenic disturbances of thinking and emotional processes. Ludwig Eidelberg[51] described the "psychotic character" and Arieti,[6] the "stormy character." Both authors referred to patients who had severe characterological deviations with outbreaks of uncontrolled, primitive, antisocial behavior.

Robert P. Knight[113] and Robert L. Arnstein[7] both have described borderline states in the young adult. These patients show an "active search" for identity, a constant, frenetic engagement with their world, in attempts either to comply or to rebel; yet, they are usually endowed with enough strength to resist psychotic disintegration. The crises of identity may continue for a long time. One of our patients, observed for twelve years, was first admitted to the hospital after quitting his successful position as a stockbroker: "I have tried everything—compulsive work, psychotherapy, drugs, alcohol, homosexuality, marriage—everything which should make people happy, but none of them works." He is successfully employed at the moment, but in the interim he underwent rehospitalization, arrests for drunken brawls, and received various courses of drug treatment. He has had numerous clear-cut but transient paranoid episodes, but he has, with fortunate environmental circumstances and support through therapy, maintained an orientation toward search and consolidation of his gains. It is obvious that there are quite formidable problems of differential diagnosis here. In general, we believe research will be advanced if the psychiatrist does not too readily conceive of such persons as "ambulatory schizophrenics" and the like. Some, but not all, recovered schizophrenics may closely resemble the border groups, but further work is required to elucidate these gray areas.

Paranoid Syndromes

Many paranoid syndromes are also border states. On one end of the spectrum is the paranoid personality, a personality variant, like the anxious and aggressive personality, and certainly not a "disease." On the other end, we encounter the previously mentioned paranoid schizophrenia, one of Kraepelin's classical types. Between these extremes lies a variety of paranoid syndromes, the rare paranoia and the more encapsulated paranoid conditions in which some schizophrenic symptoms are seen, which we will discuss below. These attempts at classification would be of little importance if they did not reflect our insecure knowledge about etiology and the essence of these disorders, whether schizophrenia and related disorders are forms of human existence or diseases. The paranoid syndromes associated with cerebral syndromes are considered in chapters 16, 22 and 23.

PARANOID PERSONALITY A paranoid personality is characterized by the excessive and permanent presence of suspiciousness, hostility, and rigidity. Since these traits variably occur in all persons, it is impossible clearly to delineate a diagnostic class of paranoid personalities. At times, everyone feels that he is discriminated against or taken advantage of and reacts with anger and fear. Everyone also has the occasional feeling that people stare at him or make remarks. Psychologically healthy persons, however, will check such experiences and reactions and, more crucially, make corrections in their relationships when they seem appropriate. In those whom we label loosely as paranoid personalities, such reality-testing is severely impaired. As N. Cameron sees it, the paranoid does not have the capacity to take the role of other persons and to assume a detached and objective view either of himself or others; the paranoid is detached, where others are involved.[39] Throughout their adult lives (and often since childhood), these persons have been unable to trust or confide; they live in fear and seclusiveness. Some are shy, withdrawn, asocial, and passive, but the majority of the patients are driving, ambitious, aggressive, and usually hostile and destructive.

Paranoid personalities have an extraordinary tendency to be severe and critical with others but are extremely sensitive if criticism is directed against them. Criticism means attack, and the paranoid personality responds with a counterattack. Any move, any gesture by others, is interpreted as unfriendly, hostile, detrimental to them, and as deliberate rejection or humiliation. The paranoid personality seems unable to distinguish between friend and foe; when friends are treated as enemies, sooner or later there are few friends left. Even these friends are constantly tested and provoked until they withdraw or actually become antagonistic, and this proves to the patient that his mistrust and expectation of betrayal were justified. Corrective and punitive measures by society are taken, of course, and only provoke further expressions of hostility. Understandably, persons with so much hostility and so little trust not only make poor friends, but also poor marriage partners or lovers. Their oversensitivity and jealousy, their inability to understand people, and their anger create trouble in close relationships. They are unlikely to recognize simply that their feelings are hurt, that they are limited and vulnerable; rather, they respond to slight rejection with automatic anger, a misreading of the motives of others, thoughts of revenge, and querulous resentment. In addition, their sexual needs are often infantile; there often is an apparent lack of interest in sex, a high frequency of adult masturbation, and an inclination to sadistic and homosexual practices. The tendency to antisocial and criminal behavior is considerable; however, in the group of paranoid personalities, we find some gifted individuals: outstanding artists, inventors, scientists, leaders and misleaders of humanity. Some of the great moralists of all times had personalities of a distinctly paranoid flavor. Perhaps they are differentiated from some borderline schizophrenias at times by their strong "identity," manifest in their "dedicated" hostility and mistrust.

PARANOIA This is a very rare syndrome. The true paranoiac suffers from more than suspiciousness and mistrust; fleeting ideas of reference and persecution have become permanent and cannot be altered. Such persons become progressively estranged and incapable of using corrective feedback (sharing the views of others). This may be related to the intensity of their destructive feelings and wishes. The patient is not merely argumentative and stubborn but becomes engaged in endless feuds and litigations. He may take up a particular mission, pursuing it relentlessly and with complete disregard of his own or other persons' interests. Of course, the boundaries between the *idée fixe* of the stubborn person, the dominant idea of the paranoid personality, and the delusion of the true paranoiac are fluid. The paranoiac is often provoked by a real or imaginary tort, which may set into motion endless lawsuits and completely unfounded accusations. It is impressive how paranoid patients find both their persecutors and their followers. Often, the character of paranoid accusations (for instance, that all judges are bribed) is easily unmasked; other paranoid accusations have led to some of the worst witch hunts, mass persecutions, and ugly prejudices in all ages and have also made martyrs of paranoiacs.

The cogency with which the paranoid can cite reality as his defense can often mislead the unwary diagnostician. The paranoiac's arguments, or at least the premises for his arguments, may stand up for a while to skillful empirical testing and to logical inquiry, but he usually sooner or later tips his hand, and we discover that the patient has a well-developed system of paranoid delusions. In the ideal case, however, these delusions are consistent and often carry a certain degree of conviction; in the true paranoiac, hallucinations and illusions are not supposed to occur. The psychiatrist, confronted with a person with a cause, or a case against some injustice, typically finds himself uncomfortably judging issues on their merit and arguments on their cogency rather than diagnosing the organization of personality forces in the patient; therefore, it requires skill to stick to patterns of behavior—to diagnose, rather than to agree or disagree. Usually, true paranoiacs are extremely hostile and, all too often, destructive and dangerous. Psychiatrists, like everybody else, shun contact with such patients. It is difficult to commit them to hospitals and to control them anywhere. Arthur Miller's play, *A View from the Bridge*, illustrates the difficulty of preventing catastrophe. Often we act after things happen—too late. Under the stresses they themselves create, most paranoiacs eventually develop cognitive and affective disturbances and then fall within the boundaries of schizophrenia. What usually defies our diagnostic ability is the onset of paranoia and its differentiation from paranoid personality. With better and more subtle clinical investigations and tests of thought disorder and personality organization, this difficulty will possibly be overcome too.

The following illustrates a case of "true" paranoia in a twenty-nine-year-old man.

> The patient was admitted for psychiatric evaluation after he was shot by a U. S. Marshal when he attempted to escape. Until about ten years before this event, he was manager of a large moving firm. He had high ambition and in general rather conventional ideas, was proud of his ability to make a good income, buy a new car every year, afford good clothes, and so forth. He then began to feel that he and his superiors disagreed, and he asked in rather rapid succession to be transferred to other sections of the firm. His sister, who became alarmed over these difficulties, could not find out what rankled him. He finally simply decided not to go to work, and when she urged him to return, he became angry. He stayed at home idly, convinced that the company would apologize and ask him to return to an even better position. He could not believe that after three years of idleness he was actually discharged. During that time he seemed depressed, spent most of the time alone, reading. Finally, he decided to learn a completely new trade and became a mechanic. He strictly avoided work in his home town in order not to embarrass his family. In contrast to his previous performance, his work record was poor. He left his jobs frequently; either he was fired or found it impossible to get along with fellow workers and bosses, although at that time during the war there was a critical shortage of workers. Increasingly, he picked quarrels with all family members, excepting his mother. Just a few months before admission, he seemed to have less difficulty and began to look like his old self and held a job. He tried to enlist in the Navy and was turned down, which hurt and enraged him. When he was notified by his draft board of his impending draft he protested the decision. He failed, however, to appear at his physical examination, saying he had an important engagement at that time. On the following day a deputy U.S. Marshal arrested him. He seemed polite and cooperative and on the way to his hearing received permission to buy cigarettes and at that time attempted to escape; the marshal's shot grazed his left leg, leaving only a superficial wound. He complained of pain, numbness, and weakness in that leg, but no structural cause could be found and his complaints continued until finally arrangements were made to have the patient transferred for psychiatric examination.
>
> The family is of Czech descent. They are Catholics but indifferent to their faith. The father, a meek friendly man, successfully operated a hardware store; the mother, a strong, stubborn woman, dominated the household. Of her four

sons and two daughters she always preferred the patient, her firstborn, and the patient was also extremely attached to her; even when she refused to put up bail, he considered her his best and only friend. Indeed, he never had any close male or female friends. Little was learned about the patient's sexual activities, except that he never had any enduring sexual or erotic attachments. He took girls to dances and dated as did everyone else. He angrily protested inquiry about homosexual practices—"such filthy business"!

During his psychiatric observation he was aloof, uncooperative, or politely evasive. Assuming that any information gathered would be held against him, he refused to take tests and constantly stressed that he was in this hospital under protest. Clinically and in psychological tests there was no disturbance of formal thinking; there were no hallucinations. His speech was stilted and over elaborate. When asked to participate in work activities, he said, "I would rather stay in my room; when one is locked up in a hospital contrary to one's wishes, it is not conducive to one's enjoyment of the society or of one's fellow men." The patient feels he has no complaints, except against society, and no loyalties, except to his mother. During his hospitalization, it was impossible to penetrate his rigid defenses and gain his confidence. After three months of unsuccessful attempts to engage him in psychotherapy, he was transferred to a public mental hospital.

Schizophrenic Paranoid Syndromes

Kraepelin differentiated the classical type of paranoid schizophrenia (with paranoid delusions and a pervasive disintegration of thinking and feeling) from *paraphrenia,* or *paranoid condition,* as it is called in the American diagnostic classification. In paraphrenia, the disintegration is limited to certain paranoid complexes. For example, such patients have hallucinations: they hear voices that abuse them and have rather circumscribed ideas of being persecuted, to which they usually respond with a certain blandness. The pervasive disturbances of thinking and feeling, which are characteristic for schizophrenia, are absent. These patients are not withdrawn, and they are reasonably efficient in their reality-testing and may be able to "encapsulate" and hide their delusional system for a long time.

A young housewife reported that her butcher attempts to have rectal intercourse with her when she buys meat. Other customers seem to overlook these obvious attempts. She is a warm and friendly woman who carries out her domestic duties quite efficiently and on the surface, at least, has a loving relationship with her husband and children. She hears voices who tell her how to protect herself against the butcher's attempts. When asked why she frequents the store, she becomes evasive.

Isolated delusions of grandiosity are rare. In some cases a megalomanic phase, when grandiose delusions abound, follows a phase of persecutory delusions. The simplistic and insufficient explanation has been made that patients who feel persecuted inevitably must reach the conclusion that they are very important persons. Ideas of grandiosity are also an expression of intense lifelong narcissism or the return to infantile notions of omnipotence. The latter is found in schizophrenics and organic deficit states with grossly impaired reality-testing.

The syndrome of *sensitive delusions of reference* was first described by Ernst Kretschmer;[118] it is characterized by erotic delusions and certain oversensitivities. It occurs not infrequently in middle-aged spinsters who develop delusions (after a life of sexual abstinence and frustration) that men have begun to pay attention to them by unmistakably expressing love either in subtle signs, which only they can understand, or occasionally in grossly obscene gestures and demands. These lovers may be one or several well-known persons (for example, famous actors), none of them realistically available. The syndrome is similar to the paranoid oversensitivity of some physically handicapped persons, and particularly those suffering from deafness.

We encounter *delusional jealousy* not only in schizophrenias but also in many different psychiatric disorders, especially in alcoholic and drug psychoses.[140] In contrast to normal jealousy, clear provocation to jealousy is lacking in the pathological form, yet some pathologically jealous patients manage to "choose" unfaithful partners and often provoke them into unfaithfulness. What is essential, however, is that the pathologically jealous person does not lose interest in his love-object even if the love is not returned; the anger and hostility over the rejection and humiliation is sustained and strong. Ambivalence, a cardinal feature of all types of jealousy, is marked. In many of the delusional forms of jealousy, we find impotence in the male patient, as well as various forms of infantile and deviant sexuality, particularly homosexual behavior. The milder but troublesome jealousies of the neurotic personality are far more frequent than the rare psychotic forms.

The psychopathology of the relatively rare syndrome of *folie à deux* or "induced simultaneous insanity" is of broad interest.[83] In the typical pair, the dominant partner is a man or a powerful woman; the inductee, invariably a woman or a very passive male, accepts the delusional system of the dominant person. *Folie à deux* has received a good deal of attention because it clearly suggests psychological modes of transmission of severe mental illness.[47] We will return to this topic in our discussion of the psychodynamics and social dynamics in the etiology of paranoid symptoms.

The Question of Etiology

The etiological problem is complex, and at this juncture our knowledge represents more of a speculative game than an opportunity to assess an array of well-verified facts. In general, we know more about what makes a schizophrenic better or worse than about the obscure events of the "premorbid era," which predisposed to the disorder or precipitated it. At this time, there is no convincing evidence that any particular biological or psychosocial event in itself produces schizophrenic behavior. The sustained endeavors of biological investigators so far have not provided convincing leads. The analytic-psychological investigators have contributed more to an understanding of the meaning of schizophrenic behavior when it occurs than to a differentiation of factors and mechanisms which induce the disorder through some psychosocial mode of transmission. In a word, we are still groping in darkness.

Biological Variables

A biological factor could initiate or maintain a state in which schizophrenia might occur, or make recovery difficult, or indeed all of these. It could, as Jung[103] believed, come into play only after a series of psychological events. What is critical is that any postulated "biological weakness" or weakness in bioadaptive functions or "quantitative factor" be specified by research. Yet, schizophrenia presents no clear and compelling path for biological investigation. Many findings are clearly secondary to the way the schizophrenic lives, although it is often forgotten that the way he lives *is* a measure of his psychobiological capacity for adaptation. If it is said that he lives under stress, the neurobehavioral definitions of such stress and its physiological consequences have also yet to be systematically made. Much investigation has been poorly designed or good investigation ignored because of a search for *the* schizophrenic factor (indeed, one worker reported a particular streptococcal toxin, which appeared to be specific!). Conceptually, a disorder of the *organization* of systems is unlikely to yield readily to a single factor; where there is a known pharmacological inducing agent (in the sense of a model psychosis), the sequences of biochemical and neurophysiological events are just beginning to be worked out for a few compounds. How much greater the task is in the case of schizophrenia! It has been remarked that when specific dysfunctions are discovered, we may simply lose a group of disorders we had been calling schizophrenia (which, about a hundred years ago, was subsumed under the "acquired idiocies"), and the remainder would comprise the continuing enigma for researchers.

Research Strategy

There is hardly a somatic function that has not, at some time, been reported to be abnormal in schizophrenics. Body weights of schizophrenics have been found to deviate from statistical averages, but as far as routine findings are concerned, the composition of body fluids has been found generally within normal limits. Many biochemical findings reviewed below have been a function of appetite, exercise, and hospital diets; similarly, physiological findings, such as the edema and cyanosis which sometimes are noted, are probably caused by orthostasis contingent on activity patterns. Where, then, is the "lead" to be investigated?

It is evident that basic links between patterns of activity and an array of psychophysiological biochemical processes must be estabished before the psychobiology of schizophrenic behavior can be comprehensible. The relationship, for example, of biological processes and sustained attention (or the capacity for goal-directed activity) is barely appreciated at the neurophysiological and biochemical levels; further, the intrinsic normal control mechanisms for biochemical and electrophysiological processes are essentially unknown. The strategy of research in this field, therefore, may be directed toward (1) attempts simply to identify regular characteristics within a schizophrenic group, which can then lead to further differentiations and suggest specific neurobehavioral mechanisms for study; (2) attempts to study model or parallel disorders (such as drug reactions, deprivation states, or psychomotor epilepsy) or presumably important etiological factors (such as the role of excitation or isolation in infancy) in order to find substances, processes, or variables to investigate in patients; and (3) elucidation of basic control mechanisms in neurobehaviorally interesting biochemical or physiological systems (such as hormonal or sleep regulation). In general, a schizophrenic patient may best be viewed as a different psychobiological organism than the normal; in fact, the most characteristic finding is a wider fluctuation or range of psychobiological measures in a group of patients than would be expected in normals. Further, correlations of, say, biochemical events with fluctuations in the course of the disorder, or with reparative processes may be as relevant as the search for causative mechanisms.

Psychophysiological Response

The Worcester group extensively studied the biology of schizophrenics in the 1930's and 1940's; and Roy G. Hoskins[98] and, more recently, H. Freeman[67] documented a number of psychophysiologic functions that differed in schizophrenic populations and normals. David Shakow's review of psychological studies has been discussed.[175] The typically sluggish response of patients is emphasized in various studies showing the "physiology of withdrawal." The blood pressure of schizophrenics was found to be lower and resistant to environmental (stress, cold) and drug-induced input. This "rigidity" is not constant and may shift with improvement. A tendency to sustained peripheral vasoconstriction has been noted, and subpapillary capillary abnormalities are still under study. From the pharmacologic response to cholinergic and anticholinergic drugs, several investigators have suggested abnormalities in these systems.[152] Such approaches require a variety of techniques; an attempt to replicate a finding of abnormal cholinesterase measures was not successful.[54]

In general, there are reports showing diminished *compensatory* physiological response: for example, a lack of cardiac hypertrophy in valvular lesions; lower temperature; decreased response to pyrogens; and decreased response (of nystagmus) to rotary and caloric stimulation. A certain lack of responsiveness to pain and to various drugs seems to exist. The biological organization underlying unresponsiveness must be differentiated in chronic and acute states.[101] Ernst Gellhorn and G. N. Loofbourrow have reviewed the problem of autonomic control in schizophrenics.[75] With newer techniques, pupillary response has been employed as a model system in which central and neurohumoral controls can be deduced,[164] and a lack of inhibition of the pupilloconstrictor nucleus has been reported for acute patients. Usually, findings of sluggish compensatory responses do not occur in patients in better contact; such findings may represent correlates of the life led by the patient or perhaps are related to his diminished capacity for organized response.

Even though few sedentary control populations have been tested, we think the noted differences both in perception and reaction time and in physiological response cannot be explained simply by diminished physical activity; rather, they seem related to an altered organization of central activation mechanisms, a physiological and psychological difference in the mode of engagement with the environment. These correlates of the disorganization (perhaps based upon an overactivation that is sustained and hence leads to rigidity or unresponsiveness) may be more aptly sorted out with better concepts, better controls, better selection of populations,[150] better measures and, most importantly in this field, replicated measures.

Brain Structure and Function

Many neuropathologists, among them Alois Alzheimer, were at one time convinced that schizophrenics show definite neuropathological changes, such as specific atrophies and degenerative changes in cortical areas three and five. None of these changes has stood up to careful re-examination. Reinvestigation with sophisticated histochemical techniques and electron microscopy are warranted not because of their novelty but because of their demonstrated power to define the chemical anatomy of ultrastructures, which hitherto eluded study. There is a possibility that some schizophrenias will turn out to be midbrain diseases, although J. E. Staehelin came to the conclusion that schizophrenia is not a diencephalosis.[179] A. D. Zurabashvili and his co-workers postulated synaptic disturbances in the ascending reticular system, so far without solid evidence for such a hypothesis.[200] Robert G. Heath and his collaborators have reported specific septal spike activities from deep electroencephalograms.[87] Such spikes have also been seen in other diseases and in various states of agitation. Hill[90] reviewed the subject of electroencephalographic changes in schizophrenia; he and others report a variety of unspecific changes but no well-defined or specific abnormalities.

If, as many workers believe, significant neural events in behavioral states are not revealed by usual EEG recordings, we shall have to await research with computer analysis of the electrical activity of the brain. C. Shagass and Morris Schwartz, employing computer analysis of scalp-recorded potentials evoked by peripheral nerve stimulation, have successfully differentiated patient populations,[174] and studies by Callaway and his co-workers of attention similarly discriminate patient groups.[35] Studies reflecting basic neural control mechanisms are important; thus, because ions change membrane potentials and activate enzymes important in energy metabolism, sodium and magnesium have been studied in body fluids and erythrocyte membranes and their fluctuation with symptoms has been noted. No generalized electrolyte defect has been established.

Endocrine Findings

Ever since the classical descriptions of the disorder were published, investigators have tried to discover endocrine and metabolic causes. Manfred Bleuler has surveyed the clinical endocrine findings in a thorough book without reaching any positive conclusions.[23] The frequency of onset of schizophrenia during adolescence (though not at puberty), and also at the time of childbirth, the puerperium, and the involutional period has been interpreted as indicating the importance of endocrine factors; of course, these events are also of great psychosocial significance. Minor endocrine symptoms,[4] for example, menstrual disturbances; feminine physique of male patients; masculine traits of women (hirsutism); and also major endocrine disease (acromegaly, hyperthyroid, and hypothyroid dysfunctions, diseases of the adrenal system), have all been observed in occasional patients, but have not thrown any light on the etiology of the disorder.[78, 138] If schizophrenia is an endocrine disease, clearly it does not fit the model of any medically known endocrine dysfunction.

In general, the student will find researchers leaping at any incongruous tissue to study in the hope of discovering even an inexplicable biochemical finding. If there is any strategy to such a "shotgun" approach, it is that a model system or a substance or process will be revealed, which could, much later, be linked to mechanisms more directly leading to the altered functions underlying schizophrenia. The reports by Mark D. Altschule of the beneficial effect of pineal extract referable to presumed anomalies of the pineal secretion have not been confirmed.[3] There is a link of this organ to tryptophan metabolism, and the aldosterone releasing hormone of the pineal and the metabolic products of the pineal skin-lightening hormone have a beta carboline structure and hence could conceivably be psychotoxic in man.[77, 134] Assays of various sex hormones in schizophrenic patients have been negative. No consistent thyroid changes have been noted, although fluctuation with changes in clinical status may be observed.[138] Studies of steroid metabolism do make it evident that schizophrenia is, by this definition, stressful, but causal mechanisms are not identified.[139,167] Investigations of Samuel Eiduson, and co-workers[52] and of E. L. Bliss, C. G. Migeon, C. H. N. Branch, and L. T. Samuels[25] have not confirmed earlier findings of Hudson Hoagland and G. Pincus,[92] who extensively studied biological changes in schizophrenics and found the adrenal cortex less responsive to stimulation. Notions of adrenal-cortical dysfunction led some workers to try unsuccessfully adrenalectomy as a possible "cure."

A vast amount of work remains to be done before we will understand the biochemistry of neuroendocrine functions generally, let alone in schizophrenia. The role of hormones in altering accessibility to enzymes and their involvement in mood and mental changes warrants further search. As in every approach reviewed, the significance of such study will not be known until laboratory methods are developed to deal with other than the most grossly evident dysfunction of a physiological system. Psychiatrists generally underestimate the importance of subcellular mechanisms, the phenomena of rate and kinetics, and their known relevance for drug-induced effects on neurobehavioral systems. Conceivable mechanisms of importance to the biology of schizophrenia may have to await technical and substantive developments in biochemical pharmacology, physiological and brain chemistry, as well as skill in patient evaluation and selection.[150]

Metabolism and Proteins

Anomalies of carbohydrate metabolism, particularly of anti-insulin activity, have been reported by Meduna, Gerty, and Urse,[135] and a persistent finding has been an abnormal oral glucose tolerance test, and the intravenous test is often reported as abnormal.[68, 89, 151] The responsible mechanism is unknown. Abnormalities in the insulin-activated phosphate metabolism of red blood cells are of continuing interest.[27, 82] Although cerebral circulation, oxygen, and glucose uptake of brain are normal, abnormalities referable to the intermediate metabolism of glucose in brain are reported.[168, 189] T. P. Detre *et al.* reported a diminished perception of high-frequency vibration, which the authors related to an unknown disturbance of carbohydrate metabolism.[44] There are many reports on pathological liver functions in the literature; none of them has been confirmed by careful replication.

J. S. Gottlieb and his co-workers[82] postulate anomalies in intermediate carbohydrate metabolism. They believe the schizophrenic is unable to use available energy to react to stress; glucose tends not to be readily metabolized via the Emden-Myerhoff scheme whereby lactose, pyruvate, and some high-energy bonds are formed under "emergency" or anaerobic conditions. Essentially, this group is attempting to identify a relationship between endogenous serum factors and the various pathways for energy metabolism. As an assay for serum activity, they employ chicken erythrocytes; these are incubated with plasma from schizophrenics and show a higher pyruvate production than normal controls;[73] this was interpreted as a reflection of the failure to mobilize ready energy. There is extensive work directed toward isolating and characterizing the alpha globulins (probably a lipoprotein) responsible for this effect. Where specific chemical identification of a substance is lacking, the problem is at least to find increasingly specific bioassays (such as the graded response of isolated smooth muscle or a quantitative change in animal behavior) and to characterize its effects on basic biochemical mechanisms. Thus, serum factors, while responsive to stress in normals, are reportedly greatly increased in about 60 per cent of schizophrenics under stress. Simply the transferring of the patient to a new ward could evoke increased activity of this serum factor. The extent to which the factor reliably occurs more frequently in schizophrenics than in other populations is uncertain. Jack Durell's laboratory produced evidence that the serum factor influences the stability of red cell membranes, rupture of which could alone account for the changes in carbohydrate measures;[166] this was also found in Gottlieb's laboratories.[122]

Other investigators, some starting from quite different standpoints, have been led to a study of similar serum proteins in schizophrenia.[18] From findings of a copper-containing globulin, ceruloplasmin, which M. Ozek[148] had found elevated in schizophrenics, several workers in the 1950's proceeded to study certain dyes or adrenaline as a substrate for ceruloplasmin. They found that schizophrenic serum oxidized these substrates more rapidly than normal. The elevations of ceruloplasmin later proved not to be specific for schizophrenia, and Roger K. McDonald [132] and others showed that increased oxidation was contingent upon dietary deficiency of ascorbic acid. M. K. Horwitt has cogently emphasized the importance of nutritional controls in such studies.[96] Robert G. Heath *et al.* confirmed these findings but reported that massive transfusions of blood from schizophrenics produced psychotoxic effects in normals,[86] and in extracting the psychotoxic factor (called taraxein), Heath believed it was closely related to, though qualitatively different from, ceruloplasmin. This substance, unlike the proteins active in assays involving carbohydrate metabolism and rat rope-climbing behavior, produced various EEG changes in monkeys and "psychotic" symptoms in man. However, investigations by Eli Robins *et al.*[159] failed to confirm the psychotoxic effects of taraxein in humans.

Whether the various stress-responsive proteins are specific for schizophrenia or are in any way linked with its pathophysiology remains to be seen. There is no a priori necessity that a defect in a biochemical system should directly produce behavioral effects; nor is it unlikely that such research could be as relevant to certain steps in the psychophysiology of stress as to the etiology or pathophysiology of schizophrenia. One problem has been to differentiate the kind of stress schizophrenia is (rather than, say, a momentary crisis). McDonald, for example,[132] found increased excretion of a methylated metabolic product of norepinephrine (VMA) in the urine of chronic schizophrenic patients. Normal subjects could begin to approximate this increased metabolism of norepinephrine only with marked physical exertion. Thus, in spite of the apparent relative motor inactivity of patients, there appears to be a great deal of activity of *some* kind in being a chronic schizophrenic; to pose a puzzle, we seem to be dealing with an "active inactivity" or an "inactive activity."

There are other approaches involving proteins; for example, various autoimmune mechanisms have been proposed,[145] and an elevation of macroglobulins has been reported by several investigators.[61,62] Investigations of the allergic reactivity of schizophrenic patients showed no difference in amnestic response or skin reactivity with the exception of histamine, which several investigations have shown produces a less intense dermal and vascular response in schizophrenic groups;[66] apart from metabolic defects (such as histamine metabolism which is under study), such findings could involve altered CNS function leading to altered protein metabolism and vascular reactivity. An inability readily to develop new immune responses in schizophrenia, if present, again would point to some factors involving protein metabolism.[193]

Biotransformations

A major current pathway of research involves the search for enzymes that could produce psychotogenic substances from bodily tissues; this approach promises less confusion than the results of previous assays (on submammalian organisms) for the presence of toxic phenolic acids and indoles in schizophrenics' urine.[161] The rationale for this approach is based on the chemical structure of a wide number of psychotogenic compounds, all of which are related to endogenous indolealkylamines, catecholamines, or beta carbolines. Exogenous compounds, such as LSD, related in structure to biogenic indoles, are now known to influence the metabolism of serotonin in the brain;[64] and the gamut of psychoactive drugs are linked to the metabolism of biogenic amines.[186] It had been proposed that products of epinephrine metabolism could be transformed into possible psychotoxic compounds[147] such as adrenochrome or structurally related psychotomimetics (such as mescaline). In general, such compounds have just begun to be investigated at the sites of critical interest.[10] Although the adrenochrome hypothesis[94] was not confirmed[187] (and its psychotoxicity was found to be unreliable), the substance is present in salivary glands.[11]

A mescaline-like derivative (3, 4-dimethoxy phenethylamine), possibly arising from the norepinephrine precursor (dopamine), was reported by A. J. Friedhoff and E. Van Winkel[72] and subsequently by others as considerably higher in the urine of schizophrenics than normals. This interesting work has stimulated interest in methylation as a possible endogenous route to psychotoxic catechols. Finally, the demonstration of enzymes in the mammal, which can produce psychotoxic tryptamines, has been of interest.[9] G. G. Brune and H. E. Himwich observed that acute exacerbations in chronic schizophrenic patients are associated with marked increases in the urinary excretion of tryptamine and associated metabolites.[33, 34] A number of other biotransformations of catechols and indoles are reported in schizophrenics.[80, 132] These current approaches are opening the path for the study of enzymes and their activity in different clinical disorders that could lead to psychotoxic effects. In other chapters, we have mentioned the search for isozymes and the various *endogenous* mechanisms involved in the transport, distribution, storage, and release of brain neurohumors. From drug studies it appears that a local change in endogenous receptor substances, as well as a psychotoxin, could critically alter neurobehavioral states.[63] For any of these changes, either genetic or reactive sequences could conceivably be involved. Whatever biochemical changes may be found to distinguish some populations, it is likely that there will still be a long path in order to connect the biochemical dysfunction to neurobehavioral operations. This is one reason that controlled studies with model systems in the laboratory are of general use, since they point to possible substances and mechanisms for clinical investigation. The critical fact is that everything we know about neurobehavioral organization would accommodate a biological factor as causative or contributory to schizophrenic behavior, and nothing we know has been, in fact, firmly linked to etiology. Several extensive and critical reviews of the neurochemical basis,[178, 195] and history of these findings may be consulted.[109, 131, 177]

Heredity and Constitution

The importance of hereditary factors in the etiology of schizophrenia cannot be disputed, but the mode of inheritance and the relative importance of genetic factors still is far from clear. So-called pedigree studies show that schizophrenias occur in certain families and that the prevalent mode of transmission is either direct or collateral and appears to be complex. In some families—for example, in the Wittelbachs, the royal house of Bavaria—schizophrenics have been noted in many generations. Jan A. Böök, reviewing the work of H. Sjögren, E. Stromgren, and others, as well as his own work, reported that expectancy figures in families with a schizophrenic proband are significantly higher than in the general population:[26] for parents, approximately 12 per cent; for siblings, 9 to 12 per cent; for grandchildren, 3 per cent; for first cousins, nephews, and nieces, 2 per cent.

The most impressive data have been collected on identical and fraternal twins. E. Slater found, in 115 fraternal and 179 sets of identical twins, a concordance rate of 14 per cent in fraternal, and 76 per cent in identical, twins.[176] F. J. Kallmann, in his monumental studies of 517 fraternal and 174 identical twin pairs, found a concordance of 15 per cent in fraternal and of 86 per cent in identical twins.[105] E. Essen-Möller,[56] and also P.

Tienari[191] and E. Kringlen, in carefully studied series, report much lower concordance figures. In a relatively small and statistically insignificant series of identical twins who were separated, Kallmann found in the separated twins a concordance of 77.6 per cent, compared with 91.5 per cent in those who were not separated. Kallmann's and Slater's twin studies do not altogether negate the influence of environment, because psychological identification in identical twins is much stronger than in fraternal twins. A very careful genetic and psychosocial study of such twins, possibly on a national scale, would be of utmost importance and might yield very important clues to why some twins are afflicted and others not; William Pollin *et al.* have begun multidimensional studies of families in which twins are discordant for schizophrenia.[154] Don D. Jackson, in a critical review of published twin research reports, concludes that the over-all finding of genetically determined schizophrenia is unconvincing.[102] (See Chapter 6.)

The mode of inheritance is an open question; different authors express differing opinions. Some, as Kallmann and H. Luxenburger, have assumed recessive inheritance; others, as Böök, assume a major simple dominant gene with a heterozygous penetrance of about 20 per cent and a homozygous penetrance of 100 per cent. Julian Huxley[100] and coworkers suggest a simple dominant gene and discuss balancing advantages and disadvantages in selection; for example, cited as favorable were an alleged resistance to most infections, diseases, wound shock, and the effects of biochemical changes (insulin, thyroxin, histamine). In all likelihood, inheritance of schizophrenia is multifactorial. Genetic studies are complicated by our inability to make precise diagnoses; yet today, more than ever, there is hope that future biochemical studies will enable us to identify both genetic carriers and potential schizophrenics.

Ernst Kretschmer found a preponderance of leptosomic, athletic, and dysplastic constitutions in schizophrenic patients.[117] Kretschmer's detailed quantitative data were not confirmed, although the over-all impression of a high percentage of leptosomic patients in the schizophrenic group is shared by many. Kretschmer also described a normal personality type, the schizothymic, and a border state, the schizoid, with leptosomic body build. The schizothymic, essentially a normal personality type, resembles Jung's introvert; the schizoid is characterized by oddness, an avoidance of close relationships, and a certain unpredictability. We believe today that Kretschmer's contribution to the schizophrenia problem is his description of these transitional personality types rather than his emphasis of correlations between body build and schizophrenia.

The Psychological Meaning of Schizophrenic Behavior

Schizophrenic behavior is most confusing and unpredictable because it contains a high proportion of unintegrated segments of behavior; however, we believe, as do many psychoanalysts and existentialist psychiatrists, that much of schizophrenic behavior is meaningful. The simplest attempt to establish meaning is by relating or comparing schizophrenic behavior to known forms of behavior. Storch's description of schizophrenic behavior[184] as archaic behavior is such an endeavor.

A schizophrenic patient fell from a third-story window when he tried to launch a contraption that would permit him to fly to the sun. Like his famous model Icarus, he failed. Is the patient's behavior more meaningful if we consider that he wanted to be close to his father and also compete with him? We believe it is. The rich symbolism of schizophrenic behavior, as in the above episode, has obviously invited equally rich interpretations as well as the abruptly "concrete" consequences! Here, of course, lies the danger of the interpretative approach, especially when it does not take into account the intensity, literalness, and incapacity to cope with reality, which characterizes schizophrenic behavior. From a practical point of view, an interpretative approach, not regarding schizophrenics as dumb and unfeeling brutes, but rather seeing them as sensitive and possibly oversensitive persons with a highly differentiated but disintegrated and idiosyncratically coded system of communication, has had an important humanizing and therapeutic impact.

The behavior of schizophrenics is more specifically meaningful if we can establish a lawful connection between such behavior and psychosocial variables. Alfred Stanton and Morris Schwartz demonstrated outbreaks of violence or periods of incontinence were related to definite upset and conflict in ward management; some aspect of staff dissension (probably a change in expected *patterns* of staff behavior as well as specific acts of commission or omission) was perceived by the patients and responded to by them.[181] We observed a severely disturbed young woman who became most upset with her therapist; he finally reminded her of what she already knew—that his mother had died recently. He hoped to account, thereby, for something of his depressed behavior, which, he correctly knew, the patient must have perceived. It was striking that she thereupon relaxed and, with no more than a perfunctory condolence, expressed her relief that she was not implicated. Both the sensitivity and the egocentricity of the patient are related and apparent in this example. Yet patients are *not* mind readers, as some accounts imply. Rather, they are unstable and egocentric and misinterpret the slightest cue indicating a change in the affective and the interpersonal structure surrounding them as crucially implicating them, their security, their rightness or wrongness, and the like; they correctly interpret an element of reality and miss the context. Patients are indeed responsive, but a patient who shows too much interest in the therapist is probably not just being friendly, but expressing a loss of his fragile identity; he loses touch with himself as he becomes too concerned with others. Such patients require a healthier self-centeredness (which requires painful effort and might appear excessive to the layman) rather than the disorganized, unsatisfactory, and vulnerable egocentric position they generally assume.

Not all schizophrenic symptoms are usefully seen as having meaning. Certain symptoms in deteriorated schizophrenics may lose their original meaning and become empty stereotypes. Stereotyped behavior shows a loss of boundaries and a false economy; the same ritual or response comes to stand for a multitude of meanings and situations.[142] But even deteriorated patients retain some ability to communicate meaningfully.

Psychoanalytic Interpretations of Paranoid Schizophrenia

Freud's[71] interpretations of the Schreber diary became a basis for psychoanalytic interpretation and explanation of paranoid schizophrenia. Just how generalizations from this one diary could be extended to interpretations of other paranoid syndromes and schizophrenia in general is not always clear. Freud assumed that Schreber's disorder was precipitated by an increase of homosexual libido, by a passive-feminine, or homosexual, wishful fantasy directed toward his physician; these were repetitions from his childhood of wishes concerning the patient's father and brother. The defense against such wishes involved projection, denial, and also hysterical mechanisms, which, according to Freud, were responsible for the hallucinations. Freud stated he did not know why these particular mechanisms were used, but it appears to have been his conviction that the increase of homosexuality was the precipitating etiological factor and that a fixation at a narcissistic level provided the disposition. In his discourse, Freud, with characteristic self-irony, had asked whether there was more delusion in his theory than in Schreber's delusion. It is clearly not easy to describe and make sense out of processes that inherently are irrational. I. MacAlpine and R. A. Hunter critically reviewed the interpretations of Freud and other psychoanalysts and added their own thought that Schreber's delusions reflected his primitive fragmented state, his preoccupation with his essential identity, and his archaic procreation fantasies rather than homosexual wishes.[128] They rightly stressed that neurotic mechanisms used to explain schizophrenic behavior do not sufficiently focus on the primitive nature and meaning of psychological processes in schizophrenia.

Henriette R. Klein and William A. Horwitz showed that homosexuality is by no means the universal factor in the history of paranoid patients.[110] As James S. Tyhurst put it simply, not all homosexuals are paranoid, nor are all paranoid patients homosexual.[192] If one considers the more likely possibility (and this is what Freud probably meant) that an increase in latent homosexuality precipitates a paranoid development, one cannot help but wonder why this happens only in some persons; after all, latent passive homosexual wishes, and defenses against them, are of universal importance, particularly for the psychological understanding of the male. Robert P. Knight made an important addition to the original hypothesis by stating that the aggression in connection with unconscious homosexual wishes is the decisive factor in producing paranoid symptoms.[112] The paranoid person suffers from tremendous unconscious hate, and he expects to be hated by the persons to whom he is attached. The importance of ambivalence in such sadistic and masochistic relationships was also stressed by Robert C. Bak.[12] It is our own opinion that presence of homosexual themes is guaranteed by the altered state and organization of mental processes in which identity is fragmented. Yet, there are a number of cases in which homosexual wishes do seem to have dominated personality development. These persons seem to us to have both a quite concrete need for, and a dread of, changing identities with the father: a patient kept his father's cap to wear in moments of panic whereupon he even called himself by the father's name; at other times, he violently rejected and competed with the father. In other words, it is the function and meaning of the homosexuality in the paranoid, not simply sexual strivings, that is significant; their identification with the same sex involves the very core of their security and identity.

Freud was the first to stress the role of projection and denial in paranoid and schizophrenic development.[70, 71] R. Waelder emphasized the significance of denial, which he considered as basic for psychosis—just as basic as repression is fundamental for neurosis.[194] Denial of reality is a more profound distortion than repression, although it may be a more primitive and simpler mechanism. The wish "I love the man" becomes a true denial: simply, "I hate him." This, in turn, may be projected, "He hates me." Denial permits no reality checks, and it sets off bizarre and primitive reworking of reality to take the place of what is excluded. The proposition: "I do not love at all; I do not love anyone," may become modified into the narcissistic formula, particularly in megalomanic delusions: "I love only myself." In paranoid jealousy occurring in males, the denial and projection of homosexual love takes the formula: "I do not love him; I love her and deny that she does not love me." This persists, even though it is clear from the patient's behavior that his interest is in the man with whom the woman is engaged. For the patient with critical identity needs, either actually to be that man (who seems more "real" than the patient) or to be the real woman loved by him could be equally important dynamically. Pronouns identify persons in their roles. The autistic child who calls his mother "I," or himself "you," shows a profound disturbance in the very beginning of development of the ability to transform roles into identity and a basis for relationships. The child must integrate what he is told. The command: "You do this" at some point genuinely must become, in effect, "Me doing this because I am told to or because I also want to." The schizophrenic patient who hears voices telling him what to do is perhaps in some sense struggling with an aspect of what was once a real event. He is improving when he learns that these inner voices are now his and that he can choose to take an attitude of listening or not listening to them. Arieti sees the dynamics of the schizophrenic as an attempt to deny that he is a bad child, something he has tried to do since childhood through compliance (which is frequently seen in the biographies of the early development of schizophrenics)[155] or withdrawal.[5] We also quite frequently encounter denial that the mother was in fact cold and unloving; worthlessness and self-abasement seem preferable to any perception that conveys the real hopelessness of obtaining wished-for love and security from the ungiving or imperceptive mother. This deep sense of shame and worthlessness is projected or denied, but with this denial there is a loss of any coherent self. Even many neurotic patients find it intolerable to express their anger and their feeling that: "I am not the bad one—you are." They often aggravate the therapist by their insistence that those with whom they are obviously in conflict are simply wonderful people; they have learned to fear and distrust their own negative feelings and to accept the myths (mother *does* love you) and tacit instructions about legitimate feelings (don't complain about being confused) that once were offered them. They see no alternatives, no chance of weighing and sorting the situation. For the schizophrenic, it has apparently been crucial throughout his development (and certainly is at the time of his disorder) that he not destroy an image of security in spite of his raging feelings. It is postulated that a persistent, lifelong craving for a symbiotic relationship (a union or "oneness" with the mothering person) is characteristic of schizophrenic patients. This is an ambivalent craving in which the patient simultaneously wants to love and destroy. Withdrawal, thereby, becomes useful; the image of security is thus preserved while separation from the actual aggravating parents or parent-surrogates is required by disturbed behavior.

Projection, as we have emphasized, is a universal defense, and what differentiates normal from abnormal projections is that most persons are able to distinguish between what is real and what is projected. One can imagine an infant with internal pain (or a person with little capacity to discriminate) identifying his stomach-ache as bad—not "me"; or the ache is part of a different self (it or the self is disowned), or it is a bad "something," (such as mother) causing the ache. Many normal adults react to illness (often before they *know* they are ill) with irritability toward others or withdrawal and avoidance of others. This failure to locate the difficulty is relatively benign. An adolescent wanting guidance may hear a casual remark and decide it is an order; this reflects his momentary need for guidance. Where there is a failure to distinguish boundaries of the self, including failure to allocate responsibility for actions and events, the importance of structure, of real or magical cues and directions is enhanced. In psychoses, the epigenetically early agents for structuring—parental instructions—become active and are hallucinated; "they" argue and cajole and compel.

Freud considered delusions as attempts of restitution. "The delusion formation, which we take to be a pathological product, is in reality an attempt at recovery, a process of reconstruction."[70] Paranoids and schizophrenics in general replace a chaotic, immensely frightening world by a more orderly apperception; it is less frightening despite being more hostile. Freud also felt that paranoid delusions contain a kernel of truth that can be discerned in the history of the patient, particularly in his childhood when he was subjected to cruelty, inconsistency, and rejection. Thus, we can see how delusions are formed and replace reality, how they are modeled on a semblance of reality and contain a biographical truth. Why reality was experienced as so unpleasant, impossible, and devastating as to compel a schizophrenic adjustment never has been answered satisfactorily.

A number of psychoanalysts expressed hypotheses about the meaning and etiology not only of paranoid schizophrenia but of schizoprenia in general. Ego weakness was stressed first by Federn.[60] Heinz Hartmann assumed a lowered ability of the weak schizophrenic ego to neutralize aggression.[85] Milton Wexler stressed the role of a pathological superego.[196] William L. Pious sees in schizophrenic behavior an archaic response (an experience of dying or emptying) to psychological deprivation to which the schizophrenic is exquisitely vulnerable.[153] Pious views the course of subsequent events—the symptoms—as a part of a progressive thrust of attempts to cope with the unstable regressed state, to "focus," and to achieve more organized levels of functioning. Many psychoanalytic investigators assume that the predisposing factors are found in traumatic events in early childhood. Melanie Klein related adult paranoid reactions to the paranoid disposition of the infant.[111] Another prominent spokesman for the theory that schizophrenia and paranoia have their origin in infancy was the influential Harry Stack Sullivan, who distinguished between dementia praecox, an organic disease, and schizophrenia, a disorder of living.[185] At some particular time, the structure of the schizophrenic's world is torn apart, and he suffers from dreadful experiences. Subsequently, the security operations become regressive, and early uncanny emotions recur. This brief mention of Harry Stack Sullivan's rich observations and speculations cannot do justice to his work; it has to be read in the original.

Schizophrenia and Social Groups

Stress in groups can produce transient thinking disturbances and paranoid behavior. We have witnessed the eruption of such behavior in one, many, or all members of small and large self-study groups. It is important to distinguish shared delusions from individual delusions. Generally, the projections of primitive man and of children, or of particular cultures, do not necessarily interfere in a major way with actual contact with reality and the disposition, capacity, and energy to deal with reality. The social context in which distortions of reality occur has to be taken into account; only this differentiates the odd and unrealistic content of certain religious, philosophical, and political systems from individual psychotic belief systems.

We owe to Norman Cameron one of the most interesting discussions of the paranoid development. In an article entitled, "The Paranoid Pseudo-community," [37] he outlined his original thesis, and in a later article, he integrated his original thoughts with psychoanalytic propositions.[38] An adult who is likely to become paranoid has not developed skills to understand other persons adequately or to communicate freely with them. This inability to put himself into another person's role may lead to the belief that he is the target of a community of real and imaginary persons who plot against him. If he swings into paranoid action against this pseudocommunity, he is apt to be in trouble with the real community. Cameron believes that the evolution of the pseudocommunity saves the patient from further aggression. The hypotheses that the paranoid patient forms are preferable because they are less anxiety-producing than the strange, unstructured, threatening world that produces such uneasiness and vigilance. In his own way, the paranoid tries to understand the threatening, inescapable events around him. The final crystallization and formulation of his fears and extremely hostile urges is the conceptual pseudocommunity that serves for the internal absorption of aggression.

The concept of induced psychoses plays a major role in the etiological speculations of those who have studied the role of family dynamics in schizophrenia.[45, 83] In *folie à deux,* the partner in whom behavior disorder is induced is usually passive and less intelligent. Ordinarily, this partner is a woman and, in rare cases where it is a man, he is impotent, homosexual, or extremely passive. The passivity and a certain readiness for identification are the key elements in induced psychosis; the importance of imitation and identification points to a certain relationship to the hysterical disorders. Actually, the careful study of any close interaction in a tightly knit group, such as some families, would reveal a number of beliefs, norms, family myths, and jargon which outsiders might not comprehend and which, strictly speaking, represent distortions of reality or at least a restricted perspective.

The small group significantly structures meaning and values; it is the arena in which the major segment of living and suffering occurs. The importance to a family or office group of the behavior of a petty tyrant, a boss, or a phobic mother is immense. Tears, tantrums, depressions, paranoid sensitivity, and suspiciousness are normally encountered when the structure of small groups changes or one of the key figures becomes disruptive. Shift the rules of the game, and in the attempt to orient themselves most people will pay special attention to events, searching for meaning, that is, new rules. People are willing to live with great discomfort if it is familiar or stable; they do not want the rules to be changed. A phobic lady had her family highly restricted in their activities because of her dirt phobia, and her husband even enlarged the attic to store the papers she refused to throw away. Participation in, and support of, the patient's symptomatology, as well as opposition to and fear of it, are regularly and inevitably seen; and this has given rise to speculation that such socially regulated support or disruption of expected roles is of etiological importance to the development of life-disrupting and crippling personality change. Whatever the merits of such speculation, a shift in rules regulating role expectations in a group can undoubtedly act as a precipitating factor for the vulnerable parties. Ernest Gruenberg calls attention to the relation of *folie à deux* to other shared forms of psychopathology, such as mass psychoses through the ages (for example, children's crusades, dancing mania).[84] Conflict between the wish for sexual and aggressive experience and the fear of such experience can be resolved by displacing the responsibilities and guilt to groups; group frenzy expresses such wishes and wards off more intimate personal experience and guilt. This type of analysis may be applied not only to *folie à deux* but also to other forms of upheaval in groups, to certain instances of mass hysteria (invasions from Mars, mass swoonings of female adolescents listening to popular singers), and to such antisocial phenomena as lynchings and rioting.

Family Studies

In general, clinicians cannot help being impressed with the family pathology of schizophrenics.[120] Further, psychiatrists and therapists who read and pay attention to these studies will have a far richer set of referents in which to place the problems of the patient. Harry Stack Sullivan found the relationship to the "Mothering One" particularly disturbed. According to D. L. Gerard and J. Siegel, schizophrenic families are more disturbed than control families.[76] L. C. Wynne and coworkers carried out a very detailed investigation on schizophrenic triplets and subsequently engaged in carefully controlled studies of families of schizophrenics, from which they conclude that relationships and communcation in families of schizophrenics are regularly and significantly disturbed.[199] Kenneth L. Artiss came to a similar conclusion by direct observations of schizophrenics and their families in their homes.[8] Intensive observations of a group of thoroughly studied families led Theodore Lidz, Stephen Fleck, and Alice Cornelison to conclude that the families of schizophrenic patients are thoroughly disturbed, unhappy, and divided, with serious breakdowns in communication.[127] The marriages were gravely disturbed; members were eccentric, intensely irrational, and suffering from severe and often overt incestuous and homosexual conflicts. Lidz *et al.* pointed out that it was not only mothers who transmitted irrationalities and facilitated faulty identifications by the patient, even during the preverbal stage; the weak, passive fathers also had their share in establishing profoundly disturbed patterns. These investigators described the failure to form a nuclear family; the existence of family schisms owing to strife and the absence of reciprocity; and family skew and the blurring of generation lines that occurs when one parent competes with a child or involves it in an abnormally erotic relationship. The whole family atmosphere becomes charged with conscious incestuous fantasies, irrational and paranoid ideation, and, importantly, the family and its way of operating with the child do not help the child toward emancipation. Yrjö Alanen *et al.* began to explore the interesting complex problem of why one particular sibling develops schizophrenia without coming to the definite conclusion that either constitutional or psychodynamic factors alone are responsible.[2] As these hypotheses find increasing support by carefully controlled studies, this material is becoming of great etiological significance. J. E. Oltman, J. J. McGarry, and S. Friedman did not find a significant difference between schizophrenics' and hospital attendants' families in the number of broken homes, but such crude sociological concepts as broken homes do not reflect the subtle disturbances that seem to count.[146] In a relatively well-controlled study of schizophrenia that also deals with such gross variables, Jerome K. Myers and Bertram H. Roberts found no specifically distinguishing characteristics of families of schizophrenics.[143]

An interesting theory, proposed by Gregory Bateson, Don D. Jackson, and their co-workers,[13] is based essentially on the assumption that in schizophrenia the metacommunicative system has broken down. Metacommunication is communication about communication; for example, the labeling of humor as humor, of play as play and not as serious business. Schizophrenics use unlabeled metaphors. These unconventional communicative habits were appropriate at one time when the pre-schizophrenic child was exposed to serious "double-bind" situations in which the child could not win no matter what he did; in adult life, these habits of obtuseness are no longer appropriate. A prototype of such a situation is the first injunction by a forbidding mother: "Don't do this or I will punish you." The second injunction is: "Don't see me as a punishing agent"; and the third forbids the child to escape. When no responses are possible, fear and rage ensue, and communication breaks down. A mother gives her son two neckties for Christmas and when the boy appears wearing one, she asks disapprovingly, "Didn't you like the other one?" Here, the boy cannot in sanity wear both, and if he wears either or none he will displease his mother. Actually, these "binds" depend upon the absence of a self which is sufficiently autonomous to take the risk and seek its own ends. It is important for the psychiatrist to learn to identify methods by which the patient is covertly pressured, and he must expect to decode the most innocuous-appearing interchanges between patient and family. For example, what kind of responsive parent could write sweetly to her desperately lonely daughter, who was just sent to a hospital, "Isn't it nice, we now have two new things in the family: your treatment and sister's typewriting lessons." The daughter's desperate promiscuity, careless self-mutilations, and bizarre liaisons, recounted in an oddly dissociated way, reflect the lack of secure self-feeling and uncertain identity of a girl who was a "thing" to her mother. Psychiatrists have become truly familiar, through close study of families, with such characteristics of parents and the consequences to the patient of consistently impervious "off the mark" parental attitudes.

Yet, as compelling as these descriptions of family behavior are, it is nevertheless likely that the patient, with the defects in identity we have noted, himself provokes and generates such conflicting messages as the double-bind and hears them where they are not intended. Parents of adolescents (and anyone who deals with passive dependency, for that matter) often find that their remarks are taken literally and that they themselves are thereby "bound" by the response of the child. The parent cannot give an order without being told, in effect, that he is a beast, unreasonable, or silly; the parent cannot "please" the child. An assistant who monitored every word spoken by his boss finally provoked the harassed authority into asking the man to be less dutiful and more sensible. It is always possible to "hear" conflicting messages if one is "set" to do so, and this is certainly the set of the schizophrenic patient. The psychiatrist learns to listen for ambivalence and covert meanings and, more importantly, to hold his "professional suspicion" in abeyance until there is clear evidence as to how these meanings operate in patterns of behavior. The patient also hears at several levels and may well reinforce parental misbehavior by listening to the unconscious of the parent—to allusions, inconsistencies, and omissions—rather than assessing the current reality or taking a remark at face value. "Why don't you visit?" a mother writes to her adult son who, we believe (having predicted the meaning of this family's codes fairly well), is correct in fearing this means "live with us forever." But it is also true that this mother, fortunately, can and does manage without her son—something he too frequently forgets. It is he who cannot visit briefly without disorganizing. In some symbiotic relationships, however, one can predict that as the child improves and gets well, the parent will react with disturbance and even disorganized behavior; mother and child have never been able to be separate and individual, and, in the psychological sense, operate as a "seesaw." A result of family studies is that the therapist can evaluate far more realistically than he otherwise might the behavior of the patient's parents and the kinds of stresses and confusing communications the patient must have experienced. This practical consequence of family studies has not been widely heralded, but we believe it already has significantly influenced practice in many centers. Nevertheless, no clear-cut patterns that generally and confidently differentiate the family pattern of schizophrenics from nonschizophrenics have as yet emerged.

Epidemiological and Cross-Cultural Studies

No definitive contributions to the etiology problem have been made by epidemiological and cross-cultural studies; this is not really surprising, since true incidence and prevalence figures are lacking. R. E. L. Faris and H. W. Dunham found that a much higher number of admissions to mental hospitals came from slum areas of big cities than from the suburbs and "golden fringes." [59] They related this distributional phenomenon to the psychological isolation and deprivation of lower-class living. Critics of the Faris-Dunham thesis claim that the schizophrenics in the slum areas have gradually, over generations, accumulated at the bottom of the social scale. August B. Hollingshead and Fredrick C. Redlich, in their study of treated schizophrenic patients, disproved this "downward drift" hypothesis.[95] The families of schizophrenics are not more downwardly mobile than the normal population; if anything, these authors were impressed with some upward mobility. Hollingshead and Redlich found that the prevalence of schizophrenic patients in the lowest social class is nine times as high as in the two upper classes. This striking finding was accounted for largely by an accumulation of chronic patients of the lowest class in public mental hospitals. No definite knowledge about the relationship of social class and schizophrenia exists, but preliminary research makes it likely that the true incidence and prevalence of schizophrenia in the lowest social class is unusually high.

Schizophrenics have been observed in all cultures and subcultures. Psychiatrists in developing countries report differences in primitive and more advanced areas; in general, however, we are impressed that symptomatology and types in different parts of the world are quite similar,[16, 180] as are accounts from other centuries.[99] Anthropologists and some psychiatrists have suggested cultural explanations of paranoia. Paranoid attitudes are more frequent in some cultures than in others; the suspicious and hostile Dobus of the South Pacific are a pertinent example.[17] It is likely that in police states, where mistrust is strongly reinforced, mildly paranoid personalities are more frequently encountered. The same may be true in poverty-stricken but highly competitive societies. Minority groups develop paranoid attitudes, and in turn paranoid attitudes have been exhibited against such groups.

Summary Remarks about Etiology

To interpret schizophrenic behavior as meaningful behavior does not explain it. Many depth-psychological concepts, for example, ego weakness and breakdown of ego functions, regression to primary processes, narcissistic fixation, are merely descriptive terms. They point to certain mechanisms and experiences without telling us what stimuli produced schizophrenic responses, or why just such responses and no others occurred. The search for meaning has not provided an answer to the quest for etiological factors. Yet, this does not negate the possibility that learned or acquired factors play an important role; in the paranoid disorders, particularly, it is quite likely. We know a good deal about the genesis of paranoid personalities and how some of them become paranoid. We also believe that many schizophrenics develop from schizoid personalities or from what Helene Deutsch described under the term of "as if" personalities, characterized by a provisional identity and lack of genuineness, warmth, and a capacity for relationships.[46]

However, such observations contribute relatively little to a comprehensive understanding of the etiology of the disorder.

Thus, no satisfactory general etiological explanation exists at present. Both "somaticists" and "psychologists" offer mostly promissory notes. No really good data on precipitating causes exist; we are impressed with the coexistence of stressful psychological experiences with the onset of many schizophrenias, and we sometimes can identify the life-crisis or impending adjustment the patient could not manage. Whether these events cause the outbreak of the psychoses or themselves are expressions of psychotic processes has not been determined. Why schizophrenics react in their specific way to psychosocial stimuli is also unknown. Among predisposing causes, our best leads lie in the field of genetics, but the mode of inheritance in schizophrenics, and particularly why certain individuals are phenotypically schizophrenics, is also unknown. Although various metabolic, endocrine, and neurological anomalies have been reported, these have not been essential to the disorder or sufficiently verified to permit etiological inferences. Depth-psychological propositions usually assume regression to early narcissistic fixations as a result of traumatic experiences and avoidance reactions to parents; they stress the role of lifelong faulty communications, particularly with mothers and fathers of schizophrenics. Although data of this kind are of extraordinary interest, they still await further confirmation. Further, they must account for why such upbringing "takes" in one case and not another, and finally, how such factors succeed in generating a world-wide incidence of disorder. Whereas factual knowledge about single and multiple etiological factors is most rudimentary, vague theories abound; some of them are judicious guidelines for current and future research, and there is no harm in such theoretical assumptions as long as tentative knowledge is not taken for established fact.

From what we have said so far, it is not surprising that there is a wide split in theories of the schizophrenias. Are they localized brain diseases? We don't think this is a sufficient answer. Are they psychologically determined narcissistic neuroses, as Freud called them on several occasions? Existentialist psychiatrists and some others look at schizophrenia as a way of life, a form of *Dasein*. Ludwig Binswanger, in his famous case histories,[21] sketches different examples of such schizophrenic existence; but every case stands alone and is removed from the consideration of natural science. Lidz, building on Freudian, Sullivanian and Meyerian ideas, has also considered schizophrenia not as a process but as a potential fate, an escape from an altering of the internal representation of reality.[127] The earliest origins of such a fate, according to Lidz, can be found in unbearable stresses of the preverbal stage. One might say that the symptomatology can be understood best as an archaic attempt at preserving individuality. But the costliness and the pain of such an adjustment is inordinately high.

There have been numerous synthesizing theories, among them Leopold Bellak's noncommittal multifactorial theory.[14] One scheme that appeals to us is the following: the schizophrenias, or at least some of them, are characterized by a constitutional defect, possibly genetic. This biological factor might be conceived as an enzyme system, which, with its substrates and cofactors, operates at some critical interneural systems, possibly in a septal-hypothalamic-midbrain-limbic circuit, which could "miscue" the organism to react to stress in the absence of major stress—a racing motor with the clutch disengaged. In any event, there is a shift in the processing of input to that range which normally is characteristic for overactivation. The normal range of input, thus, would impinge on a system near to stress levels, and integrations of input are thus weak or faulty. Such a state in childhood conceivably would render the child more vulnerable to surrounding confusions. Certain traumatic experiences in childhood, such as maternal rejection, engulfment, or aggression, would augment the person's vulnerability; conditions favoring what is called a strong ego development would increase resistance and permit the development of sufficiently stable psychological structures, boundaries, and bonds to permit a reasonable level of function. This bond-formation, nevertheless, would be intrinsically vulnerable in persons with this basic disorder. Normally, we can suppress dreamlike thoughts and states, and we also have an appetite and zest for reality and genuine gratifications. We would visualize the biological defect in some sense impairing the capacity both to deal with reality and to suppress dreamlike states; through the overactivation, such inhibitory activity is impaired, and integration of input and organization of output are made difficult. The switch from an existence in a real world to a dream world could be produced psychologically or somatically, but, once produced, the access to reality might require far more strength than is available. Once this occurs, pathological defense mechanisms (contingent on the inability to erect more satisfactory restitutive measures) become necessary for more-or-less successful adaptations to a rapidly shifting inner and outer world. Such stress could further disorganize neurochemical regulations. In any event, we believe that we will have to comprehend both biological and psychological factors and, more than we have tried before, we must stipulate their action at various junctures and phases empirically established as critical in schizophrenia from childhood to onset and exacerbation or remission of acute psychosis. The further compelling difficulty with this set of guesses, of course, is that we do not know what enzyme systems would be disturbed, nor what neural systems are involved; what precipitates the schizophrenic break; and what predisposes, psychologically or socially, to schizophrenia rather than neurosis, sociopathy, or depression.

Diagnosis and Differential Diagnosis

The diagnosis of schizophrenia is either very easy or very difficult. The typical cases, and there are very many such, can be recognized by the layman and the beginner; but some cases offer such difficulties that the most qualified experts in the field cannot come to any agreement. Such difficulties hardly can be surprising; there is no clear, fundamental definition of schizophrenia and there are marked differences in international psychiatry as to what is meant by the term. In the United States, the concept of schizophrenia is broader than in the rest of the world and includes marginal types. In general, the diagnosis of schizophrenia is made too frequently; we are inclined to believe that the less skilled the psychiatrist, the more often the diagnosis of schizophrenia. As the diagnosis still has a connotation of malignancy and grave implications for patients and their families, it encourages drastic therapies and should be made with great circumspection. It is based entirely upon psychological and rather subjective criteria. All too often the diagnosis is made without specification of stage and severity. For guidelines, we refer to our discussion of symptoms and course. The diagnosis of the first stage is most difficult because all the criteria—of subtle changes in communication and identity; alterations of ego boundaries; the appearance of beginning autism, dereism, and a general regression—are subtle and defy readily objective observation and precise description. The diagnosis of the classical symptoms, clearer in the second stage, is easier; and the third stage of deterioration offers no problems. Increasingly, we have become less concerned with the classical subdiagnoses and more concerned with the question of which schizophrenias recover. Some authors have called schizoid characters latent schizophrenics; as latency only can be proved if latent phenomena change into manifest symptoms, we consider the term latent schizophrenia meaningless unless the diagnosis is made retrospectively. The schizoids must also be differentiated from those arrested states of schizophrenia that show relatively slight defects, such as mild emotional blunting. As schizophrenias usually (if not always) develop in what appear to be neurotic personalities, it is not surprising that almost any neurotic symptom may be encountered in the history of schizophrenic patients as in other behavior disorders! The remark that the more hysterical a hysteria is, the more likely it is a schizophrenia has been attributed to Eugen Bleuler. Certain dramatic, brief, hallucinatory episodes were referred to in older texts as hysterical psychoses; some of these turn out to be schizophrenias. The presence of anxiety, of phobic, compulsive, and particularly of hypochondriacal symptoms in schizophrenia is well known. In borderline states, only observation over a long period of time may clear up the differential diagnosis; this is also true for certain psychoses occurring in prisons and under other conditions of isolation and deprivation.

The differential diagnosis from antisocial personality types also may be very difficult because schizophrenics often are impulsive, sexually infantile and deviant, and destructive against themselves and others. This propensity for lack of control makes it important to evaluate whether the patient may be dangerous, and, particularly, whether he is suicidal. The hybrid term schizo-affective psychosis reflects our difficulty of making a meaningful differentiation of schizophrenic and manic-depressive psychosis in certain patients. In general, we err by assuming too easily the presence of a manic-depressive disorder. Long-term follow-up shows that patients diagnosed early as manic-depressives not infrequently later turn out to be schizophrenics. Unfortunately, our ability to differentiate clearly between schizophrenic and manic-depressive disorders descriptively and dynamically is not so well developed as Kraepelin once assumed. The schizophrenic identity problem—disintegration of thinking and feeling and, of course, deterioration—is absent in the manic-depressive. The capacity of the schizophrenic patient for reality-testing is more clearly decreased.

Another group which at times may offer considerable difficulties in the differential diagnoses is the symptomatic psychoses. Theoretically, consciousness, memory, and orientation in schizophrenia are not disturbed. Yet, unclear cases and borderline conditions are not infrequent. We are inclined to consider both oneirophrenias and lethal catatonias as toxic-infectious rather than schizophrenic disorders. Often, particularly in psychoses of pregnancy and puerperium, only the course will establish the differential diagnosis; if the patient does not recover promptly, we assume—not always correctly—that schizophrenia exists. The organic psychoses with neurological signs offer no problem in differential diagnosis, although some early brain tumors, syphilis of the central nervous system, presenile, and other organic psychoses such as Huntington's Chorea may be mistaken initially for schizophrenias. Mistakes arise in not paying attention to the symptoms of organic deficit, particularly of memory defects and, unfortunately, in not carrying out thorough neurological and laboratory examinations. A high level of alertness in the diagnostician will help to avoid missing organic disease when it is present. The differential diagnosis between psychomotor epilepsy and schizophrenia may be difficult; however, no diagnosis of epilepsy should be made without the presence of periodic alterations of consciousness, repeated EEG examinations and, in some cases, a trial of anticonvulsants.

In a paranoid personality, the typical suspiciousness and hostility, the inability to see another point of view, and a tendency to distort reality (to project without the ability to correct such distortions) are all relatively stable and ego-syntonic character traits. In paranoid psychoses, these traits become progressively more prominent; reality distortions are more flagrant; the capacity to check hostile impulses decreases; and the patient's behavior becomes less acceptable. At times, it is impossible to make a differential diagnosis between paranoid personality and paranoid psychosis, and we then assume the existence of border states. To be sure, this requires diagnostic elegance, but border states properly include a range of disorders, previously described, which are real enough; border states need not be a wastebasket.

Whether or not paranoia belongs to the schizophrenic group, a question that is not entirely settled, is not merely a taxonomic problem. It highlights the question whether certain schizophrenias are psychologically caused. The differential diagnosis of paranoid disorders and toxic reactions is usually easy. Alcohol paranoia occurs mostly in deteriorated alcoholics; symptoms of jealousy in such patients are predominant. Most of the paranoid disorders during the involutional period belong, in the authors' opinion, to the schizophrenic group. Paranoid disorders in old age and in some chronic brain diseases probably represent latent paranoid personalities that have become manifest through organic deficit, which weakens the proper discrimination of complex social stimuli and diminishes the capacity for reality-testing. Lifelong paranoid schizophrenics, on the other hand, may be less occupied with delusions and less overactivated following arteriosclerotic and senile changes in old age.

Prognosis

With the expansion of the schizophrenia concept, and observations of relatively mild cases, the prognosis of the disorder is not considered to be ominous, as it commonly was in Kraepelin's day.[41] The difficult problem is to differentiate the severe from the mild cases, the patient who will respond to therapy from the one who will not, the malignant "true schizophrenic" type from the benign schizophreniform psychosis.[120] There are a number of catamnestic statistical studies of schizophrenics,[162] but none of these studies provides the background to make a precise prognosis in the individual case. They differentiate between bad and good cases and single out certain signs and symptoms characteristic for these groups. Patients with good prognoses, the so-called reactive schizophrenias, have adequate prepsychotic personalities with good sexual, occupational, and social adjustments. The onset, which is usually acute, can be traced to definite traumatic events. In the "process" schizophrenias, the prepsychotic personalities slide in their adolescence insidiously into progressive psychotic reactions. Although E. H. Rodnick and N. Garmezy[160] based the distinction between reactive and process schizophrenia on a relative sparse scale of measurement, the distinction has wide appeal. Confusional symptoms and manic-depressive features such as those that are seen in schizo-affective patients improve the prognosis; flatness of affect is a bad prognostic sign. Ernst Stengel observed that the presence of obsessive-compulsive symptoms usually protects the patient from disintegration and deterioration.[183] In general, we consider hebephrenic and paranoid symptomatology prognostically unfavorable and catatonic symptoms more benign. Previous stability, good intelligence, and good marital and social adjustment are all good prognosticators. Lidz,[127] Wynne,[199] and others have implicitly drawn attention to the prognostic value of relative family stability. The social class of the patient is related to prognosis: the lower-class schizophrenic becomes chronic more easily. Once committed to an institution, he is likely to stay there, gradually drifting from acute services to the back wards and their deteriorating atmosphere; his community and family have closed their doors to him.[95] Cohort studies over a ten-year period by Jerome K. Myers, L. L. Bean, and M. P. Pepper confirm this.[144] Lower-class patients who are released, on the other hand, may have less pressures and expectations to contend with, and this could influence readmission and posthospital adjustment.

Treatment

In these days of vigorous treatment, it is hardly possible to observe "spontaneous" remission; we don't bemoan this fact but merely wish to point out that we are no longer able to establish a base line for therapeutic evaluation. We can only compare different therapies of this complex fluctuating disorder. Unfortunately, we cannot predict any better which patient will respond to treatment than we could predict, in the pretherapeutic days, which patient would remit or relapse. This reservation, of course, should not curb our therapeutic enthusiasm but caution us in our inclination to overestimate our therapeutic abilities.

One of the striking phenomena of the last few decades of therapy of schizophrenia has been a strong wave of optimism. Today, many psychiatrists consider schizophrenia an eminently treatable disorder. Even those, like the authors, who feel that we are very much in the dark about etiology, believe that most schizophrenias can be helped significantly even though the organic and psychosocial methods of treatment are empirical and quite unspecific. Of the many estimates of therapeutic outcome, David McK. Rioch's statement that one-third of the schizophrenic soldiers treated in the United States Army are returned to full duty is an impressive example of how much and how little is being achieved.[158]

Three general rules are more important than specific prescriptions.

(1) As specific guidelines for treatment of schizophrenia barely exist, the therapeutic program must be flexible; it will usually include more than one approach.

(2) The program must be highly individualized, to focus sharply on the unique characteristics of each patient and his family.

(3) The personal dignity of schizophrenics, even deteriorated patients, must be respected; all too often, this is not the case.

In the following sections, some of the different therapies are discussed; we shall then consider the problem of choice and of integration of therapeutic approaches in the individual case. We reiterate that the assessment of the therapy of a disorder that is characterized by remissions and relapses is an arduous task. Furthermore, many schizophrenics are the targets of many widely differing approaches, which makes scrutiny of one particular approach very difficult.

Hospitalization

Whether or not to admit a schizophrenic patient to a hospital requires mature clinical judgment. Not much time has passed since one of us was almost dismissed from his position after stating at a staff conference that he had not recommended hospitalization for a rather harmless schizophrenic patient. At that time, hospitalization was the beginning and the end of therapy of schizophrenics; today, it is neither. We hospitalize schizophrenics if they are dangerous to themselves or to others or are regressed to the point that they need hospital care, are physically ill, have to be removed from a very stressful environment, or need the vigorous or total treatment and the reliable atmosphere that only a good psychiatric hospital can provide. It must be remembered, however, that hospitals do not always provide the best setting for psychotherapy. They may facilitate excessive regression. The therapist is cast into the role of a jailer and enemy. Even if administrative decisions are made by another psychiatrist, the schizophrenic assumes (and commonly he is not wrong about this) that administrator and therapist are really not acting independently but are working together; as he sees it, they are plotting jointly against him.

The generally laudable current tendency to discharge patients rapidly to family and community may cause trouble; some schizophrenics need prolonged active therapy in a protective setting. There is, however, probably nothing worse for schizophrenics than the isolating and humiliating experience of being on a back ward. The violence of other patients, the callousness of personnel, the ugliness of the setting, and the stultifying emptiness of the environment reinforce regression and withdrawal.

Organic Therapies

Anyone who has witnessed the rise and fall of different organic therapies cannot avoid a certain skepticism. Today, the standard lobotomies have almost disappeared. We are also past the crest of enthusiasm for the coma therapies, which have been replaced to a large extent by treatment with tranquilizing drugs. Yet brain surgery and coma therapies which have vanished have left their mark; if nothing else, they have helped to teach us that schizophrenia is not a hopeless disorder.

There are occasional schizophrenic patients who, after previous failure with drugs, have responded to insulin coma therapy. In general, however, the cumbersome technique is rarely used any more in American hospitals. Electric convulsive therapy is still employed in the treatment of schizophrenia. It has not been very effective in the schizophrenias. Even critical proponents of the method do not recommend it in general, but specifically for the treatment of stuporous and hyperactive catatonic patients. Remissions in pure catatonics may occur after a few shocks, but experienced therapists generally suggest a full course of treatment, consisting of twelve to twenty shocks. Very massive treatment with one or more shocks daily, in our opinion, is not justified. It regresses the patient, makes him apathetic, and produces temporary deficit states. In general, ECT need not be used as a routine, but rather as an emergency "sedative" with schizophrenics. Prolonged sleep therapy (*Dauerschlaf*) and the newer hibernation therapies, in which drugs produce long-lasting somnolence, are considered dangerous and ineffective and are not used in the United States.

The psychological and biological effects of major tranquilizers in schizophrenia, in spite of a great deal of research, is not clearly known; their effect on amine receptors and metabolism and on selected central sites provides the clearest directives for current research. From a psychological standpoint, the idea that tranquilizing drugs reduce anxiety and render certain pathological defenses unnecessary is just as tenable as an explanation as it was a tentative explanation of the effect of lobotomy. Scrutiny of controlled drug studies reveals that the drugs are reliably effective and that, as yet, no one symptomatic picture is preferentially benefited by particular compounds.[42] One can conclude that the majority of schizophrenic patients will tend to show some degree of improvement. Generally speaking, we recommend the judicious use of drugs, preferably in conjunction with psychotherapy and in any case with milieu therapy.

The danger of long-term psychotic episodes is quite evident in prognostic studies; this, more than any other consideration, warrants the use of drugs, since failure to learn new modes of coping and entrenchment in pathological modes of behavior are the frequent consequences of prolonged episodes of psychosis. The fact that we can and do treat a few patients with intensive psychotherapy and without drugs does not mean that in the overwhelming number of cases drugs are not indicated and useful. Indeed, adequate and sustained therapy with phenothiazines—the drugs of choice—may enhance any psychotherapeutic approach and the latter is less likely to be successful in the absence of drugs. We have been using chlorpromazine, perphenazine, trifluoperazine, and thioridizine, but a number of equally effective compounds are available. For details of techniques of pharmacological therapy and electroconvulsive treatment, the reader is referred to Chapter 11.

Psychotherapy

If one assumes that schizophrenic behavior is predominantly a learned form of behavior, a psychotherapeutic approach designed to "unlearn" such behavior is logical.[30] It is of more than passing interest that even those who assume that organic factors play a crucial role in the genesis and treatment of schizophrenia do not recommend that a relevant psychotherapy be excluded from the treatment of schizophrenia. Thus, various types of psychotherapy are at least recommended in the treatment of schizophrenia, if not actually practiced, in many of the major North American and a few South American and European psychiatric centers. Some clinicians, however, doubt that true schizophrenia can be treated by psychotherapy and milieu therapy—by which they mean the effort is unlikely to influence the outcome. This, of course, depends on consideration of goals in therapy. The authors' experiences indicate that psychotherapy and milieu therapy are very useful means of treatment and, more importantly, have brought a humane quality to the problem of schizophrenia, affecting patients, staffs, and the community at large. Psychotherapy has enlightened and enlarged our understanding of the disorder and may provide us with the basis for more sharply formulated research questions and clinical differentia. In some individual cases, psychotherapy may have provided the crucial difference between deterioration and restitution. Yet, as compared with organic therapies, there are virtually no sound evaluations or controlled catamnestic studies of schizophrenic patients in psychotherapy. We rely almost entirely on witness reports, and the principal witness is the therapist himself; if such reports are made by sound and sensitive therapists, they should not be disregarded.

Psychotherapy of schizophrenia stems from two sources: from the pragmatic, comprehensive approach of Adolf Meyer,[137] and from psychoanalysis, although Freud himself doubted that schizophrenics could be so treated.[69] He felt that psychic energies involved in the psychoses could not be altered by the analytic techniques, that the patients were not capable of transference, and that the schizophrenic ego was too weak to profit from psychoanalytic therapy. Although no one has recommended classical psychoanalysis except in periods of remission, many psychoanalysts have expressed optimism about applications of modifications of the psychoanalytic technique. Some of these modified techniques have little resemblance to classical analysis; they do, however, base their procedures on classical or neoanalytic theories. Analytic psychotherapy of the schizophrenic patient was well described by Lewis B. Hill.[91] His student, Marshall Edelson, provided us with a very good discussion of a dynamic milieu therapy.[50] The first to report his experiences and make definite recommendations was Federn;[69] Marguerite A. Sechehaye,[173] Gertrud Schwing,[171] Knight,[113] Beulah Parker[149] and others followed. Sechehaye's use of "symbolic realization" is sensitively cued to the patient's level of communication; she has written vivid accounts of the treatment of these patients. Frieda Fromm-Reichmann summarized some of the modifications of analytic therapy.[74] She insists on extreme sincerity in the therapist; only such an attitude will allay the extreme suspicion of the patient. An approach that also establishes closeness but that is radically different from the procedures of the mothering and gentle Fromm-Reichmann has been advocated by John Rosen.[163] He makes daring, forceful interpretations of the patient's unconscious processes and tries to overcome his isolation in a very direct and intense relationship. Free association is impractical because it tends to discourage coherence. Acting-out must be tolerated to a greater degree than in neurotics. There is less emphasis on interpretation than on the formation of relationship, although schizophrenics often understand unconscious processes very readily. Some schizophrenics are highly efficient eavesdroppers and know quickly what is going on in the therapist's mind, although they may misjudge the fragments of truth they apprehend. This fragmented apprehension of a piece of reality is especially relevant in paranoid cases who omit balancing judgments.

Patient and therapist usually face each other, take walks, and so forth. It is important to be seen in order to be trusted. We believe that interpretations simply give the desperately lonely patient a feeling that he is, if not understood, at least cared for. Kenneth L. Artiss[8] and David McK. Rioch[158] stress that it is important to understand the patient's major message in a given social context. Pious has noted that the schizophrenic "translates" for the therapist, and vice versa, and that this is somewhat different from interpretation.[153] He also has made the insightful observation that the patient, when talking, often is thinking out loud rather than communicating. Because they are taught that there is meaning in the schizophrenic's behavior, therapists frequently will want to interpret all that is being said. On the other hand, the patient simply may be "collecting himself," as one of our patients put it.

It simply is not possible, with a schizophrenic patient, to maintain distance at all times. As is apparent in our remarks about being seen and looked at and being present, being close to the patient means having an optimal distance with respect to intrusion, on the one hand, and imperviousness, on the other. This is an exquisitely delicate matter: what to the therapist's mind might be warmth can easily be felt as intrusiveness by the patient. Stability, availability and tolerance are most important. Bruno Bettelheim pointed out that, in working with disturbed children, "love is not enough."[20] The disturbed child's needs are far more egocentric and, in a sense, more practical as well; a little girl put it that she liked the counselors who "becared" her—they helped her tie her shoes, get her books, and keep her life in some order; the counselors who "loved" her simply hugged and kissed her like her parents but weren't what she needed. Similarly, the therapist who is concerned about the often primitive personal needs of the schizophrenic patient and can accept the patient's idiosyncratic methods of making his way through the difficulties of a day is more useful than the warm but undiscerning doctor. Therapies are not always what therapists say they are. When Albert E. Scheflin observed Rosen's "direct analysis" of patients, he found that Rosen's approach consists of many techniques that seem to work simultaneously,[169] such as control, suppression, support, and reassurance; insight-giving; and the formation of a relationship.[97] John C. Whitehorn and B. Betz commented on the special sensitivities that therapists of schizophrenics must have in order to succeed.[197] A very important qualification is the therapist's capacity for scrupulous honesty in the recognition of his own feelings; schizophrenics are particularly sensitive to alibis and lies. Another quality is the therapist's ability and courage to take the patients' cold and raw hostilities. Personal qualities for therapists of schizophrenics are possibly more important than technical training.

In order to provide psychotherapy to large numbers of patients, therapists have experimented increasingly with group methods. This also seems to have the advantage of providing the schizophrenic patient with many more direct opportunities for help in his socialization. Such methods, combined with aspects of milieu therapy, have been successful even with relatively deteriorated patients in public mental hospitals. As in all questions of individual versus group therapy, decisions as to the preferred methods must be based on the availability of personnel and especially on the specific needs and difficulties of the individual patients. Combinations of individual and group therapy, if possible with the same therapist, are to be preferred. A patient who lives in an environment where his personality is helpfully reflected to him, and where his rationalizations and avoidances may be questioned by fellow patients, brings to the therapeutic hour a much clearer image of his status and his adjustments to his life than the therapist and patient alone could reconstruct.

Milieu Therapy and Family Therapy

In addition to understanding that inactivity and isolation are detrimental to schizophrenics, modern psychiatrists believe that schizophrenics rarely get well merely by seeing a psychotherapist a few times a week and have advocated more vigorous and concerted efforts. A generation ago, Abraham Myerson introduced what he termed "total push" therapy, which consisted of vigorous and concerted efforts to treat patients with organic procedures, psychotherapy, and occupational and recreational therapy; however, little attention was paid to individual needs and conflicts of the patient. Today, we are convinced that the best therapy consists of a highly individualized system of re-education of the patient in a stable, reliable setting. Such re-education uses individual and group therapy, controlled experiences in group living, occupational and recreational therapy, and adult education; it is also coordinated with organic therapy when indicated. And it is especially important to use the help patients can give one another. Until now, such programs were possible only in hospital setting; in the very recent past, total therapy has been realized also in day- and night-wards, halfway houses, and community rehabilitation centers.

There is evidence that families can push a patient more deeply into the disorder or help him to come out of it. At the National Institute of Mental Health, Murray Bowen undertook an unusually informative experiment, although hardly a feasible general plan—simultaneous hospitalization of both patient and family.[28] Since then, family therapy of schizophrenics has been introduced in many centers and found to be useful. Patient and family are either treated by different therapists who communicate with each other, or the family and patient are seen by the same therapist in separate or joint group sessions. This is a rather radical departure from the old notion that psychiatrists cannot serve two masters well; in some cases, this method works surprisingly well. In contrast to the extreme permissiveness of early experimentation with dynamic milieu and family therapy, a more rigorous task and reality-oriented regimen recently has been recommended. The type of family therapy must vary with the needs of family members. In some cases, family members may be as much in need of therapy as the patient. In other cases, information and advice, such as preparing the family for the possibility of relapse, is sufficient. A parent who seeks help independently may be greatly supported in learning new ways to manage the difficult problems of a sick child; the blow to self-esteem that a child's illness entails can also be dealt with, and a less manipulating or manipulatable parent may be of direct value to the schizophrenic's treatment, as well as a more comfortable person in his own right. We must guard against viewing parents as culpable; rather, they are varyingly incapable because the child is baffling and disruptive to their adjustments as parents.

The following case report illustrates the course of a schizophrenic disorder in a college student who benefited from dynamic psychotherapy.

> The patient, an attractive, somewhat obese, college girl was admitted to a psychiatric hospital at age twenty-two. She had been a disturbed child at least since puberty (age fourteen), with increasingly severe episodes of restlessness and irritability, especially at the time of her menses. Her psychosis was first clearly recognized at age eighteen, when she had an acute transient manic episode, just after matriculating at a leading women's college. She transferred to a small college near her home, where, with considerable difficulty, she completed two years of study. She then reacted with a series of acute schizophrenic states requiring lengthy hospitalization, including courses of electroconvulsive and insulin coma therapy. A lobotomy had been advised, but her parents brought her to the hospital for further evaluation.
>
> Although she did not lack in charm and poise, it was hard to get to know her. When upset, she would ward people off with angry retaliations for real or imagined slights. When feeling better, she was generally bored, inaccessible, and she responded with scattered and concretistic thinking. Yet, her haughty manner and stubborn pride had their appealing aspects; her incisive wit and sarcasm could often be shared, and there were, at times, unexpected flashes of penetrating insight and a capacity for a direct and meaningful exchange. She deeply appreciated any interest shown in her and had a childlike capacity for gleeful enjoyment of small pleasures. On another level, she had a sophisticated talent for enjoying ironies and inconsistencies.
>
> She stubbornly maintained an ambition to complete her education and be-

come an interpreter of foreign languages at the United Nations. In practical terms, this ambition appeared strange, concrete, and unsuitable, in view of her limited linguistic capacities. In another sense, however, her ambition seemed to be a poignant expression of her urgent need to become an "interpreter" of her own chaotic thinking processes, as well as a desperate hope of interpreting her immediate family environment. Her parents could not communicate with each other, and they consistently overlooked her opinions in decisions and actions crucial to her welfare.

She showed a wide variety of reactions. There were acute manic episodes, in which an increasing elation and hyperactivity culminated in bitter recriminations, assaultiveness, and threats toward her mother. She also developed acute paranoid delusional states, when she would accuse people of talking against her, complain of messages transferred to her mind by radio, and express delusions of being drugged and poisoned, as well as somatic delusions such as having frostbite or her skin peeling off. Some excited states were associated with promiscuity and sexual preoccupations, and she generally found her sexual feelings to present difficult problems. There were acute episodes of estrangement, derealization and hystrionic behavior. She took a walk with her psychotherapist in the midst of one such episode and described how frighteningly unreal the world looked to her; she took his hand as if she were blind and in danger of being struck by an automobile. For periods of many months, she spoke only in typical schizophrenic language. At these times, she never responded directly but carried on a seemingly irrelevant and scattered chatter. Many of her responses were linked to important subjects, but in a concrete way in which important themes were obliquely introduced by symbols, klang and pun associations, or through the medium of some trivial detail. For example, aimless chatter about details in an advertisement became intelligible when it was recognized that the advertised product was produced by a rival to her father's firm. Working a crossword puzzle, she searched for a five-letter word meaning "multitude." She picked "show" (rather than crowd), explaining, "A multitude is a crowd; crowds go to the theater, and a theater is a show." Such shifts of boundaries and focus were characteristic. She enjoyed and cooperated with efforts to decipher her peculiar language, but she could also speak more coherently when the therapist refused to participate in this decoding.

During periods when flamboyant symptoms were quiescent, she explained that, for her, the world was constantly changing. Her delusional episodes were so disorganizing that it was hard for her to convince herself that a particular person, before, during, and after an upset, was one-and-the-same person. She struggled to overcome a distorted integration of sensory stimuli. Background noises, even the chirping of birds, could provide intolerable distractions. Her eyes were forever watchful, noting every detail to be sure it was all real. At times, she brought to her almost scientific vigilance an esthetic sensibility that added some zest to the visual preoccupation. She could also please her father, because he too was interested in details. More often, however, she simply focused on banal and tedious details of her environment to maintain some hold on reality and to ward off chaotic inner experiences. She lapsed into states of boredom and apathy, extending to despair but not to profound depression. She was seriously hampered in using her obviously superior intelligence. Her abilities to concentrate, to remember, to form abstractions, to draw conclusions, and for visual motor cordination were all impaired in one way or another to a disabling degree. She could not, for example, learn to type.

Her inner disorganization, as described above, was complemented by disturbances in her family. Very extensive information on her background was accumulated when she became a research patient for a study of families of schizophrenics.[127] Among the conclusions of this study, we note that her family "never formed a real entity which served as a protective shelter for its members." "A spirit of mistrust pervaded the home, and each person had to protect himself from derision and hurt." "The parents' preoccupation with their own defenses left little room for sensitivity to the needs of others, causing them to be impervious to emotional needs of their children." "There was intolerance of difference, blame for error, projection of one's own deficiencies onto other family members." "Not only did each person hide his real feelings and intentions, but each parent had his own strange paralogic reasoning. The mother was vague or stereotyped and seriously scattered under stress, and the father rigid and paranoid. Then the patient's vagueness, at first purposeful and later schizophrenic, added to the confusion."

The patient remained at the hospital for four years and was assigned, over the years, to four different therapists. She and her family also worked closely with a research social worker. She gradually became involved with the therapeutic community of the hospital and progressed in a carefully supervised and regulated program of activities and relationships with ward personnel and patients. Psychotherapy was attuned to her level at a given time. Generally, it was less interpretative and more one of responsive actions designed to foster trust, a sense of reality, self-respect, and to meet her concrete hunger for a stabilizing relationship. Such responsiveness involved, on a verbal level, painstaking clarification with her of areas of confusion in her life, and on a nonverbal level, activities and responses such as taking walks and feeding birds and patiently sharing her abject sense of boredom. The therapist attempted to provide external controls when she was upset, to avoid participating with her in her delusions, and to support or not interfere with her spontaneous moves toward progress. She appreciated the staff's increasingly detailed understanding of her family, and she and her parents were able to become somewhat more direct and tolerant of each other. However, she was not really able to use this understanding to gain psychological distance from a pathological involvement with her family but, rather, clung to the hope that her parents would somehow be magically transformed into the kind of parents she wanted. She also held to her hope of rescue through academic achievement and professional attainment and steadfastly refused to accept any job beneath her potential ability.

The patient has been carefully followed for seven years since she left the hospital in the care of her parents. She finished college and remains alert to the world about her. She has had infrequent acute disturbances, arising whenever she makes some premature move toward independence from her family, but she has required only one brief subsequent hospitalization. She has been maintained on phenothiazines, which appear to help her maintain an equilibrium and to dampen the fluctuation of markedly disturbed states, but fundamentally, her thinking remains seriously disturbed. She has never had a job. Her friendships are superficial. Any move toward intimacy with men, particularly in terms of sexuality, proves highly disturbing. The pettiness and banality of her parents' ostensibly "healthy" lives provide little incentive for her. They devote their available time to promoting her recreational interests, taking her on trips and to theatrical and athletic events. These activities, television, some reading, caring for her pets, shopping, driving a car, a conflicted absorption with food, and a passive involvement in the details of her parents' lives constitute the substance of her existence. She appears docile, affable, and childlike, concealing her feelings of despair. She knows that she can go on this way until the next crisis in her life when her aging parents are no longer able to care for her. Considering the fact that she had been well on the way toward indefinite hospitalization for acutely schizophrenic states, one can respect her progress.

Very few schizophrenic patients are able to avail themselves of highly skilled, dedicated therapists who carry on analytic, or interpretative, therapies geared to the patients' level of function. Luckily, there are many cases in which a warm, human and supportive approach with emphasis on the solution of everyday problems of living has helped. Such an approach can restore, to a certain extent, the patient's shattered self-esteem and also remove him from some of the worst stresses in his family or job. It should be kept in mind that schizophrenics now and again have been helped by sound, wise, and interested friends (hard to find), a good nurse or attendant, or a fellow patient. These persons may enable the patient to check his impulses to the degree that he does not get into trouble or may help him to take his delusions less seriously.

Rehabilitation

The remarkable work carried on in some mental hospitals in Europe and America has demonstrated the importance not only of carrying on a program of social therapy within the institution but also of making an active effort to rehabilitate the patient into his community. M. Carstairs[40] reported on the rehabilitation of schizophrenics in Great Britain. The core idea is to get the schizophrenic patient back into the community, even if he is not completely recovered, and help him to adjust there. In other words, a "social remission" is preferred to a lifelong existence in mental hospitals. To push patients out of their "asylums" at all costs may not always be in the patients' or families' best interests; to come to a proper decision about discharge, psychiatrists must use their best judgment. To enable the patient to live with his family may require a very skillful job by the psychiatric social worker. To enable the patient to make a living and to find some occupational satisfaction is the goal of occupational rehabilitation. This approach has been stressed by Sir Aubrey Lewis.[125] Few schizophrenics do well in jobs requiring intense interpersonal relationships and serious responsibilities.

Occasionally, the proper placement of a schizophrenic in a suitable occupational and social setting may obviate prolonged therapy. It is always a matter for discriminating judgment; should the patient rigorously avoid close family relationships, or can he be better supported in the family? Either course must be firmly worked out in terms of the patient's needs and as firmly sustained. Considerable progress has been made in the rehabilitation of the "schizophrenic masses" which have overcrowded our public hospitals. With the help of drugs, counselling and group activities by "ancillary" mental health workers, the use of halfway houses and sheltered work shops, many of these patients can be kept out of the all too often stultifying atmosphere of "continuous care" wards and be engaged in a meaningful life within the community.

Psychiatrists not infrequently are asked for eugenic advice, particularly whether schizophrenics should be permitted to marry and have children. There is little doubt that schizophrenics, generally speaking, do not contribute to marital bliss and a happy family life. Fortunately, schizophrenics, with their definite narcissistic and infantile sexual needs, are not often inclined to get married or raise families. Families with one or two schizophrenic parents are also seriously handicapped in raising children; yet, on medical eugenic grounds we are not justified in recommending sterilization. There is no evidence that such measures could lead to an elimination of the disorder, even over very long periods of time.

Which Therapy in the Individual Case?

Directive-organic psychiatrists will rarely recommend analytic psychotherapy and psychoanalysis for schizophrenics. In like manner, many analytic psychotherapists feel like traitors when they resort to drugs and shock therapy. Nonetheless, a resolute decision as to the type of therapy rarely needs to be made; rather, several methods may be employed simultaneously. Some time ago, one of the authors wrote: "When asked by students, I usually answer that my own preference—in case I developed such a psychosis—would be to obtain prolonged intensive dynamic psychotherapy carried out in a specially equipped hospital by an experienced analyst who likes schizophrenics. I hope I would be able to find and afford such a therapist and hospital, for they are extremely rare. If such a procedure failed, I would consent to shock treatment and lobotomy." [156] Clearly, times have changed. Today, we would ask for good psychotherapy in an open hospital with an active group milieu and rehabilitation program and adequate and sustained drug therapy. What remains unchanged is the fact that the research that will lead us to a truly rational therapy of schizophrenia is still ahead of us.

NOTES

1. K. A. Achté, "The Course of Schizophrenic and Schizophreniform Psychoses," *Acta Psychiat. Neurol. Scandinavica*, Suppl. 155 (1961).
2. Yrjö Alanen, J. Rekola, A. Stewen, M. Tuovinen, K. Takala, and E. Rutanen, "Mental Disorders in the Siblings of Schizophrenic Patients," *Acta Psychiat. Scandinavica*, Suppl. 169 (1963), 168.
3. Mark D. Altschule, "Some Effects of Aqueous Extracts of Acetone-Dried Beef-Pineal Substance in Chronic Schizophrenia," *New England Journal of Medicine*, 257 (1957), 919.
4. Mark D. Altschule and J. Brem, "Periodic Psychosis of Puberty," *American Journal of Psychiatry*, 119 (1963), 1176.
5. Silvano Arieti, *Interpretation of Schizophrenia* (New York: Robert Brunner, 1955).
6. Silvano Arieti, "Schizophrenia," in Silvano Arieti, ed., *American Handbook of Psychiatry* (New York: Basic Books, 1959), Vol. I, p. 445.
7. Robert L. Arnstein, "The Borderline Patient in the College Setting," in Bryant M. Wedge, ed., *Psychosocial Problems of College Men* (New Haven: Yale University Press, 1958).
8. Kenneth L. Artiss, ed., *The Symptom as Communication in Schizophrenia* (New York: Grune & Stratton, 1959).
9. Julius Axelrod, "Enzymatic Formation of Psychotomimetic Metabolites from Normally Occurring Compounds," *Science*, 134 (1961), 343.
10. Julius Axelrod, "The Formation, Metabolism, Uptake and Release of Noradrenaline and Adrenaline," in *The Clinical Chemistry of Monoamines* (Amsterdam: Elsevier Publishing Co., 1963).
11. Julius Axelrod, "Enzymatic Oxidation of Epinephrine to Adrenochrome by the Salivary Gland," *Biochem. et Biophys. Acta*, 85 (1964), 247.
12. Robert C. Bak, "Masochism in Paranoia," *Psychoanalytic Quarterly*, 15 (1946), 285.
13. Gregory Bateson, Don D. Jackson, J. Haley, and J. Weakland, "Toward a Theory of Schizophrenia," *Behavioral Science*, 1 (1956), 251.
14. Leopold Bellak, "A Multiple-Factor Psychosomatic Theory of Schizophrenia," *Psychiatric Quarterly*, 23 (1949), 738.
15. Leopold Bellak, ed., *Schizophrenia* (New York: Logos, 1958).
16. P. K. Benedict and I. Jacks, "Mental Illness in Primitive Societies," *Psychiatry*, 17 (1954), 377.
17. Ruth Benedict, *Patterns of Culture* (New York: New American Library of World Literature, 1946).
18. J. R. Bergen, R. B. Pennell, C. A. Saravis, and H. Hoagland, "Further Experiments with Plasma Proteins from Schizophrenics," in Robert G. Heath, ed., *Serological Fractions in Schizophrenia* (New York: Harper & Row, 1963).

19. Josef Berze and Hans W. Gruhle, *Psychologie der Schizophrenie* (Berlin: Springer, 1929).
20. Bruno Bettelheim, *Love Is Not Enough* (Glencoe, Ill.: The Free Press, 1950).
21. Ludwig Binswanger, "The Case of Ellen West," in Rollo May, Ernest Angel, and Henri F. Ellenberger, eds., *Existence* (New York: Basic Books, 1958).
22. Eugen Bleuler, *Dementia Praecox or the Group of Schizophrenias*, J. Zimkin, trans. (New York: International Universities Press, 1950).
23. Manfred Bleuler, *Endokrinologische Psychiatrie* (Stuttgart: Thieme, 1954).
24. Manfred Bleuler, *Krankheitsverlauf, Persönlichkeit und Verwandtschaft Schizophrener u. ihre gegenseitigen Beziehungen* (Leipzig: Thieme, 1941).
25. Eugene L. Bliss, C. J. Migeon, C. H. H. Branch, and L. T. Samuels, "Adrenocortical Function in Schizophrenia," *American Journal of Psychiatry*, 112 (1955), 358.
26. Jan A. Böök, "Genetical Aspects of Schizophrenic Psychoses," in Don D. Jackson, ed., *The Etiology of Schizophrenia* (New York: Basic Books, 1960).
27. Ivan Boszormenyi-Nagy, F. J. Gerty, and J. Kueber, "Correlation between an Anomaly of the Intracellular Metabolism of Andenosine Nucleotides and Schizophrenia," *Journal of Nervous and Mental Disease*, 124 (1956), 413.
28. Murray Bowen, "A Family Concept of Schizophrenia," in Don D. Jackson, ed., *The Etiology of Schizophrenia* (New York: Basic Books, 1960).
29. Malcolm B. Bowers, Jr., "The Onset of Psychosis: A Diary Account," *Psychiatry*, 28 (1965), 346.
30. Eugene B. Brody, "What Do Schizophrenics Learn during Psychotherapy and How Do They Learn It?" *Journal of Nervous and Mental Disease*, 127 (1958), 66.
31. Eugene B. Brody, "Borderline State, Character Disorder, and Psychotic Manifestations—Some Conceptual Formulations," *Psychiatry*, 23 (1960), 75.
32. Hilde Bruch, "Falsification of Bodily Needs and Body Concept in Schizophrenia," *Archives of General Psychiatry*, 6 (1962), 18.
33. Guenter G. Brune and Harold E. Himwich, "Biogenic Amines and Behavior in Schizophrenic Patients," in J. Wortis, ed., *Recent Advances in Biological Psychiatry* (New York: Plenum Press, 1963), Vol. V.
34. Guenter G. Brune and Harold E. Himwich, "Effects of Methionine Loading on the Behavior of Schizophrenic Patients," *Journal of Nervous and Mental Disease*, 134 (1962), 447.
35. Enoch Callaway III, R. T. Jones, and R. S. Layne, "Evoked Responses and Segmental Set of Schizophrenia," *Archives of General Psychiatry*, 12 (1965), 83.
36. Norman Cameron, "Reasoning, Regression and Communication in Schizophrenics," *Psychological Monographs*, 50 (1938), 1; Whole No. 221.

37. Norman Cameron, "The Paranoid Pseudo-Community," *American Journal of Sociology*, 49 (1943), 32.

38. Norman Cameron, "The Paranoid Pseudo-Community Revisited," *American Journal of Sociology*, 64 (1959), 52.

39. Norman Cameron, "Paranoid Conditions and Paranoia," in Silvano Arieti, ed., *American Handbook of Psychiatry* (New York: Basic Books, 1959), Vol. I, p. 508.

40. Morris Carstairs, "Industrial Work as a Means of Rehabilitation for Chronic Schizophrenics," *Congress Report, 2nd International Congress for Psychiatry, Zurich*, 1 (1957), 99.

41. Louis S. Chase and Samuel Silverman, "Prognostic Criteria in Schizophrenia," *American Journal of Psychiatry*, 98 (1941), 360.

42. Jonathan O. Cole, "Evaluation of Drug Treatment in Psychiatry," *Psychopharmacology Service Center Bulletin*, 2 (1962), 28.

43. Herman H. deJong, *Experimental Catatonia* (Baltimore: Williams & Wilkins, 1945).

44. Thomas P. Detre, R. G. Feldman, B. Rosner, and C. Ferriter, "Vibration Perception in Normal and Schizophrenic Subjects," *Journal of Neuropsychiatry*, Vol. 3, Suppl. 1 (1962), 145.

45. Helene Deutsch, "Folie à Deux," *Psychoanalytic Quarterly*, 7 (1938), 307.

46. Helene Deutsch, "Some Forms of Emotional Disturbance and Their Relationship to Schizophrenia," *Psychoanalytic Quarterly*, 11 (1942), 301.

47. Kenneth Dewhurst and J. Todd, "The Psychosis of Association—Folie à Deux," *Journal of Nervous and Mental Disease*, 124 (1956), 451.

48. Otto Diem, "Die einfach demente Form der Dementia Praecox [Dementia Simlex]," *Arch. Psychiat. Nervenkr.*, 37 (1903), 111.

49. E. von Domarus, "The Specific Laws of Logic in Schizophrenia," in Jacob S. Kasanin, ed., *Language and Thought in Schizophrenia, Collected Papers* (Berkeley and Los Angeles: University of California Press, 1944).

50. Marshall Edelson, *Ego Psychology, Group Dynamics and the Therapeutic Community* (New York: Grune & Stratton, 1964).

51. Ludwig Eidelberg, *An Outline of a Comparative Pathology of the Neuroses* (New York: International Universities Press, 1954).

52. Samuel Eiduson, N. Q. Brill, and E. Crumpton, "Adrenocortical Activity in Psychiatric Disorders," *Archives of General Psychiatry*, 5 (1961), 227.

53. Joel Elkes, "Effect of Psychotomimetic Drugs in Animals and in Man," in Harold A. Abramson, ed., *Neuropharmacology* (Transactions of Third Conference; New York: Josiah Macy, Jr., Foundation, 1957).

54. George L. Ellman and E. Callaway, "Erythrocyte Cholinesterase-Levels in Mental Patients," *Nature*, 192 (1961), 1216.

55. Jean Étienne D. Esquirol, *Mental Maladies*, translated by E. K. Hunt (Philadelphia: Lea and Blanchard, 1845).

56. Erik Essen-Möller, "Psychiatrische Untersuchungen an Einer Serie von Zwillingen," *Acta Psychiat. Neurol. Scandinavia*, Suppl. 23 (1941).

57. Henri Ey, "Unity and Diversity of Schizophrenia," *American Journal of Psychiatry,* 115 (1959), 706.
58. Poul M. Faergeman, "Early Differential Diagnosis between Psychogenic Psychosis and Schizophrenia," *Acta Psychiat. Neurol. Scandinavia,* 21 (1946), 275.
59. Robert E. L. Faris and H. Warren Dunham, *Mental Disorders in Urban Areas* (Chicago: University of Chicago Press, 1939).
60. Paul Federn, *Ego Psychology and the Psychoses* (New York: Basic Books, 1952).
61. W. J. Fessel, "Interaction of Multiple Determinants of Schizophrenia," *Archives of General Psychiatry,* 11 (1964), 1.
62. W. J. Fessel, H. D. Kurland, and R. P. Cutler, "Serological Distinction between Functional Psychoses," *Archives of Internal Medicine,* 113 (1964), 669.
63. Daniel X. Freedman, "Studies of LSD-25 and Serotonin in the Brain," (Proceedings of the Their World Congress of Psychiatry; Toronto: University of Toronto Press and McGill University Press, 1961).
64. Daniel X. Freedman and N. J. Giarman, "LSD-25 and the Status and Level of Brain Serotonin," *Annals of the New York Academy of Science,* 96 (1962), 1.
65. Daniel X. Freedman and Nicholas Giarman, "Brain Amines, Electrical Activity and Behavior," in Gilbert H. Glaser, ed., *EEG and Behavior* (New York: Basic Books, 1963).
66. Daniel X. Freedman, F. C. Redlich, and W. W. Igersheimer, "Psychosis and Allergy," *American Journal of Psychiatry,* 112 (1956), 873.
67. H. Freeman, "Physiological Studies," in Leopold Bellak, ed., *Schizophrenia: A Review of the Syndrome* (New York: Logos, 1958).
68. Harry Freeman and Fred Elmadjian, "Carbohydrate and Lymphoid Studies in Schizophrenia," *American Journal of Psychiatry,* 106 (1950), 660.
69. Sigmund Freud, "Psychoanalysis" [1926], *Standard Edition* (London: Hogarth Press, 1959), 20.
70. Sigmund Freud, "A Case of Paranoia Running Counter to the Psychoanalytic Theory of the Disease" [1915], in Standard Edition (London: Hogarth Press, 1955), 14.
71. Sigmund Freud, "Psychoanalytic Notes on an Autobiographical Account of a Case of Paranoia, (Dementia Paranoides)" [1911], in Standard Edition (London: Hogarth Press, 1955), 14.
72. A. J. Friedhoff and E. Van Winkel, "Conversion of Dopamine to 3,4-Dimethoxyphenyl Acetic Acid in Schizophrenic Patients," *Nature,* 199 (1963), 1271.
73. C. E. Frohman, G. Tourney, P. G. S. Beckett, H. Lees, L. K. Latham, and J. S. Gottlieb, "Biochemical Identification of Schizophrenia," *Archives of General Psychiatry,* 4 (1961), 404.
74. Frieda Fromm-Reichmann, "Notes on the Development and Treatment of Schizophrenics by Psychoanalytic Psychotherapy," *Psychiatry,* 11 (1948), 263.

75. Ernst Gellhorn and G. N. Loofbourrow, *Emotions and Emotional Disorders: A Neurophysiological Study* (New York: Hoeber Medical Division, Harper and Row, 1963).

76. Donald L. Gerard and J. Siegel, "The Family Background of Schizophrenia," *Psychiatric Quarterly*, 24 (1950), 47.

77. Nicholas J. Giarman and D. X. Freedman, "Biochemical Aspects of the Actions of Psychotomimetic Drugs," *Pharmacology Review*, 17 (1965), 1.

78. J. L. Gibbons, "Electrolytes and Depressive Illness," *Postgraduate Medical Journal*, 39 (1963), 19.

79. R. Gjessing, "Disturbances of Somatic Functions in Catatonia with a Periodic Course, and Their Compensation," *Journal of Mental Science*, 84 (1938), 608.

80. L. Gjessing, A. Bernhardsen, and H. Frøshaug, "Investigation of Amino Acids in a Periodic Catatonic Patient," *Journal of Mental Science*, 104 (1958), 188.

81. Kurt Goldstein, "The Significance of Special Mental Tests for Diagnosis and Prognosis in Schizophrenia," *American Journal of Psychiatry*, 96 (1939), 575.

82. Jacques S. Gottlieb, C. E. Frohman, P. G. S. Beckett, G. Tourney, and R. Semf, "Production of High-Energy Phosphate Bonds in Schizophrenia," *Archives of General Psychiatry*, 1 (1959), 243.

83. Alexander Gralnick, "Folie à Deux—The Psychosis of Association," *Psychiatric Quarterly*, 16 (1942), 230.

84. Ernest Gruenberg, "Socially Shared Psychopathology," in Alexander H. Leighton, John A. Clausen, and Robert N. Wilson, eds., *Explorations in Social Psychiatry* (New York: Basic Books, 1957).

85. Heinz Hartmann, "Contribution to the Metapsychology of Schizophrenia," in *The Psychoanalytic Study of the Child* (New York: International Universities Press, 1953), Vol. VIII.

86. Robert G. Heath, ed., *Serological Fractions in Schizophrenia* (New York: Harper & Row, 1963).

87. Robert G. Heath and W. A. Mickle, "Evaluation of 7 Years' Experience with Depth Electrode Studies in Human Patients," in E. R. Hamey and D. S. O'Doherty, eds., *Electrical Studies on the Unanesthetized Brain* (New York: Paul B. Hoeber, 1960).

88. Ewald Hecker, "Die Hebephrenie," *Virchow's Path. Anat.*, 52 (1871), 394.

89. Dorothy H. Henneman, M. Altschule, R. M. Gonez, and L. Alexander, "Carbohydrate Metabolism in Brain Disease," *Archives of Neurology and Psychiatry*, 72 (1954), 688.

90. Denis Hill, "EEG in Episodic Psychotic and Psychopathic Behaviour," *Electroencephal. clin. Neurophysiology*, 4 (1952), 419.

91. Lewis B. Hill, *Psychotherapeutic Intervention in Schizophrenia* (Chicago: University of Chicago Press, 1955).

92. Hudson Hoaglund, G. Pincus, F. Elmadjian, L. Romanoff, H. Freeman, J. Hope, J. Ballan, A. Berkeley and J. Carlo, "Study of Adrenocortical Physi-

ology in Normal and Schizophrenic Men," *Archives of Neurology and Psychiatry*, 69 (1953), 470.

93. Paul Hoch and P. Polatin, "Pseudoneurotic Forms of Schizophrenia," *Psychiatric Quarterly*, 23 (1949), 248.
94. Abram Hoffer, "The Adrenochrome Theory of Schizophrenia: A Review," *Diseases of the Nervous System*, 25 (1964), 173.
95. August B. Hollingshead and Fredrick C. Redlich, *Social Class and Mental Illness* (New York: John Wiley, 1958).
96. M. K. Horwitt, "Fact and Artifact in the Biology of Schizophrenia," *Science*, 124 (1958), 429.
97. William A. Horwitz, P. Polatin, Lawrence C. Kolb, and Paul H. Hoch, "A Study of Cases of Schizophrenia Treated by 'Direct Analysis,'" *American Journal of Psychiatry*, 114 (1958), 780.
98. Roy G. Hoskins, *The Biology of Schizophrenia* (New York: Norton, 1946).
99. Richard Hunter and Ida MacAlpine, eds., *Three Hundred Years of Psychiatry, 1535–1860* (London: Oxford Press, 1963).
100. Sir Julian Huxley, Ernst Mayr, Humphry Osmond, and Abram Hoffer, "Schizophrenia as a Genetic Morphism," *Nature*, 204 (1964), 220.
101. Walter W. Igersheimer, "Cold Pressor Test in Functional Psychiatric Syndromes," *Archives of Neurology and Psychiatry*, 70 (1953), 794.
102. Don D. Jackson, "A Critique of the Literature on the Genetics of Schizophrenia," in Don D. Jackson, ed., *The Etiology of Schizophrenia* (New York: Basic Books, 1960).
103. Carl G. Jung, "The Psychology of Dementia Praecox," *Nervous and Mental Disease Monographs* (New York: Nervous and Mental Disease Publishing Company, 1909), No. 3.
104. Karl L. Kahlbaum, *Die Katatonie oder das Spannungsirresein* (Berlin: Hirschwald, 1874).
105. Franz J. Kallmann, "Psychogenetic Studies of Twins," in S. Koch, ed., *Psychology* (New York: McGraw-Hill, 1959), 3.
106. Otto Kant, "The Relation of a Group of Highly-Improved Schizophrenic Patients to One Group of Completely-Recovered and Another Group of Deteriorated Patients," *Psychiatric Quarterly*, 15 (1941), 779.
107. Bert Kaplin, ed., *The Inner World of Mental Illness* (New York: Harper & Row, 1964).
108. Jacob S. Kasanin, ed., *Language and Thought in Schizophrenia* (Berkeley and Los Angeles: Univ. of California Press, 1944).
109. Seymour Kety, "Biochemical Theories of Schizophrenia," Parts I and II, *Science*, 29 (1959), 1528; 1590.
110. Henriette R. Klein and W. A. Horwitz, "Psychosexual Factors in the Paranoid Phenomena," *American Journal of Psychiatry*, 105 (1949), 697.
111. Melanie Klein, *The Psycho-Analysis of Children, Third Edition* (London: Hogarth Press, 1949).
112. Robert P. Knight, "The Relationship of Latent Homosexuality to the

Mechanism of Paranoid Delusions," *Bulletin of the Menninger Clinic*, 4 (1940), 149.

113. Robert P. Knight, "Borderline States," in Robert P. Knight and C. R. Friedman, eds., *Psychoanalytic Psychiatry and Psychology* (New York: International University Press, 1954).
114. Lawrence C. Kolb, "The Body Image in the Schizophrenic Reaction," in A. Auerback, ed., *Schizophrenia* (New York: The Ronald Press, 1959).
115. Claus Konrad, *Die Beginnende Schizophrenie* (Stuttgart: Thieme, 1958).
116. Emil Kraepelin, *Dementia Praecox and Paraphrenia*, translated from 8th German Edition of *Textbook of Psychiatry* (Edinburgh: Livingstone, 1919).
117. Ernst Kretschmer, *Physique and Character* (New York: Harcourt, Brace, 1926).
118. Ernst Kretschmer, *Der sensitive Beziehungswahn: Third Edition* (Berlin: Springer, 1950).
119. Einar Kringlen, "Schizophrenia in Male Monozygotic Twins," *Acta Psychiatrica Scandinavica*, Suppl., 178 (1964).
120. Ronald P. Laing and A. Esterson, *Sanity, Madness and the Family* (New York: Basic Books), 1965.
121. Gabriel Langfeldt, "The Prognosis in Schizophrenia," *Acta Psychiat. Neurol. Scandinavica*, Suppl. 110 (1956).
122. K. L. Latham, K. Warner, P. Beckett, J. S. Gottlieb, and C. E. Frohman, "The Relationship of a Plasma Factor in Schizophrenia to Membrane Permeability," Federation Proceedings, 24 (1965), 326.
123. Paul Lemkau, "The Epidemiological Study of Mental Illnesses and Mental Health," *American Journal of Psychiatry*, 111 (1955), 801.
124. Max Levin, "Hallucination: A Problem in Neurophysiology," *Journal of Nervous and Mental Disease*, 125 (1957), 308.
125. Sir Aubrey Lewis, "Resettlement of the Chronic Schizophrenic," *Congress Report* (Second International Congress for Psychiatry [Zurich: 1957]).
126. William T. Lhamon and S. Goldstone, "The Time Sense," *Archives of Neurology and Psychiatry*, 76 (1956), 625.
127. Theodore Lidz, Stephen Fleck and Alice Cornelison, *Schizophrenia and the Family* (New York: International Universities Press, 1966).
128. Ida MacAlpine and R. A. Hunter, "The Schreber Case," *Psychoanalytic Quarterly*, 22 (1953), 328.
129. I. Matte Blanco, "The Symbolic Logic Approach to Psychiatry and Psychology," Adolf Meyer Lecture 1965, *American Journal of Psychiatry* (in press).
130. W. Mayer-Gross, Eliot Slater, and Martin Roth, *Clinical Psychiatry* (London: Cassell, 1955).
131. Roger K. McDonald, "Problems in Biologic Research in Schizophrenia," *Journal of Chronic Disease*, 8 (1958), 366.
132. Roger K. McDonald and V. K. Weise, "The Excretion of 3-Methoxy-4-Hydroxymandelic Acid in Normal and in Chronic Schizophrenic Male Subjects," *Journal of Psychiatric Research*, 1 (1962), 173.

133. Andrew McGhie and J. Chapman, "Disorders of Attention and Perception in Early Schizophrenia," *British Journal of Medical Psychology*, 34 (1961), 103.

134. William M. McIsaac, "Formation of 1-Methyl-6-Methoxy-1,2,3,4,-Tetrahydro-2 Carboline under Physiological Conditions," *Biochem. Biophys. Acta*, 52 (1961), 607.

135. Ladislas J. Meduna, F. J. Gerty, and V. G. Urse, "Biochemical Disturbances in Mental Disorders," *Archives of Neurology and Psychiatry*, 47 (1942), 38.

136. Ladislas J. Meduna and W. S. McCulloch, "The Modern Concept of Schizophrenia," *Medical Clinics of North America*, 29 (1945), 147.

137. Adolf Meyer, "The Evolution of the Dementia Praecox Concept," *Collected Papers* (Baltimore: Johns Hopkins Press, 1951), Vol. II.

138. Richard P. Michael and James S. Gibbons, "Interrelationships between the Endocrine System and Neuropsychiatry," *International Review of Neurobiology*, 5 (1963), 243.

139. R. Michaux and W. G. Everly, "Action catalepsigene des ethers methyliques des mono-et polyphenolamines," *Life Sciences*, 3 (1963), 175.

140. Charles W. Miller, "The Paranoid Syndrome," *Archives of Neurology and Psychiatry*, 45 (1941), 953.

141. Benedict A. Morel, *Traité des dégénérescences physiques, intellectuelles et morales de l'espèce humaine et des causes qui produisent ces variétés maladives* (Paris: J. B. Baillière, 1857).

142. Rafael Moses and Daniel X. Freedman, " 'Trademark' Function of Symptoms in a Mental Hospital," *Journal of Nervous and Mental Disease*, 127 (1958), 448.

143. Jerome K. Myers and Bertram H. Roberts, *Family and Class Dynamics in Mental Illness* (New York: John Wiley, 1959).

144. Jerome K. Myers, L. L. Bean and M. Pepper, "Social Class and Psychiatric Disorders: A Ten Year Follow-up," *Journal of Health and Human Behavior*, 6 (1965), 74.

145. K. N. Nazarov, "Specific Brain Antigens and Autosensitization to Them in Various Mental Disorders," *Federation Proceedings*, Transl. Suppl., 23 (1964), T375.

146. Jane E. Oltman, J. J. McGarry, and S. Friedman, "Parental Deprivation and the 'Broken Home' in Dementia Praecox and Other Mental Disorders," *American Journal of Psychiatry*, 108 (1952), 685.

147. Humphrey F. Osmond and J. Smythies, "Schizophrenia: A New Approach," Part I, *Journal of Mental Science*, 98 (1952), 309.

148. Metin Ozek, "Untersuchungen über den Kupferstoffwechsel im Schizophrenen Formenkreis," *Arch. Psychiat. Nervenkrank.*, 195 (1957), 408.

149. Beulah Parker, *My Language Is Me*, "Psychotherapy with a Disturbed Adolescent" (New York: Basic Books, 1962).

150. Seymour Perlin and A. R. Lee, "Criteria for the Selection of a Small Group of Chronic Schizophrenic Subjects for Biological Studies: Special Reference to Psychological (Family Unit) Studies," *American Journal of Psychiatry*, 116 (1959), 231.

151. George M. Perrin, M. Altschule, and P. Halliday, "Carbohydrate Metabolism in Brain Disease," *Archives of Internal Medicine,* 105 (1960), 752.

152. C. C. Pfeiffer and E. H. Jenney, "The Inhibition of the Conditioned Response and the Counteraction of Schizophrenia by Muscarinic Stimulation of the Brain," *Annals of the New York Academy of Science,* 66 (1957), 753.

153. William L. Pious, "A Hypothesis about the Nature of Schizophrenic Behavior," in Arthur Burton, ed., *Psychotherapy of the Psychoses* (New York: Basic Books, 1961).

154. William Pollin, James R. Stabenau, and Joe Tupin, "Family Studies with Identical Twins Discordant for Schizophrenia," *Psychiatry,* 28 (1965), 60.

155. Curtis T. Prout and M. A. White, "The Schizophrenic's Sibling," *Journal of Nervous and Mental Disease,* 123 (1956), 162.

156. Fredrick C. Redlich, "The Concept of Schizophrenia and its Implication for Therapy," in Eugene B. Brody and Fredrick C. Redlich, eds., *Psychotherapy with Schizophrenics* (New York: International Universities Press, 1952).

157. Thomas A. C. Rennie, "Follow-up Study of 500 Patients with Schizophrenia Admitted to the Hospital from 1913 to 1923," *Archives of Neurology and Psychiatry,* 42 (1939), 877.

158. David McK. Rioch, "Introduction," in Kenneth L. Artiss, ed. *The Symptom as Communication in Schizophrenia* (New York: Grune & Stratton, 1959).

159. Eli Robins, Kathleen Smith, and I. P. Lowe, "Attempts to Confirm the Presence of 'Taraxein' in the Blood of Schizophrenic Patients," in H. A. Abramson, ed., *Transactions of the 4th Conference, Josiah Macy, Jr., Neuropharmacology Foundation* (1959), pp. 123.

160. E. H. Rodnick and N. Garmezy, "An Experimental Approach to the Study of Motivation in Schizophrenia," in M. R. Jones, ed., *Nebraska Symposium on Motivation* (Lincoln: University of Nebraska Press, 1957).

161. R. Rodnight, "Body Fluid Indoles in Mental Disease," *International Review of Neurobiology,* 3 (1961), 251.

162. John Romano and F. G. Ebaugh, "Prognosis in Schizophrenia," *American Journal of Psychiatry,* 95 (1938), 583.

163. John Rosen, *Direct Analysis* (New York: Grune & Stratton, 1953).

164. Leonard S. Rubin, "Autonomic Dysfunction in Psychoses," *Archives of General Psychiatry,* 7 (1962), 27.

165. Henrious C. Rümke, "Die Klinische Differenzierung innerhalb der Gruppe der Schizophrenen," *Nervenarzt.,* 29 (1958), 49.

166. J. W. Ryan, J. Durell, and J. D. Brown, "Stimulation of Aerobic Glycolysis in Chicken Erythrocytes by Human Plasma," *Federation Proceedings,* 24 (1965), 326.

167. Edward J. Sachar, J. W. Mason, H. S. Kolmer, Jr., and K. L. Artiss, "Psychoendocrine Aspects of Acute Schizophrenic Reactions," *Psychosomatic Medicine,* 25 (1963), 510.

168. William Sacks, "Cerebral Metabolism of Isotopic Glucose in Chronic Mental Disease," *Journal of Applied Physiology,* 14 (1959), 849.

169. Albert E. Scheflin, *A Psychotherapy of Schizophrenia* (Springfield: Charles C Thomas, 1961).

170. Kurt Schneider, "Wesen und Erfassung des Schizophrenen," *Zeitschrift ges. Neurol. Psychiat.*, 99 (1925), 542.

171. Gertrud Schwing, *A Way to the Soul of the Mentally Ill* (New York: International Universities Press, 1954).

172. Harold F. Searles, *The Non-Human Environment* (New York: International Universities Press, 1960).

173. Marguerite A. Sechehaye, *A New Psychotherapy in Schizophrenia* (New York: Grune & Stratton, 1956).

174. C. Shagass and Morris Schwartz, "Excitability of the Cerebral Cortex in Psychiatric Disorders," in Robert Roessler and Norman J. Greenfield, eds., *Physiological Correlates of Psychological Disorder* (Madison: University of Wisconsin Press, 1962).

175. David Shakow, "Psychological Deficit in Schizophrenia," *Behavioral Science*, 8 (1963), 275.

176. Eliot Slater, *An Investigation into Psychotic and Neurotic Twins* (London: University of London Press, 1951).

177. John R. Smythies, *Schizophrenia* (Springfield: Charles C Thomas, 1963).

178. Theodore L. Sourkes, *Biochemistry of Mental Disease* (New York: Harper & Row, 1962).

179. John E. Staehelin, "Psychopathologic der Zwischen und Mittelhirnerkrankungen," *Schweiz Arch. Neurol. Psychiat.*, 53 (1944), 374.

180. Edward Stainbrook, "Some Characteristics of the Psychopathology of Schizophrenic Behavior in Bahian Society," *American Journal of Psychiatry*, 109 (1952), 330.

181. Alfred Stanton and Morris Schwartz, *The Mental Hospital* (New York: Basic Books, 1954).

182. E. Stauder, "Die Tödliche Katatonie," *Arch. Psychiat. Nervenkr.* 102 (1934), 614.

183. Ernst Stengel, "A Study of Some Clinical Aspects of the Relationship between Obsessional Neurosis and Psychotic Reaction Types," *Journal of Mental Science*, 91 (1945), 166.

184. Alfred Storch, "Über das Archaische Denken in der Schizophrenie," *Zeitschrift ges. Neurol. Psychiat.*, 78 (1922), 500.

185. Harry Stack Sullivan, *Schizophrenia as a Human Process* (New York: Norton, 1962).

186. S. Szara, "Behavioral Correlates of 6-Hydroxylation and the Effect of Psychotropic Tryptamine Derivatives on Brain Serotonin Levels," in D. Richter, ed., *Comparative Neurochemistry* (Oxford: Pergamon Press, (1964).

187. Stephen Szara, J. Axelrod, and S. Perlin, "Is Adrenochrome Present in the Blood?" *American Journal of Psychiatry*, 115 (1958), 162.

188. Thomas S. Szasz, "The Problem of Psychiatric Nosology," *American Journal of Psychiatry*, 114 (1957), 405.

189. Yasuo Takahashi, "An Enzimological Study of Brain Tissues of Schizo-

phrenic Patients. Carbohydrate Metabolism. Part III. Pyruvic Acid," *Folia Psychiat. Neurol. Japonica*, 7 (1953), 252.

190. Victor Tausk, "On the Origin of the Influencing Machine in Schizophrenia," *Psychoanalytic Quarterly*, 2 (1933), 519.

191. Pekko Tienari, "Psychiatric Illness in Identical Twins," *Acta Psychiatrica Scandinavia* (Munksgaard, Copenhagen), Suppl. 171, (1963).

192. James S. Tyhurst, "Paranoid Patterns," in Alexander H. Leighton, John A. Clausen, and Robert N. Wilson, eds., *Explorations in Social Psychiatry* (New York: Basic Books, 1957).

193. Warren T. Vaughan, Jr., J. C. Sullivan, and F. Elmadjian, "Immunity and Schizophrenia: A Survey of the Ability of Schizophrenic Patients to Develop an Active Immunity Following the Injection of Pertussis Vaccine," *Psychosomatic Medicine*, 11 (1949), 327.

194. Robert Waelder, "The Structure of Paranoid Ideas," *International Journal of Psycho-Analysis*, 32 (1951), 167.

195. Heinrich Waelsch and Hans Weil-Malherbe, "Neurochemistry and Psychiatry," in *Psychiatrie der Gegenwart* (Berlin: Springer-Verlag, 1964).

196. Milton Wexler, "The Structural Problem in Schizophrenia," in Eugene B. Brody and Fredrick C. Redlich, eds., *Psychotherapy with Schizophrenics* (New York: International Universities Press, 1952).

197. John C. Whitehorn and B. Betz, "A Study of Psychotherapeutic Relationships between Physicians and Schizophrenic Patients," *American Journal of Psychiatry*, 111 (1954), 321.

198. John C. Whitehorn and G. K. Zipf, "Schizophrenic Language," *Archives of Neurology and Psychiatry*, 49 (1943), 831.

199. Lyman C. Wynne, I. M. Ryckoff, J. Day, and S. I. Hirsch, "Pseudo-Mutuality in the Family Relations of Schizophrenics," *Psychiatry*, 21 (1958), 205.

200. Arlipii D. Zurabashvili, *Theoretical and Clinical Investigations in Psychiatry* (Tbilisi: [Russian] Georgian Academy of Sciences, 1961).

CHAPTER FIFTEEN

Manic and Depressive Behavior Disorders

Basic Considerations

Manic and depressive behavior disorders make up a large group of disorders characterized by profound disturbances of affect without deterioration. It is a heterogeneous grouping, which includes disorders ranging from presumably endogenous psychoses to abnormal grief. The "melancholia" of antiquity, aptly described by Aretaeus,[2] occurred in those "who become thin of their own agitation . . . complain of a thousand futilities and desire death." Jules P. N. Falret first described manic-depressive psychosis as *folie circulaire*,[15] and Emil Kraepelin rigidly differentiated manic-depressive psychoses from dementia praecox.[30] Salient differences and similarities between grief and melancholia were noted by Sigmund Freud, and Ernst Kretschmer described cyclothymic and cycloid personalities as transitions from normal behavior to manic-depressive psychosis.[31] The pathogenesis of most of these disorders is still obscure, although advances in psychotherapy and organic therapy have made them eminently treatable.

Incidence and Prevalence

The incidence and prevalence of manic-depressive disorders are not reliably known; according to current estimates, the prevalence is three to four per 100,000 population. The rate of admissions of manic-depressive patients to hospitals is between one-tenth and one-twentieth of the rate of admission for schizophrenics. Prevalence data in the New Haven Study indicated that eight per cent of these patients were diagnosed as manic-depressive.[23] Reported findings on ethnic differences may be attributed for the most part to inadequate or biased samples. The common clinical impression that severe depressions are more frequent in Scandinavian countries, in Scotland, and in New England may not stand up under critical examination. J. C. Carothers reported a scarcity of severe depressions in tropical Africa,[9] and Edward Stainbrook felt such patients were rare in other primitive societies.[51] The incidence of mild depressions, particularly in the involutional age, is probably very high, but there are no exact data. Depressions occur at all ages; they often remain unrecognized in infants and children and are not infrequent in young adults.

The Confused Terminology

The term *affective behavior disorders* implies a primary disturbance of affect. The term *manic-depressive behavior* disorders refers to two important characteristics: the extremes of pathological affect and the repetitive, alternating, or cyclic attacks. It is desirable to reserve the word *depression,* a term first used by Adolf Meyer, for a *syndrome;* one must not confuse it with the affect of sadness. Equally, mania also refers to a syndrome and is not synonymous with euphoria and elation. Hypomania is, by definition, a milder form of a manic syndrome. The syndromes of mania and depression may occur in a wide variety of disorders, but they are found in their purest forms in the manic-depressive behavior disorders. The term melancholia is used by some psychiatrists to designate severe depressive disorders.

Most authors call manic-depressive disorders psychoses; at times, Freud referred to them as narcissistic neuroses in contrast to transference neuroses. The distinction between psychotic and neurotic depression is a problem that has remained with us. A grief reaction is a complex and characteristic response to a loss. We differentiate between normal and prolonged, intensive, or pathological inappropriate grief. *Reactive depressions* are severe and lasting reactions to stimuli that ordinarily produce grief. They are contrasted with *endogenous depressions,* a term referring to inner processes that produce the disorder; but this actually only reflects our ignorance of etiological variables. Walter Von Bayer elegantly defined endogenous psychosis as the empty space between the uncomprehended psychological phenomena and the unexplained somatic.[4] Another term, latent depression, refers to somatic or behavioral reactions that indicate a depressive affect which is not obvious.

The Symptoms of Depression

In simple severe depression, patients report that they are sad, gloomy and that nothing seems enjoyable; they feel hopeless and helpless, and their self-esteem withers. In mild cases or in prodromal stages, the harder they try to combat the mood, the worse they feel. They are apt to complain endlessly about aches and pains and vague symptoms of dreadful diseases, not yet diagnosed but apt to break out at any moment. Although sadness is the most notable affect, concomitant anxiety, tension, or hypervigilance are inferred from subjective reports and from behavioral and psychophysiological phenomena. Patients express guilt, shame, and feelings of unworthiness over past sins and failures; they feel trapped, hopeless, and desperate. Since therapy depends upon the appraisal of the pathological emotions and the events that produce them, the differentiation of guilt and grief depressions is of practical importance. Persons with "guilt depressions" have often a marked sadomasochistic sense of humor, with a tendency to tease and to be teased. Grief depressions show a painful absence of humor.[41]

In mild cases, patients complain that they tire easily and cannot work or concentrate. In severe cases, the posture of despair is paralleled by a general inhibition of intellectual and motor functions; they move and speak slowly and with effort, and their facial expressions become rigid and pained. In some, motor retardation approaches stupor. Subjective time passes slowly for these patients. On objective examination, intelligence and memory are usually intact, even though patients complain about their inability to think; inhibition and lack of confidence may influence certain test performances adversely. As we usually describe mental status, there is no disturbance of orientation, no confusion, no disturbance of thinking, except for the occasional retardation. A. T. Beck, however, feels that the depressive interpretation of reality fundamentally involves an altered cognitive function, which narrows, restricts and distorts and personalizes the world;[5] impaired judgment of values, self-image, and interpersonal situations is certainly implied in the depressive affect.

Along with the affects of despondence, guilt, shame, anxiety, and the general retardation, a number of physical symptoms can be discerned, especially disturbances of food intake and elimination. Many depressions begin with loss of appetite and gastrointestinal complaints. In severe cases, the anorexia may even necessitate forced feeding. Many complain of dryness of the mouth, presumably due to a decrease in salivary secretion; some show crying without tears. Some patients are constipated; some vomit; in most severe depressions there is weight loss, but in milder depressions the patients may eat voraciously, with weight gain. Other somatic complaints, often exaggerated and the focus of concern, also include "hot flashes," coldness of the extremities, and tachycardia with dyspnea. Many severely depressed women complain of dysmenorrhea and amenorrhea, possibly due to a decrease of gonadotropic hormones. In both sexes, there is usually a decrease in sexual desire; impotence in the male then becomes another reason for profound feelings of inadequacy. Insomnia is the rule; patients have trouble falling asleep and usually—especially agitated patients—sleep only for a few hours. As a result, they complain of exhaustion and fatigue, particularly in the morning hours; it is conjectured that the depression which lifts toward evening is related to the lessened demand for work that generally marks the day's end. Neuroendocrine factors as well as insomnia, fatigue, and the structure of daily demands or expectations may determine the diurnal variations. Early results in monitoring stages of sleep suggest that the depressive sleeps mostly in the "paradoxical" stage, has little oculomotor activity (little "scanning of the dream scene"), and little "slow" sleep, which may be required for a response of restfulness. Diurnal fluctuations of symptoms have been thought of as characteristic of "endogenous" depression; in our observation they may occur in any severe depression.

In agitated depression, the patient expresses his affect by marked restlessness, often to the point of extreme, incessant and exhausting hypermotility; unlike in the simple depressions, anxiety and anger as well as sadness can easily be discerned. A paranoid coloring and querulousness is often evident. The aggression of all depressive patients is intuitively discerned by those who interact with them; their retardation and helplessness and particularly their incessant complaints are clearly experienced as troublesome and annoying. Even the retarded seem, in their posture of deep dejection, utterly refractory to any consolation. Hypochondriacal complaints may be delusionary; such patients say they have no stomach, no brain, and that they are dead.

Neurotic traits of the premorbid personality give severe depressions their individual aspects. E. Stengel thought that obsessive traits are particularly prominent; depressions would develop when obsessive defenses did not suffice to check the anxiety generated by unacceptable ambivalent hostile and dependent needs.[53] In hysterical depressed patients, and in schizoids who become depressed, we often see marked degrees of depersonalization. A mild sense of unreality is very frequent in depressed persons. It is quite obvious that depressed patients, as much as they suffer and torment themselves, also derive some gratification by such self-torture and its impact on others. A dangerous aspect of the depressive patient's aggression, discussed later, is his self-destructive behavior.

Mania

Mania and hypomania occur more rarely than depressive states. Mania is conceived of as a mirror image of depression, a view strengthened by the cyclic alternations in the relatively rare circular disorders. The basic affect is a euphoric state of mind; in its purest form these patients feel happy, unconcerned, free of worry; according to Binswanger, they are in a playful and festive mood.[7] Such experiences may produce a feeling of envy in the ordinary mortal; but these affects are exhibited without any concern for reality or the feelings of others. Mood is often expansive, and some patients have extraordinary, though not fixed, delusional notions about their power and importance. They are apt to involve themselves in senseless and risky enterprises, but some gifted hypomanics can be very successful. Manics and particularly hypomanics (because their behavior is more organized) have a quick wit and a good sense of humor; unlike schizophrenics, they are quite capable of producing hilarity in others, including their therapists, even if their jokes are not very tactful or subtle. More often than not, the euphoric mood is accompanied by a troublesome irritability. Readily provoked by harmless remarks, patients quickly forget the alleged slight, only to be provoked anew a short while later. To such "provocations" they react with unabashed fury; they may scream, curse, abuse, and become violent, but quickly calm down, quite unlike the angry paranoid. Irritability in manic patients may be an expression of anxiety as well as of hostile impulses.

In contrast to depressed patients, manics are extremely self-confident. They are on top of the world; egocentric, their self-esteem, on the surface at least, knows no bounds. Nothing and nobody else counts. With such feelings of magical omnipotence and supreme self-esteem goes an extraordinary lack of guilt and shame, and often a denial of realistic danger. The patient's lack of guilt, his optimism, and his inability to forecast social consequences frequently drive him into fringe enterprises, irresponsible spending, expansive planning, and misdemeanors of a sexual, aggressive, or possessive nature; but serious criminal acts are rare. The leader of a federation of women's clubs appeared at a tea party in a bathing suit; so great was her prestige that she "got away with it," her friends assuming that there was some moral message in her attire, even though they could not fathom it. The male manic patient is less apt to get into sexual difficulties because potency as well as desire is usually impaired. Manic behavior, although unmistakable, is often not recognized by lay people, possibly because there is no clear-cut identity change. Persons are seen, for a time at least, as simply "acting up." Psychological tests reveal that intelligence and memory are intact. The flightiness and distractibility that characterize the performance on tasks requiring attention are related to the patient's emotionality and his lack of self-criticism.

Accompanying the euphoric, expansive, irritable mood of manics is the accelerated pace of psychomotor activity. They are always on the go, often quickly changing from one to another of their multiple enterprises. In the sphere of motility, they seem to be indefatigable, or at least not to register fatigue with all their restless agitation; they may eventually become dangerously exhausted. The increase of verbal production is striking, with logorrhea and its counterpart in thinking, flight of ideas. Except in extreme cases, the ideas usually remain sufficiently relevant to be followed without difficulty by the psychiatric examiner. Manic and depressive disturbances of affect do not always occur in pure form. Kraepelin described mixed forms, transient stuporous and perplexed states, which at one time were considered special types.

The following example of flight of ideas was recorded between a therapist and a manic patient, a Greek-American dockworker who had ten previous manic-depressive episodes:

Therapist: How do they treat you at the hospital?

Patient: Fine, fine—fine food—good American cooking—I say good American cooking because it's different from Mom's cooking—Mom was born in Greece—her meals are greasy—I'd like to go to the greasy spoon.

T: You go home for a meal once in a while?
P: Oh yeah—every day on a pass—I never pass, they don't let me out——
T: Why not?
P: I need a rest—I don't need a rest—I am a crackpot——
T: That's why you are here?
P: Naw—I checked myself in—like hell I did, I never check in at a bughouse. I was five times in Middletown (a State hospital), they give you shock treatments—stick a hose in your mouth and your body goes way up in the air.
T: You remember it?
P: I remember everything—I have a memory like an elephant—you want to see my trunk? [Laughs] They help you, like they help them old ladies with frowzy gray hair—if they help them why are they still there—I tell you it's better to treat a patient with sympathy. Now take a patient who has euthritis——
T: Arthritis?
P: Yeah, euthritis—There are two doctors and two nurses—instead of that treatment they open a book—a big doctor wrote that book—bigger than you—two heads are better than one—two pretty heads like them nurses. A man can walk better with a woman than alone.
T: I don't quite follow——
P: Oh, you're no dummy, Doc. You're following me, all right.

Characteristic physical changes can be related to the basic affect: inadequate nutrition, partly because they have no time to eat, and serious loss of weight in conjunction with their insomnia and overactivity. In severe cases, there may be dehydration, which requires prompt attention. Manic patients have a marked tendency to neglect themselves; typically they are sloppily or insufficiently dressed, ungroomed, and unwashed. More serious is their inclination to overlook and deny organic illness.

Course of Manic and Depressive Behavior Disorders

There are both cyclic and sporadic affective behavior disorders. Some cyclic affective disorders develop gradually, others suddenly. Ordinarily, early depressive and manic symptoms impress us as accentuations of patterns of the premorbid personality. Depressive patients at first show their need for love emphatically; when their expectations are not fulfilled, they will provoke rejection and fall into their characteristic self-punitive and self-deprecatory patterns. The indiscretions of manic patients also fulfill specific latent needs of the premorbid period. In the majority of patients, onset is in middle life, very rarely before the age of twenty. Not many develop their first attack after the age of sixty. The relative frequency of manic episodes is higher in younger patients; in the older age group, depressive syndromes predominate. First attacks, in Thomas A. C. Rennie's series[42] (before the days of electric convulsive therapy), lasted an average of six months; only 21 per cent had a second recurrence; 64 per cent had a third; and 45 per cent had a fourth attack. There are patients with regular alternating recurrences of manic and depressive episodes with or without an interval of normality. There are others in whom only depressions and, more rarely, only manic episodes occur. Attacks in the older age ranges usually last longer. The overwhelming number of patients (93 per cent, according to Rennie) recover from their attacks. In cases who do not recover, we often find the family constellation is so unfavorable that the patient simply has no chance to be rehabilitated.

It is more difficult to predict the course of *nonperiodic* depressions. In contrast to the cyclical disorders, there is considerable evidence that the sporadic affective disorders are responses to past and present psychosocial constellations. Certain patients respond to losses of any kind with a short-lasting depressive syndrome and usually recover from it with (and even without) therapeutic intervention. In other cases, these depressions are more enduring; there are some who suffer from permanent and even life-long, relatively mild, depressive states. For these cases we use the term, depressive character. Sporadic manic syndromes are rarely observed.

Etiology

Although etiological theories are many, our knowledge of the causative factors is scanty, and we must view affective behavior disorders as of unknown and exceedingly complex etiology. Statements about etiology in the literature often do not differentiate between severe and mild disorders, between single depressive or manic attacks and recurrent and cyclic disorders. In general, it is assumed that in severe and cyclic disorders, organic factors, and in milder and sporadic reactions, psychological events are more likely to be contributory. This clearly is a gross oversimplification. We find psychological precipitating events in very severe cases; and some mild cases, even after thorough exploration of the patient's background, personality, and recent history, seem to come out of the blue.

Biological Causes in Manic-Depressive Behavior Disorders

There is a large body of literature that asserts that genetic factors predispose to affective behavior disorders. Franz J. Kallmann,[27] Eliot T. O. Slater,[49] and others point out a marked increase in the incidence of manic-depressive psychoses in relatives of the patients, in contrast to the general population, although the figures are far from consistent. The expectancy in parents varies from 1.8 to 14.5 per cent, in children from 6.1 to 14.4 per cent, and in siblings from 2.7 to 18.8 per cent; the normal expectancy, according to these authors, is 0.8 per cent. Both Kallmann and Slater assume the existence of a single dominant gene with incomplete penetrance. In dizygotic twins, the expectancy is about 25 per cent and in monozygotes almost 100 per cent. Kallmann thinks that recurrent potentiality for extreme self-limited mood alterations is associated with a specific (but as yet undemonstrated) neurohormonal disturbance. He also assumes the existence of physiological and psychological devices that protect adults from the harmful effects of such extreme mood swings. Both Kallmann and Slater cited a high frequency of cyclothymic persons in the families of manic-depressives to support the view that the severe disorders are extreme variations of normal personalities. This is in keeping with Kretschmer's observations of the significance of the pyknic habitus to this continuum; and William H. Sheldon and his coworkers however, with more refined measurements, found that manic-depressives do not belong to a pure type, but are fat mesomorphs.[46] Although individuals seem to vary in capacity for vivid responsiveness to any mood, this impression has not been successfully objectified and linked to clinical disorder. The psychoanalyst Karl Abraham also assumed that excessive oral demands and ambivalence, which according to the psychoanalytic point of view are of etiological significance in these patients, have a constitutional basis.[1]

In a number of patients, brain pathological changes have been cited as precipitating causes of affective behavior disorders. Arteriosclerotic changes found in a fairly large number of older patients do not account directly for depression. Stengel reported cases of postencephalitic patients who had periodic depressions and an aggravation of their postencephalitic symptoms.[52] The discovery by J. Olds and P. Milner[37] of cerebral "pleasure and pain" centers leads to a purely speculative notion that manic-depressive disorders are possibly associated with long-lasting cyclic alterations of such centers. It is the impressive periodicity and intrinsic course of these disorders that suggest to many experienced clinicians an endogenous biochemical or physiological process. The fact that certain depressions lift after pharmacological therapy has further elicited arguments for an organic etiology; furthermore, our clinical impression and our review of the literature suggest that antidepressants are mildly or moderately effective in depressive disorders but that in mixed (schizo-affective) and schizophrenic disorders, where phenothiazine tranquilizers are potent, they are without effect. These impressions would argue (though not compellingly) for a distinctive pathophysiology in depression. Similar suggestive evidence lies in the studies of "sedation threshold," pioneered by C. S. Shagass.[45] The dose of amobarbital given to the point of slurred speech and EEG changes (in the direction of drowsiness) differentiated depressive disorders fairly successfully. A more precise end point—a shift in the base level of the G.S.R.—has been employed with even greater reliability. Truly solid evidence for presuming an organic and chemical etiology, however, is lacking, and many findings are not differentiating. It has been noted that in many depressions an elevation of 17-hydroxycorticosteroids occurs; but this is also found without depressions.[18]

It is likely that in psychotic depressions, catecholamine metabolism, at present under investigation, is disturbed; and it has also been noted that gastric secretion is unresponsive to histamine in some depressions.[60]

The relationship of organic illness to depressive behavior disorders is recognized by authors with such divergent views as M. Roth and George L. Engel. Roth holds organic illness to be a precipitating factor in half of all depressive patients.[43] The effect of such illness is not necessarily directly physiological, with the possible exception of some virus diseases, infectious mononucleosis, and infectious hepatitis, which are regularly accompanied by mild depression. Resistance to infection may be lowered in depression. A psychosomatic factor is present, since the enervation accompanying some diseases might not be appreciated by the patient; he does not, in fact, have the energy to appreciate and respond to his world at his usual pace, but ignoring his body, he tries to do this and further exhausts himself. With illness or with menopause and its hormonal changes, the change of structure of usual patterns of activity may be responded to by many as equivalent to a deprivation and loss; the enervation or changed reactivity may leave one to face issues normally avoided and thus lead to depression. Engel views grief as if it were a disease[13] and believes that psychogenic depressions precede the onset of many somatic and psychosomatic diseases. Although precise and convincing physiological and biochemical data about the mechanisms of affective behavior disorders in general—and depression in particular—are lacking, the expectation that cyclic and severe affective disorders have a chemical basis does appear plausible. Research will require refinement in measurements and invention in what is measured (and when it is) before these issues can be settled.

Psychological Causes of Depression and Mania

Meyer Mendelson has critically reviewed the psychodynamic theories of depression.[35] In older textbooks, we find the injunction that the diagnosis of depression must be based on the pathognomic symptom of primary despondency, and the diagnosis of mania on primary euphoria, without anydemonstrable psychological cause. Today, we seriously mistrust this statement. In a large number of well-explored cases of depression, and in some manic cases, psychological trauma preceding affective reactions can be uncovered. When Kraepelin belittled psychogenic causes of depressions and mentioned that one of his patients became depressed after the death of a pigeon, he overlooked a fact that is well recognized today: that the patient's statements do not necessarily refer to the real events but often are symbolic allusions. In all likelihood, Kraepelin's patient did not mourn for the pigeon; rather, the bird stood for an important unconscious love-object. On the other side, we must always keep in mind the danger of finding the psychological antecedents one is looking for; this makes explanations all too easy.

In any case, a good deal is known today about the psychogenesis of depression, though much less about mania.

One of the most incisive attempts to understand grief and depression and to bridge the gap between the two is found in Freud's *Mourning and Melancholia*,[16] from which much of our current knowledge stems. In normal grief, the bereaved mourns the loss of a person, property, or ideological belief; he is sad, lost, and unable to enjoy anything. Freud thought that after the loss, libido was withdrawn from the lost object and temporarily invested within the mourner. Thus, the mourner is self-centered, attends to his suffering, may feel ambivalently guilty for sins of commission and omission toward the lost person and for the anger occasioned by a painful desertion. Each act that recalls the loss again evokes some bit of mourning, gradually freeing the mourner for new ties to pleasurable activities, events, and persons. Freud spoke of the stepwise release of ties through recurrent grief as the "work" of mourning. During this period of helplessness and pain, we recognize that society assists the patient to reorient himself to the loss and toward new tasks and persons.

Normal grief shades into the abnormal. In abnormal grief, the patient behaves as if he had suffered a severe loss, although in most cases no serious objective loss has occurred, and the nature of the unconscious loss remains obscure to the patient. There is another element in pathological depression, which is relatively unimportant in normal mourning; the melancholic suffers from a much more severe and persistent fall in self-esteem. He accuses himself of nonexistent or vastly exaggerated misdeeds toward the lost person, and he also exhibits a variety of destructive and self-destructive forms of behavior. Freud,[16] asking who could be so terrible, found that these self-reproaches were actually meant for the hated lost love-object. He thought this accounted for the striking shamelessness with which patients could afford to accuse themselves. He astutely noted that melancholic criminals and worthy people show little difference in their self-recrimination and in their exaggerations of small indiscretions. It seems unimportant what people have really done; the private evaluations and fantasies are what count. Freud was able to show that these fanatsies still contain a kernel of truth. He mentioned the resentful mourning of the rejected bride. Some divorced women behave like embittered widows. There is probably no mourner who is completely free from guilt; rather than transfer interest to new ties, the old objects are clung to, often with fury and resentment. The old rule-of-thumb that mourning lasting longer than six months is suspect of melancholia cannot be taken too literally, but has some value. In the grief-denying culture of the United States, this allotted period for "legitimate" grief is shorter.[58] Analysis of depression has revealed the role of identification: the melancholic does not relate to the lost object, but a part of himself takes on attributes of that object, thus preserving an unrelinquishable tie.

Freud cited conditioning factors: from the narcissistic nature of the symptoms he inferred that the original ties of the depressive were narcissistic and ambivalent. He pointed to an oral dependency and to a sadomasochistic character of the depressive's relationships. The desperate clinging quality of depressives, their moral war with and engulfment of those about them, their "swallowing" of anger and often stubborn refusal of proffered food and love are well-known attributes. As patients, they shame and provoke the physician, proving his helplessness; as parents, they often thrive on helplessness in the child and provoke nameless guilt when the child differs from the parent's needs.

No psychiatrist before Freud and Abraham saw clearly the many psychological elements in depression. Extending these studies, Edward Bibring, in his refreshing clinical observations, looks at depression as a state of helplessness and powerlessness after experiences of illness, failure, and loneliness.[6] The aspirations to be loved, to be strong, and to be good have not been fulfilled. The systemic conflict, according to Bibring, lies in the ego itself; it cannot live up to either the expectations of the superego or to its own esteem. Developmental determinants for self-esteem may influence the dominant symptomatology; loss of love, of objects, and of nurturance are related to lonely dejection; loss of autonomy, to angry and ambivalent characteristics; and loss of approval and status, to guilt and inferiority. Edith Jacobson makes the pertinent observation that the depressive devalues his parents and destroys them in fantasies for which he pays with his guilt.[25] Sandor Rado assumes that the depressive patient has an intense need for oral gratification, the "alimentary orgasm." [39] Trivial provocations may produce a catastrophic reduction of self-esteem, maintenance of which does not depend on achievement but on love. If love is supplied (and it cannot be supplied sufficiently to satisfy the insatiable demand), the patient reacts with rebellious hostility. To reconcile the parental figure in fantasy, the depressive punishes himself, expresses remorse, and seeks new demonstrations of love by atonement. Such behavior is repetitious of analogous events in infancy; according to Rado, depression in both adult and infant is essentially an unsuccessful cry for love.

The most elaborate statements on the predisposing infantile experiences of the first year of life have been made by Melanie Klein.[28] She feels that the infant goes through paranoid and depressive phases during which strong oral, sadistic, and devouring wishes are directed against the mother whom he loves, fears, and depends upon. Fear over such hatred produces depression. Later depressions are a repetition of this early depressive position. In children, one can observe loss indiscriminately responded to by paranoid fury and projection, which is followed developmentally by a capacity to discriminate objects, to feel depression, and to internalize the fear and anger. Both reactions to loss are seen in adults, but it seems unwise to endow babies with these complicated psychological mechanisms. If and how infantile depressions, investigated by J. Bowlby,[8] G. L. Engel and F. Reichsman,[14] R. Spitz[50] and S. R. Pinneau,[38] are related to adult depressions, is still an open question. That hopelessness and helplessness are universal problems of living occurring in all ages cannot be denied.

In an outstanding study, Mabel Blake Cohen and her co-workers explored the interpersonal and familial environments of a series of manic-depressive patients.[11] The families of these patients were typically set apart from the surrounding milieu by some factor which singled them out. They belonged to minority groups, had lost money, or an important member of the family was mentally ill. The families tried to overcome this and regain a position of honor; owing to various circumstances, the patient became the chief carrier of the burden to regain prestige. The model family in this study was strict and conventional. Family authority was impersonal, and was usually vested in the mother, who was reliable but disliked; the father was weak and ineffectual. The infancy of the patient was normal. Later, the mother began to make demands on the future patient, who learned to perform accordingly, in order to be accepted, and who also became sensitive to envy and competition. Characteristically, the patient developed into a relatively well-adjusted, sociable, conventional, hard-working, and overconscientious person. He could not admit his dependency or his subtle rebelliousness. In general, he learned to disregard his own feelings and also developed massive scotomata for the feelings of others. He learned to achieve goals by techniques such as exploitation of guilt and manipulation of feelings of obligation. When these techniques to gain attention and love became offensive to others, who rejected the patient even more forcibly, the patient responded with helplessness and a psychotic state. The investigators did not have reliable controls, nor did they specifically show why severe depressions occur in some and not in other persons with similar interpersonal environment, or why some patients become manic rather than depressed. Obviously, minority problems, weak fathers, opportunistic attitudes, and excessive demands do not always produce depression; nor is it established (or claimed) that this kind of biography invariably is present.

Since Freud, it has been assumed with some conviction that depressions are reactions to losses and separations. We believe that losses and separations that occur early in life produce childhood depressions and predispose an individual to depression in adult life, which may be triggered off by a relatively minor traumatic stimulus. The already low self-esteem then completely collapses, and clinical symptoms of depression develop. Often, intense worry, irrational guilt, and isolation are the reactions of the child to a depressive parent; the child seems to feel it wrong to see the world brightly, and this identification with the ailing parent produces depressive trends as an adaptive maneuver in the child. Depression in children may be manifest in fear, hypochondriasis, or in learning and conduct problems. Mothers (and some doctors) who love to hold and "keep" infants (or patients) but cannot tolerate ambulatory children tend to evoke a feeling of guilt and "depression by identification" in the child (or patient) who leaves and "abandons" them. Guilt in depressed patients may, then, represent worry about the parent's depressed and covertly angry response; the child feels responsible and adopts the notion that it is bad to differ or to abandon. Often, such empathized or fantasized abandonment is used by the patient as a reproach to the physician who takes a vacation or is on sick leave. It is bad and intolerable for the doctor to leave him, just as he was bad for wishing to separate from a clinging parent. If marked ambivalent feelings toward the lost person or object exist, and if the self-punitive tendencies are strong, the patient develops a guilt depression rather than grief depression. It should be remembered that, although psychoanalytic propositions have contributed much to our understanding of predisposing and particularly of precipitating factors in normal and abnormal grief, they have by no means solved the problem of etiology of depression.

The same reservation can be made even more emphatically about the manic state. Freud compared the manic to the poor devil who has suddenly won a large sum of money and is relieved of his lifelong anxieties of existence. Manic celebration, of course, is too often based on a loss of reality bounds rather than on a reshaping of them; guilt and fear are temporarily replaced by omnipotence and invulnerability (as we see it in intoxication and ecstasy). But we are unable to point to psychological processes that account for the essential and necessary conditions for the genesis of the phenomenon, or for its resolution. Bertram Lewin objects to the prevalent view that the manic state is essentially a defensive reaction to an "underlying depression."[32] He assumes that the elation of the manic state is the result of a conflict of oral instincts and massive denial. Why such conflicts take the form of manic episodes in some and of milder euphoric states in others (or possibly just in a normal happy disposition) remains unclear.

Diagnosis and Differential Diagnosis

Recurrent and Cyclic Manic-Depressive Psychoses

The recognition of early stages and borderline states can present insurmountable problems. The diagnosis of all cyclic manic-depressive disorders is based on the following considerations: (1) There must be a distinct and marked phasic disturbance of affect without accompanying cerebral pathology and without intellectual deterioration and personality disintegration. Hallucinations and delusions are relatively rare, although paranoid hypersensitivity and projection are often seen. (2) The attacks must be well defined; neither very short periods of elation or depression nor lifelong depression or euphoria are characteristic. (3) The presence of other manic-depressives and cyclothymic persons in the family has been considered of diagnostic value, even though we cannot clearly distinguish between genetic and psychosocial transmission of behavioral symptoms. (4) Precipitating psychogenic factors are not conspicuous.

Types of Depression

Single attacks of severe depression are more frequent than circular psychoses or single attacks of mania. Roy Grinker and his co-workers,[17] in an important and sophisticated statistical and clinical study, arrived at five categories of feelings and concerns and ten categories of behavior in the depressed syndromes. They were able to distinguish four basic types: (1) Patients who feel dismal and hopeless, who suffer from loss of self-esteem, but who have only slight guilt feelings. They are isolated, withdrawn, and apathetic, with slowed speech and thinking and constituted about one-third of the patient group. (2) Patients who feel hopeless, have low self-esteem, considerable guilt feelings, and show high anxiety. They are agitated and make clinging demands for attention. (3) Patients who feel abandoned and unloved, with little guilt. They are strikingly hypochondriacal and also demanding and agitated. (4) Patients who feel hopeless, anxious, and notably angry and provocative. Grinker *et al.* objectified the descriptive behaviors so that reliability of rated behaviors and subsequent groupings could be achieved; they also tried to understand these types in terms of defensive and restitutive attempts.

Diagnosis of Early and Atypical Depression

Although the typical syndromes of mania and depression are easily recognized, there are many atypical cases that defy clear and simple classification. In the initial stages of a depression, some patients seem to live and work under a great strain without overt symptoms. Their behavior conveys the feeling that everything is a tremendous effort, but they themselves are unaware of their burdens and at times cover up their labors by a forced humorous attitude. Self-punitive, self-abasing acts and the patient's neglect of his own interest may point to the proper diagnosis. Other depressed patients give the impression of being physically ill, although no organic findings can be established. It is important to detect camouflaged depressives who are otherwise likely to escape our attention and live in agony if not in danger of suicide. Such people complain little, put up a good front, work hard, and have a great need to conform and to please. They may put up with the common Sunday or holiday blues but take little note of the pain they assume they must endure. Only after thorough psychological exploration is a deep feeling of dejection and despair uncovered.

The Problem of Differentiation of Neurotic Depression

In all too many cases, the boundary between psychotic and neurotic depression is blurred. It seems almost that the more we learn about these syndromes the less we are able to maintain our old diagnostic scheme. To many clinicians, neurotic depression designates a relatively mild psychogenic depression. Such states can be enduring or can show marked fluctuations. The symptoms are similar though less pronounced than in a severe depression, but obviously, it is difficult to delineate clearly the severe and mild forms.

Essentially, the patients whom we label as neurotic depressives suffer from helplessness, sadness, a lack of vitality, and often pervasive and lasting feelings of guilt. The depressive feelings are deepened by the slightest indications of a loss of love or by disappointments, criticisms, misgivings, or real threats, all of which increase the patients' helplessness. They have a pessimistic view of the world and their own worth. Mild physical symptoms of fatigability, insomnia, anorexia, constipation, and decrease of general and of sexual activity accompany these affects. They find it difficult to assert themselves. In general, there is no true retardation present. They may be irritable and intermittently reveal the underlying struggle in explosive outbursts with impulsiveness and demandingness. Many of these patients are hypochondriacal and either openly or tacitly demand attention and care on these grounds. In most such well-studied patients, we find that separations and relative neglect in infancy and childhood were responded to with depression and a significant shift in the child's views of his world and himself. The early depression, or shift in behavior or attitude, becomes a mode of response, constantly reactivated by experiences of further losses, frustrations, and humiliations.

What is called abnormal grief or reactive depression falls into the category of depression. Such patients simply cannot work through the grief after a real loss; the dynamics are identical with those of all psychogenic depressions. Two special forms of psychogenic depression are clinically important. In the first, the depressed person commits minor antisocial acts—usually of a destructive and hostile nature—and by these acts invokes punishment and disapproval. It is likely that this is repetitious of infantile behavior, by which a patient wishes to test the love of his parents but also wants to be punished and atone for unconscious aggressive and sexual acts, which produce unbearable guilt. The second type, the so-called success depression, occurs paradoxically after the patient has had a striking success. The depression usually is the result of severe unconscious guilt or rage feelings; these seem to be modeled on experiences in which an abortive attempt was made to eliminate a rival parent or sibling or in which there was resentment at being abandoned and "forced" to carry on without support.

Schizo-Affective Syndromes

Insurmountable difficulties in differential diagnosis induced Stanley Cobb to transgress Kraepelinian boundaries and postulate the existence of schizo-affective states.[10] In the clear-cut case, the schizophrenic, with his autism, dereism, and characteristic thinking and feeling disorders, is quite different from the manic-depressive, with his primary mood disorder but without any radical cognitive alterations. There are, however, borderline reactions of depression, with catatonic and paranoid symptoms, and manic and depressive patients with bizarre, fantastic distortions of their experiences. Often, such patients are originally diagnosed as manic-depressive but later are found to be schizophrenic. It is a common experience to find in the records of psychiatric hospitals a change of diagnosis from manic-depressive psychosis to schizophrenia upon re-examination of the patient a few years after admission. Mabel Blake Cohen *et al.* believe that some manic-depressives develop into schizophrenics if their defenses become inadequate;[11] their break with reality then becomes complete. Even recovery, which Kraepelin stressed as the most important differential diagnostic criterion, is, as we know today, not an infallible index. It is sometimes said that it is easy to empathize with manic-depressives in contrast to schizophrenics. There is a subjective element in such assertions, which probably are made by cyclothymic and not by schizothymic psychiatrists. Yet it is true that the psychological inhibition and retardation of depressives, or the flight of ideas of manics, are easier to understand than the profound thinking disturbances and distortions of reality of the schizophrenic patient. Commonly, the diagnosis of schizo-affective disorder is made where a strong affective component, perhaps only hypomanic, occurs in a patient with schizophrenic identity problems and mild thought disorder; with recovery from the acute disorder with its affective disturbances, borderline schizophrenic symptoms may be more clearly evident. Often the examiner, responding to the dominant mood and affective quality in some acute psychotic breaks, makes the schizo-affective diagnosis.

Manic and depressive syndromes occur in the course of acute and chronic brain diseases. Typically, the manic, hypomanic or depressive syndrome may be the characteristic expression of acute alcohol intoxication. Euphoric and expansive mood, often with speech disturbance that has superficial similarity to the speech of drunkenness, are frequent in general paresis and pseudoparetic syndromes. Epileptic equivalents and clouded states may simulate short manic or depressive episodes. Depressions and, more rarely, manic states, are well known in patients with senile and arteriosclerotic brain disease. Patients with organic deficit reactions who experience losses and separations are more likely to develop apathy than a simple depression. The occurrence of manic states in older persons can be linked, in many cases, with brain damage and subsequent defensive denial.

The Problem of Involutional Behavior Disorders

Are behavior disorders of the involutional period specific disorders, or are they related to the manic-depressive disorders, schizophrenias, or neuroses? Kraepelin felt uncertain; at one time, he incorporated involutional melancholia in the manic-depressive group; then separated it.[30] Today, again we find ardent proponents of both views. Without any specific knowledge of the etiology, such disputes are an unprofitable game in which senior psychiatrists merely assert their authority. At present, there is no good nosological or etiological reason to recognize the involutional disorders as specific entities. Actually, we are always least comfortable when we try to allocate a group of disorders to an age period. The involutional period itself is not clearly defined; in women, at least, it is marked by specific endocrine events, but the disorders that are commonly labeled involutional occur in the periods of life that precede and follow the menopause by many years.

There are four types of disorder that occur in the involutional period: (1) Manic-depressive disorders, particularly the so-called involutional melancholia; (2) Paranoid disorders, which belong to the schizophrenic group in the broad sense of the word. (3) Organic deficit states, particularly in cases with arteriosclerosis and presenile diseases. (4) Neurotic disorders, with rich symptomatology that includes all types. It goes without saying that there are many transitional states between these categories.

The typical secondary symptoms of menopause in the female (for example, hot and cold flushes, palpitation, headache, grayout and blackout, anorexia, indigestion, constipation or diarrhea, fatigability, irritability, and tension) are frequent but not invariably present in female involutional psychotic behavior disorders. Some of these symptoms also occur in some male patients and are sometimes called the male climacteric syndrome; whether they can be attributed directly to endocrine changes is not established.

Manic conditions in the involutional period are rare. Paranoid disorders, particularly paraphrenic reactions, are not infrequent; and often, fantastic, self-accusing, and hypochondriacal delusions coexist with paranoid delusions. In general, the paranoid delusions of involutional patients are less bizarre, less apt to undergo disorganization than those of a younger group. Depressive patients in this age period are likely to be agitated. Every student of psychiatry encounters the middle-aged, haggard, ungroomed lady with stringy gray hair, who ceaselessly paces the floor of a ward; her face is marred by the frown of dejection, anxiety, and anger. She whines and pours out terrible self-accusations of threatening to end her miserable life, complaining querulously of dreadful disease, and demanding endless attention. It has also been said that there is relatively little psychological retardation in this disorder; of course, agitated depressions are not apt to be retarded, but over a period of time, many involutional patients with depressions show some degree of apathy.

We know as little about the specific etiology of these involutional disorders (including the role of endocrines) as we know about the etiology of manic-depressive disorders in general. A. Stensted reports that genetic factors seem to play a smaller role in involutional than in manic-depressive disorders.[55] The concurrence of psychoses in the involutional period of identical twins is only 60 per cent, considerably lower than in schizophrenias and manic-depressive disorders in the narrow sense of the word; this does not, of course, answer the open question of the etiological role of physiological changes. Psychological factors are documented, however. Although, according to A. C. Tait *et al.*,[57] actual bereavement is found in only a few patients, experiences of loss of love; of social and occupational status; threats of security loss; realistic or unrealistic concern over illness; and, last but not least, feelings of true or imaginary inadequacy over sex functions can be found in most histories of these patients. J. Barnett *et al.*[3] pointed specifically to the presence of rigid, obsessive characteristics in the premorbid personality of patients with involutional psychoses and consider them as decompensated obsessional personalities whose defenses have collapsed. In our opinion, whatever the contributing or causal factors may be, the dynamics of the disorders of the involutional period are not essentially different from the dynamics of the basic disorders to which they may belong.

Suicide

Of the various symptoms of depression, suicide and suicidal attempts are the most alarming. Grinker and his co-workers found that documentable suicidal preoccupations were not frequent in their study;[17] nevertheless, we believe that the threat of suicide must be considered in all serious depressions. Rennie reported that suicidal attempts were made in 30 per cent of all his cases.[42] The threat of suicide, of course, is not limited to depressions; it occurs in other behavior disorders, particularly in schizophrenics, in many neurotics and sometimes in relatively normal and mature persons. Closer examination reveals that the so-called rational suicide in Western culture, for example, in incurable illness, often has irrational motivations that are not obvious on superficial inspection. Yet, in view of the total number of suicides, the percentage of suiciding patients with very severe behavior disorders is small.

The total number of suicides is high. In the United States, approximately ten thousand persons commit suicide each year, which brings suicide to the eleventh place in the race toward death.[61] Men commit suicide four times as frequently as women, and the frequency of suicide increases with age for both sexes. However, three hundred teen-agers commit suicide every year in the United States. It has also been established that, in the United States, whites kill themselves more frequently than do Negroes; the suicide rate of female Negroes is particularly low. Suicide is more frequent in metropolitan than in rural areas. J. M. A. Weiss reported that persons of the upper and middle classes suicide more frequently than members of the lower classes.[59] To conceal suicide for personal, cultural, and, particularly, for religious reasons, is very common and presents a problem for accurate epidemiology. Quite probably this explains the commonly cited figure that Protestants commit suicide seven times as frequently as Catholics. In any event, the primary data are unreliable, and international statistical comparisons must be viewed with great caution. Of course, there are always handy though rarely confirmed explanations to explain differential figures. The highest rate of suicide in the world supposedly occurs in West Berlin. In the United States, San Francisco has the dubious distinction of leading suicide statistics. Austria, Germany, Switzerland, Japan, and Denmark are said to have high suicide rates; in Spain, Ireland, and Egypt low rates are reported. The United States is in the middle.[61] Eighty per cent of all suicides are committed by the common methods: firearms (in males), drugs, gas, hanging, and drowning. The notion is unproven that choice of method depends less on cultural variables than on unconscious motivations. The personal factor does seem predominant in some cases, particularly depressives and schizophrenics, who employ irrationally cruel methods, for example performing ghastly self-mutilations. In both categories, the suicide of the patient may also follow homicidal acts. Unfortunately, it is not rare with the demanding and possessive narcissism of depression and the failure to distinguish self and others, for an afflicted mother to take her children into death with her.

The obvious precipitating causes for suicide are severe disappointments in love, business, or social life; secret humiliations and failures; or dread of a painful and hopeless existence, as in chronic illness, regardless of whether the reasoning is well founded or not. On the surface, it seems that persons commit suicide when they see no other way out. The rational suicide of the soldier who is a member of an aristocratic caste and who feels that he or his group has lost honor is no exception to this. We know, however, that the external desperate situation alone usually does not lead to suicide. Émile Durkheim, in a classical study at the turn of the century, considered psychosocial isolation and a confusion of norms, or normlessness, which he called "anomie," as decisive causes.[12] Herbert Hendin, studying suicide in the three Scandinavian countries, found suicide rates high in Sweden because Swedes are rigid performers who hate themselves for failure.[19] The aggressive Norwegians suffer from an inverted aggression type of suicide, and the Danes a "dependency loss" type of suicide. Whether Hendin's imaginative conclusions stand up under rigorous scrutiny remains to be seen. Flurries of suicide (following the suicide of a celebrity) and favorite sites for suicide point to a factor of identification and suggestibility, a looseness of the self-boundaries, as well as loneliness in the psychology of some suicides.

Freud emphasized that suicide is homicide turned against the self. Many persons who commit suicide demonstrate their unconscious murderous hatred of a person. Suicide, then, may be considered an act of ultimate self-punishment and expiation. In times of war, when destructive drives have a more legitimate outlet, suicides are rare. The suicidal are unconsciously absorbed in killing. It is less certain whether they want to die. For the child, death may be an arbitrary extreme punishment, which is seen as temporary and reversible. This magical view of mortality is often discovered in serious suicidal attempts; the patient does not take into account the fact that, if the act is successful, it is not just final for now, but forever. In his discussion of Freud's death instinct and man's unconscious desire to destroy himself, Karl Menninger points to the many forms of partial or larval suicide: chronic invalidism, drug addiction, crime, and, in a certain sense, most mental disorders.[36]

Erwin Stengel, in a study of survivors of suicidal attempts, reported that the factor of unconscious hatred and self-punishment is not the only important variable.[54] Attempted suicides are nine times more frequent than suicides, and there is the ever-present question whether such attempts are bona fide. Stengel showed that suicide attempts have a very incisive social effect; they may bring about a dissolution of severe and seemingly insoluble conflicts in interpersonal relations. There are few events that have such dramatic and drastic effect on the survivor and the persons who interact with him; the threat of death evokes re-evaluation of personal ties and values. Even histrionic attempts have a cathartic effect. R. Rubenstein, R. Moses, and T. Lidz similarly see in clear suicidal gestures an effort not to die, but to improve a relationship with another person.[44]

The danger of suicide is always present in uncommunicative, self-destructive patients. In a depressive patient, it is greater when the general psychological inhibition and retardation begins to lift than when the patient is at the depths of his depression. The shift from a stable mental state, while welcome, may create unanticipated instabilities. What has been called the "four D's" represents a possible sequence related to the correlation of suicide with apparent improvement: "depression, doubt, decision, and death." A covert decision for death, resolving all doubt, is presumed to release the grip of depression; now cheerfully determined and bent on concealing his aims, the patient lulls suspicion and commits suicide following hospital discharge or relaxation of vigilance. The presence of very sadistic-masochistic fantasies is also a danger signal. The following case of an agitated depression illustrates aspects of the narcissistic and sadomasochistic elements in some suicides.

> The patient, a lonely, disillusioned, though successful sculptress of 27, married "to keep myself from drifting," but her lifelong moodiness persisted. She shifted from resentful dejection (in a spiteful pout at age five, she ate a toadstool "to die") to periods of energetic cheerfulness. To her quite passive husband she related in a somewhat smugly possessive and bullying manner. She felt little fondness for her infant, forcing herself to care for him, and with a second pregnancy remained angrily depressed (attempting suicide with aspirin) until her husband relinquished his opposition to an illegal abortion. On learning of a homosexual affair of his, she did not recognize the marital disharmony or his disturbance, but felt "this is better than his running around with other women." Nevertheless, she became jealous, dreamed of shooting two men

and a woman, and the following day, after an unanticipated display of temper by her husband (who slammed the door and left for the evening), she attempted suicide with gas, protecting her son in this and leaving herself to be found by the errant spouse.

Her father, a farmer who yearned to be a musician, was, like the patient, unpredictably violent and dominated the oversensitive, ineffectual mother. Fearing him, the patient had contempt for the mother; attractive, she hated being a girl and felt deserted by her two older sisters who left her to her loveless parents. In the hospital she tried to touch and embrace therapists and nurses; she pleaded and teased for little favors. Gaining some insight, she still could not control her impulses and made several attempts to elope when rebuffed. Forcibly returned, sedated and placed in an "isolation room" she was briefly visited by her therapist (who felt helpless with her tantrums and teasing); she was furious and contemptuously angry and agitated with him. He left, and only 15 minutes after she had been observed by the nurse on duty (her blanket over her head, seemingly quietly asleep), she set fire to the mattress and was found dead of suffocation in her self-made tent.

It is commonly assumed that announcements of suicide plans are usually harmless and that agitated depressives are more likely to commit suicide than quiet ones; both assumptions are wrong. All too often, we are misled in our predictions and misjudge suicidal cues.[56] Unfortunately, the fact is that short of brutally depriving patients of any freedom, suicides are bound to occur, even in the best-run hospitals. When they do occur, those even remotely related suffer sorrow, guilt, anxiety, and anger: Why? What could I have done differently? What did I miss? Such reactions attest to the narcissism in the depressive disorders in which self-esteem (of the patient, as well as his loved ones) is brutally attacked, and both the helplessness and omnipotence of the self and others is mercilessly exposed. Expertise can somewhat narrow the margin for error; but to hold bitter post-mortems in the belief that we could always, or even frequently, have surely known the truth in advance of the patient's choice or impulse, only reflects our inherent illogical omnipotence upon which the suicidal transaction invariably touches.

We are struck not only with the guilt which suicide leaves in its wake but also by the bitter inheritance—the model bequeathed to surviving children and relatives. We see some depressed patients who as children have been critically abandoned in the aftermath of a parent's death (whether natural or self-inflicted). Such a patient may identify with that person in his current depression and act out— rather than talk out—his ancient grief, guilt, and fantasy of reunion. The consequential childhood losses may also be symbolic and not readily apparent. Considering the sardonic logic of the depressive, we would caution the psychiatrist to be aware of the anniversaries of such departures and beginnings (for example, birthdays, when patients have been known to give back their birthrights to well-wishers who failed them through the grim reunion of suicide). In all cases where identifications are primitive and narcissistic, "anniversary reactions" may be significant.[20] A popular honors student, feeling that to his parents he was only a collection of prizes, sent them (with unconscious self-contempt) his own awards to keep; just prior to graduation he left his death notices for them as well.

Another morbid factor is the history of previous attempts. This portends a grave prognosis; it indicates a mode of solution for problems, often vigorously denied and beyond conscious perception, which is lying "rehearsed" and ready to be executed when there is any severe disruption or dissociation in a current crisis. A schizoid or hysterical capacity for dissociation, or for the loosening of ego boundaries which accompanies a depressive state, seems to us particularly ominous. Although we do not always know the harsh, sadistic fantasies and rules that unconsciously underlie suicide, we are impressed with the loss of a focus upon the "sentient self"; the person who will actually be injured seems to disappear. One of our patients (called sweet and responsible by her family) just escaped death through no effort of her own. She told of her feeling that as she cut her wrists she did not exist; her childishly intrusive mother was paramount in her mind ("There's not room inside me for both of us."), and the patient felt like an observer who did not really think "who was being killed." We talked one patient to safety from his perch on a window ledge by forcibly reminding him that it was *he* who stood there: "Joe, *you* are the one who is going to be hurt." Besides loss of self, a split or concealment of the "true self" may be observed, as will be discussed below.

Obviously, the seriously suicidal patient needs to be hospitalized, but in spite of rigid safety measures (such as elimination of "sharps," drugs, matches, cords, twines, curtains, glass, and even clothing), the determined suicidal patient often finds a way to "outwit his enemies." He often shows a life history (learned about too late to help) of significant concealment, a muted double life, more an internalized trick than a flagrantly acted out episode. "You thought I was always a good girl—I fooled you," said one patient who recovered; she viewed her successes in life as based on a pose of compliance that worked while a secret part of her was rebelling. It is our impression that conflicts among hospital personnel may lead to a relaxation of vigilance with these persons and thus facilitate suicide. A diffusion of responsibility (probably evoked by the patient's approach) is strikingly observed in hospital suicides; it is as if the patient's loss or concealment of "self" is acted out and reflected in the staff's loss of focus upon the patient who then quietly does his work.

The depressive suicidal patient often lulls judgment; we are disturbed, touched, and moved to rescue him *after* the fact. His needs for unquestioned attention and incessant love without regard for the needs of others are covert. In contrast, other narcissistic patients, childlike, wistful, and provocative, strike beyond our normally intact judgment directly to our primitive yearning to rescue and protect (or to be rescued); they become not only staff pets, but compelling centers of concerned attention. They re-evoke quite personal erotic longings and response to abandonment—feelings that may partially have determined the professional caretaker's choice of work. We can, in fact, often diagnose the patient by our response. T. F. Main, for example, felt he could tell from the response of his normally rational staff (who suddenly were in all sorts of turmoil based actually on their passion to rescue an appealing and perplexed young girl), the character diagnosis of the person evoking this storm.[34] Rescue fantasies or guilt reactions in professional persons are irrationally powerful and commonly seen in our field. These patients (as well as many actors and public personalities) communicate to us, as to themselves, by feelings rather than more rational signals, and it is an advance in psychiatry to be aware of these mechanisms and the earlier mentioned "depressive techniques" for compelling response and bypassing the usual filters of judgment and perspective.

E. S. Shneidman, N. L. Farberow and L. Calista have established a suicide clinic in the Los Angeles General Hospital, where patients who make suicidal attempts can be referred and treated.[48] The most effective method of preventing suicide is to provide opportunity for close contact and discussion of destructive and self-destructive impulses and to maintain a clear focus on the status of such patients. If the therapist feels teased or in doubt and cannot resolve this directly with the patient, he should examine his own extratherapeutic anxieties (his fear of losing face with colleagues, for example) and then act clearly, firmly, and directly, perhaps to hospitalize the patient, or openly to accept the risk of failure. We must respect the ultimate fact that it is the patient who must "decide to live" and thus we try to reinforce his true autonomy; the patient, on the other hand, requires us, often as his only tenuous bond to life, to consider if he is sufficiently able to risk this choice at a given time. It is not an easy task for anyone.

Therapy of Affective Behavior Disorders

Well-systematized therapies of manic and depressive behavior disorders were developed in the nineteen thirties. Until then, psychiatrists could only do their best to prevent the patient from destroying himself, use drugs that were far from specific, and wait for spontaneous remissions. In all but the mildest cases, a custodial regime of hospitalization was mandatory. In a discussion of modern methods of treatment, it is important to keep in mind that, quite apart from vigorous treatment, these disorders have always been observed to remit and to have a tendency to recur without any identifiable cause. Results of therapy in manic depressive patients are difficult to evaluate.[47] Why, then, do we treat them, particularly, by rather drastic methods? The reasons are obvious. "Spontaneous" remissions are very slow at best. Treatment shortens the course of the psychotic episode, alleviates great suffering, and reduces the danger of destructive and self-destructive behavior. It is also known that some manic-depressive patients (as well as some neurotic depressives) who are grossly neglected, brutally mistreated, or forced to return to very unfavorable psychological situations do not recover at all.

In general, treatment with both organic and psychosocial methods has been found to be highly successful. There is no general agreement as to preference of organic or psychosocial methods of therapy; even in the individual patient, it is often difficult to come to a decision. Our over-all recommendation is to treat mild depressions by psychotherapy and severe cases by a combination of psychosocial and biological treatment. In manic patients, we are more likely to use organic methods. In many severe cases, a fast remission can be initiated by organic therapy but sustained only by psychosocial treatment. We are also increasingly impressed by the importance of family therapy in patients with affective disorders, where concrete patterns of emotional blackmail, of behavior reinforcing the patient's pathology (such as denial and withdrawal) can be demonstrated.

HOSPITALIZATION OR OFFICE TREATMENT Although in general we have become less ardent about hospitalization of manic-depressive patients (and all psychiatric patients for that matter), the danger of suicide alone forces us to recommend hospitalization for many patients. In severe cases, it is also necessary to remove the patient from the pressure of hostile and destructively dependent interaction in his natural environment. By permitting more direct expression of his needs and feelings in the controlled and protective hospital setting, a psychotherapeutic relationship becomes possible, not merely between the patient and psychiatrist for a few hours a week, but in an enduring interaction with nurses, attendants, and other patients. Manic-depressive patients should be hospitalized whenever this is possible (and in many situations it is impossible) if electric convulsive treatment is contemplated. We have always been reluctant to recommend electric convulsive therapy outside of a hospital, although it is not an infrequent practice. Depressed patients who are so severely ill that such therapy is indicated need a therapeutic environment around the clock; even when suicide is not feared, such patients tend too easily to deny illness and avoid the chance for a reorientation of ties and habits that clear-cut hospitalization provides. There are, of course, cases in which special circumstances may make office or clinic treatment desirable or necessary. One example was the recommendation of ambulatory shock therapy in a patient who was in danger of being deported if he required hospitalization; in another case, we administered such therapy to a patient who would have been disqualified for a government position, not if he were treated, but if he were hospitalized. For both depressed and manic cases, the usual patient is insured a better chance of consolidating his gains by late, rather than early, discharge from the hospital.

Electric Convulsive Therapy

Electric convulsive therapy has found a wide application in manic-depressive disorders. In severe and particularly in agitated depressions, it is the method of choice: it is relatively simple; fatality is low; and complications are not severe. L. B. Kalinowski recommends six to twenty treatments producing convulsions and coma.[26] Barbiturates should not be given during this therapy. For details of technique, we refer the reader to Chapter 11.

It seems that the immediate recoveries from depression after electric convulsive therapy exceed untreated remissions. In recurrent depressions, successes are less spectacular than in single depressions of the involutional period, and some evidence points to a shortening of the interval between bouts. Huston and Locher found that 80 per cent of their involutional patients recovered after electric convulsive therapy, in comparison with 46 per cent of spontaneous recovery.[24] It has been felt by some, however, that improvement is not always sustained. Although shock therapy is of little fundamental help in manic states, it is an efficient sedative in states of excitement. Whenever possible, electric shock treatment should be supplemented by individual and group therapy and by occupational and social rehabilitation.

PHARMACOLOGICAL THERAPY Phenothiazines, especially high doses of chlorpromazine, have been used with success in manic states. With the exception of agitated depressions, tranquilizers can occasionally aggravate depressions or produce confused states. In all likelihood the effect of drugs depends on the severity and type of depression. In very mild depressions, a wide variety of agents are used. The combination of amphetamine with chlorpromazine occasionally has been useful, as have amphetamine and a barbiturate. In general, however, we avoid amphetamine combinations and employ chlorprothixene, or amitryptaline, treating sleep disturbances when indicated with hypnotics such as chloral hydrate. Nathan S. Kline has recommended MAO inhibitors and reported a specific energizing effect.[29] According to many experienced clinicians and some controlled studies, the results with drugs in severe depression have been less good than in electric shock therapy, and changes clearly do occur more slowly.[22] The currently best-established drug therapy in mild and severe depressions employs imipramine in doses of 75 to 150 mgm. per day; initial effects are usually first observed within 5 to 14 days. Such doses may be maintained over a period of weeks or months. Although the toxicity of imipramine or amitryptaline is considerably less than that of some of the MAO inhibitors, there are characteristic side effects and contraindications as discussed in Chapter 11. Chlordiazepoxide and congeners may be used in combination with antidepressants when anxiety is a persistent component.

PSYCHOTHERAPY Mild depressions should be treated by psychotherapy whenever this is feasible. The opinions on indications for intensive psychological treatment in the severe case are divided: some therapists think it is useful; some do not. We have treated severe manic-depressive patients by analytic techniques and helped them to resolve certain problems of living. It was observed, while the patients were under treatment, that their depressions lifted and gradually developed into manic states, to lapse later into new depressions. Our strong impression is that severe circular manic-depressive disorders do not yield to psychotherapy only. Paul Hoch reports recurrences that took place in patients who were considered successfully treated by psychoanalysis and related methods.[21] Yet, for the prevention of future relapses few rational approaches are available; occasionally the use of such a difficult, lengthy, and costly undertaking as prolonged intensive psychotherapy is warranted and successful.

To help bereaved persons, support, sympathy, and companionship are the common-sense methods. In the atypical case of enduring grief, Erich Lindemann recommends psychotherapy beyond support and reassurance.[33] It is important to share the patient's grief; to review the relationship with the deceased and doubts or guilt about what could have been done; to help the patient face the altered reality and, in Lindemann's words, "repeople the empty space." He also feels that, in some acute grief reactions, medication may be indicated. In the mild and simple depression, any sensitive person knows what to do; as with simple bereavements, we know that time is a very powerful curative agent.

In the treatment of "psychogenic" depressions, support and sympathy are not enough. Patients thirst insatiably for such support and show great resistance to a vigorous exploration of their conflicts. The psychiatrist who does not want to be used as a wailing wall may respond with annoyance to such behavior, and a satisfactory psychotherapeutic relationship then becomes difficult. But even kindness may upset the patient by increasing his guilt, as Rado pointed out.[40] Mabel Blake Cohen *et al.* observed that the depressives annoy us with their manipulations and exploitations, in contrast to schizophrenics, who frighten us.[11] We have also been impressed with the ambivalence of such patients and their many subtle, covert, and overt expressions of hostility.

A deliberately stern and firm approach sometimes relieves the patient's self-punishment, but this merely illustrates the pathology; some therapists encourage projection of the internalized anger. The paranoid quality spontaneously evident in many depressions indicates the ambivalent need to find an object of love and hate, but overt expression of hostility must be kept within bounds lest it disorganize and overwhelm the patient.

The first goal in therapy is to help the patient feel accepted despite his symptoms but *not* because of them; later, the goal is to provoke him to wonder why he damages himself even more than others and to help him see, if possible, the familial ties and commands that, through his symptoms, he automatically obeys. Often what the patient requires from the doctor, others once asked of him. When the patient is ready, one may demonstrate how he undercuts his already abysmally low self-esteem. Beck advocated helping the patient identify his automatic self-deprecatory thoughts and when they recur to question their validity.[5] Once the self-esteem stops spinning downward, the first round is won. Gradually weaned from his insatiable quest for love and support, the patient learns to use more mature techniques for gratification; in part, this entails close attention to his current modes of relating with and manipulating others. The moderately or severely depressed patient is, in a sense, an addict for love; and addicts are notoriously difficult to treat; they interpret "weaning" and withdrawal as rejection. The ultimate aim of therapy is both the development of coping techniques and the sufficient exploration of the narcissistic injury underlying the depression to prevent recurrence. This ultimate goal is not frequently reached.

It is worth noting in passing that depressive patients strike at the vanity and self-esteem of the therapist; over and over again they assure us of our helplessness and limitations. This is provocative, but should be taken as a reflection of their own wounded vanity, their self-centered need to have a "stellar position at the bottom of the ladder." The fact that we unconsciously identify with the patient's attack (and are aggravated) only reflects the role of narcissism in the disorder and the identification by the patient with the harsh demands of a loved parent. Insensitivity, not only to others but also to their own rights and limitations, characterizes the relationships of such patients; sacrifice, compliance, and responsibility are interpreted at the level of coercion, fear, and guilt, not choice.

Psychotherapeutic difficulties with manic patients are even greater, and a truly rational psychotherapy is nearly impossible. To spend an hour a day with a manic patient, letting him associate freely (which he does all too readily) can be more a filibuster than treatment. The hypomanic patient usually is not motivated to undergo therapy because he feels too well, and such a patient may be more accessible to therapy when he is depressed or in a normal interval. If the therapist becomes a significant person to any of these patients, he is, in any event, in a position for the patient to use his support and sense of reality when the patient is ready for it. In recovery, the majority deny problems; therefore, psychotherapeutic contact established during illness can provide a more enduring bond to inner realities that must be dealt with at some point in an extended treatment program.

NOTES

1. Karl Abraham, "Notes on the Psychoanalytical Investigation and Treatment of Manic-Depressive Insanity and Allied Conditions," in *Selected Papers* (New York: Basic Books, 1953).
2. Aretaeus, *The Extant Works of Aretaeus, the Cappadocian,* edited and translated by Francis Adams (London: Printed for the Sydenham Society, 1856).
3. Joseph Barnett, A. Lefford, and D. Pushman, "Involutional Melancholia," *Psychiatric Quarterly,* 27 (1953), 654.
4. Walter von Bayer, "Zur Psychopathologie der endogenen Psychosen," *Nervenarzt,* 24 (1953), 316.
5. Aaron T. Beck, "Thinking and Depression: I. Idiosyncratic Content and Cognitive Distortions," *Archives of General Psychiatry,* 9 (1963), 324; "Thinking and Depression: II. Theory and Therapy," *Archives of General Psychiatry,* 10 (1964), 561.
6. Edward Bibring, "The Mechanism of Depression," in Phyllis Greenacre, ed., *Affective Disorders* (New York: International Universities Press, 1953).
7. Ludwig Binswanger, *Über Ideenflucht* (Zurich: Orrell-Fussli, 1933).
8. John Bowlby, "Childhood Mourning and Its Implications for Psychiatry, *American Journal of Psychiatry,* 118 (1961), 481.
9. J. C. Carothers, "A Study of Mental Dereangement in Africans and an Attempt to Explain Its Peculiarities, More Especially in Relation to the African Attitude to Life," *Psychiatry,* 11 (1948), 47.
10. Stanley Cobb, *Borderland of Psychiatry* (Cambridge: Harvard University Press, 1943).
11. Mabel Blake Cohen, G. Baker, R. A. Cohen, F. Fromm-Reichmann, and E. V. Weigert, "An Intensive Study of Twelve Cases of Manic-Depressive Psychoses," *Psychiatry,* 17 (1954), 103.
12. Émile Durkheim, *Suicide* (Glencoe, Ill.: The Free Press, 1951).
13. George L. Engel, "Is Grief a Disease?" *Psychosomatic Medicine,* 23 (1961), 18.
14. George L. Engel and F. Reichsman, "Spontaneous and Experimentally Induced Depressions in an Infant with a Gastric Fistula," *Journal of the American Psychoanalytic Association,* 4 (1956), 428.
15. J. P. Falret, *Des Maladies mentales et des asiles d'alienes* (Paris: J. B. Baillière, 1864).
16. Sigmund Freud, "Mourning and Melancholia" [1917], in *Standard Edition* (London: Hogarth Press, 1955), 14.
17. Roy R. Grinker, J. Miller, M. Sabshin, R. Nunn, and June C. Nunnally, *The Phenomena of Depressions* (New York: Paul B. Hoeber, 1961).
18. David A. Hamburg, "Plasma and Urinary Corticosteroid Levels in Naturally Occurring Psychological Stresses," in S. Korey, ed., *Ultrastructure and Metabolism of the Nervous System* (Baltimore: Williams & Wilkins, 1962), p. 406.

19. Herbert Hendin, *Suicide and Scandinavia* (New York: Grune & Stratton, 1964).

20. Josephine R. Hilgard and M. F. Newman, "Anniversaries in Mental Illness," *Psychiatry*, 22 (1959), 113.

21. Paul H. Hoch, "Psychodynamics and Psychotherapy of Depressions," *Canadian Psychiatric Association Journal*, 4 (1959), Special Suppl. S24.

22. Hans Hoff, "Indications for Electro-Shock, Tofrānil, and Psychotherapy in the Treatment of Depressions," *Canadian Psychiatric Association Journal*, 4 (1959), Special Suppl. S55.

23. August B. Hollingshead and Fredrick C. Redlich, *Social Class and Mental Illness* (New York: John Wiley, 1958).

24. P. E. Huston and L. M. Locher, "Involutional Psychosis," *Archives of Neurology and Psychiatry*, 59 (1948), 385.

25. Edith Jacobson, "Contribution to the Metapsychology of Cyclothymic Depression," in Phyllis Greenacre, ed., *Affective Disorders* (New York: International Universities Press, 1953).

26. Lothar B. Kalinowsky and Paul H. Hoch, *Shock Treatments, Psychosurgery, and Other Somatic Treatments in Psychiatry* (New York: Grune & Stratton, 1952).

27. Franz J. Kallmann, *Heredity in Health and Mental Disorder* (New York: Norton, 1953).

28. Melanie Klein, *New Directions in Psychoanalysis* (New York: Basic Books, 1957).

29. Nathan S. Kline, ed., *Psychopharmacology* (Washington, D. C.: American Association for the Advancement of Science, 1956).

30. Emil Kraepelin, *Clinical Psychiatry*, translated from seventh German edition by A. Ross Diefendorf (New York: Macmillan, 1923). [Original: *Psychiatrie: ein Lehrbuch für Studierende u. Ärzte*, 7. AUFL. (Leipzig: Barth, 1923)].

31. Ernst Kretschmer, *A Text-Book of Medical Psychology*, translated by and with an introduction by E. G. Strauss, (London: Oxford, 1934), [Original: *Medizinische Psychologie*, AUFL (Leipzig: Thieme, 1926)].

32. Bertram Lewin, *The Psychoanalysis of Elation* (New York: Norton, 1950).

33. Erich Lindemann, "Symptomatology and Management of Acute Grief," *American Journal of Psychiatry*, 101 (1944), 141.

34. T. F. Main, "The Ailment," *British Journal of Medical Psychology*, 30 (1957), 129.

35. Myer Mendelson, *Psychoanalytic Concepts of Depression* (Springfield: Charles C Thomas, 1960).

36. Karl Menninger, *Man against Himself* (New York: Harcourt, Brace, 1938).

37. James Olds and P. Milner, "Positive Reinforcement Produced by Electrical Stimulation of Septal Area and Other Regions of Rat Brain," *Journal of Comparative Physiology and Psychology*, 47 (1954), 419.

38. Samuel R. Pinneau, "The Infantile Disorders of Hospitalism and Anaclitic Depression," *Psychological Bulletin*, 52 (1955), 429.

39. Sandor Rado, "The Problem of Melancholia," *International Journal of Psycho-Analysis*, 9 (1928), 420.
40. Sandor Rado, "Psychodynamics of Depression from the Etiologic Point of View," *Psychosomatic Medicine*, 13 (1951), 51.
41. Fredrick C. Redlich, J. Levine, and T. P. Sohler, "A Mirth Response Test," *American Journal of Orthopsychiatry*, 21 (1951), 717.
42. Thomas A. C. Rennie, "Prognosis in Manic-Depressive Psychoses," *American Journal of Psychiatry*, 98 (1942), 801.
43. Martin Roth, "The Phenomenology of Depressive States," *Canadian Psychiatric Association Journal*, 4 (1959), Special Suppl. S32.
44. C. Robert Rubenstein, R. Moses, and T. Lidz, "On Attempted Suicide," *Archives of Neurology and Psychiatry*, 79 (1958), 103.
45. Charles S. Shagass, J. Naiman, and J. Mihalik, "An Objective Test Which Differentiates between Neurotic and Psychotic Depression," *Archives of Neurology and Psychiatry*, 75 (1956), 461.
46. William H. Sheldon, S. S. Stevens, and W. B. Tucker, *The Varieties of Human Physique* (New York: Harper, 1940).
47. Michael Shepherd, "Evaluation of Drugs in the Treatment of Depression," *Canadian Psychiatric Association Journal*, 4 (1959), Special Suppl. S120.
48. Edwin S. Shneideman, Norman L. Farberow, and Calista V. Leonard, *Some Facts about Suicide* (U.S. Public Health Service Publication; Washington, D. C.: Government Printing Office, 1961).
49. Eliot T. O. Slater, "The Inheritance of Mainic-Depressive Insanity and Its Relation to Mental Defect," *Journal of Mental Science*, 82 (1936), 626.
50. René A. Spitz, "Anaclitic Depression," in Ruth S. Eissler, ed., *Psychoanalytic Study of the Child* (New York: International Universities Press, 1946), Vol. 2, p. 313.
51. Edward Stainbrook, "A Cross-Cultural Evaluation of Depressive Reactions," in Paul H. Hoch and Joseph Zubin, eds., *Depression* (New York: Grune & Stratton, 1954).
52. Erwin Stengel, "Über ein periodisch auftretendes Syndrom: Steigerung der Speichelsekretion, Parkinsonistische Motilität, Melancholische Depression," *Archiv für Psychiatrie* 106 (1937), 726.
53. Erwin Stengel, "A Study of Some Clinical Aspects of the Relationship between Obsessional Neurosis and Psychotic Reaction Types," *Journal of Mental Science*, 91 (1945), 166.
54. Erwin Stengel, "Enquiries into Attempted Suicide" (Proceedings of the Royal Society of Medicine, 45 [1952], 613).
55. A. Stensted, "A Study in Manic-Depressive Psychosis," *Acta. Psychiatrica Scandinavia* (1952), Suppl. 79.
56. Alan A. Stone, "A Syndrome of Serious Suicidal Intent," *Archives of General Psychiatry*, 3 (1960), 331.
57. A. C. Tait, J. Harper, and W. T. McClatchey, "Initial Psychiatric Illness in Involutional Women," *Journal of Mental Science*, 103 (1957), 132.

58. Edmund H. Volkart and Stanley T. Michael, "Bereavement and Mental Health," in Alexander H. Leighton, John W. Clausen, and Robert N. Wilson, eds., *Explorations in Social Psychiatry* (New York: Basic Books, 1957).
59. James H. A. Weiss, "Suicide: An Epidemiologic Analysis," *Psychiatric Quarterly*, 28 (1954), 225.
60. Harold G. Wolf and S. Wolf, "Studies on a Subject with a Large Gastric Fistula," *Transactions of the Association of American Physicians*, 57 (1942), 115.
61. World Health Organization Report, *Epidemiological and Vital Statistics Statistical Report* No. 9 (1956), 243.

CHAPTER SIXTEEN

Behavior Disorders Associated with Brain Diseases

Relevance of Brain Diseases for Psychiatry

The behavior disorders associated with diseases or dysfunctions of brain tissue are of practical and theoretical importance for psychiatry. It is distinctly unwise to surrender their diagnosis and therapy to internists and neurologists; but some psychiatrists, on the grounds that the profession should concern itself with purely psychotherapeutic approaches, are inclined to do so. Clinical investigation of these disorders touches on the basic questions of the biological organization of drives, affects, and cognitive processes. The practical importance of accurate diagnosis is evident when exclusively psychotherapeutic treatments are misapplied, or when specific organic treatments are required for organic dysfunctions. These organic disorders constituted about 10 per cent of all patients in the New Haven area; the total prevalence is probably higher. The changing picture of modern medicine is reflected in a decrease of behavior disorders associated with infections and an increase of drug psychoses and behavior disorders associated with atrophic, degenerative, and vascular changes of the central nervous system, some of which are discussed in Chapter 21.

Problems of Diagnosis and Classification

The presence of brain damage and dysfunction often can be deduced from the observation of behavior, but the *absence* of cerebral impairment cannot be diagnosed by the clinical observation of behavior patterns. Clinical classifications of behavior disorders associated with brain syndromes are based on correlations of characteristic behavior patterns with medical and neurological findings. The simple correlation of certain behavioral patterns with neuropathological processes does not really explain the course of a clinical disorder or the behavior present in it with anything approaching a desirable degree of precision. In practice, the physician depends upon the total clinical context, including history, physical and laboratory findings, as well as the positive presence of particular patterns of behavior.

The behavioral features of cerebral impairment have been recognized for centuries. There are three major behavioral syndromes that are commonly correlated with cerebral dysfunctions. These are the various stages of *delirium*, the *dysmnesic syndrome*, and *organic dementia*. *Delirium*, an old term, which has gained little in precision over time, refers to a disturbance of consciousness and manifestations of severe anxiety; it is associated most frequently with febrile diseases, metabolic and vascular disturbances, toxic reactions, and the immediate sequelae of trauma. The *dysmnesic syndrome* is characterized by memory defeats associated with deep cerebral lesions of various kinds; Korsakoff's syndrome is the best-known representative (see also Chapter 23). *Dementia* is encountered with a large number of relatively unchanging or slowly progressive lesions produced by trauma, neoplasm, and by vascular, metabolic, atrophic (senile), degenerative, and chronic inflammatory diseases. Put more succinctly (and not quite correctly), delirium is associated with acute brain syndromes, organic dementia with so-called chronic syndromes; the dysmnesic states may be associated with either. The student must be wary of terminology employed in these disorders, since it has not evolved from a satisfactory view of brain function and neurochemical changes. For example, there is the implication that acute syndromes are reversible and that chronic syndromes are irreversible. Yet it is not always clear whether it is meant that the *behavioral* syndrome is irreversible or the underlying neurophysiological and neurochemical changes. If we are to oversimplify, it is frequently the case that certain active, transient, and general cerebral processes cause delirium and that less active, more focal processes result in cerebral deficits and produce general deterioration. It is well known, however, that delirious syndromes change into chronic deficit states or into a dysmnesic syndrome. Often, delirious syndromes and chronic deficit states coexist. As far as it is known, enduring damage to neuronal elements is irreversible, since regeneration does not occur; however, this anatomical fact does not define functional organization, and behavioral deficit states associated with chronic encephalopathies are not necessarily irreversible. In fact, behavioral improvement may be observed in these conditions. The determining factors are both behavioral (prior personality, learning, motivation, and so forth) and organic (the extent, nature, locus of the cerebral pathology, and the rate of reparative and compensatory changes of nervous, glial, and vascular tissues).

Behavior disorders associated with *acute cerebral pathology* have also been called symptomatic psychoses, acute toxic confusional states, and delirious syndromes. Karl Bonhoeffer grouped these syndromes, in a classical work, as "exogenous reactions," in contrast to the schizophrenias and manic-depressive psychoses, which he assumed were produced by endogenous processes.[8] This is misleading since toxins are, of course, exogenous but largely act through alterations of endogenous neurochemical mechanisms; "endogenous" endocrine intoxication might produce a syndrome similar to an exogenous toxin. There are poisons such as amphetamine that produce behavioral syndromes and lack "organic" behavioral characteristics.[20] The dilemmas of classification are the result of our lack of knowledge of pathophysiological sequences and of the relationships of brain and behavior generally.

Similarly, the syndromes associated with *diffuse chronic brain syndromes* have been referred to as organic dementias or deterioration, and as organic deficit states, and also diffuse cerebral *psychosyndrome.* It is often not clear whether the *diffuseness* referred to is neuropathological or neurobehavioral characteristics and whether it is demonstrable in terms of cellular damage and dysfunction. *Small localized lesions* may produce general and pervasive effects on personality along with deficits in specific skills; large diffuse lesions of brain parenchyma may produce minor specific deficits and only slight alterations in intellectual or personality functioning.

Brain and Behavior Deficit States

A few generalizations concerning our basic and objective knowledge about neurobehavioral correlations are relevant before we review the clinically encountered disorders. A number of primitive responses as well as input channels of the brain appear to be built in. Yet it is apparent that learning and conditioning also partially determine the "localization" of functions and thereby the consequences of lesions, a fact relevant to the variable "functional repair" observed following lesions. Hans-Lucas Teuber presents the view, with which we agree, that specific cerebral systems mediate not only their own activity but also the activity of other areas and systems and that the highest and most complex levels of neural control cannot be organized without interactions of both higher and lower cerebral areas.[90] He finds *both* specific, isolated sensory and neurobehavioral defects and nonspecific or general intellectual impairments in various groups of brain-injured persons.

In general, then, how do specific and general behavioral defects relate to local and general areas of the brain? There appears to be a "gradient toward specialization" of local areas of the brain, which varies with respect to specific functions and areas; Malcolm Piercy proposed that the steepest gradient was probably for language function and reading, and, therefore, small local lesions might be quite damaging to function.[70] Karl Lashley proposed two principles to account for the effects of volumes of tissue, on the one hand, and for specific areas of brain tissue on the other.[53] The principle of "*mass action*" would mean that the more tissue lost, the more function lost; maze-learning ability in rats has been shown to be dependent not on specific areas ablated but on the amount of tissue lost. The second principle, *equipotentiality* of function, applies when it can be shown that there are areas other than the focal lesion that are fully equipped to carry on the behavior; a localized lesion would not then necessarily overtly impair behavior. The principle of *double dissociation,* enunciated by Teuber, applies where different and separable functions are represented, for example, in similar anatomical areas of the two sides of the brain.[90] Depending on the specific neurobehavioral functions studied, one or more of these principles have been found to be operative with brain lesions. For human intelligence as measured by I.Q., large volumes of cerebral tissue can be lost without significant change; thus, mass action does not play a large role. On the other hand, certain aspects of intellectual operations can be selectively impaired by focal lesions, so that the brain is only "somewhat" equipotential for intelligence.[70] It is possible, although not proven, that the greater the level of initial intelligence in man, the greater the protection against the effects of the lesion, although the psychosocial consequences of aphasia to a linguist and to an equally intelligent laborer would clearly be more drastic for the skilled man.

Donald O. Hebb noted that a larger mass of brain is used to develop intellectual abilities than to sustain them.[41] Lesions outside the "language area" have a greater effect on the development of vocabulary in children than in adults; but children recover more rapidly from dysphasias after injuries to local language areas. The principle of mass action appears to be involved in the development of skills; but once skills are highly developed, they then appear vulnerable to focal disruption. Prior learning and experience affect localization of brain functions and their response to injury. The maze-learning of rats raised in a restricted environment was vulnerable to large, nonspecific frontal lesions but not to small occipital lesions, which affected rats reared in a highly visual environment. Neurobehavioral studies also show that the organization or complexity of a learned habit is important. Animals learn to solve problems by discriminating, say, visual stimuli; one problem may be "overlearned," or the animal may "learn to learn" rapidly by wide experience with discrimination problems, thereby acquiring a "learning set."[37] Such sets, even more than specific overlearning, protect animals with focal temporal lobe lesions from the expected impairment both in performance and new learning. The "learning set," however, is lost with highly focal lesions and thus appears to be more focally and complexly organized (and more vulnerable to disruption) than the simple overlearned habit.[70]

Confining our discussion solely to man, we can note a few general facts. Perhaps the only specific objective effect common to a wide gamut of organic lesions in man is that found by Teuber with a test for recognition and discrimination of "hidden figures"; this test identifies brain injury rather than intellectual impairment.[91] Teuber also noted the resiliency and flexibility of the so-called higher functions following brain injury; there may be "intellectual recovery" but a persistence of deficits in the more elementary forms of sensation.[90] In general, posterior cortical lesions affect intellectual and language functions more than anterior lesions, which may be involved in such "dyspraxias" as the inability to start and stop and subtly regulate or modify behavior. For a wide range of functions, the left side of the brain of both left- and right-handed individuals is usually dominant for language. Bilateral lesions of the hippocampus and adjacent deep areas appear specifically vulnerable to producing effects on "consolidation" of input, or the retention aspects of immediate memory. The exceptions and differences in detail from these broad generalizations are great; some will be cited in the discussion of specific problem areas. The student should be aware of the rapid progress that is being made in relating both neurobehavioral and neuroanatomical factors to special and clinical behavioral observations and should recognize that explanations and observations derived from clinically distinguished syndromes have yet to be integrated through basic and clinical research with this developing knowledge in neuropsychology.

The Major Syndromes

Delirium

Disturbance of consciousness is the cardinal symptom of delirium. We can distinguish three different facets of disturbed consciousness: a decrease of vigilance, a disturbance of focussed attention, and a general perplexity and bewilderment. The "clouded consciousness," disorientation, and confusion in delirium are usually quite apparent. Many patients are seemingly slow and dull (they find questions difficult to cope with); they are more or less episodically in a haze and "out of it." They may be outright somnolent but sleep poorly. Many seem in the twilight zone between sleep and wakefulness, and only restricted segments of their ongoing experiences seem to matter; we speak then of a constriction of consciousness. In some cases with a malignant course, the clouding of consciousness may change to coma or subcoma; on the other hand, in cases with a favorable course, the initial coma may be followed by increasing awareness and periods of agitation, until a stable apprehension of the environment is reached. Occasionally, underreactivity is concomitant with psychomotor agitation, which can cycle the patient into a confused panic. Although the majority of patients show a dullness in grasping details, some show an increased alertness. This, to an extent, may be compensatory, an expression of the severe anxiety that is a regular concomitant of these behavior disorders. Whether this is a true hypervigilance (with the exception of delirium tremens) is questionable and, generally, the slowed EEG correlates with the confusion and underresponsiveness.[77] A frequent symptom is distractibility, a shifting of attention to varied elements in the environment, and an inability to concentrate on any one of them. A baffled, dazed, perplexed state, in which recognition of other persons and events seems difficult, is characteristic. Grasp of reality is poor; the unfamiliar is treated as if it were familiar—the hospital staff become members of the family—and hallucinations are common. Familiar persons and sights calm the patient. Disturbances of concentration, memory, and attention may be overshadowed by confusion, disorientation as to time, place, and, finally, person. The hallucinations in deliria are visual and auditory and are not infrequently elaborated by wish and primitive imagery. They often tend, however, to be more social than autistic; for example, the patient may speak to his absent family.

Such patients, whether agitated or underactive, are always anxious and seem haunted and harassed. Whether such anxiety is a direct consequence and primary effect of the basic cerebral changes or whether it is secondary to the altered ability to process input, to the bewildering and frightening perception of the environment, is an open question. Often, delirious patients suffer from severe physical illness, and one component of the anxiety could be in reaction to this unclearly perceived threat to life and limb. Actually, denial of illness in the presence of its objective manifestations is striking, and such denial is frequently observed in such patients.

Severe cases of delirium with rapid onset and a dangerously progressive course are referred to as *acute deliria.* In such cases the patients suffer from very serious illness or from extensive brain injuries; they rapidly become exhausted, dehydrated; and they often develop hyperpyrexia, convulsions, and, subsequently, coma with a high probability of a fatal outcome, the pathogenesis of which is obscure. Just as important as the recognition of this acute and dangerous condition is the recognition of mild or abortive forms of delirium. This is seen in short episodes of febrile delirium in children and in the mild degree of transient confusion in a great many toxic or infectious diseases. Such syndromes are very frequent and escape the attention of physicians, unless they have been trained to recognize them. The symptoms are mild anxiety, some restlessness, oversensitivity to light and noise, emotional lability, transient changes of body feelings or body image, and irritability. The patients find it difficult to concentrate, but they also say that they cannot rest and complain about insomnia. When faced with specific tasks such as tests, they become panicky, seem uncooperative, and become easily disorganized. They also seem briefly not to hear questions (rather than being preoccupied or avoiding questions). They have nightmares, fleeting hallucinations, and a tendency to transient delusional thinking.

Shifts in attention and concentration are the prodromal symptoms and the last to disappear in the natural course of a major delirium. They reflect most sensitively the loosened grip on reality and occur before disorientation, dysmnesia, and a hallucinatory syndrome. Max Levin points out that disorientation as to person, place, and time (in that order) generally clears up before the hallucinatory syndrome, which, in toxic states, can occasionally persist for some weeks.[54] He reasons that orientation is a simple and basic function, but that the ability to think abstractly (that is, without hallucinating) is more complex. Confused states can last for months and should be differentiated from the more active phase of delirium. The Viennese school of psychiatry refers to such states as amentia; the word is inept, but the condition exists.

We distinguish core disorders without difficulty but find cases of acute brain syndrome that are clinically indistinguishable from other major behavior disorders. Many symptomatic psychoses have a striking resemblance to schizophrenic and paranoid syndromes. In some patients, we observe *catatonic syndromes* such as excitement or stupor and mannerisms, perseverations, and characteristic changes of motility. *Epileptiform states* occur and include not only the typical seizures but also the great variety of epileptic equivalents such as "psychic seizures" and dreamlike states—which are described in Chapter 18. Frequently, sweeping mood changes like those in manic-depressive psychosis occur; mild depressions, often quite prolonged, cannot always be differentiated from the underresponsiveness of patients whose sensorium is slightly clouded; such apathy, for unknown reasons, is characteristic of a large class of illnesses such as virus infections, infectious hepatitis, and mononucleosis.

Dysmnesic Syndrome

This syndrome, first mentioned in Syergei S. Korsakoff's classical description,[51] is characterized by a defect in retention and reproduction of newly acquired mnemic material. In severe cases, such things as a simple name or one or two digits cannot be recalled even after a short period of time. Memory for events of the more remote past is usually intact. Of course, in severe dysmnesic cases, the capacity for new learning is grossly diminished. Patients with such defects are generally disoriented and understandably often have a tendency to fill memory gaps with confabulations and a general defensive attitude, which induces them to remain disengaged and uncommitted in most areas of living.

G. A. Talland and coworkers, in extensive clinical and psychological studies of the Korsakoff syndrome, emphasized a marked lack of spontaneity and blandness of affect and observed that confabulation is not a necessary sign of the syndrome.[89] Since the retrieval of old memories prior to illness is generally available, the defect in memory lies in the retaining of new information; new information is registered but, even if affectively significant, is usually not retained. Perceptual changes independent of the memory impairment can be observed; the patients' discriminations are liable to be blunt, and they are prone to miss cues relevant to their tasks; they tend to perseverate and have difficulty in changing their original set. Generally, they perform well on motor tasks, unless given latitude or choice situations, in which case their reaction times are slower. Although reasoning and judgment show no characteristic impairment in tasks where memory function is not involved, the characteristic defect is impairment in serial tasks and failure to resume uncompleted tasks. The defect is evident where sequential integration of information would be necessary for problem-solving, since patients forget both visual and verbal information, losing more with the passage of short periods of time. Talland ascribes all of these defects in dysmnesic patients to "an insufficiently sustained activation," which leaves the patient unable to complete the processes necessary for anything but the most immediate acts of perception. The defect apparently affects the sustaining of an emotional involvement as well as the retrieval of previously registered information.

Wilder Penfield and his associates link the temporal lobe with memory storage.[69] They report interpretive illusions with electrical stimulation of the temporal lobe in conscious patients; *déjà vu* and paramnesias, as well as organized visual hallucinations (which such patients call memories), are elicited. Yet remote memories are generally intact after bilateral hippocampal damage. The hippocampus, in Brenda Milner's opinion, may be concerned with consolidating the immediate memory input rather than serving as a filing cabinet for engrams of past events.[60] In view of the links of the hippocampus with midbrain and diencephalic areas, the pathophysiology of the amnesic syndrome may involve either or both of these structures.

Organic Dementia

Patients with organic dementia suffer cognitive, emotional, and motivational impairment. The essence of the thinking disturbance in organic dementia or deterioration lies in a loss of ability to handle complex and multiple relationships. Kurt Goldstein, in fundamental studies, showed that the patient with chronic brain syndrome is able to handle only concrete but not abstract relationships.[33] Such a patient will stop at a red light but becomes confused and panicky (Goldstein's "catastrophic anxiety") when the light is out of order; to him the light is a concrete event and not one of several imperfect devices used to regulate traffic. We might say the patient is "stimulus bound" and lost without it. The inability to handle symbols of varying complexity in life situations or various sorting tests is seen as a fundamental cognitive deficit of patients with chronic brain syndromes.

It cannot be said that all the behavioral changes are always secondary to the cognitive changes; it is probably best to think of a synchronous deterioration to a lower level of operation of affectively linked cognitive functions. As mentioned previously, we are impressed in a clinical sense more with a general disorganization, desocialization, and regression of the behavior of such patients than with a simple deficit of intellectual functions. Patients functioning at a lower neurobiological level find it difficult to control their emotions and their infantile drives. Their disproportionate anxiety, irritability, dejection, or euphoria is impressive. In some, aggressiveness seems more marked; in others, an unrealistic passive and clinging dependent behavior is evident. In many severely affected patients, primitive, uncontrolled sexual behavior becomes prominent. Masturbation without restraint, oral and anal sexual behavior, exhibitionistic and voyeuristic traits can appear. Thus, the clinical syndromes depend on the degree of intellectual deficit as well as the appearance of pathological affects, the regression of drive behavior, and the nature of the defenses the patients are able to muster. Just how defense mechanisms are related to the many different specific sensorimotor and cognitive defects and general impairment of intelligence is not well appreciated; denial of unpleasant or fearful reality is commonly seen, and a pseudoreligiosity and rigidity are not uncommon mechanisms of control over instinctual wishes and troublesome affects.

From a clinical standpoint, it is important to view intellectual deterioration as a process with differences in severity and progression. Subjective awareness of a loss of function occurs in many normal persons during the years of decline, but this is the exception in pathological deterioration. Early symptoms are apt to be depressive mood swings, a feeling of general inadequacy, and a sense of the effort required for work, rather than recognition of specific intellectual defects. During this *early stage*, patients complain of fatigue, of overwork, and of harassment. Their failures are most conspicuous when they are faced with multiple tasks under pressure or when they are in novel situations and cannot fall back on routine performance. There is frequently a decrease in cultural interests and signs of a coarsening of interpersonal relations. In the educated and refined person, there seems to be a disappearance of the higher individual intellectual and esthetic characteristics, a leveling of the personality. Unexpected outbursts of anxiety and anger and an excessive need to be considered, taken care of, and reassured often puzzle those who are close to them. In organic deficit states, in contrast to behavior disorders in old age (where the family is perhaps overalert for signs of impairment), this first stage usually passes unnoticed.

With inccreasing severity of the process—during the *second stage*—the patient's inefficiency (though not its cause) becomes obvious to everyone but himself. When faced with failure, he is apt to use excuses and alibis: his hearing is failing; the problem was not properly explained to him; or there is an outright refusal to see the failure and its consequences. Patients try to extricate themselves from various obligations or challenges by any number of techniques. When not under pressure, they still appear reasonably normal. Finally, gross impairments in social and intellectual function appear, such as crude, tactless, and impulsive behavior and a resurgence of infantile sexual and aggressive needs. With the deterioration of intellectual aptitudes, there is a decrease in ability for reality- and value-testing; suspicious, paranoid, and megalomanic attitudes and misinterpretation of personal relations and of social or occupational status are common. Memory, attention, and concentration may be impaired; there may be paraphasias and changes in speech as well as a tendency to perseverate and difficulty in changing or maintaining a set.

With the most severe dementia—the *third stage*—the patient is helpless, unable to take care of himself. Intellectual deterioration has reached the point that even the simplest tasks in tests and in everyday living cannot be carried out. Speech and ideas are grossly impoverished; stereotyped or perseverating speech is not uncommon, and in the worst cases no communication at all is possible. The patient, incontinent, now has to be cleaned; he also has to be clothed and fed and requires constant nursing care. The danger of infection and injury is great, and extremely regressive behavior, such as playing with excreta and eating of feces, may occur. Such severe adaptive failures challenge the resources even of hospitals prepared to protect the patient.

Etiological Mechanisms

Causes of Delirium

Delirious syndromes are the result of acute exogenous, noxious physical and chemical factors as well as of certain psychosocial events. If constitutional factors play an etiological role, they are difficult to assess. The noxious factors produce what John Romano and George L. Engel call, in analogy with dysfunctions of other organs, a cerebral insufficiency.[77] The postulations of these investigators rest largely on EEG findings of a general slowing of brain waves, which is correlated with the underawareness or clouding of consciousness. R. Adams and M. Victor, however, reported normal EEG tracings in some cases of delirium.[1] In any event, at this time we are neither able to measure the degree and speed of physical-chemical damage to the brain which produces delirium, nor to identify the biochemical systems involved and the interneural systems affected. There has been a search for the effects of toxins on various aspects of energy metabolism (substrates and steps in electron transport), which could influence efficiency of neuronal function. The active protein and amino acid metabolism of brain, the function of the glutamic acid cycle, and the role of the latter in utilizing endogenous ammonia (which can be psychotoxic) has been under investigation. Similarly, shifts in the metabolism, concentration, and localization of presumed neurotransmitters and neuromodulators (modulating synaptic transmission or neural thresholds) are under study. In general, none of these approaches yields a unitary explanation of cerebral insufficiency. The point is that the neurochemistry of febrile, metabolic, endocrine, and drug psychoses is not just incompletely understood, but what we do understand points to different pathways and mechanisms specific to the different psychoses. In clinical fact, there are differences in course, intensity, onset, and direction of cerebral insufficiency symptoms. With experimental intoxications, different successions and arrays of symptoms with different doses or different drugs may be seen. The tendency for clinical psychiatry to lump all toxic-infectious psychoses into a single behavioral syndrome has unfortunate implications and leads to unwarranted generalizations. The varied symptomatology of these psychoses has been exhaustively reviewed by Werner Scheid.[80]

In general, the acute cerebral processes that produce delirium are correlated with diffuse lesions, but the existence of acute psychotic reactions with mesencephalic and diencephalic lesions is well established. On gross pathological examination, edema (swelling), hyperemia, and multiple small hemorrhages of the brain are found in some cases. On histological examination, acute degenerative changes in the ganglion cells, myelin sheath, and glia are noted. In many cases, in spite of evidence of behavioral symptoms associated with infection or poisoning, no structural or physiological changes of the brain can be demonstrated with current techniques. Sleep deprivation and deprivation of "fast sleep" that accompanies nocturnal dreaming (dream deprivation) combine to produce irritability, illusions, and, occasionally, symptomatic psychoses;[104] the neurophysiological and neurochemical bases for these changes as well as those of pyrexia are now approachable by experimentalists; their results should be of great interest.

Psychosocial Factors in the Etiology of Delirium

Although most symptomatic psychoses can be viewed as cerebral insufficiencies, it would be a grave error to underrate psychosocial events as significant precipitating factors. The previously held assumption that delirious-confused syndromes are only associated with acute anatomically demonstrable brain damage must, in the light of present experimental and clinical evidence, be rejected. The most important precipitating psychosocial event is so-called sensory deprivation. When patients are isolated, immobilized, and understimulated, delirious symptoms are likely to worsen. Typically, these exacerbations occur at night with patients who are in single rooms rather than on wards. They also may occur after operations when patients are unable to move, to see, or to hear. As we indicated earlier (Chapter 6), in the case of the damaged or inefficient brain, actual sensory decrement or motor restraint are important factors. Analogous disturbances can take place under conditions of combined sensory and social deprivation in solitary confinement in prison, on long voyages, and on monotonous drives and flights.[87] The use of isolation and fear as components of the complex procedures by which individuals confess crimes of which they are innocent testifies to the powerful need we have for recognition and stability through social interactions; even punishment and rejection is preferable, perhaps, to isolation. There is no doubt that isolation, coupled with extreme physical and psychological stress (high anxiety), may produce psychotic-like reactions.

Ignorant of speculative advances that lump all isolation, deprivation, and drug effects into one mechanism (such as "loss of ego autonomy"), investigators have continued to sort out different mechanisms for changing contact with the environment and to test for specific and sequential effects. Experimental work in man and animals reveals a number of ways of rearranging those coordinations that normally *prevent* disorientation and illusions and indicate how we keep in tune with a shifting environment while actively moving in relation to it.[92] With phylogenetic complexity there is a greater complexity of feedback systems and an increased dependence on central components of feedback. In man there are regulatory operations (structures or schemata) that anticipate change and "smooth out" discrepancies and variations of input. Discoordination of such mechanisms produces difficulties in adaptation. For example, if man's visual world is inverted by wearing prismatic lenses, he eventually learns to orient. But when such spectacles are removed, he acts as if the world were distorted; presumably, a central compensatory schema, which operated during the world of inverted images, still dominates vision for a time. People coming off a boat often see the world as if it were moving and walk accordingly; the pattern of adjustment to the movement of waves continues to operate while they are on land. Generally, objects as well as expected input-patterns have constancy for us and remain about the same size whatever their distance. The retinal image of a distant object is actually small, but its perceived size is usually constant. If one's hand is held eight inches in front of the eye, and the eye is fixated at a distant object, the hand (which should be larger) will appear diminished in size (and enhance the sense of perspective), indicating the orderly rearrangements of actual retinal projections for perceptual convenience. Micropsias and macropsias are characteristic illusory distortions in deliria, in LSD states, in sleep, and in sensory deprivation; Teuber suggests that they represent the unchecked operation of these normally compensatory processes.[92] What we perceive is generally "unreal," but it *is* ordered and constant and hence can be responded to in an orderly fashion. The lack of coordination of these central schemata with related ongoing sensory and motor processes can produce not only an unreal but also a maladaptive world. These considerations point to man's dependence upon structured and expected inputs that are meaningful in terms of his intentions, directions, and manipulations; this dependence is comprised of complex feedback systems that are crucial for normal operations and vulnerable to impairment at a number of points in altered states.

It is postulated that for every self-induced movement, there is a set of corollary central interneural discharges that inform and "prepare" central sensory systems for the input that is to be anticipated as a result of the movement. When movements of the organism and sensory input are correlated—when the anticipatory structures are correct—constancy and smoothness of performance occurs. Future study may reveal the importance of such interneural "lead" systems, or internal schema, in regulating psychological functions other than the spatial organization of perception and in introducing confusion when "unhooked" from their input-output controls.

Given the impaired cognitive and orienting capacity of the person with cerebral insufficiency, any severe psychological stress, but particularly those which produce strong fear, is apt to contribute to the outbreak of a delirium or to aggravate it. The most important fear of such patients is the fear produced by the severe illness: the threat of invalidism and death. Often, symptomatic psychoses are precipitated when vulnerable patients, especially old people, are merely brought to a new, complex, and confusing environment, which is also frightening, such as a hospital or exposure to threatening medical-surgical procedures. Whereas strangeness and anxiety have a disintegrating effect, familiarity with supporting and interested persons in a friendly environment quite impressively helps the patient's reorganization. Personality factors predisposing to delirium are poorly understood. In all probability, considering the range of pathways and symbolically meaningful transactions that support integrity of function, there are few persons with a uniform "general" vulnerability to any toxic state. Vulnerability depends on the nature and strength of the various precipitating and conditioning factors, together with the psychological adaptations that are ready to be mustered for such states. D. X. Freedman and A. J. Benton, for example, found no greater sensitivity to the usual effects of LSD in alcoholics with a history of several episodes of delirium than in normals.[27] The changes of consciousness, arousal, and orientation observed in deliria are conceivably the result of impaired function of activating systems and altered feedback to central regulatory functions. Such cerebral dysfunction can be produced by chemicals, by an alteration of sensory inputs, and possibly even by extreme anxiety and denial of reality or by a combination of all these factors. The dysmnesic syndrome is usually the result of severe and more lasting brain damage, frequently in the diencephalic and mesencephalic regions. It cannot be clearly allocated either to the acute or chronic encephalopathies.

Causes of Organic Dementia

Enduring brain damage is the necessary and essential cause of organic deficit states, but we are far from understanding completely how the destruction or impairment of cerebral cells produces deterioration. Besides the neural factors, there are very important contributing behavioral factors that shape the clinical picture of every case. The neurological diseases causing deficit states are neoplastic, inflammatory, vascular, or degenerative. In general, they are diffuse, involving cortical and subcortical areas. The importance of the size of the lesion and of compensatory cerebral mechanisms was stated previously.

It is usually difficult to distinguish between behavior contingent upon primary cerebral deficit, release mechanisms, and restitutive processes. It is almost equally difficult to establish the primary behavioral loss and distinguish it from secondary reactions such as denial of illness and attempts to adjust at a lower level of function and to relearn new responses. Furthermore, there are reactions as the result of the new social role of a person with behavioral deficit that complicate the picture. As in all illnesses, the psychosocial factors of the patient's life situation have a bearing on symptoms and the course of the organic syndrome. The course of these illnesses is adversely influenced if organic deterioration is particularly threatening, as in persons whose livelihood depends on an exceptionally well-functioning brain; or when the patient has had a previous history of precarious adjustment; or if the desirable social support of the patient by family and friends is lacking; or if medical personnel are insensitive to the patient's needs.

Local Brain Damage Associated with Behavior Disorders

So far, our discussion has centered on behavior disorders largely associated with diffuse or extensive brain damage. There is also substantial evidence for the existence of behavior pathology associated with local brain damage; indeed, as we have indicated, strategic lesions affecting midbrain, hypothalamic, limbic, or frontal circuits may be quite effective in altering personality.

Manfred Bleuler assumes that patients with local brain damage suffer from relatively mild personality disorders, which he called *local cerebral psychosyndrome.*[7] He describes this as characterized by an increase or decrease of basic drives such as hunger, thirst, sexuality, and aggression. Changes of mood, such as mild depressions and hypomanic states, are frequent and occur in an unpredictable fashion. Patients are either impulsive or apathetic. Intellectual changes are not found. Such persons impress their fellow human beings, not as mentally ill, but as odd, queer, strange, and bizarre personalities. Certainly the syndrome is extraordinarily broad; Bleuler assumes that it also occurs in local brain damage after head injuries, in epileptics, and in patients with endocrine diseases. The latter group Bleuler calls the *endocrine psychosyndrome.* Certainly, many sociopathic personalities and patients with severe character neuroses show the above characteristics without any biological evidence of cerebral damage. Detailed correlations between such hypothetical or proved local brain damage and behavioral changes have not been established. In our experience, some of the behavioral changes, such as mood changes, may be partially explained in well-studied patients by a minute knowledge of the psychosocial dynamics. In spite of these reservations, many patients, for example, some patients with endocrine diseases, show the pathological behavior Bleuler mentions. Other syndromes have been described, such as low frustration tolerance and enhanced impulsivity in postencephalitic disorders and the "minimally damaged" hyperkinetic child with distractability and perceptual disturbances. Finally, it should be noted that compensatory personality developments—rigidity, suspicion, isolation, or whatever—may occur when there is an underlying chronic and covert deficit in perception and affect. For example, the odd sensory experiences of mild, undetected psychomotor epilepsy may generate such reactive developments. Generally, neuropsychologists warn that where clinicians subsume an array of symptoms into broad syndromes, specific patterns of defects are obscured. The only manifestations of behavior deficit that seem clearly linked with local cortical damage are the aphasias, agnosias, and apraxias. Even in these disturbances, we are now inclined to assume that specific and general loss of function coexist and are intrinsically interwoven.

Aphasias, Agnosias, and Apraxias

Aphasia is a cerebral disturbance of symbolic linguistic function that must be distinguished from anarthria, which is caused by peripheral, nuclear, and supranuclear lesions of the phonetic apparatus. *Agnosia* refers, in the usage of most experts, to an impairment of recognition and of cerebral perceptual organization in the absence of impairment of the sense organs. *Apraxia* is a cerebral dysfunction in which patients without any impairment of the subcortical and peripheral motor system are unable to plan and carry out motor acts. The differentiation between general deterioration and the foregoing dysfunctions, however, is by no means simple or clear. Actually, our knowledge of aphasias, agnosias, and apraxias is still (as Henry Head put it, decades ago[39]) in a chaotic state. There are several reasons for this: We lack a good and universally accepted theory of speech, language, and of higher mental function. We rely totally in this field on clinical observations of development and impairment of speech, gnosis, and praxis; animal observations, although pointing to a variety of principles concerning the analysis of brain function, have taught us relatively little about these human functions of speech. Until recently, there have been no statistically reliable approaches to the vast and varied clinical material.[101] For all these reasons, we are still struggling with the most basic problems, particularly whether the aphasias and related disorders can be viewed as the dysfunctions of an instrumental skill or whether the impairment of speech is invariably linked with a more general impairment of higher mental function.[32] Today more than ever we are inclined to assume the latter, although R. M. Reitan has currently argued to the contrary, showing data from some nonverbal tests in which aphasics do comparatively better.[75] Hebb, on the other hand, pointed out that implicit verbalization is usually required in many of the tasks psychologists devise and that simply increasing the complexity of tasks can, per se, impair the performance of the aphasic.[40] The location of the specific lesion and the type of aphasia as well as initial skill and intelligence appear differentially to affect the extent of "general impairment." Aphasias usually involve lesions of the left hemisphere with some latitude in the areas involved; the left hemisphere appears generally to dominate verbal activity. Injuries to this hemisphere produce diminished performance on verbal tests whether or not aphasia is present. Milner developed an intracarotid amytal test: injection in the artery ipsilateral to the injured hemisphere produces aphasia.[62] Such techniques, she found, give convincing evidence that the left hemisphere is dominant for language, especially in right-handed persons and in the majority of left-handed individuals. However, recovery from aphasia in left-handed individuals is more rapid, and there is also evidence that partial bilateral representation of language in left-handed or ambidextrous persons is present. Psychiatrists should be competent to carry out a brief and simple examination of aphasic, agnosic, and apractic patients. A listing of the essentials of such a procedure follows:

1. Recording of spontaneous speech and comprehension of patient in ordinary conversation. Note complete or incomplete ability to speak; paucity of speech or increased production of speech; telegram style, aggramatism; echolalia; perseveration; searching for words; inability to remember words, particularly those not of practical importance to the patient.
2. Testing of comprehension by simple commands.
3. Testing of ability to repeat words.
4. Naming of objects. This is particularly important for the diagnosis of amnestic aphasia.
5. Testing for reading and comprehension of written material.
6. Testing of ability to write spontaneously or on dictation and ability to copy words, letters, simple drawings.
7. Ability to understand figures and carry out simple calculations.
8. Recognition of familiar objects, either by naming them or by pointing at them. Recognition of forms and colors.
9. Recognition of such physical defects as hemiplegia, blindness, deafness, and aphasia; recognition of parts of one's body, particularly extremities and fingers.
10. Ability to carry out simple, meaningful acts such as buttoning one's clothing, lighting a match, winding a watch, shaking hands.
11. Recognition of music; pitch, rhythm, chords and melodies.
12. Determination of a change in experience of time; slow or fast motion experiences.

In motor or expressive aphasia, first described by Paul Broca,[13] patients are unable to speak spontaneously; they utter only a few words, usually when they are excited, and these are generally stereotyped or overlearned phrases; for example, expletives. Often these patients have insight to their difficulty. Repetition of words spoken by the examiner may be possible, particularly during recovery. Unvocalized speech and ability to comprehend are relatively intact. (For instance, such patients can tap syllables.) Sometimes an inability to write (agraphia) is present. Self-initiated verbal articulation, *dyslexia,* and difficulties in reading tend to be most correlated with discrete and localized lesions. In classical cases, the lesion is located in the foot of the third frontal gyrus of the left hemisphere, but any lesion in the lower Rolandic area may produce motor aphasia.

Sensory or receptive aphasia is an inability to understand words and sentences, invariably accompanied by severe impairment of motor speech. Speech becomes unintelligible (jargon speech) and agrammatical; at times patients speak in a telegram style, but more often there is an increased flow of speech. Ordinarily, patients are unaware of the defect. *Agraphia* and an inability to read (*alexia*) are invariably present. The lesions first described by Carl Wernicke were in the anterior part of the first and second temporal gyrus of the dominant hemisphere.[102] Localization of these aphasias is by no means reliable. In lesions involving the temporoparietal region and the Island of Reil, the defects are severe. These *central or global aphasias* are characterized by a complete inability to speak and understand and by agraphia and alexia. These patients usually appear confused and deteriorated.

Amnestic aphasia is the inability to recall names of familiar objects. At one time, such a defect was thought to be caused by lesions of the dominant angular gyrus, but we know that such a precise localization is not possible. Kurt Goldstein showed that patients with an amnestic aphasia are able to name objects correctly in a concrete but not in an abstract context;[34] for example, when he is about to drink coffee, a patient will name the cup correctly but will be unable to do so in a hypothetical or test situation.

Semantic aphasia is a term coined by Henry Head, referring to the language disorders of patients with organic deterioration.[39] It cannot be localized; all language modalities are disturbed: speaking, understanding, and recall of words. Speech is generally impoverished, and such patients often perseverate markedly.

The lesions underlying most *agnosias* cannot be precisely localized. In fact, the concept has come under sharp attack from neuropsychologists working with special tests to identify specific defects and analyze their underlying interrelationships. If one ponders the question, the existence of specific centers in which "knowing" or recognition is truly a specialized function would substantially rearrange our concept of consciousness and its neural basis. Head pointed out that in most agnosias, visual field defects were present as well as dementia; in any event, if true agnosia exists at all, it is quite rare. Apparent cases of agnosia show abnormally rapid fading or adaptation in those parts of the visual field that appear normal under conventional testing. H. L. Teuber and M. B. Bender[93] reported defects in flicker-fusion threshold and defects of perception of movement and of dark adaptation; altered tachistoscopic thresholds of contour recognition have been noted in the intact field. Therefore, "primary" defects in the receptive apparatus may be involved, although the analysis of receptive and recognition defects requires further animal and human study. Clinically, it is particularly difficult in patients with agnosias to differentiate the general deterioration from specific deficits. A large number of agnostic syndromes, with lesions in the major occipital lobe, have been described: the different alexias, the inability to recognize geometric forms, an agnosia for colors, and the agnosia for objects and pictures, as well as an agnosia for mathematical symbols.[67] Among the auditory agnosias, an inability to recognize musical sounds and tunes, usually combined with a musical apraxia, has aroused interest. In such cases, lesions in both temporal lobes, but especially of the right side, have been found.

J. Babinski described an agnosia in which patients with a hemiplegia and a lesion of the subcortex of the marginal gyrus of the minor hemisphere do not recognize their own limbs and assume that they belong to someone else.[3] A related phenomenon, denial of blindness, described first by G. Anton, was found to occur in lesions of association fibers between occipital, temporal, and lower parietal lobes.[72] Edward A. Weinstein and Robert L. Kahn showed that such denial of illness cannot be strictly localized and that it actually serves a very broad defensive psychosocial function of patients who are severely threatened by dysfunction and illness.[100] Similar explanations may be applied to the complicated and interesting phenomenon of phantom limb, in which patients continue to experience the vivid existence of a lost part of their bodies; however, in this instance, explanations based on the activation (or unchecked persistence) of central schemata by unconscious self-induced attempts to move the missing limb must be considered.[50]

Among the *apraxias*, the inability to plan and execute simple skilful acts and gestures was described by Hugo Liepmann as ideokinetic apraxia.[56] The loss of the ability to write, or agraphia, is the most important apractic syndrome. Ideomotor apraxia refers to inability to imitate or execute hand movements and ideational apraxia to the loss of ability to use common objects; for example, matches are picked up but the rest of the sequence is forgotten; a loss or agnosia of the concept for habitual movements is implied. A syndrome of acalculia, confusion of right and left, finger agnosia and agraphia was described by J. Gerstmann and placed in the major angular gyrus;[28] Arthur L. Benton and others have challenged this concatenation of "parietal" defects.[4]

At the conclusion of this brief excursion into aphasias, agnosias, and apraxias, we wish to emphasize that new approaches are emerging. In extension of the fundamental contributions of Head, Goldstein, Teuber and A. R. Luria, sophisticated psychophysiological explorations show that specific localized loss of function is always associated with more general behavioral deficit and that the dissociation of "higher and lower" functions is conceptual rather than grounded in the facts of neurological organization. Better statistical evaluation and correlation of psychological and neuropathological material has begun to raise doubts about much of the previously held interpretations and localizations.

Special Syndromes

For a time, in a literal extension of Jackson's evolutionary theory, all that was distinctly human and "higher" was ascribed to frontal lobe dominance. More recently acquired clinical and experimental knowledge has required a different definition of "higher," since frontal lobe lesions have little impact on purely intellectual functions. Rather, they may produce variable alterations in behavior, in judgment, motivation, and social involvement and appropriateness, and this has led to such laudatory epigrams as the frontal lobe being the lobe of culture and civilization. In animals, the chief specific effect localized to lesions of the frontal and not other lobes is a failure on delayed response; in a version of the shell game, one of two cups is baited in full view and a shield briefly interposed before the animal chooses the baited cup. Animals with frontal lobe lesions, with otherwise intact memory, do not make the correct response. This is thought to represent a defect in visual kinesthetic integration, and some special defects related to this have been shown in man.[94] Milner has identified a tendency to perseverate, an inability to change a previously successful set, even though errors are apparent to the patient; this dysfunction may be linked to motivational factors.[61] The striking deficits are in the behavior of patients; they become insensitive and unconcerned in their social relations and careless of their appearance. They may neglect duties at work and with family and friends; they are tactless and rude, more with apparent lack of concern than with aggression. In some patients, this is combined with a silly euphoria referred to by its German designation as *Witzelsucht*, a tendency to stoop to practical joking with disregard of the feelings of others and social taboos. In other patients, a lack of incentive or lack of control has been noted. Luria[57] observed that speech cannot be effectively used for control; he observes a defect related to set and activation, since what he calls the "prestarting" mechanism is disturbed. In expanding lesions, memory and recall are relatively intact, and there is usually no clouding of consciousness. Psychological changes often appear before such frontal lobe signs as forced grasping and sucking reflexes and dysphasic, dyspractic symptoms. After removal of the expanding lesion, considerable restitution of functions occurs in most patients, provided no diffuse damage exists. With unilateral lesions, neither psychological nor neurological signs may be apparent. It should also be clear that the indifference, carelessness, and shortsightedness of mild frontal lobe states are not mandatory but probable; the factor of the prior personality must be taken into account. The extent to which the lobe is concerned in particular kinds of anticipation (such as the anticipation of anxiety), as well as the use of imagination for planning, is not at all clear. The links of the frontal lobe with the hypothalamus and activating systems still require further investigation; some of the effects of frontal lobe surgery for intractable pain have been compared to those of morphine, that is, inducing indifference to pain during the recognition of its presence. Given these observations, it is likely that affective evaluation and appreciation of input are impaired; the overanticipation—normally linked to pain and distress—is diminished.

Recently there has been a strong interest in temporal lobe lesions, particularly those correlated with convulsive seizures and altered subjective states (see Chapter 18). After cardiac-resuscitation and after the use of dialysis, the "artificial kidney" in severe poisoning with barbiturates or following open cardiac surgery in which there has been cardiac arrest, a *syndrome of decerebration* has been noted when the patient awakens from coma. All complex psychic activities, as well as the most primitive orientation reactions, are extinguished; these patients have an entirely "vegetative" existence. On occasion even such patients have shown considerable improvement, regaining primitive speech and memory and the ability to perform in a simple and concrete manner.

Diagnosis of Behavior Disorders Associated with Cerebral Syndromes

The diagnostic procedures in behavior disorders associated with cerebral disease follow very definite steps: (1) The psychiatric interview examination to detect delirium, dysmnesic state, or organic deficit. (2) Psychological testing, particularly special tests designed to detect confusion, memory defects, intellectual and emotional impairment at an early stage when clinical scrutiny can only raise "suspicions" of pathological organic processes (see Chapter 8). (3) Physical and especially neurological examination to determine localization and type of cerebral lesions, and relevant laboratory procedures. In many cases, radiological and EEG examinations are necessary; in a few deficit reactions, air encephalograms and angiograms are also indicated. The intravenous amytal test can bring out residual defects but is not applicable in initial diagnosis.

Assessment of the emotional and social factors that contribute to the syndrome and the understanding of the psychodynamics of delirious and deteriorated patients is a difficult task; it calls for much sensitivity and ingenuity. Grasp of the social environment of the patient, particularly his relations with his immediate family, is essential. Because the latter data are so difficult to obtain with patients who suffer from acute and chronic brain syndromes, our workup, formulation and conclusions often remain woefully inadequate. This is regrettable because very often proper therapy depends on the understanding of psychosocial factors. The behavior of these patients is not a meaningless kaleidoscope of weird symptoms but reflects capacities, stresses, and conflicts as well as immediate and remote needs.

Fully developed delirious syndromes are easily diagnosed; early and atypical syndromes often defy definitive diagnosis. Alteration of consciousness, which undoubtedly is the cardinal symptom, may be very difficult to detect. The differential diagnosis of delirium from schizophreniform psychoses (such as oneirophrenia with its dreamy states) can, as we have indicated, be extremely difficult. In some delirious-confused syndromes, as in certain psychoses of pregnancy and puerperium, a diagnosis can be established only after prolonged observation. In some cases, deficit states develop after deliria; in others schizophrenic syndromes emerge. A precise differentiation of delirium and deficit states also is not always possible. Figuratively speaking, the damage of deficit reactions can be clearly discerned only after the storm has passed.

Theoretically, chronic organic deficit states are easily diagnosed. Intellectual deficit must be present. In incipient cases and in those cases for which M. Bleuler postulates local brain damage, the diagnosis may be difficult or impossible. Only repeated careful clinical observations and special tests can establish such early behavioral and neural deficits. Clinicians generally have not acquainted themselves with the studies of the microanatomy of behavior that occupy neuropsychologists who have devised special tests of discrimination and sensorimotor function, or tasks demanding different levels of problem-solving. To an extent, the clinical psychological tests employed in personality diagnosis (see Chapter 8) suggest correlations with brain damage generally; sometimes, however, the data correlate with specific syndromes. Reitan,[74] who employs a battery of neuropsychological tests derived from Ward C. Halstead's tests,[35] has had a degree of success in identifying not only the presence of lesions but also whether that lesion is diffuse or localized, and on which side of the brain it is located. Obviously, such tests do not have the capacity to define neuropathological processes or the intricate neurochemistry of the lesion. Even though there is precision in describing specific defects, it is generally not easy to "explain" the clinical phenomena and the consequences to the personality from such test data. Much of the differential diagnostic efforts, of course, are concerned with the differentiation and localization of the underlying cerebral and general disease. In general, however, the basic neurological and general illness does not have a rigidly specific impact on the clinical picture.

The differential diagnosis from schizophrenia is not always simple. We tend to describe the disturbances of attention and primitive thought of the schizophrenic in terms of motivations and alteration of complex coding operations (such as identity and symbolization), which have to do with meaning, object relations, and communications. The schizophrenic's austistic distortions of person, time, and place do not appear to be simple confusional defects nor confabulations or attempts to "cover up" an inability to perceive the environment. The schizophrenic lacks a goal directed "set"; he generally is not perceived to be struggling to approximate a reality that the patient with organic disease, due to aphasia, confusion, memory deficit or deterioration appears to be reaching for, if he is at all able. But such distinctions do not hold as precisely either for the acute schizophrenic (who may occasionally appear basically well preserved but "toxic") nor for the symptomatic psychosis or the dementing organic, whose regression may be bizarre. The schizophrenic is also said to be "trying" (his symptoms are "restitutive") even though the motivation toward reality is impaired. In fact, we find too many gray areas, and this convinces us that such comparisons will not replace the careful study of pathogenic sequences over time; for example, the rate and suddenness of change in organic conditions could, among other factors, account for some of the behavioral differences in the two disorders. The use of words and symbols in a wide range of organic and schizophrenic thought disorders has not yet been sufficiently distinguished by formal tests and clinical observation and needs to be defined by further research.

Principles of Therapy of Behavior Disorders Associated with Brain Disease

Treatment of Symptomatic Psychoses

As most acute symptomatic psychoses are concomitant with disease, injury, or poisoning, treatment of the underlying pathological process is of paramount importance. The milder forms are rarely seen by psychiatrists but rather by other medical and surgical specialists and by general practitioners. In treating the basic disease, therapists often must face the dilemma that certain drugs, effective for the treatment of the underlying illness, will possibly aggravate the symptomatic psychoses; for example, cortisone used in the treatment of lupus erythematosis may in itself produce a symptomatic psychosis.[58, 71] When such treatment is vital, the therapist has no choice but to risk aggravation of the psychosis. Most patients with symptomatic psychoses require medication with sedating and tranquilizing drugs. Paraldehyde and chloral hydrate are preferable to barbiturates. The phenothiazines and chlordiazepoxide are effective. Proper dietary measures and care in avoiding dehydration, hyperthermia, and physical exhaustion are important. Delirious patients need skilful nursing and constant supervision. Patients are apt to injure themselves; they may fall out of bed or wander off the wards; all too often they are seriously suicidal. They are invariably anxious, often panicky and agitated, but, in general, we have learned to use physical restraint most sparingly. Nurses and other hospital personnel must try to alleviate the aggravating feelings of fright and strangeness. In some respects, delirious patients must be handled as children with nightmares; a light should be left on at night, and close contact with warm, reassuring, mothering persons is important. Such patients can handle only relatively simple messages and should be kept, whenever possible, in settings with which they are familiar. Exposure to stressful procedures (for example, enemas) may throw some delirious patients into a panic. Some postoperative deliria, particularly in elderly patients, can be avoided by skillful psychological preparation and expert supportive handling during and after the feared procedures.

Treatment of Patients with Chronic Organic Deficit States

Apart from specific medical or surgical therapies, which require cooperation with other specialists, certain general principles are important for the treatment of behavior disorders associated with chronic brain disease. Most of these patients suffer and make others suffer, not just because of their deterioration, but because they are anxious, angry, and suspicious and because they are often mistreated and badly handled. The psychotic reactions of such patients are the consequences of neurological lesions as well as responses to social and interpersonal stresses. If the deteriorated patient is kept in a job he cannot manage; if he is abruptly discharged from his responsibilities; or if he is made to feel that he is a burden or disgrace to his family and humiliated in his helplessness and his rational and irrational need for affection he will respond with inappropriate behavior. All patients with organic brain disease need psychotherapeutic guidance based on a grasp of the environmental stresses and the patient's abilities. It is essential to pay attention to hypochondriacal responses and to a defensive denial of illness; denial need not necessarily be combated, but its presence should be appreciated by the caretaking staff. An important decision is that of determining when it is desirable to hospitalize a patient with behavior disorder associated with brain disease. Apart from the hospitalization required for a thorough examination and workup, the present trend is to hospitalize only the very sick, helpless, and deteriorated patient with deficit reactions. Treatment of any patient with organic brain disease requires close work with family members. We believe that in many patients with chronic organic brain disease, psychotic reactions can be avoided or substantially reduced by individual and group counseling of family members. Patients will do best in an environment which is supportive and stable. Lest we forget, families of such patients also require support and information.

Three recent developments in the therapy of patients with organic behavior deficit must be stressed. The first is the use of phenothiazines and chlordiazepoxide in some patients, which has helped not merely to "subdue" them chemically, but in many cases to reduce overwhelming anxieties and to establish contact, a prerequisite for further therapy. The second advance is the recent progress in retraining patients with localized brain damage; for example, patients with the aphasias, motor and sensory deficits, as well as patients with diffuse encephalopathies and severe behavior disorders. The third advance is the prevention of the patients' regression, whenever this is possible. These measures make the theraputic outlook for patients with all types of organic behavior disorder more hopeful than a short time ago. Even when specific therapy is not available, it is more rewarding to use a psychosocial approach with such patients than to view them in detached fashion as interesting specimens of cerebral pathology.

Symptomatic Psychoses in Infectious Diseases

Cerebromeningeal Infections

The symptoms of behavior disorders associated with infectious diseases of the central nervous system vary from very slight clouding of consciousness, barely noticeable except to a careful and experienced observer, to extremely severe and fatal syndromes. Delirious symptoms accompanying the different types of suppurative and non-suppurative leptomeningitis, brain abscess, and sinus thrombosis are frequent.[80] Meningococcus septicemia produces a severe delirium. Mental retardation and antisocial behavior disorders as sequels to suppurative, viral, and tuberculous meningitis in infancy have been observed; invariably in these diseases, of course, not only the meninges but the brain is affected. Apart from their occurrence in tuberculous meningitis, symptomatic psychoses in tuberculous patients are rare unless associated with drug psychosis. The emotional lability, oversensitivity, apparent overconcern, and also denial of illness observed in tuberculosis are primarily the result of the peculiar conditions of living and therapeutic treatment to which a number of tuberculous patients are still subjected.

ENCEPHALITIS The most important category in this group is lethargic encephalitis, first described by Constantin von Economo in his classic work *Die Encephalitis Lethargica*.[24] Economo studied the acute and subacute cases of a pandemic that circled the globe between 1916 and 1917. At present, there are no acute cases. Patients suffer from various disturbances of the sleep mechanism, which include not only drowsiness but also insomnia and reversal of sleep rhythm. Another characteristic symptom is dysfunction of the internal and external eye muscles. The most important of these are a disturbance of convergence and the occurrence of so-called oculogyric crises or involutionary rotating of the eyes. With oculogyric crises, which occur mostly in the subacute and chronic stage, the patient often experiences obsessive thoughts of an aggressive nature. Other frequent symptoms are choreiform and myoclonic twitching and generalized convulsions. The major disturbances are explained by the crucial inflammatory lesions in the regions of the oculomotor nuclei, the tectum, and the central gray of the sylvian aqueduct. The acute phase lasts from a few days to several weeks, with a mortality rate varying from 5 to 75 per cent. Among the sequelae, the symptoms of postencephalitic Parkinsonism and certain enduring behavior disorders are most important. The psychiatric symptomatology is rich and varied, running the gamut from severe organic deficit states to paranoid, catatonic, schizophreniform, and manic-depressive symptoms.[12] Some patients have shown a marked tendency to develop obsessive symptoms. Impulsive, aggressive behavior is frequently observed. In children, mental retardation as well as extremely asocial aggressive and sexual behavior have been noted as sequelae.

In other forms of encephalitis, such as *St. Louis encephalitis, Japanese encephalitis,* and *inclusion encephalitis,*[11] symptoms of delirium and stupor have been found. Any neurotropic virus—and new varieties continue to be found—may produce an aseptic meningitis or encephalitis, some with only transitory mental signs. Postencephalitic changes vary from mild behavior syndromes of poor impulse control to severe symptomatic psychoses and organic deficit states; the symptoms, as in Economo's encephalitis, depend on the location of the lesion. Acute rabies encephalitis produces in man apathy, drowsiness, and delirious reactions; hyperirritability has been noted but, contrary to legend, not biting. These patients have painful and excruciating spasmodic contractions following food and water intake (hence the term *hydrophobia*). A symptomatic psychosis has been described in *toxoplasmosis* with lesions in the regions of the Ammon's horn and the mammillary bodies. Delirious reactions have also been noted in *acute chorea*. The behavior disorders in syphilitic infections of the central nervous system, which rarely take the form of acute symptomatic psychoses, are discussed in a later section.

General Infections

In cerebromeningeal infections the brain is directly affected, but its involvement in other infections associated with behavior disorder is indirect. Symptomatic psychoses in various forms of *pneumonia* are not infrequent, although modern methods of treatment have helped to reduce the severity and frequency of this complication. In pneumonococcus pneumonia, delirious reactions are more typical, whereas depression and apathy are characteristic symptoms of virus pneumonia. Although delirium usually occurs during the height of the febrile period, it may be seen in the period of defervescence, particularly in older, physically weak patients. The prognosis in such defervescence and *exhaustion psychoses* may be quite serious. Many severe bacterial diseases such as *streptococcal infections, typhoid fever, typhus* are accompanied by delirious reactions. French psychiatry still assumes that intestinal infections—*les encéphalites coli bacillaires*—have a special significance in the etiology of symptomatic psychoses. In the French literature, there are numerous reports of symptomatic psychoses associated with *ascarides* and *echinococcus infestations*. Another disease group that is still of great epidemiological importance and that produces symptomatic psychosis is *malaria*. In acute cases, particularly of tropical malaria, delirious reactions occur; in the subacute and chronic patients, apathy and depression are characteristic. Some psychotic reactions occurring in malaria are not produced by the infection but by atabrine; paranoid, depressive, and schizophreniform symptoms have been observed. Symptomatic psychoses occur in *rheumatic fever;* they have been ascribed to hyperpyrexis but may have other causes.

Symptomatic Psychoses in Internal Diseases

H. B. Rome and D. B. Robinson reviewed the symptomatic psychoses in severe *cardiac, hepatic, pancreatic, renal, and metabolic diseases*.[78] The symptoms in these diseases vary from mild, fleeting states of confusion and underawareness to panic, agitation, and delirium. In certain decompensated cardiac diseases, particularly in aortic stenosis and mitral insufficiency, psychotic reactions are relatively frequent. Just what the pathophysiological processes are is not known; hypoxia is undoubtedly an important factor, but the significance of psychosocial factors is also quite apparent. Any stressful stimuli that produce general anxiety or specific fear of death or of being incapacitated, humiliated, provoked, or deserted may contribute to the eruption of a delirious episode in such patients. The behavior disorders in arteriosclerosis and hypertensive brain disease are discussed in Chapter 21.

Symptomatic psychoses contingent upon severe *diabetes* are rare. Usually they are delirious episodes, although in chronic and terminal cases permanent organic deficit reactions have been noted. The neurochemical basis for such states is not clear, although the vascular disease associated with severe diabetes cannot be an insignificant factor. Symptomatic psychoses in *spontaneous hypoglycemic states* are usually of short duration and correspond closely to the altered brain metabolism.[19] Altered states of consciousness; changes of body image; dizziness or anxiety; or autonomic symptoms and complaints referred to the body that are episodic and show a periodicity sometimes related to food intake should alert the physician to this condition. The psychiatric and neurological symptoms of these reactions have become familiar to psychiatrists since the introduction of insulin therapy for schizophrenia and have been described in Chapter 11. Delirious psychoses associated with internal diseases also occur when patients are debilitated, partially exsanguinated, or in terminal conditions. Such reactions have been referred to as *exhaustion deliria*. The term has also been applied to deliria following prolonged exertion, sleep deprivation, and starvation. The following case illustrates a typical symptomatic psychosis associated with pancreatitis.

A fifty-year-old, white, married attorney was admitted to a community hospital with the chief complaint, "My stomach has been hurting." Approximately forty-eight hours prior to admission, following an alcoholic binge on New Year's Eve, the patient developed midline epigastric pains unrelieved by milk or alkali and associated with nausea and vomiting. The patient had a long history of intermittent colicky right upper quadrant pain associated with fatty food intake. Physical examination at the time of admission was compatible with the diagnosis of acute pancreatitis. Serum amylase on admission was 291 units and rose to 595 the following day. Forty-eight hours after admission, the patient became increasingly agitated and on the third day after admission developed auditory and visual hallucinations, sweating, and tremulousness; he heard accusatory voices and hallucinated judges and lawyers arguing about his fate. Further, the hospital staff were seen as disguised FBI personnel involved in a master plot to imprison him. On the fourth hospital day, the patient became combative, because: "I'm being held against my will and I have legal rights to leave. Who are you, the FBI?" He refused liquid by mouth, saying,

"I'm sure it would be poison." He complained, "I think I'm being taken to the state prison." The patient told the psychiatric resident, "Get out of here, you S.O.B. . . . I want to see a fire marshal." He jumped past two aides and pulled a fire alarm in the hospital corridor, "in order to stop the train and get the firemen so that I can be free."

Transferred to the psychiatric service, he received 2.5 mg. of perphenazine intramuscularly and calmed down considerably within a half-hour. On the following day he was fully oriented and felt quite contrite about his previous behavior which, in part, he attributed to his guilty concern over repeatedly breaking his physician's stern prohibition of drinking. The patient was maintained on perphenazine, 4 mg. q.i.d., plus chlordiazepoxide 30 mg., t.i.d., in decreasing dosage, the drugs finally being discontinued on the twelfth day after admission.

He was transferred back to the surgical service, at which time he was fully alert and oriented. His liver and pancreatic tests were within normal limits, and he was soon discharged as much improved.

Prior to hospitalization, the patient had had no psychiatric contact. Although he had been drinking three to six cocktails a day for many years, there had been no decrease in his work performance, which was satisfactory. The events surrounding his New Year's binge and his need for daily intake of alcohol were not revealed, nor was his rebellion against the medical regimen directed toward pancreatitis readily explained.

Symptomatic Psychoses in Nutritional Deficiencies

It is difficult to assess the role of general malnutrition in psychotic reactions. Most such reactions cannot be explained by malnutrition alone. They often occur under extreme and complex conditions—in prisons and in areas of starvation, where other psychological and biological stresses are abundant. After experimental starvation, with its constriction of attention and drives, its evoked dreams of food associated with irritability and mood changes, six weeks of treatment were required for recovery.[81] Psychotic reactions in individuals who for various reasons inflict extreme diets on themselves, wonderfully portrayed in Franz Kafka's *Hungerkünstler*, certainly cannot be attributed simply to malnutrition. Besides psychoses associated with general malnutrition, certain psychotic reactions caused by specific nutritional deficiencies have been described. These generally are not acute brain syndromes, being more insidious and chronic.

The most important deficiency psychosis occurs in *pellagra*, in which niacin and possibly the amino acid tryptophan (the precursor for endogenous niacinamide) are implicated. Before preventive dietary measures were introduced, psychoses due to a deficiency of the Vitamin B complex made up 10 per cent of the admissions to state hospitals in the southern United States. Since the introduction of niacin therapy by J. Goldberger these have been virtually eradicated.[31] Pellagra psychoses still exist, particularly in some of the African countries. The avitaminosis is characterized by a dermatosis, particularly of hands and feet; stomatitis and glossitis; and vomiting; diarrhea and the very general symptoms of headaches, dizziness, fatigability, and weakness are noted. Patients occasionally develop tremors and myoclonic twitches. The pellagra psychosis is usually a delirium preceded by depression and anxiety. Hallucinosis and schizophreniform syndromes have also been described. Therapeutic doses of 500 mg. of niacin (nicotinic acid) per day orally and Vitamin B complex, thiamine, and tryptophan combined with a high caloric-balanced diet lead to prompt response. Another psychosis, which is phenomenologically and etiologically similar, was described by N. Jolliffe as *Nicotinic Acid Deficiency Encephalitis,* seen to follow febrile deliria and severe illness where malnutrition was a problem.[46] An acute reaction, this disorder may be accompanied by frontal lobe symptoms, such as forced sucking and grasping reflexes and cogwheel rigidities. It responds favorably to nicotinic acid therapy.

Thiamine (B_1) *deficiency* (*beriberi*), still endemic in Southeast Asia, is characterized in mild forms by irritability, fatigability, anorexia, and insomnia. Neurological manifestations in severe cases are peripheral bilateral polyneuropathy of the lower extremities (numbness of the toes, paresthesias, calf tenderness, muscular atrophy, and diminished vibratory sensation and reflexes); encephalopathy may follow. *Wernicke's encephalopathy* is the most serious form of B_1 deficiency.[103] It produces delirious or dysmnesic syndromes with disturbances of consciousness and ophthalmoplegias. Seen mainly in alcoholics, the disorder can occur wherever vitamin deficiency (starvation) or poor absorption (for example, gastric carcinoma, pernicious anemia) are found or extensive intravenous replacement therapies are required (see also Chapter 23). Vitamin-enriched foods have, since 1942, led to marked reduction of the incidence of these disorders. Treatment in all psychoses associated with Vitamin B deficiencies consists of vitamin supplements and a corrective diet. Otherwise, psychiatric therapy follows the general principles that apply to the treatment of symptomatic psychoses.

Depressions have also been described in Vitamin C deficiency, or *scurvy.* In *Kwashiorkor,* a tropical protein deficiency disease in young children, depression is an early symptom. Children suffering from Kwashiorkor die unless they are treated with a high protein, high vitamin diet; however, even if the metabolic deficiency is corrected, they usually become mentally retarded.

A number of metabolic diseases associated with mental deficiency have been described; they require prompt dietary control but do not constitute a clinical problem in usual psychiatric practice. On the other hand, they do (as with the gamut of nutritional disorders) raise important questions concerning the role of amino acids, amines, and vitamins (as cofactors in amine metabolism or as involved in carbohydrate metabolism and methyl transfer systems) in the maintenance of normal brain function. The neurochemical and neurobehavioral relevance of these substances and disorders is receiving renewed research interest (see chapters 6 and 20).

Organic Reaction Types in Patients with Endocrine Diseases

Many of the behavioral syndromes associated with endocrine diseases are complex and obscure. More often than not, one cannot decide whether the behavior pathology in such patients is the result of psychosomatic or somatopsychic processes or whether it is caused by cerebral pathology. In this chapter, behavior disorders which primarily seem to be produced by brain pathological processes associated with certain endocrine diseases will be reviewed. Some are delirious syndromes; others, organic deficit states. We have already mentioned M. Bleuler's endocrine psychosyndrome, which is identical with his local cerebral psychosyndrome.[7]

Cretinism as a result of endemic goiter or thyroid aplasia has become a rare disease since the introduction of iodized salt as a preventive measure. Cretins are mentally retarded; their irritability and the occurrence of paranoid traits are probably the result of mistreatment and neglect.[14] In *adult myxedema,* usually occurring after thyroidectomy and in climacteric women, paranoid and depressive syndromes are common.[2] In postoperative and spontaneous *tetany* delirium, depression, and schizophreniform symptoms were observed.[76]

Most patients with *hyperthyroidism* show a high level of anxiety; they are oversensitive, irritable, emotionally extremely labile, and frequently suspicious and paranoid. A considerable number of hyperthyroid patients develop psychoses.[55] In some patients, a delirium-confusional syndrome accompanies the metabolic crisis. In the majority of patients, disturbance of consciousness is absent or slight; the patients exhibit manic excitement, depressive mood swings, schizophreniform symptoms with visual and auditory hallucinations, and frequently paranoid and somatic delusions.[15] These symptoms may persist even if the patients develop hypothyroid symptoms in the course of medical and surgical treatment. More often than not, we are unable to differentiate between toxic psychoses and nontoxic psychoses, which are possibly the result of severe interpersonal stresses (see Chapter 13). The complex interplay of psychological and biological factors is demonstrated by the following case history of a patient with hyperthyroidism:

> The patient, a forty-one-year-old married housewife, was admitted to the psychiatric service in a state of agitation and anxiety. She seemed bewildered and deluded, stating she died three days ago. The psychotic behavior followed difficulties with her aged and ailing father. She had nursed him for his cardiac condition with a firm hand until two days before admission, when he started to breathe peculiarly. When a physician could find nothing wrong, she rebuked her father for his behavior and a fussy argument ensued. When the physician explained that her father might live for years but become a complete invalid, she fainted. She awoke claiming she had died and said, "I breathed for him." She felt her father also was dead and that her husband had remarried. She

began to see peculiar-looking people staring at her and was increasingly confused.

Five years before admission, the patient noted a gradual swelling of her neck, a bulging of her eyes, and she suffered from palpitation, sweating, and diarrhea. At that time, she became increasingly anxious and interpreted this as signs of early menopause. She finally consulted a physician who made the diagnosis of hyperthyroidism. She received Lugol's solution and radiological treatment; temporary remissions followed. There was one earlier psychotic episode, which occurred when the patient nursed her mother, who suffered from cancer, with exaggerated devotion until she finally could not go on any longer. At about this time she developed fears that both parents would die and for a while believed both were dead. When her mother did die, she began to improve.

The patient comes from Anglo-American stock. The father, a cabinet maker, used his myocardial disease to dominate the family. The mother was a retiring, reserved person who could not express her affection. One brother left the home early and was thereafter not heard from, dying finally of tuberculosis. The patient, a shy, seclusive child, had a mediocre school record. After leaving school she worked in factories where she met her husband, a clerk. Their early marital life was happy. The patient was fearful of having children but also wanted them. Since the birth of the two girls, now fifteen and twelve, sexual intercourse had become uninteresting. Occasionally, she masturbated after intercourse to achieve an orgasm and felt guilty over it.

On admission, she was sedated, and her initial agitation and extreme anxiety changed to an irritable reluctance to communicate; at times, she rambled irrelevantly and giggled, and then would be preoccupied with her guilt and anxiety. There seemed to be no gross deterioration, but judgment was grossly inadequate. Physical examination revealed a slightly diffuse, enlarged thyroid and elevated pulse and pressure. Laboratory findings were compatible with hyperthyroidism. After about two weeks of antithyroid medication, the patient became quieter but was still bewildered. In the third week, she was found unconscious after trying to strangle herself with gauze from a vaginal pad, the only residual being subconjunctival hemorrhages. She said she did not want to kill herself but to save other people on the ward. She became increasingly agitated, refused to take food and medication and had to be tube-fed. After six weeks, she was transferred to a state hospital where, three months later, she began to improve. She still felt that she had to atone for her father's death. Gradually her mood lifted and the self-accusations were no longer expressed. Six months after admission, she seemed to be free from psychotic symptoms and was discharged, although there was still evidence of mild hyperthyroidism.

Behavior disorders in *pituitary diseases* range from mild to severe syndromes and are usually unspecific. Patients with *Simmond's disease* or *pituitary cachexia* invariably exhibit depressive symptoms and apathy, which, in the terminal stage of the disease, are followed by stupor, coma, and death. Delirious symptoms with hallucinations, paranoid delusions, and psychomotor agitation leading to quick exhaustion occur. As therapy with cortisone in itself may produce toxic delirium, the task of treating the symptomatic psychosis may be very difficult. The syndrome of anorexita nervosa is discussed in Chapter 13.

In *acromegaly* and in *gigantism* caused by eosinophil adenoma, symptomatic psychoses with rather unspecific paranoid and depressive symptoms occur.[6] For psychosocial rather than biological reasons, homosexuality and other forms of sexual immaturity seem to be frequent in such patients. In patients with diabetes insipidus, hysterical mechanisms augmenting the excessive fluid intake and excretion have been noted. In some cases of *adiposogenital dystrophy* (Fröhlich's syndrome) unspecific symptomatic psychoses and organic deficit states have been observed.

Many experienced endocrinologists find that most patients with *diseases of the adrenal cortex* have marked personality changes; they are irritable, moody, show fluctuations of lethargy and impulsiveness, and usually have uneasy and often paranoid interpersonal relations. Psychiatrists have also been concerned with the effect of abnormal epinephrine and norepinephrine output; the impact of medullary hormones on normal and abnormal behavior has dominated neurobehavioral theories for some time. In his original description of *chronic adrenal cortical insufficiency,* Thomas Addison mentioned severe mental derangement. Together with the characteristic symptoms of asthenia, anorexia, nausea, weight loss, changes of skin pigmentation, and hypotension, patients often suffer from moderate depression, anxiety, and irritability.[18] Not infrequently, delirious and hallucinatory psychoses are present, which are not always correlated with the severity of the clinical symptoms or the level of insufficiency of the adrenal cortex, reduction of 17-ketosteroids, hypoglycemic symptoms, or changes of mineral balance. In very acute cases, however, delirious reactions are generally present. In some cases with a more prolonged course, psychoses with severe organic deficit reaction have been observed; in such patients, atrophy of the frontal lobes has also been found. The milder psychotic reactions are usually transient and respond well to corticoid therapy.[88] About 20 per cent of patients with *Cushing's syndrome,* which is caused by hyperfunction of the adrenal cortex and not a pituitary disease, develop severe behavior disorders.[96] It seems that most patients with Cushing's syndrome suffer from personality difficulties, such as marked introversion, a high degree of irritability or apathy, and depressive mood swings. Their interpersonal relations are markedly disturbed. So far, no thorough psychodynamic study establishing the etiological basis for such disturbed relationships has been reported.

In women suffering from *adrenogenital syndrome,* invariably the symptoms of masculine appearance, hirsutism, deep voice, amenorrhea, enlargement of the clitoris, and, if symptoms appear before puberty, absence of breast development, are accompanied by problems of sexual identity and severe conflicts that may reach psychotic proportions.[86] A lack or decrease of sexual desire is usually noted; in some cases, homosexual attachments develop. It is important to know that in cases produced by tumors, physical and psychological symptoms disappear after successful operations. In such cases, delirious symptoms may be caused by electrolyte imbalance as a result of a dysfunction of aldosterone, a water and mineral metabolism-regulating hormone. The rare *pheochromocytomas* are attributed to medullary hyperfunction, with symptoms of paroxysmal or lasting hypertension. These paroxysmal attacks of hypertension may be accompanied by severe attacks of anxiety, headaches, nausea, and palpitation.[44] The clinical picture is very similar to the reaction produced by injection with a large dose of epinephrine.

Behavior Disorders in Diseases of the Sex Glands

Hypogonadism

Underdevelopment of the genitalia and genital malfunction may be the result of chromosomal aberration, of pituitary and adrenal dysfunction, or of gonadal diseases and malformations resulting in insufficient secretion of androgens and estrogens after maturation. Usually these hormonal disturbances do not produce brain diseases in the narrow sense of the word; hence, symptomatic psychoses are rare. Clinicians, however, encounter many somatopsychic and psychosomatic reactions. Endocrinologists differentiate between a complete absence of function, or eunuchism, which is rare, and a partial absence of function, or eunuchoidism.[105] The most frequent cause of eunuchoidism is undescended testes or cryptorchism. In the adult male, the symptoms vary depending on whether the underlying disease or injury occurred before or after puberty. If it develops before puberty, a characteristic appearance results: the male patient has an infantile penis and scrotum, a beardless face, smooth skin, and underdevelopment of hair of the pubic region, trunk, and axilla; no sperm are produced; the extremities are long, and the voice is high-pitched. In the female, the genitalia remain infantile; breasts are underdeveloped; pubic and axillary hair are scant; ovulation is absent; menstruation is absent or scant and irregular; and hormonal assays reveal an underproduction of androgens and estrogens. Usually, but not always, the sex drive in such patients is diminished or absent. Many of these patients are depressed and feel inadequate and insecure. Some are, on the surface at least, well adjusted and serene, functioning well socially and occupationally. After hormonal therapy, growth of genitalia and secondary sexual characteristics and increase of sexual drive are noted. When hypogonadism develops after puberty, as a result of diseases or injuries, bodily changes are slight or do not occur, but in the male impotence invariably develops; this is caused probably by the psychological rather than the hormonal impact of castration. After ovariectomies, menopausal signs and symptoms appear; the sexual drive is decreased in some women but not in others, which again can probably be explained by psychological rather than by physiological factors.

Psychosexual development and gender role—identification with parents of the same sex—proceed somewhat independently of glandular activities in humans, although glandular dysfunctions, contingent upon their obvious effects on secondary characteristics, produce problems in such development and may influence strength of sexual drive.

PUBERTAS PRAECOX Sexual precocity, or pubertas praecox, is defined as the premature development of genitalia and secondary sex characteristics before the age of ten, often during the third or fourth year of life. In spite of the mature appearance of the genitalia, these patients are sterile and as a rule do not have the sexual drive characteristic of normal adults. The symptoms are caused by obscure diseases of the gonads and also of the adrenal, pituitary, and pineal glands and by hypothalamic lesions. The occurrence of signs and symptoms of the illness are invariably very alarming for the families of such children; and in the patient they provoke subsequent anxiety and neurotic conflict, which require sensitive psychotherapeutic handling.

Hermaphroditism

According to Lawson Wilkins,[105] and to John Money, J. G. Hampson, and J. C. Hampson,[63] one has to differentiate a number of variables that determine gender and sexual role: chromosomal sex; gonadal sex; hormonal sex; external and internal genital morphology; and the psychosexual role, which is largely the result of life experiences. In the rare case of true hermaphroditism, gonads of both sexes are present; most so-called hermaphrodites, however, have gonads of one sex with genital characteristics of both sexes and are properly termed pseudohermaphrodites. The endocrine and genital symptomatology of the various syndromes is rich and varied. Discrepancies between development of the external genitalia and breasts and growth of hair in male and female pseudohermaphrodites, and also in some cases of hypogonadism, or cases of *Klinefelter's syndrome*, are particularly apt to produce identity problems. The psychotic reactions, which usually resemble schizophrenia, seem to be the result of the severe conflicts and interpersonal stresses to which these patients are subjected. Hormonal therapy and reconstruction of the malformed genitalia, along with a carefully planned program of child-rearing, can produce astounding positive results. Money, Hampson, and Hampson[64] recommend that the assignment of sex in neonates and young infants be made primarily on the basis of the appearance of the external genitalia and the prospect of repair by plastic surgery. In order to avoid serious psychiatric consequences, once the sex is assigned, no changes should be contemplated.

Psychoses of Pregnancy and Puerperium

This group includes symptomatic psychoses of all types. The psychological and endocrine aspects of the cycle of events—conception, pregnancy, delivery, infant care—are invariably involved. Delirious anxious-confusional syndromes and stuporous reactions occur. There is also a relatively high incidence of schizophrenic and schizophreniform as well as manic-depressive reactions. Existing affective and schizophrenic psychoses are often exacerbated during pregnancy; and this is taken by some as an indication for therapeutic abortion. In many cases, it is impossible at the time of onset to diagnose what course the psychosis will take. Because of the unpredictable course, many psychiatrists feel that the biological and psychosocial aspects of pregnancy, childbirth, and puerperium simply precipitate a latent psychosis. Such a statement reflects the feeling that many factors contribute to the genesis of these disorders and that we are essentially in the dark about the relative significance of the etiological factors.[107] In general, schizophreniform reactions are most frequent during pregnancy and puerperium; the psychoses occurring shortly after delivery are more frequently delirious syndromes. Postpartum psychoses, disorders psychologically or perhaps endocrinologically linked with delivery, may occur within the first few days or as late as three to twelve months following delivery.[36] The principal factors which are considered to be of etiological importance are: (1) Toxic and metabolic processes (actually these psychoses occur more frequently in eclampsias and other toxic disturbances of pregnancy; for example, in severe hyperemesis). (2) Existence of a latent psychosis. (3) Psychological stressful factors. We will discuss the psychological problems of normal pregnancy more fully in Chapter 25. Here we shall mention only that, in a large percentage of women who develop generative psychoses, a negative attitude to the pregnancy and to the child is apparent. These patients are typically fearful of pregnancy and often opposed to it; they have ambivalent, hostile feelings toward the child. In many patients there is a history of actual or attempted abortion. Death wishes toward the child may be overt; if covert, they are often easily uncovered. Such death wishes occur both in highly anxious, guilt-ridden mothers and in patients who seem bland and unconcerned.

In the opinion of experienced clinicians, these psychoses seem less prevalent today than they were a generation ago. Improved obstetrical, medical, and, last but not least, modern psychological management are surely responsible for this decrease. In many cases, a combined organic and psychological therapeutic approach is indicated. Often a pure psychological approach in patients with symptomatic psychoses does not produce any change; with a few electric shocks added, however, a symptomatic psychosis may be stopped and a protracted course prevented. There is no contraindication to electric convulsive therapy during a normal pregnancy. As psychological problems loom very large in these patients, the best psychotherapeutic approach is one that combines support and reassurance with working through the problems of the mother—her hostile, ambivalent, and guilty feelings toward the child, and the child's father, the associated conflicts (about motherhood, femininity) and fears (of birth, bodily damage, responsibility) that are relevant.

Postoperative Psychoses

Delirious, hallucinatory, and paranoid reactions have been observed in connection with many surgical illnesses and procedures. Two basic types can be distinguished theoretically: (1) Symptomatic psychoses (in the narrow sense of the word) associated with cerebral dysfunction, as in operations where cerebral damage occurs. (2) Operations that produce extreme anxiety reactions with disorganization of behavior. In clinical practice, this distinction may be blurred. Symptomatic psychoses are particularly frequent after brain surgery, cardiac surgery, surgery of male and female reproductive organs, and ophthalmic surgery.[83] In cerebral operations, the direct trauma to the brain is followed by cerebral edema, swelling, hemorrhages, and thromboses; in addition, neurosurgical procedures are apt to provoke very strong anxieties. In operations on the external genitalia, hysterectomies, mastectomies, or prostatectomies, stress is also great.[95] Other factors that contribute to the precipitation of postoperative psychoses are prolonged anesthesia with possible brain damage, loss of blood, and infection. Postoperative psychoses in children and very old patients are more severe and frequent than in the middle age range.

The psychological stress of surgery, apart from that contributed by poor preparation of the patient, can be understood only by empathic scrutiny of the role the surgical intervention plays in the life situation, the meaning of organ dysfunction, and the fantasy and fears of death, mutilation, and dependency that are inevitable when one exposes oneself literally to the knife. Anesthesiologists could considerably enlighten our profession with detailed reports of their observations of anxiety and its effects on the physical as well as psychological adjustment of the surgical patient. The prognosis for postoperative psychosis in general is good. In treatment, apart from psychiatric therapy of the symptomatic psychosis, preoperative reduction of unrealistic anxiety by proper communication and sensitive emotional support of patients is of importance.

Drug Psychoses

These reactions are on the increase because modern medicine has been using more potent drugs. In making a diagnosis of a drug-induced psychosis, one must investigate the possibility that the illness being treated is the principal causative factor and not the drug. Drug-induced intoxication, drug withdrawal, drug-induced activation of latent psychosis or weakening of vulnerable personality defenses, idiosyncratic "drug fever" with associated delirium, and directly and regularly induced symptomatic psychoses represent different mechanisms and pathways to drug psychosis. Drug reaction should be differentiated, when possible, and not indiscriminately "lumped" into one category. Each and every drug that induces mental changes acts through different specific "initiating pathways," and the course, duration and mode of termination of drug-induced behavioral changes will differ with the particular drug and dosage schedules as well as with personality and environmental variables. For example, a single class of compounds—barbiturates—can produce a range of different mental states: intoxication, sedation, or withdrawal psychosis, or idiosyncratic rage reaction, depending on multiple variables. The major psychoses produced by alcohol, opiates, barbiturates, bromides, amphetamines, tranquilizers, antidepressants, are taken up in Chapters 22 and 23. The model psychoses produced by psychotomimetics and psychedelic drugs are discussed in Chapter 11. In general, drugs produce the gamut of the symptomatic psychoses. Delirious reactions, and schizophreniform and manic-depressive syndromes are most frequent. Some of the more commonly encountered drug psychoses, other than those mentioned above, are caused by digitalis,[48] atropine,[43] and atabrine.[60] Cortisone, in most cases, produces mood changes, usually euphoria and even mania, with flight of ideas and not infrequently with changes in body image and delusionary elaborations of a paranoid or grandiose nature. Occasionally, however, a depressive reaction is seen. Cortisone may produce rather long-lasting psychoses but no permanent organic deficit reaction. There has been a great deal of speculation about the mechanism of cortisone psychoses without any definite conclusion; practically, it is not yet possible to predict such psychoses excepting in obviously prepsychotic persons, and even here the evidence is not firm. Cortisone seems to have a greater propensity to produce psychoses than ACTH.[71]

Behavior Disorders in Industrial Poisoning

In a rapidly industrializing world, one would expect an increase in industrial poisoning. Fortunately, however, the dangers of industrial poisoning are well recognized and usually prevented. Compared with psychological hazards in industry and business, the risk of poisoning is slight and possibly overemphasized in the literature. The following is a brief discussion of industrial poisons of some importance for psychiatrists. Due to modern hygienic measures, *lead encephalitis*, with symptoms of headache, insomnia, apathy, or irritability, occasionally convulsions, and a dysmnesic syndrome, and even lasting organic deterioration, rarely comes to the attention of modern clinicians.[68] The same is true of *mercurial encephalopathy poisoning,* described so well in the case of the Mad Hatter by Lewis Carroll.

Symptomatic psychoses occur after poisoning with *industrial solvents* such as trichlorethylene, trichlormethane, toluol, benzene, benzol, xylol, carbon tetrasulfide, hydrogen sulfide, carbon tetrachloride, and carbon disulfide. After several weeks of exposure to toxic doses, patients develop headaches, nausea, and mood changes with both manic and depressive syndromes and states of excitement and delirium.[9] In some cases, dysmnesic syndromes appear. Usually, patients with such psychoses have a good prognosis.

Carbon monoxide and *illuminating gas* are common industrial and domestic poisons. The difference between innocuous and dangerous inhalation is small. Its accessibility makes "gas" a popular means of suicide. Clinically, we are usually concerned with acute poisoning, but there is increasing evidence of chronic poisoning (with irritability and fluctuating mental clouding) through exposure in garages, hangars, and heavy traffic.[29] After severe poisoning, which is always accompanied by coma, varyingly reversible residuals of acute and chronic brain damage, delirium, agitated and catatonic states, lingering dysmnesic syndromes have been observed.[85] In severe cases, patients suffer from a deficiency state. Lesions of the basal ganglia are manifested by Parkinsonism, choreiform, and decerebrate rigidity and occasionally by prolonged alteration of consciousness. In acute cases, treatment is artificial respiration, adequate oxygenation, perhaps use of dialysis, and the administration of antibiotics to prevent pneumonia. Even patients with severe cerebral damage are apt to improve, sometimes after months and years.

Psychiatrists have become very familiar with psychiatric and neurological symptoms in therapeutic electric coma treatment. Such symptoms as convulsions and delirious and confusional states after accidental electric shock are rare. After exposure to high-voltage currents, many neurological and psychiatric syndromes have been observed. Delirious syndromes also have been reported after heat exhaustion and heat stroke.

Behavior Disorders Caused by Cerebral Anoxia

Cells of the central nervous system are exceedingly sensitive to even brief and slight diminution of oxygen supply.[21] Cerebral anoxia, caused by severe anemia, by marked and sudden decrease in blood flow as in some cardiac and vascular diseases, by antenatal and neonatal asphyxia, or by decrease of oxygen in the atmosphere, rapidly produces a necrosis of cerebral tissue. The globus pallidus and the nuclei of the cranial nerves are particularly sensitive to anoxia. Slow and prolonged anoxia may produce cerebral atrophy. Cerebral damage may occur after anoxia in anesthesia or exsanguination. A clinical syndrome very similar to the one seen after carbon-monoxide poisoning has been observed after suicidal and homicidal attempts by *hanging or strangulation*. When patients wake up from coma, they often develop delirious and dysmnesic syndromes. In severe cases, there are various dyskinesias, tremors, and choreiform and myoclonic twitching; generalized convulsions are also seen. Lasting intellectual deficit may occur. The mechanism for such dysfunction is prolonged interference with the oxygen supply of cerebral tissues and subsequent cell damage.

In *altitude sickness*, patients complain of dyspnea, headache, fatigue, anxiety, and irritability. There is also evidence of diminished efficiency in mental and physical tasks, but no severe behavior disorders have been reported. In *decompression illness*, no lasting psychoses have been reported. When severe cerebral damage is survived, brief delirious and confusional states occur. More important are the mild confusional states caused by rapid decompression, which quite possibly are responsible for a number of otherwise inexplicable blunders in flying and diving. With about 85 per cent oxygen saturation, normal individuals will show unexpected emotional outbursts; in controlled experiments, emotional lability usually precedes intellectual impairment. The complex hazards of extremely rapid flights at very high altitudes have become the subject of the new speciality of space medicine. The effects of decompression, acceleration, low oxygen supply, extreme variations in temperature, cosmic radiation, weightlessness, and buffeting on physiological and behavioral processes, as well as the extreme psychological stresses and sensory deprivations occurring in space flight, are currently being explored.[79]

Behavior Disorders Associated with Brain Tumors

Brain tumors are found in two per cent of all autopsied cases. They are encountered in all ages; and gliomas, which make up nearly half of all brain tumors, are by no means rare in children. Symptoms and signs of brain tumors may be general or local. The general symptoms may be attributed mostly to the effect of long lasting increased intracranial pressure; the local signs are due to localized destruction of cerebral tissue by the tumor and functional restitution by healthy cerebral tissue. The most important general neurological signs and symptoms are convulsions, visual disturbances such as diplopia and blurred vision, headaches, nausea, and vomiting. Convulsions occur in 50 to 80 per cent of cases and are of the *grand mal* type; there may be focal seizures and Jacksonian seizures. Headaches are severe though intermittent and are usually frontal or occipital. Diplopia is caused by eye muscle paralysis; the diminished vision by papilledema or optic atrophy. The well-known triad of headache, vomiting, and choked disc may occur so late that it is not of great diagnostic value. Localized symptoms depend, of course, on the location, size, and rapidity of growth of the tumor. The significance of various seizures is dealt with in Chapter 18.

In many instances, the psychiatrist is the first to see a patient with brain tumor because psychiatric disturbances may be the only presenting symptoms. Not infrequently, psychiatrists and general practitioners who are not alert to such a possibility will miss the diagnosis or delay it,[73] a serious and possibly fatal mistake in operable tumors. In 100 brain tumors verified by operation or autopsy, the following neuropsychiatric symptoms were first to appear: "neurotic" complaints in 21; speech difficulties in 19; complaints of memory and intelligence deficit in 18; character changes in 15; fatigue in 14; drowsiness in 12; "psychotic" complaints in 8. On objective neuropsychiatric examination, speech disturbances were discovered in 19; psychotic syndromes in 18; intellectual deficit in 12; and personality changes in 10. The most frequent false diagnoses were: personality disorder, epilepsy, and "no disease." We know that in mental hospitals a fairly large number of clinically undetected brain tumors is discovered by post-mortem examinations, among them many patients with meningiomas who could have been saved. Routine EEG's should be done in mental hospital patients to detect brain tumors and also obscure epilepsies before clinical symptoms are present.[98] We believe that no test is superior to a good clinical examination, but in large patient populations that cannot be thoroughly examined, such a screening may be effective. Even cursory neurological examinations will aid in detecting brain tumors and other serious neurological diseases. Of course, superficial examinations are not without danger; if they yield only negative results, the examiner may feel satisfied not to search further and may thus overlook important data. Nevertheless, even a brief neurological examination is better than none. Ophthalmoscopic examinations, which are so rarely done by psychiatrists and general practitioners, are especially helpful.

Mark Kanzer, who studied the symptoms of 250 patients with brain tumors, states that the mental disorders found in patients with brain tumors are essentially the same as in patients with other types of organic disorder.[47] The mental symptoms and signs may be divided into general and local symptoms and signs. The general symptoms are caused by increased intracranial pressure or can be understood as general cerebral reaction to expanding and destructive lesions. They are intellectual deterioration; defects of memory, recall, and attention; somnolence and stupor; coarsening of the personality; appearance of asocial and antisocial traits; and apathetic or euphoric reactions. Delirious and confused episodes and disturbances of consciousness are usually the result of rapid changes leading to cerebral edema or swelling, hemorrhages in the tumor, or sudden rises of intracranial pressure. These general changes are usually intertwined in a complex way with more specific changes, particularly aphasias, agnosias, and apraxias, and the result of seizures and focal neurological lesions.

In other patients, however, the syndromes are less fulminant, and the disorder can be mistaken for a hysterical or hypochondriacal reaction. Misinterpretation of symptoms such as headaches and dizziness and the existence of severe anxiety or very palpable defenses against such anxiety contribute to this error. A famous patient whose brain tumor was at first overlooked and who was referred for intensive psychotherapy was America's great composer, George Gershwin. The psychiatrist suspected an organic lesion, but the family physician and neurologist missed the correct diagnosis and insisted on psychiatric therapy.[25] The opposite error, that of operating on neurotic patients, also occurs.

Many tumors will produce only general signs of organic behavior deficit. Certain psychiatric syndromes, however, are frequent enough in brain tumors to deserve mention in this chapter. *Parasagittal meningioma* frequently produces personality changes that are characteristic for frontal lobe syndromes associated with deterioration: inconsiderate, crude, antisocial behavior different from premorbid personality, sloppiness, untidiness, and a silly euphoric mood. Some *frontal lobe tumors,* however, produce only minimal behavior symptoms or remain psychologically asymptomatic. In *parietal and temporal tumors* of the major hemisphere, aphasic, agnosic, and apractic disturbances together with hemiparesis, hemihyperesthesias, and hemianopsias dominate the clinical picture; in lesions of the minor hemisphere, anosognosia is usually present. In temporal tumors, the most varied types of psychic seizures have been observed, although psychic fits also occur with tumors in other parts of the brain. In *occipital tumors,* psychic fits with visual hallucinatory aura have been described. In *diencephalic and mesencephalic tumors,* disturbances of consciousness; clouded states; delirium; hallucinatory and confused episodes; somnolence and marked apathy; and akinetic mutism have been reported. Neoplastic as well as degenerative diseases of the corpus callosum, such as *Marchiafava's disease,* produce similar psychiatric and neurological symptoms, such as general intellectual deterioration, hemiparesis, apraxias, and also anosognosias. General paresis, hypertensive brain disease, and Pick's and Alzheimer's diseases may produce many of the psychiatric and neurological signs found in brain tumors. Subdural hematoma, in patients for whom a history of head injury often can be obtained only with difficulty, produces essentially the same symptomatology as neoplasm. In many cases, only neurosurgical exploration establishes the differential diagnosis.

Therapy of tumors is in the hands of neurosurgeons, with whom radiotherapists, neurologists, speech therapists, and psychiatrists, as members of a therapeutic and rehabilitative team, cooperate. Psychiatrists and other practitioners who are interested not only in the pathology of the case but also in their patients may find that patients with brain tumors, particularly if they are not deteriorated, can be aided in their rehabilitation by a psychotherapeutic approach. The following case illustrates progressive deterioration and the syndrome of denial of blindness in a patient with a glioblastoma multiforme in the left parieto-occipital region.

A forty-five-year-old man of Irish-American extraction was admitted to a general hospital because one week before admission he had complained of severe frontal headaches and dizziness and had become slightly confused. He reported seeing yellow lights on his left side. The past personal history was not contributory. He graduated from high school. For thirteen years he had been a widower; he was a successful manager of a small mattress factory. It was reported that he had always been a stable, pleasant, outgoing person and had shown no peculiarities or maladjustment in his behavior.

On admission, the patient was pleasant, cooperative, conscious, and oriented. There was no evidence of intellectual deterioration. Motor speech and comprehension were normal except for occasional difficulties in naming objects. There was a noticeable dyslexia and a dysgraphia. Right homonymous hemianopsia was present. The fundi showed bilateral papilledema of 3 D. The pupils were normal. The other cranial nerves and the motor and sensory systems and reflexes were intact. A roentgenogram of the skull showed convolutional atrophy and displacement of the pineal gland to the right. The EEG revealed a focus of slow waves in the left temporal lobe. The diagnostic impression was that of a cerebral neoplasm in the left parieto-occipital region. Following a ventriculogram, a craniotomy revealed a soft, fleshy, reddish tumor in the subcortical portion of the inferior parietal and posterior temporal region on the left side, extending toward the occipital lobe. A specimen measuring 6 cm. by 4 cm. by 5 cm. was removed. The histologic diagnosis was glioblastoma multiforme.

The patient recovered rapidly, lost his aphasia, dysgraphia, dyslexia, and hemianopsia and was asymptomatic for six months following the operation, until he reported two incidents of glassy vision. One month later, he had one attack of complete disorientation while driving a car, and three months later experienced three attacks of complete blindness, each lasting several hours. At that time, his symptoms of amnestic aphasia reappeared. His memory for recent events and recall were impaired. He was unable to write and could barely detect movements of a hand in front of his eyes. The discs were unchanged. Another ventriculographic examination and craniotomy on the right side were carried out. The tumor had spread through the posterior part of the corpus callosum; a 2.5 cm. specimen of solid tumor was removed from the right occipito-parietal region. The postoperative course was uneventful, but at that time it was noted that he pretended to see, although he was obviously blind.

One year after the first admission, the patient was transferred to the Psychiatric Clinic. He was moderately restless but cooperative, although he finally had to be helped in eating and with care of his body. He knew he was in the hospital, but he was unable to remember the operation unless he was reminded of it. Memory for the remote past was fair. He showed pronounced amnestic aphasia and agraphia. He was paranoid toward his family and persistently demanded to be discharged. On all clinical examinations, he was completely unable to distinguish strong lights from darkness. The only examination that revealed a trace of vision was the psychogalvanic skin test. Both discs showed signs of secondary atrophy. The pupils were equal and regular; they reacted promptly and extensively to light and in convergence. The cranial nerves were intact. Muscular strength and tone of the extremities were normal. There were bilateral action tremor and past pointing in the finger to nose tests and slight ataxia in the heel to shin test. Position sense and vibration sense of the trunk and the extremities were definitely impaired. Touch, temperature, and pain senses, topognosis and two-point discrimination were normal, as was body perception. There was no finger agnosia. Recognition of materials was good, but recognition of forms was impaired beyond that due to his amnestic difficulty. All deep tendon reflexes were normal. The abdominal and cremasteric reflexes were absent; the plantar reflexes were of flexor type.

The patient's ability to cooperate in formal testing procedures was extremely limited, owing to his distractibility, confusion, and aphasia. He showed difficulty in comprehension, greater at some times than at others. In the Binet vocabulary test which, under the circumstances, was hardly valid, the patient succeeded in defining the average number of words for adults. This was, however, not achieved under standard conditions: words were repeated for him when necessary, and he was given several trials unless his response indicated that he did not know the word to be defined. On the Wechsler-Bellevue test, he could answer a few of the questions relating to general information and comprehension but succeeded with only one problem in arithmetic and failed completely to grasp the similarities test. He showed a notable deficiency in all tests involving memory, repeating only three digits forward and two in reverse with many repetitions and instructions. He could remember only one item from a paragraph immediately after it had been read to him. He frequently forgot the question asked before he was able to complete his answer. It was noticed that his memory improved when distractions were reduced to a minimum during the period of delay preceding recall. The patient showed perseverative tendencies at times. He seemed to become fixed on a certain type of response and to be unable to change unless distracted by some irrelevant stimulus. The over-all impression was that of considerable intellectual deterioration.

At all times when he was asked, the patient said that he was able to see. He moved about in his room as if he could see but constantly bumped into objects. When this was pointed out to him, he used excuses such as: "It is a little dark"; "This is not a bright day"; or "I'm tired." When asked directly whether he was blind, he vigorously denied it, although at times he would say: "I don't see as well as I did before, but I can see all right. I need new glasses." He made constant false guesses about the location of windows and doors and the appearance of persons in his environment. His memory for forms and colors was correct. The syndrome of denial of blindness remained constant as long as the patient could be reliably tested.

The patient became steadily worse; both cranial flaps showed considerable ballottement, which gave his head a grotesque appearance. He had episodes of severe excitement, often yelling at the top of his voice "Murder! Murder!" Gradually he became incontinent and progressively stuporous. At that stage, a slight hemiparesis, with increased deep tendon reflexes, was noted on the right side. During the last thirty days of his life, his temperature was elevated, the pulse rapid and small, and respirations stertorous. He died in deep coma nineteen months after his first admission. Pathoanatomic diagnosis: glioblastoma multiforme, involving both the parieto-occipital region and the basal ganglia (left); herniation of the brain (right); and aspiration pneumonia.

Behavior Disorders Caused by Syphilis of the Central Nervous System

Psychiatrists are primarily concerned with late manifestations of cerebral lues. Although the central nervous system may be invaded early by spirochetes, there are, with the exception of rare luetic meningitis, no corresponding early clinical manifestations. The two types of central nervous system lues causing severe behavior disorders are syphilitic meningoencephalitis and cerebral meningo-vascular syphilis. Other forms of central nervous system lues, such as tabes dorsalis or luetic atrophy of the optic nerve, do not cause behavior disorders. Cerebral gumma has disappeared. In asymptomatic lues of the central nervous system, the spinal fluid and serum show findings typical for parenchymatous, meningeal and vascular pathology without any clinical symptoms. Such cases are not the concern of the psychiatrist but, of course, need vigorous treatment.

Syphilitic Meningoencephalitis

The most important psychiatric illness caused by syphilis is syphilitic meningoencephalitis, also called general paresis, or progressive paralysis of the insane. Before the discovery of a really effective therapy for syphilis, general paresis was a common disease; figures of admission varied between one-tenth and one-third of all admissions to mental hospitals. Today, the disease, which occurs twice as frequently in men as in women, has become rare, mostly because syphilitic patients are vigorously treated. It always has been rare in tropical countries (where malaria is endemic).

PSYCHIATRIC SYMPTOMS AND COURSE Early symptoms are headaches, tremors, and forgetfulness; fatigability; and a rapidly progressive intellectual deficit, which reveals itself in work and social relations but remains unnoticed by the patient. Many patients develop a silly euphoria; some have expansive, grandiose ideas; for example, they are enormously wealthy and brag about colossal sexual achievements and great power. Stefan Hollos and Sandor Ferenczi assumed that delusions and euphoria are a denial of a terrifying reality and impotence by uncritical deteriorated patients.[42] Their unusual crudeness and their silly practical jokes are often socially embarrassing: one of our patients asked his wife to strip so he could show off her breasts to his friends. A few patients are depressed or paranoid. They become neglectful of appearance and habits; they fail in their occupations. They show a marked intellectual deficit on tests such as in performing simple comparisons and differentiations, and they have difficulty carrying out simple calculations such as a serial subtraction test. Attention, memory, recall, and endurance are also severely impaired. Untreated patients show a progressive course and die one to three years after the first symptoms appear. In so-called galloping paresis, the end is reached within a few months.

PHYSICAL AND LABORATORY FINDINGS Patients are generally weak and become exhausted quickly, especially as they pay little attention to signs of fatigue. Their lowered resistance to infection and disease is abetted by poor hygiene and nutrition; decubital ulcers are frequent. Carelessness also accounts for fractures and head injuries with subdural hematomas. The facial expression of the patients is empty, with occasional myoclonic twitches of the face, which German neuropsychiatrists poetically call *Wetterleuchten*. There are general or focal seizures and usually short-lasting hemiplegias and monoplegias, as well as aphasias and other higher gnostic and practic disturbances. Speech is usually slurred and tremulous. Words are mispronounced, letters and syllables omitted, a tendency which is demonstrated by letting the patient repeat test phrases like "third riding Massachusetts artillery brigade" or "Methodist Episcopal." Dysarthria is paralleled by a disturbance of handwriting, which is tremulous and irregular, with gross mistakes in spelling. The pupils are unequal, irregular, and react to convergence and accomodation but not to light (Argyll Robertson's sign). Deep tendon reflexes are usually hyperactive; only in taboparesis are they absent. Some paretics also suffer from optic atrophy, often denying their blindness. Frequent convulsions are seen in *Lissauer's type* of general paresis. *Congenital and juvenile paresis* is an extremely rare disease today, although a short while ago it still merited a monograph by W. C. Menninger.[59] The disease is found in children with congenital syphilis; these children appear clinically mentally retarded and also suffer from interstitial keratitis, nerve deafness, Hutchinson's teeth, and a saddle nose.

Complement fixation and flocculation tests for lues are invariably positive in blood and spinal fluid in untreated patients. The fluid is under normal pressure. Protein is increased (100 to 150 mgm./100 cc.). There is a moderate lymphocytosis (15 to 100 cells) and a first-zone gold sol curve. Other laboratory findings, including the diffusely abnormal EEG, are not helpful.

PATHOLOGY AND ETIOLOGY Recognized in the nineteenth century, the histopathological picture was described in 1904 by A. Alzheimer and F. Nissl; in 1913, by J. W. Moore; and later H. Noguchi demonstrated the treponema pallidum in brain. There is always moderate-to-severe atrophy of the brain. The meninges are cloudy and thickened, and granular ependymitis is invariably found. The meninges show evidence of a chronic luetic inflammation with perivascular infection of lymphocytes and plasma cells. The small vessels and capillaries proliferate and are often obstructed, leading to multiple areas of softening. There are also diffuse degenerative changes of ganglion cells and proliferation of glia in the form of so-called rod cells.

Although we know more about the etiology of general paresis than any other severe behavior disorder, there are still many unsolved problems. As usual, "constitution" was early considered to be an etiological factor, without specifying just what such constitution was. A specific strain of treponema pallidum was made responsible after the observation of several cases who all developed general paresis and were infected by one person; however, there were also observations that contradicted such a conclusion. Most important, however, is evidence that general paresis does not develop in patients with adequate antisyphilitic therapy.

DIAGNOSIS AND DIFFERENTIAL DIAGNOSIS The diagnosis rests on the typical syndrome, profound progressive deterioration, typical neurological changes, and laboratory findings. Without serological findings in blood and spinal fluid in the presence of the characteristic changes, the diagnosis is, of course, asymptomatic syphilis of the central nervous system. The differential diagnosis from meningo-vascular lues is discussed later. There are a number of syndromes of a profound organic deterioration, which, at times, were referred to as "pseudoparesis." They occur in brain tumors, chronic alcoholism, chronic bromide intoxication, vascular brain disease, certain traumatic encephalopathies, and in Pick's and Alzheimer's diseases.

Therapy: The development of a reasonably effective therapy and the prevention of general paresis comprise one of the glorious chapters in the history of medicine. Julius von Wagner-Jauregg, in 1917, after working on the problem since the end of the last century, developed malaria treatment of general paresis, which was, until the 1950's, the accepted method of therapy for general paresis all over the world.[99] He was awarded the Nobel Prize in 1928 for his achievement. Von Wagner-Jauregg is also the only psychiatrist who is remembered by his native country on a postage stamp—a high test of immortality! Wagner-Jauregg felt that malaria changed the malignant course of general paresis into a more benign meningeal and vascular lues, which responds to As and Bi therapy. Actually, full remissions were rare after malaria therapy, but social remissions frequent. A certain deterioration, residual paranoid trends, and other personality defects often persisted; yet, patients with simple occupations could often be rehabilitated, although the method was complicated and not without danger. Malaria therapy was increasingly replaced by other methods of producing fever, such as diathermy. All these therapies became obsolete after the introduction of penicillin by J. F. Mahoney in 1943.

Standard therapy today is to give patients 18 to 20 million units of penicillin in doses of 600,000 units over a period of four to six weeks. If patients are allergic to penicillin, equivalent doses of aureomycin, streptomycin, erythromycin, chlortetracycline and oxytetracycline may be administered. It is felt that results of this method are equal or superior to malaria therapy and far less dangerous. Jarish-Herxheimer reactions after penicillin treatment have been observed. More important even than therapy of late syphilis has been the effect of penicillin on the early syphilis, preventing the dread metaluetic diseases. About half the patients with general paresis treated with antibiotics show social recovery; and for a larger number, the symptoms and disease picture are arrested.

Cerebral Meningo-Vascular Lues

In contrast to luetic meningoencephalitis, the cerebral parenchyma is relatively uninvolved in meningo-vascular lues. The course of the various types of meningo-vascular lues is slower and less malignant. There are spontaneous remissions, and the illness reacts quite favorably to energetic antiluetic therapy. Usually, the illness is either meningeal or vascular; mixed forms are less frequent. The anatomical picture is a chronic syphilitic meningitis or syphilitic arteritis which leads to occlusion of the vessels. One sees thickening and clouding of the meninges; histologically, perivascular infiltration is present. At times, there is internal hydrocephalus caused by obliteration or compression of the sylvian aqueduct. There are chronic inflammatory changes of all three layers of the blood vessels and also proliferation of the intima with formation of thrombi and cerebral infarction.

The clinical picture of the meningeal form is characterized by headache, involvement of cranial nerves, and pupillary changes typical for central nervous system lues. Convulsions are frequent. In acute forms, there may be delirious episodes, but more frequently patients show relatively mild deterioration and rather unspecific paranoid, depressive, or euphoric syndromes. In the vascular forms, the clinical syndrome is characterized by the size and location of infarction. Hemiplegias, hemianesthesias, hemianopsias, aphasias, and higher gnostic and practic disturbances are frequent; they are short-lasting and relatively mild. Convulsive seizures of the *grand mal*, focal, and Jacksonian types occur in many patients. The psychological picture is usually that of a relatively mild intellectual deficit and unspecific paranoid, depressive or euphoric syndrome.

In the meningeal form, the cell count of the spinal fluid may be quite high (100 to 1000 lymphocytes), the protein markedly elevated (75 to 200 mgm.). Serological reactions in blood and spinal fluid are positive; mid-zone or end-zone gold sol reactions are frequent. In the vascular forms, the serological reactions in spinal fluid are positive in 80 per cent of the patients; cell count and protein are normal or only slightly elevated, the gold sol reaction may be normal.

Pharmacotherapy of meningo-vascular lues today is the same as the treatment of general paresis. Most patients react to such therapy either by disappearance of neurological and psychiatric symptoms or by marked improvement. Social and occupational rehabilitation of such patients is essential.

Behavior Disorders Associated with Demyelinating Diseases

Multiple sclerosis is the most common disease with disseminated demyelinizing lesions of the central nervous system. The characteristic plaques of multiple sclerosis are areas of demyelinization and glial proliferation and occur throughout the brain and spinal cord. The main symptoms are blurred vision, weakness of the lower extremities, incoordination, parasthesias, and sphincter disturbances. Retrobulbar neuritis, nystagmus, scanned speech, coarse tremor at intentional movement, spastic paraplegia of lower extremities, and urinary sphincter disturbances are typical. The etiology of the disease is unknown in spite of much searching, speculation and many claims. Onset of chronic progressive illness, with a tendency to remissions and exacerbations, is usually in young adulthood. The progress of the disease varies; the economically privileged, who get better care, run a milder course.

Many observers have been impressed with the intellectual and emotional changes in these patients; S. Carter, D. Sciarra, and H. H. Merritt report that about half of the patients show emotional changes.[16] Carter *et al.* found that 26 per cent of their patients were grossly deteriorated, but they were dealing with a population of institutionalized patients. In well cared for patients, intellectual deterioration is rare. O. R. Langworthy, L. C. Kolb, and S. Androp found that of 199 patients who required hospitalization, only 16 had psychotic changes.[52] Francis J. Braceland and M. E. Griffin think that the reported changes are not typical for multiple sclerosis in general but reflect the stage of the illness; the changes vary depending on whether a patient has just become ill or is in an intermediate or late stage.[10] The bland, euphoric, and infantile hysterical attitude of many multiple sclerosis patients is striking. Molly R. Harrower and J. Kraus found that patients are dependent, show little concern over bodily symptoms, seem compliant to an extreme degree, and are excessively cordial.[38] Again, it seems that denial is the most important defense in these organic patients. Harrower and Kraus also noted significant differences between patients who are institutionalized and those who are at home. What has been observed as typical for multiple sclerosis seems largely characteristic for chronically ill patients who have been institutionalized for a long time. In patients with remissions, there were more with higher intelligence and a realistic willingness to allow anxiety to register consciously. Harrower and Kraus think it is unlikely that there is a psychological predisposition to multiple sclerosis but that the disease imposes a certain standard condition, which leaves its mark depending on the characteristics of the premorbid personality.[38]

No specific therapy of multiple sclerosis exists, but a judicious balance between rest and activity, good nursing, and a prevention of invalidism through rehabilitative efforts are essential. A psychotherapeutic orientation of the treating physician is of great importance; the cooperation of the patient with the physician's general therapeutic efforts will depend to a large degree on such an attitude. It would be a mistake to consider as helpful the dependent compliance of many patients with multiple sclerosis. The compliant patient is not always the "good" patient, although at times it is wise to let nature erect its defenses in an illness that offers relatively little hope for a lasting cure.

Another demyelinating disease characterized by severe and progressive deterioration is *diffuse sclerosis,* or *encephalitis periaxialis diffusa.* Paul Schilder has described this rare disease, which is characterized by a diffuse cerebral demyelinization with cranial nerve signs; hemiplegias and quadriplegias; aphasias; the characteristic blindness; forced laughing and crying; associated with massive bilateral lesions of the basal ganglia; and progressive intellectual deterioration.[82]

Behavior Disorders with Other Brain Diseases

Macrocytic anemia, at one time a truly *pernicious anemia,* is characterized by the occurrence of macrocytic red cells; megaloblastic hyperplasia of bone marrow; glossitis; gastric achlorhydria; and changes in the central nervous system. It is caused by a gastric factor, which is responsible for the inability of the organism to produce vitamin B_{12}. Neurological symptoms are referrable to the pyramidal tracts and posterior columns, with spastic-ataxic paraplegias, anesthesias, and hyperesthesias to touch and pain; vibration sense and depth perception are impaired.[26] Cerebral changes consist of unspecific atrophic and degenerative affective ganglion cells, glia, and cerebral vessels. The severe psychoses and deficit states which were reported at one time are no longer seen, because patients can be treated effectively with liver extracts and vitamin B_{12}. Now of historical interest, H. W. Woltmann had found psychoses and organic deficit states in less than 10 per cent of patients;[106] but apathy, irritability, and somnolence were found in more than one-third. The relationship of pathological lesions of the brain to psychic symptoms was reviewed by Armando Ferraro, Silvano Arieti, and W. H. English.[26] It is our impression that a slight intellectual deficit is found in many such patients. From a practical standpoint, the uncooperative behavior of many patients with pernicious anemia, with and without deterioration, must be kept in mind. As these patients need constant therapy, cessation of therapy inevitably leads to a relapse that must be considered self-destructive behavior, needing an appropriate psychotherapeutic approach. Psychotic reactions have also been observed in other primary and, in rare instances, secondary anemias. Organic deficit reactions and psychoses in *porphyria,* associated with the typical syndrome of abdominal pain and peripheral neuropathy, have been described.[84] The neurological and psychiatric syndromes may be triggered after sulfonamide and barbiturate medication.

Organic deficit states and schizophreniform and paranoid psychoses are occasionally observed in *basal ganglia diseases.* Emotional stress has definitely been found to aggravate symptoms of *torsion spasm* and *torticollis;* but whether such reactions are related to the basic neurological syndrome has not been ascertained. *Gilles de la Tourette's syndrome* is characterized by bizarre choreiform and athetoid movements of face, trunk, and extremities; convulsive seizures; and uncontrollable copriolalia.[30] In *Wilson's dis-*

ease, a hereditary hepaticolenticular degeneration manifested by liver cirrhosis, a basal ganglion syndrome, corneal changes (Kayser Fleischer's ring), and progressive deterioration and organic psychotic syndrome have been observed.[49] *Lupus erythematosus* is a diffuse systemic disease affecting the brain, in which depressive syndromes,[58] symptomatic psychoses, but also organic deficit reactions have been noted.[17] Mental symptoms may be aggravated by life-saving cortisone therapy. In some families with *Friedrich's ataxia*, and also in *dystrophic myotonia*, paranoid episodes and organic deficit have been reported.[22] Patients with *periarterosis nodosa* and similar vascular collagenous disease often suffer from acute and chronic cerebral behavior syndromes.

HUNTINGTON'S CHOREA In 1872, an American general practitioner, George S. Huntington, reported a progressive chronic degenerative brain disorder that later was named after him.[45] About a hundred years ago, he described in clear, simple language the three main characteristics of the illness: 1) its hereditary nature; 2) a tendency to insanity and suicide; and 3) its manifesting itself as a grave disease only in adult life.

Huntington's chorea is a rare disease that has intrigued neurologists and psychiatrists mostly on account of its striking heredity. It is attended by all the symptoms of common chorea, such as incessant jerking, twisting movements of the neck, trunk and extremities, and grimacing of the face. Movements have been aptly called dancing; hence the name, chorea. The shaking movements may be relatively mild, giving the appearance of restlessness and "nervousness," or very severe, seemingly pulling and pushing the patient around as if he were driven by demons. Two hundred years ago, in New England, these patients, as well as some twitching-and-jerking hysterical patients, were actually thought to be possessed by the Devil. There is no muscular paralysis in Huntington's chorea; pyramidal and extrapyramidal signs are absent. Usually patients have a severe progressive dysarthria. The characteristic movements cease while the patient is asleep.

Severe mental changes appear in the great majority of patients, usually after the onset of the neurological symptoms. Although occasionally a patient does not deteriorate, there is usually a progressive deterioration of an organic type, aggravated by the fact that speech often becomes incomprehensible because of the dysarthria. In addition to the deterioration, patients often become paranoid and severely depressed. Of course, in an illness of this sort, development of a psychogenic depression and paranoid traits can be readily expected, but we do not believe that these symptoms are psychogenic. Surprisingly, there are no detailed psychodynamic studies of such patients and their unaffected family members. The disorder usually begins in middle life. Onset in the twenties or after the sixties is rare. The course of the illness is progressive, but there is considerable variability in its duration, ranging from five to ten years from onset to death.

There is agreement that the illness is transmitted by a dominant gene. Skips and modifications are explained by incomplete penetrance of the gene. Most of the cases in New York and the New England states can be traced back to three men who sailed for America with John Winthrop in 1630. P. R. Vessie traced a family with Huntington's chorea for 12 generations.[97] Based on recent knowledge of other dominant hereditary traits, we assume that these patients suffer from undetermined metabolic disorders; further investigation would be of importance.

Neuropathologists have found severe atrophy of the brain with particular involvement of the caudate and lenticular nuclei and the cerebral convolutions. Chronic leptomeningitis is present; the ganglion cells show signs of degeneration with lipid pigmentation. The myelin sheathes are damaged, and there is proliferation of glia. Diagnosis and differential diagnosis in such patients is easy if a combination of neurological signs, psychiatric symptoms, and familial occurrence is kept in mind. Yet, as Newton Bigelow *et al.* noted, such patients are often mistaken for catatonic schizophrenics and alcoholic psychotics.[5] In the early stage, their symptoms are often mistaken for hysterical reactions. The differential diagnosis from other basal ganglia disturbances, such as torsion spasm and torticollis, is possible because these illnesses are not familial, and the latter patients do not deteriorate. There is no effective treatment of Huntington's chorea. Sedatives, neurotropic drugs, and synthetic belladonna drugs have only very limited and temporary effect.

NOTES

1. Raymond D. Adams and Maurice Victor, *The Effect of Alcohol on the Nervous System, Association for Research in Nervous and Mental Proceedings,* 32 (1953), 526.
2. R. Asher, "Myxoedematous Madness," *British Medical Journal,* 2 (1949), 555.
3. M. Joseph Babinski, "Contribution à l'etudes des troubles mentaux dans l'hemiplegie organique cerebrale (anasognosie)," *Rev. Neurol.,* 27 (1914), 845.
4. Arthur L. Benton, "Gerstmann Syndrome," *Journal of Neurology, Neurosurgery and Psychiatry,* 24 (1961), 176.
5. Newton Bigelow, Leon Roizin, and Mavis A. Kaufman, "Psychoses with Huntington's Chorea," in Silvano Arieti, ed., *American Handbook of Psychiatry* (New York: Basic Books, 1959), Vol. II, pp. 1248–1259.
6. Manfred Bleuler, "The Psychopathology of Acromegaly," *Journal of Nervous and Mental Disease,* 113 (1951), 497.
7. Manfred Bleuler, "Endokrinologische Psychiatrie," in Hans W. Gruhle *et al.,* eds., *Psychiatrie der Gegenwart* (Berlin: Springer, 1964), Vol. I/1B, p. 161.

8. Karl Bonhoeffer, "Die Exogenen Reaktionstypen," *Arch. Psychiat., Nervenkr.*, 58 (1917), 58.
9. Francis J. Braceland, "Mental Symptoms Following Carbon Disulphide Absorption and Intoxication," *Annals of Internal Medicine*, 16 (1942), 246.
10. Francis J. Braceland and Mary E. Griffin, *The Mental Changes Associated with Multiple Sclerosis, Multiple Sclerosis and the Demyelinating Diseases, Association for Research in Nervous and Mental Disease Proceedings*, 28 (1950), 450.
11. W. Russell Brain, "Subacute Inclusion Encephalitis," *Brain*, 71 (1948), 365.
12. Henry Brill, "Postencephalitic Psychiatric Conditions," in Silvano Arieti, ed., *American Handbook of Psychiatry* (New York: Basic Books, 1959), Vol. II, pp. 1163–1174.
13. Paul Broca, *Traité Des Tumeurs* (Paris: Asselin, 1866).
14. Hilde Bruch and D. McCune, "Mental Development of Congenitally Hypothyroid Children," *American Journal of Diseases of Children*, 67 (1944), 205.
15. Benjamin Bursten, "Psychoses Associated with Thyrotoxicosis," *Archives of General Psychiatry*, 4 (1961), 267.
16. Sidney Carter, Daniel Sciarra, and H. Houston Merritt, The Course of Multiple Sclerosis as Determined by Autopsy Proven Cases," *Multiple Sclerosis and the Demyelinating Diseases, Association for Research in Nervous and Mental Disease Proceedings*, 28 (1950), 471.
17. Edward C. Clark and A. A. Bailey, "Neurological and Psychiatric Signs Associated with Systematic Lupus Erythematosus," *Journal of the American Medical Association*, 160 (1956), 455.
18. Robert A. Cleghorn, "Psychologic Changes in Addison's Disease" Editorial, *Journal of Clinical Endocrinology*, 13 (1953), 1291.
19. Jerome W. Conn and H. S. Selker, "Spontaneous Hypoglycemia," *American Journal of Medicine*, 19 (1955), 460.
20. Philip H. Connell, *Amphetamine Psychosis* "Maudsley Monograph" No. 5 (Oxford: Oxford University Press, 1958).
21. Cyril B. Courville, "Cerebral Anoxia," in Abe Bert Baker, ed., *Clinical Neurology* (New York: Hoeber-Harper, 1955), p. 555.
22. D. L. Davies, "Psychiatric Changes Associated with Friedreich's Ataxia," *Journal of Neurology, Neurosurgery and Psychiatry*, 12 (1949), 246.
23. John M. Davis, W. F. McCourt, and P. Solomon, "The Effect of Visual Stimulation on Hallucinations and Other Mental Experiences during Sensory Deprivation," *American Journal of Psychiatry*, 116 (1960), 889.
24. Constantin von Economo, *Die Encephalitis Lethargica* (Berlin: Springer, 1929).
25. Noah Fabricant, *13 Famous Patients* (Philadelphia: Chilton Company, 1960).

26. Armando Ferraro, Silvano Arieti, and W. H. English, "Cerebral Changes in the Course of Pernicious Anemia and Their Relationship to Psychic Symptoms," *Journal of Neuropathology and Experimental Neurology*, 4 (1945), 217.
27. Daniel X. Freedman and A. J. Benton, "Response to LSD-25 in Alcoholic Patients" unpublished data.
28. Josef Gerstmann, "Finger Agnosie und Isolierte Agraphie," *Zeitschrift für Ges. Neur. und Psychiat.*, 108 (1927), 152.
29. Gordon J. Gilbert and Gilbert H. Glaser, "Neurologic Manifestations of Chronic Carbon Monoxide Poisoning," *New England Journal of Medicine*, 261 (1959), 1217.
30. Gilles de la Tourette, *Lecons de clinique thérapeutique sur les maladies du système neureux* (Paris: Plon, Nourett, 1898).
31. Joseph Goldbergre, *Pelloyra: Its Nature and Prevention* (Washington: Government Printing Office, 1927).
32. Kurt Goldstein, *The Organism* (New York: American Book, 1939).
33. Kurt Goldstein and Martin Scheerer, *Abstract and Concrete Behavior, Psychological Monographs*, 53 (1941), No. 2; whole No. 239.
34. Kurt Goldstein, *Language and Language Disturbances* (New York: Grune & Stratton, 1948).
35. Ward C. Halstead, *Brain and Intelligence* (Chicago: University of Chicago Press, 1947).
36. James A. Hamilton, *Postpartum Psychiatric Problems* (St. Louis: Mosby, 1962).
37. Harry F. Harlow, "The Formation of Learning Sets," *Psychological Review*, 56 (1949), 51.
38. Molly R. Harrower and J. Kraus, "Psychological Studies on Patients with Multiple Sclerosis," *Archives of Neurology and Psychiatry*, 66 (1951), 44.
39. Henry Head, *Aphasia and Kindred Disorders of Speech* (Cambridge: Cambridge University Press, 1926).
40. Donald O. Hebb, "The Effect of Early and Late Brain Injury upon Test Scores and the Nature of Normal Adult Intelligence," *Proceedings of the American Philosophical Society*, 85 (1942), 275.
41. Donald O. Hebb, *The Organization of Behavior* (New York: John Wiley, 1949).
42. Stefan Hollos and Sandor Ferenczi, *Psychoanalysis and the Psychic Disorder of General Paresis* (New York: Nervous and Mental Disease Publishing Company, 1925).
43. F. Hopkins and J. Robyns-Jones, "Psychoses Associated with Atropine Administration," *British Medical Journal*, 1 (1937), 663.
44. John E. Howard and W. H. Barker, "Paroxysmal Hypertension and Other Clinical Manifestations Associated with Benign Chromaffin Cell Tumors (Phaeochromocytomata)," *Bulletin of the Johns Hopkins Hospital*, 61 (1937), 371.

45. George Huntington, "On Chorea," *Medical and Surgical Reporter*, 26 (1872), 317.
46. Norman Jolliffe, K. M. Bowman, L. A. Rosenblum, and H. D. Fein, "Nicotinic Acid Deficiency Encephalopathy," *Journal of the American Medical Association*, 114 (1940), 307.
47. Mark Kanzer, "Personality Disorders with Brain Tumors," *American Journal of Psychiatry*, 97 (1941), 812.
48. John T. King, "Digitalis Delirium," *Transactions of American Clinical and Climatological Association*, 61 (1949), 65.
49. C. A. Knehr and A. G. Bearn, "Psychological Impairment in Wilson's Disease," *Journal of Nervous and Mental Disease*, 124 (1956), 251.
50. Lawrence C. Kolb, *The Painful Phantom* (Springfield: Charles C Thomas, 1954).
51. Syergei S. Korsakoff, "Über eine besandere Form psychischer Störung, combinirt mit Multipler Neuritis," *Arch. Psychiat. Nervenkr.*, 21 (1890), 669.
52. Orthello R. Langworthy, Lawrence C. Kolb, and S. Androp, "Disturbance of Behavior in Patients with Disseminated Sclerosis," *American Journal of Psychiatry*, 98 (1941), 243.
53. Karl S. Lashley, *Brain Mechanisms and Intelligence* (Chicago: University of Chicago Press, 1929).
54. Max Levin, "Toxic Psychoses," in Silvano Arieti, ed., *The American Handbook of Psychiatry* (New York: Basic Books, 1959), Vol. II, pp. 1222-1230.
55. Theodore Lidz and John C. Whitehorn, "Life Situations, Emotions and Graves' Disease," *Psychosomatic Medicine*, 12 (1950), 184.
56. Hugo Liepmann, "Das Krankheits bild der Apraxie (Motorische Asymbolie) auf Grund eines Falles von einsutiger Apraxie," *Mschr. Psychiat. Neurol.* (8, 1900), 102; (17, 1905), 289; (19, 1906), 217.
57. Aleksandr R. Luria, *Restoration of Function after Brain Injury* (New York: Pergamon Press, 1963).
58. Allan R. McClary, E. Meyer, and E. L. Weitzman, "Observations on the Role of the Mechanism of Depression in Some Patients with Disseminated Lupus Erythematosus," *Psychosomatic Medicine*, 17 (1955), 311.
59. William C. Menninger, *Juvenile Paresis* (Baltimore: Williams & Wilkins, 1936).
60. Brenda Milner, "The Memory Defect in Bilateral Hippocampal Lesions," *Psychiatry Research Reports*, 11 (1959), 43.
61. Brenda Milner, "Effects of Different Brain Lesions on Card Sorting," *Archives of Neurology*, 9 (1963), 90.
62. Brenda Milner, C. Branch and T. Rasmussen, "Study of Short-term Memory after Intracarotid Injection of Sodium Amytal," *Transactions of the American Neurological Association*, 87 (1962), 224.
63. John Money, J. G. Hampson, and J. L. Hampson, "Hermaphroditism," *Bulletin of the Johns Hopkins Hospital*, 97 (1955), 284.

64. John Money, J. G. Hampson, and J. L. Hampson, "An Examination of Some Basic Sexual Concepts," *Bulletin of the Johns Hopkins Hospital*, 97 (1955), 301.
65. Joseph E. Moore and C. F. Mohr, "Penicillin in the Treatment of Neurosyphilis," *American Journal of Syphilis*, 30, (1946), 405.
66. H. Whitman Newell and Theodore Lidz, "The Toxicity of Atabrine to the Central Nervous System," *American Journal of Psychiatry*, 102 (1946), 805.
67. J. M. Nielsen, *Agnosia, Apraxia, Aphasia* (New York: Paul B. Hoeber, 1946]).
68. *Occupational Lead Exposure and Lead Poisoning* (Report of the Committee on Lead Poisoning [New York: American Public Health Association, 1945]).
69. Wilder Penfield and Lamar Roberts, *Speech and Brain Mechanisms* (Princeton: Princeton University Press, 1959).
70. Malcolm Piercy, "The Effects of Cerebral Lesions on Intellectual Function: A Review of Current Research Trends," *British Journal of Psychiatry*, 110 (May 1964), 310.
71. Gardner C. Quarton, L. D. Clark, Stanley Cobb, and W. Bauer, "Mental Disturbances Associated with ACTH and Cortisone," *Medicine*, 34 (1955), 13.
72. Fredrick C. Redlich and J. F. Dorsey, "Denial of Blindness by Patients with Cerebral Disease," *Archives of Neurology and Psychiatry*, 53 (1945), 407.
73. Fredrick C. Redlich, R. H. Dunsmore, and Eugene B. Brody, "Delays and Errors in the Diagnosis of Brain Tumor," *New England Journal of Medicine*, 239 (1948), 945.
74. Ralph M. Reitan, "Certain Differential Effects of Left and Right Cerebral Lesions in Human Adults," *Journal Comparative Physiological Psychology*, 48 (1955), 474.
75. Ralph M. Reitan, *The Effects of Brain Lesions on Adaptive Abilities in Human Beings* (Indianapolis: University of Indiana Press, 1959).
76. Carl P. Richter, W. M. Honeyman, and H. Hunter, "Behavior and Mood Cycles Apparently Related to Parathyroid Deficiency," *Journal of Neurology, and Psychiatry*, 3 (1940), 19.
77. John Romano and George L. Engel, "Physiologic and Psychologic Considerations of Delirium," *Medical Clinics of North America*, 28 (1944), 629.
78. Howard P. Rome and David B. Robinson, "Psychiatric Conditions Associated with Metabolic, Endocrine and Nutritional Disorders," in Silvano Arieti, ed., *The American Handbook of Psychiatry* (New York: Basic Books, 1959), Vol. II, p. 1260.
79. George E. Ruff, "Psychiatric Problems in Space Flight," *Diseases of the Nervous System*, 21 (1960), Monograph Supplement p. 98.
80. Werner Scheid, "Die Psychischen Störungen bei Infektions—und Tropenkrankheiten," in Hans W. Gruhle, ed., *Psychiatrie der Gegenwart* (Berlin: Springer, 1960), Vol. II.

81. Burton C. Schiele and Josef Brozek, "Experimental Neurosis Resulting from Semistarvation in Man," *Psychosomatic Medicine*, 10 (1948), 31.

82. Paul Schilder, "Zur Kenntnis der sogenannten diffusen Sklerose," *Ztschr. f.d. ges. Neurol. & Psychiat.*, 10 (1912), 1.

83. Paul Schilder, "Über eine Psychose nach Staroperation," *Intern. Z. Psychoanal.*, 8 (1922), 35.

84. P. R. Schmidt, "Neurologische und psychische Störungen bei Porphyrin-Krankheiten," *Fortschrift Neurol. Psychiat.*, 20 (1952), 422.

85. Frederick H. Shillito, C. K. Drinker, and T. J. Shaughnessy, "The Problem of Nervous and Mental Sequelae in Carbon Monoxide Poisoning," *Journal of the American Medical Association*, 106 (1936), 669.

86. Louis J. Soffer, *Diseases of the Adrenals* (Philadelphia: Lea and Febiger, 1946).

87. Philip Solomon, P. H. Leiderman, J. Mendelson, and H. Wexler, "Sensory Deprivation," *American Journal of Psychiatry*, 114 (1957), 357.

88. Werner A. Stoll, *Die Psychiatrie des Morbus Addison.* (Stuttgart: Thieme Verlag., 1953).

89. George A. Talland and M. Ekdahl, "Psychological Studies of Korsakoff's Psychosis: IV. The Rate and Mode of Forgetting Narrative Material," *Journal of Nervous and Mental Disease*, 128 (1959), 391.

90. Hans-Lukas Teuber, "Physiological Psychology," *Annual Review of Psychology*, 6 (1955), 267.

91. Hans-Lukas Teuber, "Ability to Discover Hidden Figures after Cerebral Lesions," *Archives of Neurology and Psychiatry*, 76 (1956), 369.

92. Hans-Lukas Teuber, "Sensory Deprivation, Sensory Suppression and Agnosia: Notes for a Neurologic Theory," *Journal of Nervous and Mental Disease*, 132 (1961), 32.

93. Hans-Lukas Teuber and M. B. Bender, "Perception of Apparent Movement across Acquired Scotomata in the Visual Field," *American Psychologist*, 5 (1950), 271.

94. Hans-Lukas Teuber and M. Mishkin, "Judgment of Visual and Postural Vertical after Brain Injury," *Journal of Psychology*, 38 (1954), 161.

95. James L. Titchener and Maurice Levine, *Surgery as a Human Experience* (New York: Oxford University Press, 1960).

96. William H. Trethowan and Stanley Cobb, "Neuropsychiatric Aspects of Cushing's Syndrome," *Archives of Neurology and Psychiatry*, 67 (1952), 283.

97. P. R. Vessie, "On Transmission of Huntington's Chorea for 300 Years," *Journal of Nervous and Mental Disease*, 76 (1932), 553.

98. Raymond W. Waggoner and B. K. Bagchi, "Paroxysmal Convulsive Disorder Variants," *Research Publication of the Association for Research in Nervous and Mental Disease*, 26 (1946), 328.

99. Julius von Wagner-Jauregg and Walter L. Breutsch, "The History of the Malaria Treatment of General Paralysis," *American Journal of Psychiatry*, 102 (1946), 577.

100. Edwin A. Weinstein and Robert L. Kahn, *Denial of Illness* (Springfield: Charles C Thomas, 1955).

101. Joseph M. Wepman and Lyle V. Jones, *Studies in Aphasia* (Chicago: Education Industry Service, 1961).

102. Carl Wernicke, *Der Aphasische Symptomencomplex* (Breslau: Schletter, 1874).

103. Carl Wernicke, *Lehrbuch der Gehirnkrankheiten für Studierende und Ärzte* (Berlin: Fischer, 1881).

104. Louis J. West, H. H. Janszen, B. K. Lester, and F. S. Corneilisoon, "The Psychosis of Sleep Deprivation," *Annals of the New York Academy of Medicine*, 96 (1962), 66.

105. Lawson Wilkins, *Diagnosis and Treatment of Endocrine Disorders in Childhood and Adolescence* (Springfield: Charles C Thomas, 1957).

106. H. W. Woltmann, "The Nervous Symptoms in Pernicious Anemia," *American Journal of Medical Science*, 157 (1919), 400.

107. Gregory Zilboorg, "The Clinical Issues of Postpartum Psychopathological Reaction," *American Journal of Obstetrics and Gynecology*, 73 (1957), 305.

CHAPTER SEVENTEEN

Behavior Disorders after Head Injuries

Types of Head Injuries

According to S. Brock, 6 per cent of all injuries are head injuries.[3] In the United States alone, there are forty thousand fatal head injuries each year. A considerable number of head injuries result in acute and chronic behavior disorders. Henry W. Brosin[4] states, as does Bertholt Brecht in the *Threepenny Opera*, that we overestimate the importance of our heads, but the above figures can hardly be minimized. Psychiatrists need to know something about these disorders because, together with neurosurgeons and neurologists, they are called upon to treat such patients. This chapter focuses primarily on the behavioral manifestations of head injuries. Cranial injuries are commonly divided into closed and open injuries. In closed injuries, there is no fracture or only a linear fracture of the skull; in open injuries, there are compound and depressed fractures. In both open and closed injuries, the brain and its covering membranes may be damaged. Acute cerebral injuries are divided into (1) concussion; (2) contusion and laceration; and (3) subdural and epidural hematoma.

Concussion

This syndrome is characterized by a short loss of consciousness following a closed head injury. It is usually caused by a blow or a fall, or both, with a broad surface impact; if the head was not held in a fixed position by the neck muscles, considerable acceleration and subsequent sudden deceleration of the brain occur which presumably produces the syndrome. The typical knockout blow in boxing probably belongs to the category of concussion syndromes, although some consider the unconsciousness after knockouts a vagal reflex. After the patient awakens, the typical symptoms consist of a diffuse headache, which can be quite severe. Patients report dizziness and not infrequently they are nauseated and vomit. Most patients with a simple concussion are stunned, confused, and disoriented when they wake up: they cannot tell where they are, how they got there, and are confused about time and sequence of events. They respond slowly and are either unable to identify the persons they see or can do this only with great effort. Most patients suffer from a short amnesia, which covers the accident and the immediate period preceding it (retrograde amnesia). T. Lidz observed that patients can recover their memories of the retrograde amnesia if they receive help in reconstructing the events.[15] Usually there is also a brief disturbance of recall and retention after the patient awakens from his coma (anterograde amnesia) from which the patient does not recover fully, because he was unable to integrate the experiences of this period. During this period of awakening, patients seem emotionally labile, anxious, and suspicious. They are apt to cry or to try to defend themselves and fight because they feel threatened. In mild cases, the symptoms are fleeting, abortive, and hardly more pronounced than in sudden awakening from a deep sleep, except for the retrograde amnesia, which is a constant symptom. In most cases, these symptoms persist for a few days to a week and, with increasing severity, imperceptibly blend into an acute posttraumatic psychosis, to be discussed later in this chapter. The neurological examination does not yield any positive findings. A lumbar puncture is not indicated in concussion syndromes unless there is evidence of an open injury or suspicion of subdural hematoma. EEG and X-rays of the skull should be taken whenever feasible. EEG may show a temporary decrease of amplitude, some general slowing, and occasional spike activity. There are no macroscopic or microscopic pathological findings of the brain after concussion.

Although a number of views have been expressed, the nature of concussion is not clear. One well-grounded theory, based on experimental evidence advanced by D. Denny-Brown and W. R. Russell,[5] assumes that the force of the blow temporarily deforms the brain and results in a reflex loss of consciousness. These investigators think that the loss of consciousness is caused by a sudden inhibition of the reticular activating system. Evidence that there is a release of acetylcholine, measurable by bioassay techniques in the cerebrospinal fluid, is of particular interest, since cholinesterase inhibitors, which elevate these levels, produce changes of consciousness and amnesic defects.

Therapy of a simple concussion consists of a short bed rest. During this time, patients should be carefully observed (without being made anxious or overly concerned) for possible development of neurological and psychiatric complications. Patients may require medication for the headache; if possible, nothing more than aspirin, caffein, and phenacetin and mild sedatives for anxiety and insomnia should be administered. Heavy sedation is contraindicated. The patient should be realistically informed about his injury and prognosis. He should have an opportunity to express his fears and anger about the accident. Quick return to ordinary activities is of importance to prevent the development of invalidism.

Blast injuries in which patients are hurled through the air and lose consciousness are also essentially concussion syndromes, even when patients do not land on their heads. To make a diagnosis of blast concussion, it is necessary to establish that the patient was thrown by the blast, became unconscious, has ruptures of the eardrums, and also injuries to his lungs.[6] In most cases in which a behavior disorder follows a blast injury, the mechanisms are psychogenic rather than somatic. The frequent diagnosis of shell shock during World War I was a misnomer in practically all cases.

Contusions and Lacerations

Tears and crushing of tissue are the results of local injury to the brain, either at the point of impact or at its opposite pole by *contrecoup*. Contusions and lacerations produce more severe symptoms and a higher mortality rate than concussion. Contusions and lacerations of the brain are usually associated with compound or depressed fractures of the skull, with scalp wound and bleeding from skull openings, especially ears and nose. The coma after such injuries and also the periods of anterograde and retrograde amnesia are more prolonged than in simple concussion. The length of the coma is significant for the prognosis of the case.[19] After prolonged coma, sequelae are more lasting and serious. Immediately following the trauma, the patient not infrequently exhibits the signs of cranial nerve injuries and other focal signs of brain damage, as well as convulsions of a generalized or focal type. These convulsions, according to Wilder Penfield and H. Jasper, are mostly due to cortical irritation by pial bleeding.[22]

The EEG contributes remarkably little to the diagnosis and understanding of the pathophysiology of concussion and contusion. General bilateral and occasional unilateral slowing of the rhythm are the rule in acute post-traumatic psychosis; occasionally, fast activity is seen, but none of these changes reliably reflects the course of the injuries or even the alteration of consciousness after the trauma.

Radiological examination of the skull, lumbar puncture, and EEG are essential but may have to be delayed if the patient is in surgical shock or is extremely disturbed. Therapy of such patients is primarily in the hands of the neurosurgeons. Convulsions and epileptic status are treated as outlined in Chapter 18. Great caution must be exercised when patients need to be sedated. The use of opiates is contraindicated. Attention must be paid to the possibility of a serious rise of the intracranial pressure, often manifested by increased dullness, apathy, and somnolence. Bladder and bowel may have to be emptied by catheterization and enema.

Acute Post-traumatic Psychoses

Acute post-traumatic psychoses are frequently associated with contusions and lacerations, more rarely with concussion. In general, they are indistinguishable from the clinical picture of other symptomatic psychoses. Confused, delirious syndromes predominate, but temporary catatonic or manic-depressive symptoms are not infrequent. The characteristic course, as E. Gamper outlined it,[8] leads from coma to and through a delirious-confused syndrome to recovery or to a post-traumatic reaction which is described later in this chapter. Some patients develop acute dysmnesic syndromes. The dysmnesic syndrome may be very slight and of brief duration, barely noticeable except when the opportunity for careful examination exists. The typical post-traumatic psychosis develops abruptly when the patient begins to regain consciousness and gradually diminishes in severity. This type of course distinguishes it from psychoses associated with meningeal and encephalitic infections or fat embolism, in which symptoms increase in intensity. Fat embolism may be diagnosed by subcutaneous petechiae and yellowish deposits of fat in the retinae; the spinal fluid may also contain fat.[7] A significant number of such patients suffer from generalized and focal convulsive seizures that further contribute to temporary clouding of consciousness and confusional states.

Uncomplicated concussion psychoses last from one to two weeks. Some of them clear up without sequelae; others develop post-traumatic reactions. Obviously, psychoses associated with contusions and lacerations are more severe and last longer; when extensive damage to diencephalic and mesencephalic centers occurs, severe intellectual and characterological changes of an organic reaction type may persist; this, however, is quite exceptional. Schizophreniform syndromes, which rarely develop, may appear after a delirious syndrome. Whether a latent psychosis existed before the head injury in such cases often remains unclear. The mechanisms that produce acute post-traumatic psychoses are obscure. In the German literature, these psychoses are frequently called edema psychoses, and the temporary cerebral dysfunction is thought to be produced by noninflammatory cerebral edema following the trauma. A pneumoencephalogram with diminution of the size of the lateral ventricles to a slit or date-pit-like opening has been cited as evidence for this assumption. Treatment follows the established principles of therapy of the symptomatic psychoses, with special attention to careful supervision of the confused and agitated patients who are apt to hurt themselves or wander off the wards. As cerebral edema is not considered the essential pathology, the use of dehydrating agents such as concentrated dextrose is not indicated. The general rule is to maintain a normal water and mineral balance. Prophylactic measures against pulmonary and bladder infections and decubital ulcers in bedfast patients are necessary.

CONCUSSION PSYCHOSIS WITH DYSMNESIC CONFABULATORY SYNDROME

A seventeen-year-old high school student, the son of a real estate man, was admitted to a local general hospital in comatose condition after an automobile accident; the car had struck a telephone pole, and it took two hours to extract him from the wreck. He had fractures of the maxilla and mandible, fractures of the left ulna and radius, avulsions of the left ala nasae, and a severe laceration of the tongue. Oral bleeding required a tracheotomy. There was no clinical or radiological evidence of a skull fracture. Lumbar puncture revealed normal pressure and normal cerebrospinal fluid findings. There were no localizing neurological signs, and no abnormal somatic signs except for a pulse rate of 120. He remained in coma for seven days. When he gradually recovered consciousness, he assaulted nurses and tore their uniforms, but was not belligerent toward physicians and male hospital personnel. He masturbated openly, was untidy in his habits, and disoriented about time and place. He knew he was a high school student but did not know his grade. He could remember events for several moments prior to his accident. The examining psychiatrists noted an inability to name objects correctly, to understand speech and a jargon aphasia. His ability for immediate recall was severely impaired. He tired easily during an examination, but in more lucid moments talked about what the examiner interpreted as initiation rites. The patient was transferred to the neurosurgical service and later, because of his psychosis, to the psychiatric ward of a general hospital.

The parents of the patient supplied the following background information. They described him as a physically healthy boy who did well in school until he reached the seventh grade. At that time, his parents were divorced. The patient's mother, who had financed her husband's unsuccessful business enterprises, wanted the divorce, but was so depressed over it that she entered a psychiatric hospital. Neither parent really wanted the responsibility of maintaining a home for the boy, who had become quite unmanageable. Just before the accident he had been told that his school grades were not good enough for him to be accepted at college; according to psychological tests, his aptitudes were in the bright normal range. He was popular socially, had many friends, and was considered a good driver.

On the psychiatric service, he remained disoriented; he said the President's name was Johnson (it was Kennedy). He could not remember the doctor's name, even for a moment, and had no memory for the dates of his hospitalization. When his parents visited him, he recognized them and seemed glad to see them. The wide gaps in memory were filled in with confabulation. He was impulsive and prone to angry attacks against nurses, whom he called teachers. He constantly tried to remove his cast, screamed to be "taken out of the machine," and thought the Russians were after him. The patient was incontinent. There was a definite change in sleep rhythm; he alternated between short periods of sleep and wakefulness both day and night. Because of the possible development of a subdural hematoma, he received sedation and phenothiazines only sparingly. Lumbar puncture, cerebrospinal fluid, and skull X-ray were normal. There were slow waves in both temporal regions but the interpretation of this finding remained uncertain.

A definite change occurred when the patient's cast was taken off eight weeks after the accident. Until that time, he had required special nurses. On removal of the cast, his confabulation ceased, and he began to say that he had been told about certain events which he could not remember. The mental status now revealed that he was completely oriented; he could do serial sevens, remembered five digits forward but not backward. On intelligence tests, he did well on standard information, understanding proverbs and similarities. Psychological testing corroborated the impression that there was only relatively slight organic deficit. He began to participate in ward activities. At the first group meeting, he politely asked everyone's name and remarked that he found himself in the hospital after drinking excessively. When corrected, he became upset and wanted to leave. At other meetings he also showed some of his earlier impulsive behavior; for example, he asked a lady to remove her dress so he could see her breasts. It was decided not to force the patient into group meetings but to help him individually to restructure his social and physical world. Twelve weeks after the accident there was no evidence of organic brain damage. EEG was repeatedly normal. He drank excessive amounts of water, but the diagnosis of diabetes insipidus was excluded. The aphasia had cleared up. Recall and intellectual functions were normal. The memory for events prior to the accident returned in patches, but an amnesia covering one week prior to the accident remained. The psychological problems facing the patient, parents, and staff were to decide with whom the patient should live and to what school he should go.

Subdural and Epidural Hematoma

Subdural hematoma develops when the trauma causes venous bleeding into the subdural space. In many cases, but not always, fractures of the skull are found. In senile, very ill, and deteriorated patients often no history of trauma can be obtained. The ordinary history in *acute subdural hematoma* is one of initial head injury, coma, anterograde and retrograde amnesia. There may be a temporary return of consciousness, a so-called lucid interval, after which the patient lapses into deepening coma. Such a course is particularly characteristic for *epidural hematoma* due to arterial bleeding from the middle meningeal artery. After the patient awakens, he may show a certain unresponsiveness, dullness, and apathy; he is often irritable and antagonistic. Delirious and confused states identical to those of other acute traumatic psychoses occur. The patient invariably complains of headache. Most frequent signs are hemiplegia, hemianesthesia, and hemianopsia, with aphasic disturbances if the lesion is on the major side. Unequal pupils are not a reliable sign. Convulsions occur in acute subdural hematoma but are more frequent in chronic subdural hematoma.

Chronic subdural hematoma develops more slowly from small acute hematoma. The dura thickens and forms a membrane on the organized clot, which then expands in size by accumulation of fluid and repeated bleeding. The clinical effect is then the same as in a neoplasm. The diagnosis of acute and chronic subdural hematoma is not easy; in acute subdural hematoma, contusions and lacerations often are present as well, and they obscure the clinical syndrome. The spinal fluid is bloody; in less acute cases, xanthochromic. EEG's, which should be carried out repeatedly, often show depressed activity over the afflicted hemisphere. Sometimes cerebral arteriography is helpful, but often only neurosurgical exploration will permit the diagnosis. The behavioral symptoms of chronic subdural hematoma resemble those of other expanding lesions of the brain. General intellectual deterioration, apathy, and, more rarely, agitated and impulsive behavior and a lack of concern for the needs and sensitivities of fellow human beings are characteristic. There are, however, many cases of chronic subdural hematoma, particularly in some of our public mental hospitals, in which the signs remain unnoticed during the patient's life and become apparent only on autopsy.[27]

In both acute and chronic subdural hematomata, the only effective therapy is operative removal of the clot. In patients in good general health, the chances of successful surgery are good. In epidural hematoma in which blood of a meningeal artery pours into the epidural space, symptoms are more dramatic and the outcome much less favorable; the mortality is 100 per cent in untreated cases of epidural hematoma and about 50 per cent after neurosurgery.[20]

Late Sequelae of Head Injuries

The most frequent enduring symptoms are headaches and dizziness. The neurological signs of late sequelae of head injuries consist of cranial nerve injuries, hemiplegias, hemianesthesias, and hemianopsias, which are usually caused by focal lesions. Focal and generalized convulsive seizures caused by scar tissue occur in some five per cent of all head injuries and are discussed in Chapter 18. It is advisable to carry out EEG examinations, which may reveal diffuse or focal abnormalities, but in a remarkable number of cases the EEG may be normal. The syndromes of special concern for the psychiatrist are: (1) General and specific psychological deficit. (2) Personality changes after head injuries. (3) The so-called post-traumatic syndrome.

Intellectual Deficit after Head Injuries

As a rule, severe intellectual deterioration of an organic type is rare in patients with circumscribed trauma. It occurs in patients with decerebrate syndromes after extensive damage to the diencephalon and mesencephalic region. In patients with less extensive damage to the diencephalon, weight gain and changes in water and mineral metabolism and thermal regulation have been described.[2] There is no strict relation between the extent of the injury and degree of intellectual deterioration,[10] but length of coma and anterograde and retrograde amnesia are correlated with deterioration. In studying a series of patients with head injuries, Ruesch used relatively simple tests, such as serial subtraction, and found, on the average, only slight deficit.[24] Halstead and other investigators found that frontal lobe injuries show more deficit than other lesions. But we are inclined to agree with W. Birkmeyer, who reported that patients with frontal lobe injuries showed less deficit than those with occipital, parietal, and temporal lobe injuries.[2]

According to Donald O. Hebb, there are no tests that clearly show intellectual deficit after frontal lobe lesion to be greater than that following destruction of other parts of the brain.[11] Routine tests are of little value in the assessment of intellectual function after brain injuries.[26] Probably the nature of the tests employed determines differences in reported findings. Ward C. Halstead, who used batteries of complicated nonverbal tests such as flicker-fusion tests, dynamic visual field tests, sound perception tests, and tactile performance tests for speed, recall, and localization, found very definite deficits, such as disturbance in foreground-background discriminations in assimilating new material, and disturbances in abstraction.[10] Similar findings were obtained by R. N. Reitan.[20] As in other types of cerebral lesion, it is a mistake to view intellectual deficit as apart from other personality functions; the clinical syndromes are the composite result of cerebral defect, psychosocial pressures, and defensive operations.

Severe Personality Changes after Head Injuries

To say precisely what kinds of intellectual deficit occur after diffuse or circumscribed brain injury is far from easy, but it is much more difficult to state the nature of post-traumatic personality. K. Schneider, in a purely descriptive approach, delineated three types:[25] (1) The euphoric, loquacious, circumstantial, and obtrusive type. (2) The apathetic, dull, and slow type. (3) The irritable, undisciplined type. It is obvious that such types cannot be easily differentiated, and it is also difficult to establish significant deviations from the pretraumatic personality. In discussions of personality changes after cerebral trauma, most authors stress lack of initiative or spontaneity, impulsive irritability, explosiveness, and emotional lability, and, in severe cases, a silly euphoria as most characteristic. Modern psychiatry, however, does not regard such traits in isolation but considers them in a dynamic and social context. Depressive or euphoric moods, impulsiveness, and irritability may then be understood as reactions in the context of interpersonal relations in a particular social setting. The clowning, hysterical, and dependent behavior of patients with head injuries is not merely the result of cerebral pathology but a response to a situation where patients are rewarded for infantile and demanding attitudes. When brain-injured patients are restricted socially, it is only to be expected that they will react in infantile ways. Most of all, however, such patients have a need to deny their anxiety and concern over the real and imaginary sequelae of the injury by disengaging from social contact and refusing to accept the seriousness of their situation.

The study of brain injuries has contributed significantly to our knowledge of cerebral structure and function. K. Kleist described a large number of different syndromes deriving from an equally large number of localized lesions.[12] Today, there is disinclination to accept such a phrenological approach.[9] It seems that, in the course of new clinical, neurophysiological, and statistical knowledge of brain injuries, the time-honored syndromes of an older neurology have become less specific. Neither Hans-Lukas Teuber[26] nor A. R. Luria,[16] pioneers in the study of brain trauma, has completely relinquished the diagnosis of specific syndromes; for example, the various aphasias, apraxias, and agnosias; but rather they reinterpret them in the light of theories that view the brain as a dynamic communications system (see chapters 6 and 16).

Diffuse Post-traumatic Encephalopathies

A special type of post-traumatic encephalopathy is the "punch-drunk" syndrome first described by H. S. Martland.[17] It is seen in professional prize fighters who suffer many knockouts. These sluggers first show some incoordination of movement, staggering gait, and coarse tremors; in later stages, they suffer from marked intellectual deterioration and organic personality changes. Martland felt that the many blows to their heads led to multiple punctate hemorrhages and destructions of cerebral ganglion cells. More recent neuropathological examination of brains of punch-drunk fighters has revealed neuropathological syndromes similar to Pick's disease.[21] It is not easy to determine in the individual case whether the fighter is suffering from alcoholic brain disease, from a presenile psychosis, or has sustained brain damage. There is no doubt, however, that professional boxing may cause permanent and severe damage to the brain and the retina[13] as well as to other organs.

Post-traumatic Syndrome

Psychiatrists and neurologists use this rather vague label as a shorthand description of a complex, long-lasting reaction following head injury. There are no objective signs. The EEG does not show characteristic changes and is usually entirely negative. About one-third of all patients suffering from head injuries develop this syndrome, which may be relatively mild and annoying, or quite severe and disabling. The most pervasive symptom is headache, which is often severe, intermittent, throbbing, and which may occur day or night. Patients also complain of insomnia, frightening dreams, fatigability, weakness, and sweating. There is no doubt that anxiety plays a central role in the genesis of such symptoms; many patients complain of anxiety or of being jumpy, easily startled, and they are also hypersensitive to bright light and noise. They are irritable and feel that performance of work is difficult, especially if concentration and precision are required. They also complain of lapses of memory or attention, although no abnormalities are detected by objective testing. All these changes reveal themselves in social relations; and the patients are reported to be unpleasant, inconsiderate, and uninterested in others; some patients are aware of such changes, others not. They may develop almost immediately after the injury or weeks or months later; they may persist for weeks, months, and years.

The etiology of the post-traumatic syndrome is obscure. A division into physiogenic and psychogenic causes is not justified on the basis of present knowledge. We certainly cannot point to definite physiological changes; yet, the connection with the original trauma is undeniable. In all likelihood, premorbid personality is more important for the genesis of the syndrome than the physiological aspects of the head injury. It has been claimed, but not substantiated, that sociopathic and alcoholic patients develop more serious post-traumatic states than others. Accident-proneness has been found in the history of patients with post-traumatic syndromes. Clinically, one has the impression that very aggressive or very passive persons, particularly those who are conflicted over passive-aggressive impulses, are likely candidates for the syndrome; anger over both the physiological-psychological injury and dependency needs seems to play a role in the genesis of the syndrome and in the inability to overcome it.

Alexandra Adler found that patients who were intoxicated at the time of injury were less prone than others to develop post-traumatic syndromes.[1] According to her, post-traumatic reactions occur in certain occupations with a professional expectation of hazards (such as firemen and policemen) more often than in others. This investigator also reported that occupational difficulties in such patients are apt to occur if the pretraumatic occupational adjustment was precarious. Secondary gains, as we encounter them in compensation neuroses, are known to contribute to the syndrome. J.-E. Meyer pointed to the frequency of sexual disturbances, such as impotence, after head injury;[18] in all likelihood, psychological factors are primarily responsible for this kind of symptom.

It is easy to diagnose the typical syndrome; unfortunately, however, there are few typical cases. Aubrey Lewis, in a discussion of a neurological report on head injuries by C. P. Symonds, remarked how difficult it is to differentiate post-traumatic syndromes from the usual neurotic reactions to head injuries.[14] The great fear of having one's head injured, and the subsequent false expectations of damages and of gains, may precipitate all kinds of neurotic behavior, especially hysterical and hypochondriacal exaggerations of symptoms. Often, there is a complaint of constant headache, and there is also a therapeutic response to waking or hypnotic suggestion in such patients. In genuine post-traumatic states, there is rarely a complaint of incessant headache. Outright malingering of the syndrome, either in wartime or peace, is rare.

Psychiatric Treatment of Late Sequelae of Head Injuries

Neurological, neurosurgical, and psychiatric therapy of the chronic behavioral and neurological symptoms after head injuries is a challenging but difficult task. There have been remarkable successes with physical retraining of impaired motor function, training of aphasic patients by speech therapists, and careful occupational and social rehabilitation in many military, veterans, and civilian hospitals. Except in time of war, American psychiatrists have not concerned themselves to any large extent with these patients and have thus missed opportunities for exciting studies and rewarding therapy. Many difficulties can be prevented if patients are properly oriented about their injuries and quickly and vigorously rehabilitated. Unfortunately, physicians often contribute to the development of post-traumatic states by not paying attention to the patient's anger, anxiety, and dependency needs or by fostering an invalid attitude. Once the syndrome has developed, prolonged and patient individual psychotherapy is recommended. Experiences with group therapy are promising. The patient must have an opportunity to work through his anger, anxiety, and dependent needs. He must also be brought to the understanding that secondary gains are far less advantageous than a realistic attitude to his needs and responsibilities. Prolonged hospitalization and emphasis on analgesic or sedative medication should be avoided whenever possible; compensation claims and related matters should be speedily settled in a satisfactory manner. A vigorous and persistent program of occupational rehabilitation can be of great value. Yet it should be remembered that psychosocial measures will not always be successful because there is always the possibility of undetected lasting structural and physiological damage.

NOTES

1. Alexandra Adler, "Mental Symptoms Following Head Injury," *Archives of Neurology and Psychiatry*, 53 (1945), 34.
2. Walther Birkmeyer, *Hirnverletzungen* (Wien: Springer, 1950).
3. S. Brock, ed., *Injuries of the Brain and Spinal Cord and Their Coverings* (3rd ed.; Baltimore: Williams & Wilkins, 1949).
4. Henry W. Brosin, "Psychiatric Conditions Following Head Injury," in Silvano Arieti, ed., *The American Handbook of Psychiatry* (New York: Basic Books, 1959), Vol. II, pp. 1175–1202.
5. Derek Denny-Brown and W. R. Russell, "Experimental Cerebral Concussion," *Brain*, 64 (1941), 93.
6. Howard D. Fabing, "Cerebral Blast Syndrome in Combat Soldiers," *Archives of Neurology and Psychiatry*, 57 (1947), 14.
7. H. Felten, "Die Zerebrale Fettembolie," *Fortschritt Neurol. Psychiat.*, 26 (1958), 443.
8. E. Gamper, "Zum Problem der Commotio Cerebri," *Mschr. Psychiat. Neurol.*, 99 (1938), 542.
9. Kurt Goldstein, *Aftereffects of Brain Injuries in War* (New York: Grune & Stratton, 1942).

10. Ward C. Halstead, *Brain and Intelligence* (Chicago: University of Chicago Press, 1947).
11. Donald O. Hebb, *The Organization of Behavior* (New York: John Wiley, 1949).
12. Karl Kleist, "Gehirn und Seele," *Dtsch. Med. Wschr.*, 76 (1951), 1197.
13. L. E. Larsson, K. A. Melin, C. Nordström, G. Oehrberg, B. P. Silfverskiöld and K. Oehrberg, "Acute Head Injuries in Boxers," *Acta Psychiatrica Neurologica Scandinavia*, Suppl. 95, 1954.
14. Sir Aubrey Lewis, "Discussion of Different Diagnosis and Treatment of Post-contusional States," (Proceedings of the Royal Society of Medicine, 35 [1942], 607).
15. Theodore Lidz, "The Amnestic Syndrome," *Archives of Neurology and Psychiatry*, 47 (1942), 588.
16. Alexandr R. Luria, *Restoration of Function after Brain Injury* (New York: Pergamon Press, 1963).
17. H. S. Martland, "Punch Drunk", *Journal of the American Medical Association*, 91 (1928), 1103.
18. J.-E. Meyer, "Die Sexuellen Störungen der Hirnverletzten, *Arch. Psychiat., Nervenkr.*, 193 (1955), 449.
19. B. E. Moore and Jurgen Ruesch, "Prolonged Disturbances of Consciousness Following Head Injury," *New England Journal of Medicine*, 230 (1944), 445.
20. Donald Munro and G. L. Maltby, "Extradural Hemorrhage," *American Surgeon*, 13, (1941), 192.
21. K. T. Neuburger, D. W. Sinton, and J. Denst, "Cerebral Atrophy Associated with Boxing," *Archives of Neurology and Psychiatry*, 81 (1959), 403.
22. Wilder Penfield and H. Jasper, eds., *Epilepsy and the Functional Anatomy of the Human Brain* (Boston: Little, Brown, 1954).
23. R. N. Reitan, *The Effects of Brain Lesions on the Adaptive Abilities in Human Beings* (Indianapolis: University of Indiana Press, 1959).
24. Jurgen Ruesch, "Intellectual Impairment in Head Injury," *American Journal of Psychiatry*, 100 (1944), 480.
25. Kurt Schneider, "Über den psychischen Zustand Schädelverletzter," *Allg. Z. Psychiat.*, 101 (1934), 236.
26. Hans-Lukas Teuber, "Some Alterations in Cerebral Lesions in Man," in *Evolution of Nervous Control* (Washington, D. C.: American Association for the Advancement of Science, 1959).
27. S. B. Wortis, M. Herman, and J. London, "Mental Changes in Patients with Subdural Hematomas," in *Trauma of the Central Nervous System*, (Research Publication Association of Nervous and Mental Disease, 1943), Vol. 24, p. 274.

CHAPTER EIGHTEEN

The Epilepsies

◆ Clinically the epilepsies are characterized by recurrent seizures with motor, sensory, and autonomic signs and symptoms. In terms of the bioelectrical activity of neurons, they are described as cerebral paroxysmal discharges. In some cases, epilepsies are associated with demonstrable chemical and structural changes of the central nervous system. A variety of disturbances of consciousness constitute a correlate of seizures, and some patients suffer from behavior disorders. Since we need a term, it is at least preferable to speak of seizures rather than of convulsions, because many types of paroxysmal neuronal discharge (electrically monitored) are not manifested in tonic and clonic muscular movements, as the term convulsion implies. Obviously, "seizure" does not truly describe the operative mechanisms either; most neurologists speak interchangeably of seizure, fit, convulsion, or *ictus epilepticus* (*ictus* meaning stroke or blow). The epilepsies are of considerable clinical importance; of one thousand persons five suffer from epilepsy. The epilepsies are of primary interest to the neurologist; however, the behavioral manifestations are often so striking that, for both practical and theoretical reasons, these diseases concern psychiatrists.

Epilepsy has been known to man since time immemorial: the *sacred disease* always created a feeling of awe, and it still does. It was mentioned in the Code of Hammurabi (2080 B.C.) and was beautifully described as a natural disease by Hippocrates.[37] John Hughlings Jackson was the first to describe focal seizures, and some of his dynamic ideas, based on clinical and anatomical observations about the epilepsies and the central nervous system in general, are still unsurpassed.[35] Many of his propositions have been substantiated by one of the most important technical discoveries in the field, the development of the electroencephalographic (EEG) technique by Hans Berger in 1924.

Diagnostic Classification

No diagnostic classification of the epilepsies is universally accepted. The simple classification based on the symptomatology of seizure is, as is true of all purely descriptive groupings, rather unsatisfactory. In many patients, not just one type of seizure, but a combination of different seizures, occurs. Attempts to classify the epilepsies according to their EEG findings alone have not been practical, since these phenomena often are unspecific. Etiologically, the epilepsies may be divided into two groups. (1) *The symptomatic epilepsies:* In this group the seizure is the result of a demonstrable structural or physiological alteration of the central nervous system, as by tumor, scar, malformation, chemical disorders such as hypoglycemia, hypocalcemia, and certain types of poisoning. (2) *The cryptogenic epilepsies:* This group is composed of epilepsies of unknown etiology, that is, no causal agent or mechanism can be demonstrated. These epilepsies have also been called genuine, essential, or idiopathic epilepsies. With increasing knowledge of mechanisms, this group shrinks.

Some modern classifications are based on topographic principles. The data underlying these classifications are derived from tracking the spatial and temporal characteristics of the EEG, as well as from associated neurological signs and symptoms, and neurosurgical procedures (ablation and local stimulation). Wilder Penfield divides the epilepsies into (1) focal cerebral seizures, which begin with a neuronal discharge in the vicinity of a demonstrable abnormal focus in the central nervous system; (2) centrencephalic seizures, which originate in the central upper brain stem, mesencephalic, and diencephalic regions;[29] the latter include some of the cases of so-called idiopathic or cryptogenic epilepsies manifested by *grand mal* and *petit mal*, behavioral automatism, or psychomotor seizures; and (3) cerebral seizures, which are unlocalized and caused by diffuse abnormalities of the brain, such as toxic or metabolic diseases.

Henri Gastaut, on the other hand, has proposed a two-part division: (1) Generalized seizures with bilateral EEG abnormalities; these are initiated in the subcortex; there are no clinical localizing signs; and the discharge occurs throughout the gray matter. (2) Partial or focal or localized seizures. These seizures are unilateral, initiated in cortical or subcortical centers with a limited discharge. Henri Gastaut does not divide discharges into cortical and subcortical discharges; he believes that both systems are involved in most discharges.[9] The exact mechanisms by which the discharge obtained from scalp or cortex are generated have not been settled. It is obvious that a vast number of cellular activities are concealed in the wave forms monitored by usual techniques; and theories, as yet inconclusive, favor various "sources" (cortical and subcortical systems) for components of the scalp EEG. The complexity of electroneural events is enormous, and computer techniques have made possible analyses that may be far more discriminating with respect to behavior than our clinical EEG tools.

Symptomatology of Generalized Seizures

GRAND MAL SEIZURES The typical *grand mal* attack is a tonic-clonic seizure with a loss of consciousness. Many *grand mal* seizures are heralded by prodromata, which may precede the actual attack by hours or even days. The prodromata consist of vague, uncomfortable, and anxious feelings;

mood changes such as depressions, elation, or a histrionic lability of mood; headaches; minor gastrointestinal difficulties such as lack of appetite, flatulence, or epigastric pain; sweating; and cold or hot sensations. The prodromal symptoms ought to be differentiated from the *aura,* which does not precede the seizure but is a part of it. About half of all epileptic patients report an aura. In a number of cases, the aura is of diagnostic importance because it suggests a cerebral localization; it also has practical significance because it enables the patient to protect himself. Aura literally means breeze, but the symptoms are by no means confined to skin sensations; they may comprise motor, vegetative, and psychological phenomena as well. The most frequent types of aura before *grand mal* seizures are epigastric discomfort, dizziness, faintness, and such elementary sensory phenomena as seeing brilliant dots and lines, hearing sounds, and experiencing strange and usually disagreeable odors and tastes. The major tonic contraction may be preceded by a few muscular twitches. The actual tonic phase consists of extreme rigidity of the muscles of head, neck, trunk, and extremities. The extremities are in maximal extension; the trunk is in opisthotonus; the neck and head are thrown back. Respiration may stop for as long as a minute. At times, the last forceful expiration produces a loud cry—*le cri épileptique.* Contraction of the respiratory muscles usually causes cyanosis. When the patient loses consciousness and falls in a rigid position he is apt to hurt himself. The tonic phase ends with general trembling of the muscles, which initiates the violent contraction of the clonic phase. During this phase, the patient often bites his tongue, passes urine, or, more rarely, feces. At the end of the clonic phase, the patient is in a deep coma; the eyes are turned upward; pupils are dilated and do not react to light. Babinski's sign is usually present. Often, the patient sweats profusely. Most patients wake up gradually; they are dazed and slow as they begin to recognize their environment; they complain about sleepiness, haziness, headaches, and amnesia for the attack. Normally, recovery may take from one to several hours. The typical EEG during a seizure consists of bilateral and generalized fast spikes of high amplitude that begin during the tonic phase. During the clonic phase, these are interrupted by slow waves and even periods of electrical silence. In ordinary scalp EEG's of unanesthetized, uncurarized patients, muscular discharges obscure the typical seizure patterns. In the interictal phase, abnormal slow and fast waves are frequently seen.

PETIT MAL ATTACKS William Lennox described the so-called *petit mal triad* as consisting of the following subtypes: (1) a simple lapse of consciousness for fifteen to thirty seconds with slight twitching of facial muscles, a vacant stare, and subsequent amnesia for the attack; (2) a similar lapse of consciousness with myoclonic twitches; and (3) an episode of sudden loss of muscular tone and consciousness.[21] Typical *petit mal* seizures begin in childhood and often persist into adult years. Ordinarily they do not begin in adult life, and remission frequently occurs after adolescence. The typical EEG pattern shows bilateral and generalized bursts of three cycles-per-second spike and dome patterns concomitant with these attacks, but also frequently occurring without seizures. (See Figure 18–1.) Gastaut and

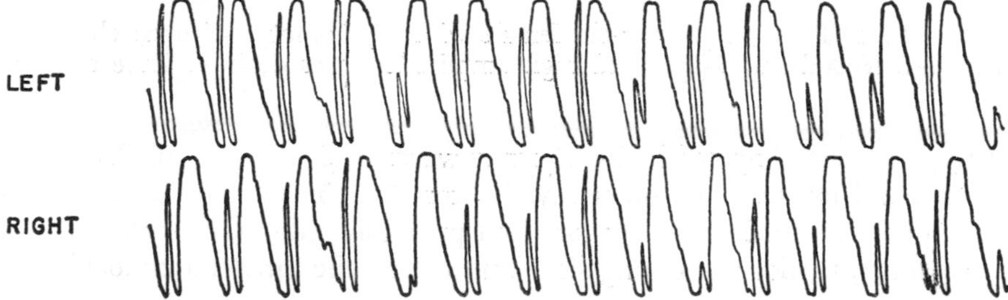

Figure 18–1. Six-year-old child with *petit mal* seizures. Characteristic 2–4 second spike and wave discharges associated with momentary lapse of attention and eyelid fluttering.

others doubt the justification of including the second and third subtypes because the typical EEG of the pure *petit mal* attack is never seen in seizures that are characterized only by loss of muscular tone or myoclonus.

Epilepsy with frequent *petit mal* seizures during childhood and a relatively benign prognosis has been termed pyknolepsy. Many observers agree that children with *petit mal* often are timid, passive, gullible, and given to day-dreaming. Frequently hysterical symptoms occur, but the *petit mal* attacks themselves cannot be induced, modified, or stopped by such psychological means as hypnosis. The seizures may increase in frequency, however, during periods of emotional stress. In some patients, a *petit mal* status may occur, producing a prolonged confusional state. A. Jus and K. Jus demonstrated that *petit mal* patients suffer from a brief preictal retrograde amnesia.[19]

PSYCHOMOTOR EPILEPSY William G. Lennox used this term very broadly and included in the psychomotor triad: (1) increased tonicity of muscles with adversive movements of head and swallowing movements and also complete arrest of motion with masticatory movements (these seizures are of longer duration than a *petit mal* attack); (2) automatic behavior such as unbuttoning of clothing, walking, or running with complete amnesia, although consciousness may be preserved; and (3) more complex "psychic seizures" (to be described in the next section) with disturbances of awareness and memory.[24] These seizures, according to F. A. Gibbs, E. L. Gibbs and W. G. Lennox, are accompanied by slow 4–6 second high-amplitude

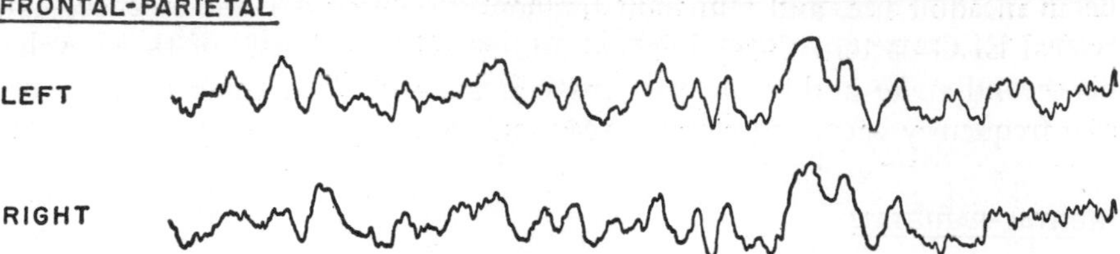

Figure 18–2. Twenty-eight-year-old female with psychomotor seizures: characteristic 1–2 second and 5–6 second high amplitude waves during seizure activity.

waves with superimposed high-frequency waves.[11] (See Figure 18–2.) It was later found by these and other investigators that, in patients with psychomotor epilepsy, such waves are localized predominantly in one or both temporal lobes, particularly during sleep and during the interictal periods.

PSYCHIC SEIZURES Psychic seizures, also called by some clinicians epileptic equivalents, refer to the paroxysmal occurrence of certain complex behavioral acts and experiences. In order to classify such events as epileptic, the patient must also exhibit other clinical and electrical manifestations of epilepsy; if no other seizures occur or if the electroencephalogram is not clearly abnormal, the diagnosis of psychic seizures remains on shaky ground. Psychic seizures occur relatively frequently. Penfield and others listed the following categories: forced thoughts, hallucinations, illusions, and delusions.[26] In some patients with localized lesions, it was possible to elicit such symptoms by electric stimulation.[17] The patients themselves refer to the paroxysmal occurrence of certain experiences and thoughts as forced thoughts; often, the patients have forgotten these memories and are startled by their emergence into consciousness. Usually, these experiences have a special symbolic significance, which can be demonstrated by the use of psychoanalytic techniques. Based on his experiments and observations, Penfield boldly assumed that the temporal lobe is the seat of memory.[27] But as yet, the engrams have not truly been pinned to a local area. In some psychic seizures, these experiences are very lively, and the patient experiences them somewhat like an observer at a play. In other cases, they take on the form of a *déjà vu* or a *déjà entendu* experience. Often the experiences are very vague and bizarre, and the patients report them as trancelike or dreamlike. The unreal character of such experiences may become very marked; some patients become unable to distinguish between fantasy and reality and suffer from visual, acoustic, olfactory, gustatory and skin hallucinations, as well as from illusions and various delusions. Another type of psychic seizure is not so much a feeling of unreality as a feeling of depersonalization with extreme anxiety and intense feelings of displeasure. A feeling of ecstatic happiness is much rarer; Fyôdor Mikhailovich Dostoyevsky, himself an epileptic, described this in *The Idiot,* the greatest literary account of epilepsy. Signs of disturbed consciousness are subtle; for example, a certain vagueness, inattention, or very fixed attention on irrelevant matters are typical. These patients are not completely amnesic but show partial memory defects; they remember things vaguely and do not develop a later amnesia for these experiences. However, distinct amnesia may occur after some psychic seizures, for example, after a period of extreme anxiety, running fits, and even rather complex attacks of aggressive, uninhibited sexual and infantile behavior. The aggressive and antisocial nature of such episodes can be very marked. Most psychic seizures have an ictal character and are of short duration. Some episodes, however, involve more complex and enduring psychotic behavior. In such cases we are usually not able to classify the episode as ictal, postictal, or interictal behavior; and all too often we are uncertain whether the behavior is in fact a manifestation of epilepsy.

The following illustrates the psychosocial problems of a patient with *grand mal* and psychomotor seizures:

A twenty-six-year-old divorced woman was admitted for diagnosis and treatment of her seizures and psychological problems. She was told that she had a seizure lasting all day when she was two; the family had assumed that this was either caused by fright or teething. The first seizure she remembers occurred at the time of her early menarche, at the age of nine. She has had three to four seizures a month since, usually before or during menses. The seizures begin with a "funny electrical feeling" in her stomach, which spreads to the upper and lower extremities after which she blacks out for two to three minutes. According to observers, she usually screams, tries to hold on to something, squeezes someone's hand, becomes slightly stiff, and, after a few seconds, lapses into a confused state during which she may be amorous, talk without realizing it, or even light a cigarette. She also has become quite pugnacious during these spells and once tried to choke her mother. There were some spells in which she wandered around the house without remembering what she did. Her mother viewed these spells as temper tantrums and did not bring her to a physician until she was sixteen; however, only one year before admission, she was seen by a neurologist and treated with mesantoin and later with dilantin. Six months before admission she developed generalized convulsions, which occurred once or twice a month. In these seizures, she had bitten her tongue and was incontinent of urine.

The patient is the fifteenth child in a French-Canadian Catholic family. The father, an unskilled laborer whom she remembers as a kindly man, died from a stroke when she was six. The mother dominates the household and still tells the patient that she has to be home at a certain hour. Of the fifteen siblings, two died of unknown illnesses; one sister has high blood pressure and suffered from a cerebral hemorrhage; four brothers are reported to be chronic alcoholics; and one sister has "spells" in which she loses her voice. One brother, with whom the patient is living, has a gastric ulcer. The patient finished the elementary grades and then dropped out of school to help with the children of the older sister. She always has felt very insecure and excluded in her social relations. She was married to a brutal man whose insatiable sexual demands disgusted the frigid patient. He beat her, openly carried on sexual affairs with other women, and forced her to take care of his invalid father. When he returned from overseas service, he divorced her against her protests. In the meantime, she started an affair with an illiterate borderline mental defective, who is quite understanding of her problems and kind to her.

The patient was found to be of average intelligence (verbal I.Q., 94; performance I.Q., 104); there was no evidence of psychological deficit. The general physical examination was negative except for a moderate hypertrichosis. Neurological findings were negative. Blood sugar, NPN, serum calcium, and phosphorus and 17– ketosteroid excretion, and routine laboratory findings were within normal limits. Skull X-rays were negative. The EEG examination showed 11–12 second frequencies predominating in the occipital leads, superimposed on much 6/sec. activity in the frontal and parietal leads. In addition, there was moderate 4/sec. and some 18/sec. activity in these leads. There was no change on hyperventilation. The EEG was interpreted as suggestive but not diagnostic of epilepsy. The hospitalization was used to stabilize the medication and to give the patient, her boyfriend, and the brother with whom the patient lives, a better orientation to her psychological problems associated with the seizures. She was put on dilantin, .1 gm. tid. She decided to go ahead with a second marriage in spite of being unable to obtain dispensation by the Catholic Church. The social worker referred her to a rehabilitation agency to help her change jobs, because she was working on a machine job, which was potentially dangerous on account of her seizures. She had not informed her employer that she is an epileptic. The therapist thought her masochistic behavior was related to an inability to express her strong aggression. An attempt was made to control both self-destructive and aggressive tendencies and to help her to express her feelings more adequately and to communicate more meaningfully.

Symptomatology of Focal Discharges

Focal or partial discharges are classified according to the localization of the epileptogenic focus and the dysfunctions that are the result of the abnormal discharge. The typical focal seizure is not accompanied by a loss of consciousness. However, unconsciousness and generalized convulsions may follow; the characteristic focal pattern is still preserved at the onset of the seizure and may be considered an aura. EEG abnormalities cover a wide range of phenomena; rapid localized spikes with increase of amplitude are rather characteristic; these discharges may remain localized or become diffuse and spread, usually from cortical to subcortical areas. The focal motor seizures, described by Jackson and named after him, begin with twitching of a muscle group, such as the muscles of the face and lips, and then spread according to the central representation of muscles in the prerolandic gyrus to neck, upper, and lower extremities; this is referred to as the *Jack-*

sonian march. Often seizures start in the fingers, more rarely in the lower extremities. In certain types of seizures, a turning of eyes, head, or trunk occurs. Such adversive seizures originate in frontal areas 6 or 8.

When skin sensations are involved in focal seizures, we speak of sensory seizures. Patients report tingling and formications in a localized region of the body. These seizures originate in the postrolandic area; a diffusion of sensory seizures has also been observed. Visual seizures, originating in areas 18 and 19 of the occipital lobe, consist of the seeing of bright, fiery spots, stars and lines, of color sensations, of scotoma, and momentary blinding as well as of micropsia and macropsia, which are similar to sensations that precede migraine attacks. Auditory partial seizures originating in the temporal lobes may consist of elementary sounds and noises, or of hyperacusis, although in most cases of temporal lobe seizures (see below) the discharge patterns are more complex. Attacks of vertigo have been observed in lesions of Heschl's gyri. Olfactory and gustatory sensations, such as foul and disagreeable odors, were reported by Jackson as an aura of so-called uncinate fits. Autonomic symptoms cover a wide range of phenomena, such as nausea, belching, urge to defecate, sighing, feeling weak, perspiration, hot or cold sensations, fear, as well as blanching and flushing, pupillary changes, sexual symptoms and experiences such as priapism and orgasm, and anxiety. These symptoms could be referred to wide parts of the rhinencephalic and limbic systems.[12]

TEMPORAL LOBE EPILEPSY Under this term, the literature describes a large group of seizures caused by temporal lesions with a highly diversified symptomatology. Ever since some neurologists equated temporal lobe epilepsy and psychomotor seizures, there has been no real agreement about what is meant by the former. This confusion has been at least partly clarified in a critical review by Gastaut.[8] The term temporal lobe epilepsy should be used with caution; many cases involve pathology not only of the temporal cortex, but also of the Island of Reil and the deeper rhinencephalic structures. In addition, other portions of the limbic system may be involved, such as the subfrontal and cingulate cortex as well as diencephalic and hypothalamic structures. There are also clinical reasons for the diffuseness of the term, temporal lobe epilepsy. The symptoms that have been associated most readily with temporal lobe seizures include the psychomotor seizures and virtually all forms of psychic seizures mentioned earlier; yet, about half the patients with temporal lobe epilepsy also have *grand mal* seizures. Denis Hill stressed the relative frequency of severe, lasting behavior disorders, such as psychotic reactions and impulsive antisocial behavior, in patients with true temporal lobe epilepsy as compared with other epilepsies.[18] We are far from a thorough understanding of these highly interesting behavior disorders, which are described more fully in the section on interictal behavior. Among the rare symptoms of focal epilepsy are transient aphasias, agnosias, and apraxias. The diagnosis of temporal lobe epilepsy depends on the demonstration of focal pathological discharges.

POSTICTAL STATES Epileptic seizures, and especially *grand mal* seizures, have been compared to electrical brain storms, which come and go quickly and usually leave no sequelae except for injuries inflicted during the seizure and a certain fatigue and depression. The depression after a *grand mal* seizure is not only an aftermath of the violent physical exertion and spent energy but also involves a psychological reaction of shame and disgust. The reorientation of the patient to his surrounding world and himself takes time, at least as much time as awakening from a very deep sleep, and usually longer. When the patient awakens, he is slightly confused and disoriented as to time and place; he thinks and speaks slowly. This mild confusion is the rule after *grand mal* seizures and also after electrically or chemically produced convulsions. If the confusion is more lasting we speak of *clouded states* or *twilight states.* Usually there is a diminished reactivity to external stimulation, a constriction of consciousness and a diminution of higher mental processes. Patients in these states will carry out some of their everyday acts, urinate, defecate, dress or undress, and cooperate with other persons. But they seldom speak spontaneously and usually only in monosyllables. They can also be extraordinarily impulsive and react with violent and aggressive behavior. During these states, epileptics have performed highly antisocial and criminal acts, which seem incompatible with their conscious strivings and attitudes.

Fugues

The concept of fugue is by no means clear.[33] Descriptively, the term is applied to prolonged drastic alterations of behavior which are characterized by pathological psychomotor activity and amnesia for the event. In a typical state of fugue a patient may wander or travel for days and weeks without any clear purpose or goal. When he recovers from the episode, he is surprised at what he has done; the behavior is not compatible with his conscious intentions. In the fugue, his consciousness does not seem disturbed on superficial examination; if stopped or questioned, he may give clear answers about his identity and seem oriented. On closer examination, however, it can be seen that attention is narrowed; when pressed for a logical account of his behavior, he becomes evasive, anxious, or angry. Fugues may be considered epileptic when seizure activity and abnormal EEG findings occur in such patients. Some epileptic fugues are epileptic equivalents; others appear to be postictal states.

Postepileptic delirium should be distinguished from fugues; it may be characterized by very severe motor hyperactivity, severe anxiety, hallucinations, and delusions. The hallucinations of such deliria are aural and visual and frequently of a religious character, with appearances of the Lord, the Virgin, Saints, or the Devil. Similarly, the delusions often center around themes of death, the hereafter, guilt, and redemption.

Epileptic fugue states should be differentiated from psychogenic fugue states. The majority of fugues are neurotic; even in epileptic fugues, neurotic, and particularly hysterical, symptoms are frequent. Many fugues are related to alcoholism; excessive and even moderate alcohol intake may precipitate the fugue. The content of the fugue is invariably related to unconscious impulses of the patient. Impulsive wandering or "poriomanic" behavior may be an escape from stress; on deeper exploration it can sometimes be demonstrated that it is a repetition of an infantile neurotic conflict. This is also true for some of the fugues characterized by extremely antisocial behavior such as arson, murder, or aggressive sexual crimes.

On careful exploration, it was found that the poriomanic, with or without epileptic disease, is running away from a dangerous experience, usually a threatening or seductive relationship.[32, 34] One such patient was insulted at the slightest suggestion of a feeling of hostility toward his wife; nevertheless, he left her on several occasions in fugue states in which he undertook long senseless trips during which he had amnesia for his identity (and his relationship to his "lovely wife"). In some adventurous globe-trotters and old salts, running away and the yearning for the frontier or the endless ocean become a more or less acceptable pattern of living.

Interictal Behavior

In the older neuropsychiatric literature, three basic forms of interictal behavior were thought to be characteristic for the epilepsies: (1) certain basic personality characteristics; (2) psychotic behavior; and (3) deterioration. In well-treated epileptics, these conditions are rare. This view, unhappily, has not yet reached the general public; even professional persons still think many epileptics are demented, psychotic, dangerous, and evil. It has not been commonly accepted that deterioration and mental deficiency are usually not the result of epileptic seizures, but of other demonstrable organic cerebral changes. One must also distinguish between basic behavioral changes and secondary changes; the latter result from the handicaps of stigmatization the epileptic experiences, which impress on him—unjustly in the overwhelming number of cases—that he is different and inferior. Even intellectual deterioration and mental deficit may be a secondary psychosocial handicap. Howard Fabing told us about the case of a young boy, considered mentally deficient, who had many seizures daily and hence was virtually unable to learn. After the introduction of anticonvulsant drug therapy, the boy acquired enough freedom from the seizures so that he could be tutored and later attend school. His "mental deficiency" disappeared.

Notwithstanding, it must be said that certain character traits are seen with some frequency in epileptics, particularly in severe and institutionalized epileptics. In mild forms, such traits as a certain stubbornness, obsequiousness, and inertia may also be observed in the intelligent and socially well-adapted epileptic. In the more severe forms, there is a tendency to perseveration of thoughts and a certain stickiness of affect. A number of epileptics also have a peculiar inclination to exaggerated piety and a preoccupation with orthodox and rigid religious, philosophical, and political ideas. Possibly this inclination for metaphysical rumination is related to the interest of some epileptics in death, rebirth, and the hereafter, concerns that likely stem from the experience of startlingly and episodically altered contact with reality which seizures entail. As in other obsessive and rigid behavior, such symptoms might be thought of as defenses against the basic anxiety and the helplessness engendered by the epileptic seizure. We have much to learn about the problems of aggressiveness, impulse control, and religiosity, and what determines and conditions these; whether they are a correlate of the seizure diatheses, a consequence of living with interruptions of consciousness, or a psychodynamically motivated reaction to these factors is unknown. Impulsive and aggressive criminal behavior in epileptics has been shown to be only slightly more frequent than in a nonepileptic control population.[2] Such actions may occur as seizure equivalents and as interictal behavior.

There is no specific epileptic psychosis between attacks, just as there is no specific ictal psychosis. Some psychoses in the interictal and postictal periods are referred to as epileptic deliria; others have the character of schizophreniform reactions. In connection with the last group, we should draw attention to two polar and contradictory statements. At one time, L. Meduna held that epilepsy and schizophrenia were mutually exclusive; this assumption led to his theory that artificial convulsive seizures are therapeutic in schizophrenia. Currently, however, we are faced with reports by Robert G. Heath and others that subcortical electrical discharges in schizophrenia and certain forms of epilepsy are similar.[15] It is quite possible that certain schizophreniform psychoses, often with a paranoid coloring, are related to the epilepsies. E. Slater and E. Glithero[31] and Glaser and coworkers[14] found such psychoses in patients with temporal lobe lesions; their affectivity was less impaired than in true schizophrenias. Patients with episodic perceptual disturbances or altered subjective awareness should be diagnostically investigated for psychomotor epilepsy.

Deterioration of epileptics without demonstrable cerebral lesions has not been reliably observed. However, secondary lesions may occur after status epilepticus. Even in cases with cerebral lesions, deterioration usually is not simply the consequence of an underlying neuropathological process, but rather the result of deprivation and neglect. This is particularly evident in epileptic children raised in so-called epileptic colonies.

Etiology

From clinical observation, neurosurgical therapeutic procedures, and pharmacological and experimental work, a great deal has been learned about the pathology of the epilepsies. Much is known today about what happens in ganglion cells and in transsynaptic propagation in and from epileptic foci to produce the spread of a seizure. Although a differentiation between cortical and subcortical epilepsy is made by many investigators, Gastaut thinks that both the cortical and subcortical systems are invariably involved.[10] The loss of consciousness is always produced by an initial subcortical discharge or spread of cortical discharge to a subcortical center. Such assumptions have been supported by experimental findings.

A potential seizure discharge is the universal property of the central nervous system. With sufficiently strong stimulation, any animal or human will respond with a seizure: as Hill simply put it, anybody can have a fit.[18] Lennox compared the organism to a reservoir fed by several pipes; overflow means seizure.[23] If the reservoir is shallow (that is, if there is genetic predisposition), it will overflow more easily. This will also happen if the flow from one or several pipes, symbolizing epileptogenetic stimuli such as trauma or infection, is strong.

Although the ultimate causes of the idiopathic epilepsies are obscure, much is known about certain predisposing and precipitating factors and pathological mechanisms. In the cryptogenic group, the role of heredity has been stressed—probably overstressed. In a survey of 4,231 patients with 20,000 near relatives (parents, siblings, and children), Lennox found that the prevalence rate of epilepsy in relatives is 3.6, compared with 0.5 in the general population. According to Lennox, however, the chance that one epileptic parent will produce epileptic children is only one in forty.[23] C. H. Alström found the prevalence rate of parents of epileptics was 1.3, of siblings 1.5, and of children 3.0 per cent.[2] In epileptic twins with brain damage, Lennox found a concordance rate of 84 in identical twins and of 10 in fraternal twins.[22] Alström assumes the existence of a simple monohybridism of dominant and recessive traits. The main dominant epileptic gene is modified by recessive polygenes.[2]

Complications of pregnancy, fetal diseases, malformations, birth injuries, and infectious diseases are considered to be the important causes of all seizures in infancy and early childhood.[25] In later childhood and adult life, cerebral injuries leading to scar formations and brain tumors are the most important contributory causes for symptomatic seizures. In old age, vascular diseases of the brain become important causes. Convulsions can be precipitated by many chemical substances above a certain threshold (for example, camphor, metrazol, acetylcholine), by a variety of physical stimuli (electrical current, photic stimulation), or by changes in the protein, carbohydrate, mineral, and fluid balance of the body, as we observe them in many febrile and metabolic diseases (hypoglycemia, hypocalcemia, uremia). Whether chronic excessive intake of alcohol and barbiturates can produce seizures is not certain. In all likelihood, seizures in chronic alcoholics and barbiturate addicts are caused by sudden withdrawal. In many patients, seizures are related to the menstrual cycle, but it has not been established whether hormonal, metabolic, or psychological variables are accountable.

Sensory input may also precipitate seizures; cases have been reported in which simple sounds or music produced seizures (musicogenic epilepsy).[5] Other interesting forms are photogenic epilepsy and the related reading epilepsy. There have been some reliable reports of seizures evoked by traumatic incidents producing fright and rage. We observed one patient in whom the first seizure occurred after sexual intercourse with her father and another whose seizures diminished and then stopped after hypnotically "reliving" a violent attack on her mother by her father when the patient was eight. B. Bandler, I. C. Kaufman *et al.* stressed the role of sexual conflicts in thirty epileptic women whom they studied.[3] In most cases, however, we must rely on conjectures about unconscious affects that precede seizures and possibly produce them. Pathological affects, particularly rage and anxiety, undoubtedly can contribute as precipitating and predisposing causes to the genesis of the seizures, but we are unable to discern the precise role played by affects and conflicts. We know more about the psychological meaning of the epileptic seizure than about its psychogenesis; a rich field for future exploration exists here.

Diagnosis

Every patient suffering from seizures should be given a careful medical, neurological, and psychiatric anamnesis and examination. Furthermore, the examiner should obtain in all cases an EEG record, X-rays of the skull, blood counts, urinalysis, determination of blood sugar, blood calcium, nonprotein nitrogen, and serological reactions for syphilis. Lumbar or cysternal puncture (with care), examination of the spinal fluid, pneumoencephalogram, ventriculogram, and angiogram should be carried out in certain cases when space-occupying or atrophic cerebral processes are suspected. A good social history must be obtained, and the patient should receive a battery of psychological tests with particular attention to intellectual functions and personality integration.[1]

Such a diagnostic approach permits the division of cryptogenic from the symptomatic epilepsies and the establishment of underlying causes, which, of course, is of great importance for a therapeutic program. It should be determined whether behavior disorder, intellectual deficit, or subnormality exist and whether such changes are primary or secondary. The patient's environment, as well as his attitudes and the attitudes of his family should be fully explored. Many behavioral changes, at one time thought to be characteristic of epilepsy, are recognized today as reactions to the seizures and to the related social stigmata. The contribution of the EEG to the diagnosis is extremely important. At one time, particularly under the influence of the earlier discoveries by the Gibbses, the characteristic changes of brain waves were considered to be of pathognomic significance for the diagnosis of epileptic types. Today, the localization of foci by EEG is considered even more important since it permits a more refined diagnosis and also enables us to propose neurosurgical intervention when this seems to be indicated. Special activation techniques, such as hyperventilation, drugs, sleep (in which seizures frequently occur), and deep electrode placements, are sometimes required for full EEG exploration of a paroxysmal disorder. It should also be remembered that there is a fair-sized group (for example, some family members) with EEG changes but without seizures, just as there are some suspect seizure-states with normal interictal records.

The diagnosis of epilepsy with typical symptoms and signs is easy; atypical forms, particularly those with behavioral and autonomic manifestations, may be extraordinarily difficult to diagnose. Frequent and ticklish diagnostic problems are the separation of *grand mal* from hysterical attacks and the recognition of epileptic equivalents, fugues, epileptic psychoses, and delirium. Epileptic seizures are rarely psychogenic; in hysterical seizures, precipitating psychological events may usually be found without much difficulty. The seizures in *grand mal* epilepsy follow a typical tonic-clonic pattern; in hysterical patients, they seem more purposive; movements are thrashing and have a dramatic quality. Hysterical patients do not hurt themselves seriously, never have severe tongue-bites, and rarely are incontinent. They sob and scream, and their seizures nearly always occur before spectators. In *grand mal* seizures, the loss of consciousness is complete and is followed by total amnesia; in hysterical seizures, patients do not become completely unconscious, and many remember the experience vaguely. In spite of these characteristic features, the differential diagnosis in atypical cases may puzzle even experienced clinicians. As hysterical traits in epileptics are frequently encountered, the term hysteroepilepsy was used in the older literature.

The differentiation of various forms of psychic seizures may be even more difficult, especially if we include in this group psychotic behavior which is often accompanied by unspecific and vague electroencephalographic symptoms. It is the writers' opinion that, at our present stage of knowledge, psychotic behavior should be classified as epileptic only if it is paroxysmal, characterized by clearly demonstrable abnormalities of the EEG, and associated with other seizure phenomena. In children, the differential diagnosis may impose unsurmountable problems; at times only a therapeutic trial with anticonvulsant drugs will provide the answer. In infants and young children, tics and breath-holding may occasionally make for difficulty in the differential diagnosis from atypical seizure.

Classical *petit mal* attacks are easily recognized by clinical observation and through the typical electroencephalographic pattern. Occasionally, narcolepsy and cataplexy may be confused with epilepsy.[36] Narcolepsy is a condition marked by attacks of an overwhelming need to sleep. Cataplexy is a loss of muscular tonus following strong emotions, especially after laughter; hence the German term *Lachschlag.* Autonomic symptoms and the syndrome of diencephalic epilepsy may be confused with migraine and migraine variants, particularly abdominal migraine. The close relationship of migraine to the epileptic disorders is well known. At times, patients with syncopal attacks are mistaken for epileptics. EEG and the clinical and laboratory findings of various types of syncope and of typical seizures are helpful in the differential diagnosis. The differential diagnosis of the group of myoclonic epilepsies—mostly rare familial diseases—exceeds the competence of the ordinary psychiatrist. Patients with cerebral vascular disorders often have short-lasting aphasias, agnosias, apraxias, sensory and motor disturbances, and confusional episodes. These disturbances must be differentiated from seizures because the episodic symptom of cerebral insufficiency in patients with vascular brain disease requires a different therapeutic approach.

Course of the Epilepsies

The onset of cryptogenic epilepsy usually occurs in childhood, the onset of symptomatic epilepsy during the adult years. Whercas *grand mal* and psychomotor seizures are observed in all phases of life, *petit mal* attacks are more frequent in childhood.[13] It is of practical importance to keep in mind that the course of epilepsies varies greatly. Epilepsy may be a relatively harmless disease that neither progresses nor seriously handicaps the patient socially or occupationally and does not lead to complications. A few patients with frequent seizures, however, suffer from psychoses, mental deficiency, and deterioration. In some cases, such states and antisocial conduct may be attributed to improper management rather than viewed as a direct consequence of the epilepsy. It is not correct to call a patient who has had one or even several seizures an epileptic. Rather than be awed by a seizure, the physician should decide what is the cause and what is the consequence of a seizure. Is a seizure in itself necessarily harmful? Most clinicians feel that it is the underlying pathology and the side effects, both psychosocial and physical (such as injuries or aspiration occurring during the seizure), which are noxious. Seizures in febrile diseases, especially in infancy or childhood, are frequent; and the chance that such children will develop epilepsy later is only slightly greater than that of children without a history of febrile disease. The *petit mal* attacks of childhood have a fair prognosis and tend to disappear in later life. Certain rare types, such as familial myoclonic epilepsies occurring mostly in children, which have been described by H. Unverricht,[38] have a particularly poor prognosis. Traumatic epilepsies are often thought to have an unfavorable prognosis; but this is not correct. D. Denny-Brown pointed out that early post-traumatic seizures have a worse prognosis than late seizures.[6] A. Earl Walker showed that one-third of post-traumatic seizures recover without treatment; one-half improve after conservative therapeutic methods.[39] In general, the prognosis of the patient and his general efficiency depend on the frequency of the seizures, age of onset of seizures, the absence or existence and severity of organic deficit, and most of all on the patient's therapeutic management. In neglected patients with early onset of seizures and evidence of cerebral damage, the prognosis tends to be unfavorable.

Treatment

As in all diseases, a therapeutic attempt must be made to treat the epilepsies causally. Space-occupying lesions must be removed, chemical abnormalities such as hypoglycemia, hypocalcemia, or pyridoxine deficiency corrected. In most of the cryptogenic and symptomatic epilepsies, however, only symptomatic therapy is possible. This consists of medication with anticonvulsant drugs, general hygienic measures, social and occupational rehabilitation, psychotherapy, and, in selected cases, surgical therapy; only rarely is institutionalization of epileptic patients necessary.

TREATMENT WITH ANTICONVULSANT DRUGS In the majority of epileptic patients, this is the treatment of choice and the most important therapeutic approach. The three most useful drugs have been phenobarbital, diphenylhydantoin, and trimethadione; more recently, primidone and the succinimides have been added. In no more than, perhaps, one-third of the patients whose seizures are controlled may the drugs be discontinued, even when the patient has a normal EEG. In any case, drug treatment should be continued for at least two years after the last seizure. The dosages listed below are for adults; obviously they must be reduced for children, according to weight. Allergic reactions to all these drugs have been noted, particularly in children. In most cases, the physician must experiment with the available drugs and dosages until the seizures are controlled.

Phenobarbital is still the most important anticonvulsant drug. It is most useful for *grand mal* seizures, psychic equivalents, psychomotor attacks, and myoclonic seizures. The recommended dose is 0.1 gm. at bedtime; if necessary, it may be increased to 0.3 gm. Drowsiness, a frequent result of the medication, tends to disappear on prolonged usage; ataxia and other toxic symptoms, such as confusional states, are rare. Addiction in epileptic patients almost never occurs. If phenobarbital is not tolerated, 3-methyl-5-ethylbarbital may be used. It is said to have a less soporific effect than phenobarbital; it is, however, demethylated quickly into a phenobarbital equivalent after intake. Phenobarbital can be combined with other drugs, particularly those which produce less drowsiness and are thus more suited for daytime medication. The danger of barbiturate addiction in epileptics is small.

Diphenylhydantoin is a valuable anticonvulsant drug that was introduced by T. J. Putnam and H. H. Merritt.[30] It is very effective in *grand mal* seizures and particularly in psychomotor attacks and psychic equivalents. It is less sleep-producing than the barbiturates. The average dose is 0.1 gm. t.i.d., which may be increased to a total of 0.6 gm. per day. Disagreeable side-effects are nausea and gastric irritation caused by its alkaline properties; in addition, a hypertrophy of the gums may be cosmetically quite disturbing. The hypertrophy may be reduced by massage and also can be treated surgically. Dermatitis has been reported. Many patients feel restless while on diphenylhydentoin medication. Toxic psychoses have been observed only very rarely; irritable and paranoid reactions occur and disappear with reduction of dosage. Ataxia is rather frequent with high dosage. Leukopenia is rare, but a megaloblastic anemia may occur, secondary to an induced folic acid deficiency.

Trimethadione (0.3 to 2.0 gm. daily) is considered particularly effective in *petit mal* attacks.[21] It is not without danger: dermatitis, aplastic anemia, leukopenia, and chronic nephrosis have been reported as the result of such medication. Other drugs, which are used more rarely, are pirimidones (1.0 to 1.5 gm. daily) and succinimides (0.5 to 2.5 gm. daily). Amphetamine sulfate in doses of 5 to 20 mgm. per day has been prescribed in *petit mal*, usually in conjunction with barbiturates.

Seizures in rapid succession that do not permit the patient to recover from one seizure before the next begins are referred to as *epileptic status*. This dangerous condition may terminate fatally and requires prompt and expert treatment. Therapy consists of intravenous injections of high doses of aqueous 10 per cent solutions of sodium phenobarbital. This medication is quite effective; a dose of 3 to 5 cc. may be given and repeated, if necessary, after three hours. If these measures fail, general anesthesia with ether, chloroform, or intravenous sodium pentothal may be tried.

HYGIENIC MEASURES Epileptic patients should live a life that is as normal and healthy as possible. They should have an adequate, balanced diet; ketogenic and other diets have not proved to be of real value. It is best to avoid alcohol, especially distilled liquor, completely. Epileptics should be encouraged to participate in the daily activities of the household and the community but must avoid overstimulation and fatigue. They should not be permitted to assume an invalid role or be pushed into such a role. They may participate in sports; but some activities, such as boating, swimming, horseback riding, and skiing should be carried out under supervision or in company with others. Opinions differ about whether an epileptic should drive a motor vehicle. Obviously, patients who suffer from frequent seizures with little warning should not drive. Nor should those patients drive alone who have rare seizures without definite aura. Still, it seems reasonable, given normal intelligence and personality, to permit an epileptic who has not had a seizure for at least one year to drive again.

A question frequently posed by adult epileptics and family members is the choice and suitability of the patient's occupation. With very few exceptions, epileptics are capable of carrying on any occupation commensurate with their intellectual and emotional capacities.[1] The only reservation involves occupations that would endanger patients who suffer from sudden seizures, and particularly from *grand mal* attacks. Unhappily, it is usually found that neither the patient, his family, nor the community at large has rational views on such matters. Many employers are opposed to hiring epileptics, even in jobs for which such patients are eminently suited. Only systematic enlightenment by psychiatrists, neurologists, and organizations such as the American Epilepsy League will be able to alter this widespread bias.[7] These prejudices center not only on the working capacity but also personality of epileptics. Many unenlightened people still believe that epileptics in general are insane and dangerous.

In seventeen of the United States, marriage of epileptics is legally forbidden. Such laws are atrocious and should be amended.[4] Epileptics who contemplate having children, however, may wish to get judicious advice from their physicians. This requires careful weighing of clinical and electroencephalographic findings, determination of intellectual performance, social adjustment, and family history.[20] When cryptogenic epilepsy occurs on both sides, and when the electroencephalograms of both partners are abnormal, prospective parents should certainly be cautioned; the decision, however, is up to them. It is of great importance to dispel these erroneous notions about epilepsy not only in the general population but particularly in the epileptic patients themselves and in the members of their families. In some measure, this can be undertaken by the therapist who works in a process of clarification and interpretation with the individual patient and his family. Alteration of attitudes can be achieved effectively in group therapy sessions of patients and family members who attend epileptic clinics. The realistic orientation of patients and their families is in a sense the most important contribution psychotherapy can make in the therapy of epileptics. Claims have been made that epileptic seizures can be treated causally by analytic psychotherapy;[16] possibly this is correct in the rare case in which important psychogenic factors are clearly demonstrable. In the authors' opinion, psychotherapy is an important auxiliary treatment in a comprehensive therapeutic program for epilepsy; nonetheless, if we could increase the frequency of visits of patients and families to the treating physician to "talk out" the fears, hidden questions, and theories by abolishing the term "psychotherapy" for such help, we would gladly do so.

SURGICAL PROCEDURES Neurosurgical procedures are the method of choice in symptomatic epilepsy caused by removable tumors. Penfield and other neurosurgeons reported improvement after removal of atrophic cerebral scars in patients with focal epilepsies who were not helped by anticonvulsant medication.[28] It should be emphasized that this represents a select group, because over half of such patients are rendered seizure-free by medication. Half of the patients who underwent subpial resection or partial lobectomy improved. However, adverse effects, such as intellectual deterioration, severe memory defects, and psychoses, were so threatening that very strict criteria for such operations are indicated. Hill lists the following contraindications to neurosurgical intervention: multiple and bilateral electrical foci, failure to obtain clear seizure patterns after electrical focal stimulation, high intelligence, involvement of the major hemisphere, and hysterical personalities.[18] Obviously, neurosurgical procedures should be recommended only after all conservative approaches have been exhausted.

INSTITUTIONALIZATION Epilepsy has become an eminently treatable disease, and since the great majority of epileptics have the capacity to live useful lives in their communities, the recommendation of admission to an institution for epileptics has become the exception. This step is usually reserved only for epileptics with very frequent, intractable seizures or for those who suffer from mental deficit, severe neurologic handicaps, and severe mental disorders, which often are not even related to epilepsy. However, for some severe epileptics who are brutally treated in their family or community, who cause their families great suffering, or who have no one to take care of them, the well-run epileptic colony may be a haven and boon. Epileptic children should be encouraged to attend ordinary schools; few need to go to special institutions.

NOTES

1. Cosimo Ajmone-Marsan and Bruce L. Ralston, *The Epileptic Seizure, Its Functional Morphology and Diagnostic Significance* (Springfield: Charles C Thomas, 1957).
2. C. H. Alström, "A Study of Epilepsy in Its Clinical, Social, and Genetic Aspects, *Acta Psychiat. Neurol. Scand.*, Suppl. 63 (1950).
3. Bernard Bandler, I. C. Kaufman, J. W. Dykens, M. Schleifer, L. N. Shapiro, and J. F. Arico, "Role of Sexuality in Epilepsy, *Psychosomatic Medicine*, 20 (1958), 227.
4. Roscoe L. Barrow and Howard D. Fabing, *Epilepsy and the Law* (New York: Hoeber-Harper, 1956).
5. Macdonald Critchley, "Musicogenic Epilepsy," *Brain*, 60 (1937), 13.
6. Derek Denny-Brown and E. G. Robertson, "Observations on Records of Local Epileptic Convulsions," *Journal of Neurology and Psychopathology*, 15 (1934), 97.

7. Arthur N. Foxe, "The Antisocial Aspects of Epilepsy," in Paul H. Hoch and Robert P. Knight, eds., *Epilepsy* (New York: Grune & Stratton, 1947).
8. Henri Gastaut, "So-Called 'Psychomotor' and 'Temporal' Epilepsy," *Epilepsia*, 2 (1953), 59.
9. Henri Gastaut, *The Epilepsies* (Springfield: Charles C Thomas, 1954).
10. Henri Gastaut, G. Ricci, and H. Kugler, "Sur la Signification des Déscharges neuroniques multiples et consécutives observées dans des régions différentes au cours des crises psychomotrices," *Rev. Neurol.*, 89 (1953), 546.
11. Frederick A. Gibbs, E. L. Gibbs, and William G. Lennox, "Electroencephalographic Classification of Epileptic Patients and Control Subjects," *Archives of Neurology and Psychiatry*, 50 (1943), 111.
12. Gerald H. Glaser, "Visceral Manifestations of Epilepsy," *Yale Journal of Biology and Medicine*, 30 (1957), 176.
13. Gilbert H. Glaser and M. S. Dixon, "Psychomotor Seizures in Childhood," *Neurology*, 6 (1956), 646.
14. Gilbert H. Glaser, Richard J. Newman, and Roy Schafer, "Interictal Psychosis in Psychomotor Temporal Lobe Epilepsy: An EEG-Psychological Study," in Gilbert H. Glaser, ed., *EEG and Behavior* (New York: Basic Books, 1963).
15. Robert G. Heath, S. M. Peacock, Jr., and W. Miller, Jr., "Induced Paroxysmal Electrical Activity in Man Recorded Simultaneously through Subcortical and Scalp Electrodes," *Transactions of the 78th Annual Meeting of the American Neurological Association*, Atlantic City (1953).
16. John W. Higgins, "Psychotherapy in the Epileptic Patient," *Diseases of the Nervous System*, 11 (1950), 142.
17. John W. Higgins, G. F. Mahl, José M. R. Delgado, and H. Hamlin, "Behavioral Changes during Intracerebral Electrical Stimulation, *Archives of Neurology and Psychiatry*, 76 (1956), 399.
18. Denis Hill, "Cerebral Dysrhythmia," *Proceedings of the Royal Society of Medicine*, 37 (1944), 317.
19. Andrzej Jus and K. Jus, "Retrograde Amnesia in *Petit Mal*," *Archives of General Psychiatry*, 6 (1962), 163.
20. William G. Lennox, "Marriage and Children for Epileptics," *Human Fertility*, 10 (1945), 97.
21. William G. Lennox, "*Petit Mal* Epilepsies," *Journal of the American Medical Association*, 129 (1945), 1069.
22. William G. Lennox, "66 Twin Pairs Affected by Seizures," in *Epilepsy, Research Publication of the Association for Nervous and Mental Disease*, 26 (1947), 11.
23. William G. Lennox, "The Heredity of Epilepsy as Told by Relatives and Twins," *Journal of the American Medical Association*, 146 (1951), 529.
24. William G. Lennox, "Phenomena and Correlates of the Psychomotor Triad," *Neurology*, 1 (1951), 357.
25. Benjamin Pasamanick and A. M. Lilienfeld, "Maternal and Fetal Factors in the Development of Epilepsy," *Neurology*, 5 (1955), 77.

26. Wilder Penfield, "Psychical Seizures," in *Psychiatric Research*, Harvard University Monograph in Medicine and Public Health (1947), No. 9.
27. Wilder Penfield, "Memory Mechanisms," *Archives of Neurology and Psychiatry*, 67 (1952), 178.
28. Wilder Penfield and Herbert Jasper, eds., *Epilepsy and the Functional Anatomy of the Human Brain* (Boston: Little, Brown, 1954).
29. Wilder Penfield and K. Kristiansen, *Epileptic Seizure Patterns* (Springfield: Charles C Thomas, 1951).
30. Tracy J. Putnam and H. H. Merritt, "Experimental Determination of the Anticonvulsant Properties of Some Phenyl Derivatives," *Science*, 85 (1937), 525.
31. Eliot Slater and E. Glithero, "The Schizophrenia-like Psychoses of Epilepsy," *British Journal of Psychiatry*, 109 (1963), 95.
32. Erwin Stengel, "Studies on the Psychopathology of Compulsive Wandering," *British Journal of Medical Psychology*, 18 (1939), 250.
33. Erwin Stengel, "On the Aetiology of the Fugue States," *Journal of Mental Science*, 87 (1941), 572.
34. Erwin Stengel, "Further Studies on Pathological Wandering," *Journal of Mental Science*, 89 (1943), 224.
35. James Taylor, ed., *Selected Writings of John Hughlings Jackson* (New York: Basic Books, 1958).
36. Rudolf Thille, *Beiträge zur Kemtnis der Narcolepsie* (Berlin: Karger, 1933).
37. Owsei Temkin, *The Falling Sickness* (Baltimore: Johns Hopkins Press, 1945).
38. Heinrich Unverricht, *Die Myoklonie* (Leipzig: Deuticke, 1891).
39. A. Earl Walker, *Posttraumatic Epilepsy* (Springfield: Charles C Thomas, 1949).

CHAPTER NINETEEN

Mental Subnormality

Seymour B. Sarason

The Challenge of Subnormal Behavior

Questions of definition and classification have long occupied those who have been concerned with the problem of mental subnormality. Since 1919 there have been five attempts on the part of the American Association on Mental Deficiency to achieve uniformity in terminology and classification. We define mental subnormality as behavior characterized by subnormal intellectual performance, manifesting itself during early development, with subsequent difficulty in maturation, learning, and psychosocial adaptation. Some of the problems arising from such a definition were recognized by the Special Committee of the American Association on Mental Deficiency:[19]

"Since adequate population norms and highly objective measures of the various aspects of adaptive behavior are not yet available, it is not possible to establish precise criteria of impaired functioning in these areas. At present, the most precise statement that may be made is that, for a judgment of inadequate or impaired social adjustment, learning, or maturation, an individual's behavior in these areas must be clearly inefficient or subnormal as judged by the best standards available for the comparison of a person's performance level with that of the general population. The inclusion of criteria of impaired adaptive behavior in the definition demands that objective measures of general intelligence be supplemented by evaluation of the early history of self-help and social behavior, by clinical evaluation of present behavior, and by whatever measures of academic achievement, motor skills, social maturity, vocational level, and community participation are available and appropriate.

Because of the different roles of maturation, learning, and social adjustment for the pre-school, school, and post-school aged groups, the definition specifies that it is necessary for the sub-average intellectual functioning to be reflected by impairment in only one of these three aspects of adaptive behavior in order to confirm a diagnosis of mental retardation. In actual practice, however, it will be found that a great percentage of individuals diagnosed as mentally retarded will be impaired, or have a history of impairment, in all three areas of adaptation.

Within the framework of the present definition mental retardation is a term descriptive of the *current* status of the individual with respect to intellectual

> functioning and adaptive behavior. Consequently, an individual may meet the criteria of mental retardation at one time and not at another. A person may change status as a result of changes in social standards or conditions or as a result of changes in efficiency of intellectual functioning, with level of efficiency always being determined in relation to the behavioral standards and norms for the individual's chronological age group.

As might be expected this formulation did not meet with unqualified approval or acceptance.[3, 4, 8, 9] Regardless of criteria employed, it should be emphasized that mental subnormality represents a staggering number of people. Estimates of incidence range from 1 and 1.5 to 3 per cent of the population. For example, in 1958 Richard L. Masland stated:[19]

> To be specific, of the 4,200,000 children born annually in the United States, 3% (126,000) will never achieve the intellect of a 12-year-old child. 0.3% (12,000) will remain below the 7-year intellectual level, and 0.1% (4,200), if they survive, will spend their lives as completely helpless imbeciles, unable even to care for their own creature needs.
>
> The U. S. Department of Health, Education and Welfare reports, "The mental and neurological diseases which are not among the leading diagnoses in terms of case frequency, may account for more days of disability in the younger age groups than any other kind of illness" . . . "and continue as the leading cause of days of disability until old age."

Despite the fact that mental subnormality involves so many people, it has only been in the last decade or so that this problem area has become of increasing interest to a wide variety of scientific and professional groups. One factor in this growing interest in mental subnormality reflects the experiences of the armed forces in World War II, during which 716,000 men between the ages of eighteen and thirty-seven years were rejected from service on the basis of intellectual inadequacy.[10] Another and perhaps important factor was the formation of a nationwide parent group (The National Association for Retarded Children), devoted to improving facilities for the care, education, and vocational training and adjustment of the mentally subnormal. The National Association for Retarded Children has stimulated basic and applied research in this area. The efforts of this organization and President John F. Kennedy's interest in the mentally retarded were responsible for the establishment in 1962 of a National Institute of Child Health and Human Development within the National Institutes of Health.

In this chapter, we shall adhere to a terminology that distinguishes between mental deficiency and mental retardation, the term mental subnormality being the general term to cover all cases.[22, 28] The term *mental deficiency* refers to those individuals who have demonstrable central nervous system defects. In contrast, *mentally retarded* individuals presumably do not have central nervous system pathology. Almost invariably these latter come from the lowest social classes; in fact, the frequent practice of labeling these individuals "subcultural" or "environmentally deprived" reflects the fact that their functioning involves cultural rather than constitutional variables. The need to differentiate between what we have called mental deficiency and mental retardation has been recognized by many workers in the field.[13] It is, unfortunately, still the case today that contributors to the literature in this field use terms (for example, mental retardation, mental subnormality, mental deficiency, feeblemindedness) in such a variety of ways that the reader must assume the responsibility for determining the referents for these terms in each publication.

Criteria of Mental Deficiency

The term mental subnormality, then, refers to individuals who are by no means homogeneous in behavior, intellectual level or efficiency, or in physical characteristics, socioeconomic status, or cultural background or development. Within this large and heterogeneous group a major category consists of the mentally defective, who meet the following criteria: (1) They possess a degree of social incompetence, which makes an independent existence in the community dubious or impossible. (2) This social incompetence is a reflection of an intellectual deficit or subnormal rate of intellectual development, which has characterized the individual from, or shortly after, birth. (3) There is underlying central nervous system pathology of a nature and degree that (a) produced the intellectual deficit and social incompetence and (b) is irremediable.

One of the more obvious implications of these criteria is that their evaluation requires the combined efforts of different professional fields: social work, neurology and other medical specialties, and clinical psychology. It is clearly not within the competence of any one specialty to obtain the data appropriate to the evaluation of all criteria. Unfortunately, and despite the warnings contained in the research and clinical literature, the most frequent basis for the diagnosis of mental deficiency is a low I.Q.

It cannot be emphasized too strongly that a low I.Q. score does not enable one to state in what ways a particular individual may be different from others with an identical score, or what his differential reactions are to a variety of situations. The low I.Q. score does not reflect his attitudes toward himself and others, what effects he will produce on what kinds of people in what kinds of situations, or the relation of all the foregoing not only to the presence or absence of central nervous system impairment but also to the familial-cultural background in which he developed. It is extremely simple, although logically naive, to "explain" a defective child's behavior on the basis of his low I.Q., as if there were in the child a force varying inversely with the I.Q., "causing" him to behave as he does. For example, it is not unusual for people who know that a particular child has a low I.Q. to say in regard to a "stupid" act of his: "What can you expect from someone as low as that? If he had more brains he wouldn't have done it." It does not occur to ask why *this* child—and not others with identical I.Q. scores—behaved in the particular way; why *this* situation and not others elicited the "stupid" response; and why, when superior children behave in the same way, the fact of their superior intelligence is not blamed for their behavior.

It follows that subdividing the defective group according to I.Q. score, that is, idiots, I.Q. 0–25; imbeciles, I.Q. 25–50; morons, I.Q. 50–70, simply increases the number of labels without adding to knowledge. Labeling an individual an imbecile does not tell us any more about him than when it is known that he has an I.Q. of 30, and knowledge of his I.Q. raises many more questions than it answers.

In many cases the nature of the medical findings are clear-cut; there is no doubt that a CNS involvement has resulted in social incompetence and intellectual deficit. *Yet it does not follow that the degree and even the nature of the social-intellectual deficits are wholly explainable by constitutional factors.* Because there is a relation between variables A and B does not mean that all of B is explainable by A. Although we shall return to this problem later, it should be here stated that the presence of a mentally defective child (or any markedly atypical child) in a family sets in motion a variety of interpersonal processes, attitudes, and relationships that help shape the development of the child. To view the behavior and personality organization of the mentally defective individual as a simple derivative of a brain defect is to ignore the understanding gained in psychiatry over the past several decades about the complex interactions between bodily dysfunctions, interpersonal relationships, and personality organization. When the psychiatrist deals with children with heart defect, physical handicap, diabetes, asthma, or epilepsy, he does not make the mistake of "explaining" behavior and personality organization only in terms of these somatic afflictions. Too often, however, the psychiatrist does make this mistake when he has to deal with the mentally defective child, almost as if the psychological principles underlying psychiatric practice do not here apply. Although some psychiatrists recognize this obvious view, the attitude is sometimes expressed that, since there is really little one can do for these children, the matter of how one tries to understand them is not of crucial significance.

The diagnosis of mental deficiency involves a prediction, that is, at maturity the condition will not have changed in a way so as to enable the individual to maintain himself independently in the community. There are several reasons why this predictive diagnosis should be made with caution. First, the validity of the clinical evaluation of intellectual functioning increases with the age of the child; in general, the validity of such an evaluation in a one-year-old child, say, is less than in a four-year-old child. Second, in many cases the diagnosis of mental deficiency is not an etiological one; it is not possible to point to antecedent factors that gave rise to the condition. And when the etiological picture is ambiguous and the child is young, the clinician must feel very sure of his grounds before rendering a diagnosis that involves a prediction of future status. The third reason why this diagnosis should be made with caution is that very frequently it results in a pervasive change in the environment of the child. That is, the perception of him by family and others may change radically, with a consequent change in overt behavior toward him. Such changes may reflect a more realistic conception of the child's condition and potentialities. However, particularly in those instances where the diagnostic picture lacks clarity, the environmental changes may effectively prevent change of which the child was capable. It cannot be overemphasized that the diagnosis of mental deficiency is as serious a diagnosis as can be made; it should never be made without the combined efforts of the appropriate specialists.

Etiological Groupings among the Mentally Defective

In the 1959 Manual on Terminology and Classification of the American Association on Mental Deficiency, eight etiologic groupings are described. These eight classifications, with some illustrative conditions for each, are given below.

(1) *Diseases due to infection:* for example, encephalopathy associated with prenatal infections, congenital rubella, congenital toxoplasmosis, congenital syphilis. (2) *Diseases due to intoxication:* for example, maternal toxemia of pregnancy, bilirubin encephalopathy, postimmunization encephalopathy. (3) *Diseases due to trauma or physical agent:* for example, encephalopathy due to prenatal injury, mechanical injury at birth, asphyxia at birth, postnatal injury. (4) *Diseases due to disorders of metabolism, growth or nutrition,* leading to mental consequences at various periods of growth, depending on the particular pathophysiology. Some of these are: infantile cerebral lipoidosis (Tay-Sach's disease); late infantile cerebral lipoidosis (Bielschowsky's disease); lipid histiocytosis of phosphatide type (Niemann-Pick's disease) and kerasin type (Gaucher's disease); hepatolenticular degeneration (Wilson's disease); rarely, porphyria (in late or preadolescence); galactosemia; hypothyroidism; gargoylism (lipochondrodystrophy, Hurler's disease); immunological disorders (Rh or ABO incompatibility; athyreotic cretinism identified by maternal antithyroid antibodies); aminoacidemias such as phenylketonuria, Maple Syrup Urine disease (with an accumulation of branched-chain amino acids, leucine isoleucine, valine, and methionine and associated disorders of tryptophan metabolism); and a growing variety of aminoacidurias, some due to changes in renal tubular reabsorption (for example, Hartnup's disease associated with a pellagra-type rash, ataxia, and either mental deficit or personality disorders in adults; and Lowe's disease with mental deficit, buphthalmos, hypotonia, and renal tubular acidosis).

(5) *Diseases due to new growths:* for example, neurofibromatosis (von Recklinghausen's disease); trigeminal cerebral angiomatosis (Sturge-Weber-Dimitri's disease); tuberous sclerosis. (6) *Diseases due to unknown prenatal influence:* for example, anencephaly; malformations of gyri; congenital porencephaly; craniostenosis; congenital hydrocephalus; hypertelorism (Greig's disease); macrocephaly; microcephaly; Laurence-Moon-Biedl syndrome; Mongolism. (7) *Diseases due to unknown or uncertain cause* with the structural reactions manifest: for example, diffuse sclerosis of the brain; acute infantile diffuse sclerosis (Krabbe's disease); progressive subcortical encephalopathy (Schilder's disease); spinal sclerosis (Friedreich's ataxia). (8) *Mental retardation due to uncertain* (*or presumed psychologic*) *cause* with the functional reaction alone manifest: for example, cultural familial retardation; psychogenic mental retardation associated with environmental deprivation; mental retardation associated with psychotic (or major personality) disorder.

In recent decades the major research developments in the field of mental deficiency have been in the genetic-biochemical-neurological aspects. The reader interested in gaining a view of these developments is referred to the volume edited by Laurence C. Kolb, R. L. Masland, and R. E. Cooke,[16] the Conference on Diagnosis of the Training School of Vineland,[26] the survey article by Masland,[19] the volume on medical genetics edited by Arthur G. Steinberg,[25] and publications by Bronson Crothers and Richmond S. Paine[5] and Eric Denhoff and Isabel Robinault.[6] It is clearly impossible within the confines of a single chapter to give clinical descriptions of other than a few conditions. Those described below are taken in part from the 1959 manual and have been chosen either in terms of their frequency of occurrence or significance in determining the direction of future research.

MONGOLISM Since 1866, when Langdon Down first described this disease, a voluminous literature has accumulated, much of it focused on possible etiological factors. When one considers that Mongolism represents approximately ten per cent of institutionalized defectives, it is not surprising that this disease has stimulated much study and discussion. In the 1959 Manual of the A.A.M.D. appears the statement that in the case of Mongolism "though there are a number of untested hypotheses the etiology of this condition remains obscure." Since then, a genetic factor in Mongolism has been identified. Mongolism, according to J. Lejeune and R. Turpin,[17] is a constitutional disease. There is concordance in monozygotic twins and discordance in dizygotic twins. In the rare instance when Mongolian mothers have children, some of these have been found normal, others Mongolian. Lejeune and Turpin express doubt that a dominant mutation exists. They suggest a polygenic inheritance because recurrence in siblings, although low, is higher than chance would explain. Slight Mongolian stigmata have been found in the relatives of Mongolian defectives. The principal factor in

Mongolism is the mother's age.[2] All hypotheses of fetal injuries have remained unsubstantiated. Mongolism occurs in all races. Lejeune and Turpin view Mongolism as the result of a regressive evolution. The palm-prints resemble those of low monkeys and are not characteristic for anthropoids.

In 1959 Lejeune and Turpin, together with M. Gautier,[18] published the first solid evidence indicating the presence of a chromosomal factor in this syndrome. In contrast to the 46 chromosomes of the normal somatic cell, they demonstrated that the Mongolian cell has 47 chromosomes. Cytological findings show a trisomy of the number 21 autosome. This "standard" chromosomal anomaly, occurring in approximately 1,700 babies, is ascribed to failure of the two chromosomes of pair 21 to separate (meiotic nondisjunction) during gametogenesis, producing an abnormal ovum. It is not known why older mothers are vulnerable, although hormonal factors have been implicated. About 5 to 10 per cent of Mongoloids are attributed to a "translocation," in which the extra chromosome 21 material is attached to another autosome; occurring independently of parental age the etiology is thought to be genetic, one of the parents being a carrier. A rarer type of Mongolism shows mosaicism in which some cells have the extra chromosome 21 and is ascribed to an intrauterine event—an error in mitosis of an early embryonic cell. Tests of some Mongoloids may show normal cytological findings. Etiological factors thus range from the molecular or genic to genetic or adventitious circumstances producing altered chromosomal structure in the gamete, to intrauterine events leading to altered chromosomal patterns. Further work is required to identify the pathogenesis of these genetic and chromosomal defects as well as the mechanisms by which mental and behavioral functions are affected. A number of other chromosomal anomalies have been described; gonodal anomalies generally manifest at puberty and occasionally associated with mental and emotional disturbance are seen in Klinefelter's syndrome in males (in which an extra X, or female, chromosome is generally found) and Turner's syndrome (in which the absence of an X chromosome leads to 45 chromosomes rather than the normal 46).

PHENYLKETONURIA Although the number of defective children exhibiting biochemical disturbances is very small, the findings in these cases are of importance because of the direction which they have given to an ongoing and future research. As H. Harris[11] has said: "In most cases of mental defect in which a gross characteristic metabolic disturbance has been found, the abnormality has been shown to be genetically determined in a relatively simple way. It seems probable that in each case one is dealing with a very specific kind of biochemical disorder due to a single gene substitution." This poses in each instance two kinds of problems. Why does the abnormal or mutant gene result in the characteristic disturbance in metabolic pattern that we observe? How does this biochemical disturbance lead to defect in mental development or function? One of the most studied metabolic defects is phenylketonuria. The findings in phenylketonuria, described in 1934 by A. Foelling,[7] demonstrated that certain severely defective individuals excreted large quantities of phenylpyruvic acid in their urine. Further study indicated that approximately .5 to 1 per cent of institutional populations had this disorder, and that the syndrome was genetically determined. Harris[11] has speculated that the abnormal concentrations of phenylalanine and other metabolites in the body fluids, due to the absence of phenylalanine hydroxylase in the liver, somehow so modify the intracellular milieu in the brain that normal metabolic processes are impeded. Possibly most of the damage is done in the first few weeks or months after birth; failure of myelinization is often observed. However, exactly how this is brought about and what the critical factors are is quite obscure. The deficiency of phenylalanine hydroxylase (converting phenylalanine to tyrosine) may be accompanied by defects in the metabolism of other amino acids and amines as well as the production of toxic metabolites such as methoxylated phenethlyamines related to mescaline. Competition of phenylalanine with tryptophan derivatives for transport into the brain may account for the altered serotonin metabolism found in phenylketonuria.

As compared with normals, phenylketonuric children tend to be less pigmented. There is usually some degree of microcephaly present; the incisors are broad and spaced widely; and there is often an odd posture in which the head and trunk are bent and the arms and legs held partially flexed. The patient walks on a broad base and in an awkward manner with rather short steps. Apart from brisk tendon reflexes, neurological findings are absent except in severe cases, which may show extrapyramidal signs—cogwheel rigidity, hypertonicity, and hyperkinesis. EEG studies suggest frontal lobe atrophy in some cases. Some phenylketonurics are hyperactive, and many show digital mannerisms. Though they range from mildly to severely defective, the greatest percentage of cases demonstrate severe deficiency. The diagnosis of phenylketonuria is easily confirmed by testing for phenylpyruvic acid in the urine (ferric-chloride test) or for elevation of serum phenylalanine, although a few instances of elevated serum levels may be encountered in normal children. Urine tests may not be positive in the first six weeks of life, but Guthrie has developed a bioassay with bacteria that shows promise for detecting excess serum phenylalanine from a few drops of blood.

GALACTOSEMIA Besides phenylketonuria, galactosemia bilirubin encephalopathy, and one form of goitrous cretinism are also now believed to reflect a single specific enzyme defect resulting in mental deficiency. Although these conditions are relatively rare, their significance resides in the basis they provide for Harris' statement that "it is obviously reasonable to suppose that among the many patients with clinically undifferentiated forms of mental defect there are a large number with similar highly specific metabolic syndromes which remain to be uncovered."

Galactosemia is characterized by a congenital disorder of carbohydrate metabolism, which results in an accumulation of galactose in the blood. The infant appears normal at birth but on a milk diet soon begins to show symptoms. Jaundice and vomiting are common and, in spite of an insatiable appetite, the child shows evidence of malnutrition. Histological changes are found in the liver and in the lens of the eye. An enlarged liver, cataracts, and severe mental deterioration become evident. The death rate is high, and persons who survive generally show some cirrhosis of the liver. The high galactose blood level produces an increased output of insulin from the pancreas and a reduced release of dextrose from the liver, which results in hypoglycemia. In infants on a milk diet, a reducing substance is found in the urine with Benedict's reagent. This may be identified as galactose by chromatography or fermentation tests.

BILIRUBIN ENCEPHALOPATHY (KERNICTERUS) Kernicterus may follow severe jaundice in the newborn and is characterized pathologically by a yellow bilirubin staining of brain areas, especially the basal ganglia, cerebellar nuclei, hippocampus, and medulla. Advanced stages of the condition are marked by demyelinization, gliosis, loss of cells in the cortex, globus pallidus, and corpus Luysii. Chreoathetosis and mental deficiency are common sequelae.

This condition is frequently due to Rh incompatibility between fetus and mother but also may be caused by A, B, O, or some of the more rare blood-type incompatibilities. In the absence of blood incompatibility, kernicterus may result from prematurity and severe neonatal sepsis, or any condition producing a sufficiently high level of serum bilirubin.

POSTIMMUNIZATION ENCEPHALOPATHY Innoculation with serum, especially tetanus antitoxin, or vaccines such as smallpox, rabies, and typhoid may result occasionally in nervous system reactions. Such a reaction usually involves the peripheral nerves but, in rare instances, takes the form of an encephalitis. When this is the case, signs of meningeal, focal cerebral, cerebellar, and cord involvement may be present. Convulsions, stupor, coma, and motor dysfunction are common during the acute phase. Permanent neurological impairment may be represented in behavior disorders, dyskinesias, convulsions, and mental deficiency in young children.

INFANTILE CEREBRAL LIPOIDOSIS (TAY-SACH'S DISEASE) This is a progressive lipid dystrophy predominantly affecting the nervous system and characterized by an accumulation of lipid substances in the nerve cells.

The disease is transmitted as a single recessive gene. The parents are normal but both are carriers with a probability of having one child out of four affected. The carrier state can be detected by the absence of the enzyme fructose-l-phosphate adolase, normally present in the serum. Marriages producing affected children show a high incidence of consanguinity.

The majority of cases are found in Jewish families with ancestors from the eastern part of Poland, although non-Jewish families occasionally are affected also.

The infant usually appears normal at birth, but clinical signs of the disease become apparent between three and ten months. Often, the first manifestation of the illness is hyperacusis. In the usual clinical course, the child who has been developing normally for perhaps three to six months becomes apathetic, shows muscular weakness, is unable to maintain his posture or to hold his head steady, and regresses in his ability to grasp objects. This motor loss is accompanied by progressive visual deterioration, leading to squint and nystagmus. Examination of the retina shows degeneration in the macular area through which the choroid vessels are seen—the pathognomonic "cherry-red spot." Blindness usually develops, giving rise to the name infantile amaurotic family idiocy. Convulsions and progressive muscle-wasting appear, and death usually ensues within one to three years of onset.

GARGOYLISM (LIPOCHONDRODYSTROPHY, HURLER'S DISEASE) This disease is manifested by the deposition of an intermediary metabolite, probably a mucopolysaccharide, in almost all tissues of the body, but especially in brain, liver, heart, lungs, and spleen. A variety of cells are involved: neurones at all levels; cells in the liver, pituitary, and skin; and reticuloepithelial cells in lymph nodes and spleen. The widespread connective tissue involvement is responsible for the skeletal deformities that characterize this condition. The urine has increased amounts of polysaccharides. Two forms of gargoylism are usually recognized, one form owing to autosomal recessive gene transmission and the other to sex-linked recessive gene transmission.

Clinically, some signs may be evident at birth. These include head enlargement, limitation of joint movement and, later, cloudy corneas. At three months, X rays may show beginning deformity of the upper lumbar vertebrae and some loss of tubulation of the long bones. Kyphosis of the lumbar spine may become evident about the same time. The characteristic features may be present as early as six months. The gargoyle has a large head with a protruding forehead that is far out of proportion to the stunted body; the eyebrows are bushy; and the nose is saddle-shaped. The features are coarse and heavy with a deep crease between lower lip and chin, thick lips, large tongue, short neck, and double chin.

Mental deficiency that ranges in degree from minimal to severe is usually evident by the time the child is two years of age. By five years, wedge-shaped vertebrae and a variety of other bone abnormalities may be distinguished on X ray. The trunk is short, even in relation to the diminished limbs. The belly is protuberant, and there is usually an umbilical hernia. Except during infancy there is a characteristic deformity of the hands in which the fingers are short and partially flexed. There may be limitation of movement at all joints. The hips and knees are usually partially flexed when the child stands. Examination of the abdomen may show considerable enlargement of liver and spleen. Clouding of the cornea, especially in the deeper layers, is usually found in the autosomal recessive cases. Examination with the slit lamp reveals multiple punctate dots of varying size.

The prognosis is particularly poor in the autosomal recessive cases, most affected children dying before their teens. A few survive into the third decade before succumbing, usually to heart failure or respiratory disease.

TUBEROUS SCLEROSIS This disease, transmitted by a dominant gene with reduced penetrance, is characterized by multiple gliotic nodules irregularly disposed through the cerebrum and central nervous system. These are associated with adenoma sebaceum of the face and with tumors in other organs.

The cardinal clinical features are the butterfly-shaped rash of adenoma sebaceum, epilepsy, and variable mental disorder. The butterfly-shaped rash may develop at any time from birth to adult life but usually begins as a few small whitish or brownish nodules or pink spots. The rash spreads from the cheeks to the forehead, head, and neck over a wide butterfly-shaped area. Small yellowish-white nodules or phacomata may be seen on the retina. Tumors are also found in other parts of the body including rhabdomyomata of the heart, kidney tumors, and periosteal thickening of the bones, especially the phalanges. Nodules under the nails are not uncommon. The pathology may involve the lungs resulting in symptoms of respiratory disease.

Sometimes adenoma sebaceum may be present without cerebral involvement or mental deterioration. In other instances, the external skin manifestations may be absent, and the case may not be diagnosed until autopsy. In absence of the characteristic rash, the calcified cerebral nodules may be visualized on X ray with the cranial vault presenting a "moth-eaten" appearance.

Retarded development and convulsions may appear very early. Though these infants may show fair motor development, retardation in social and adaptive behavior will be apparent. Progressive tumor growth and accompanying severe convulsions generally shorten the lives of these patients. They may, however, survive to adulthood, in which case they commonly become psychotic.

MACROCEPHALY Macrocephaly is a rare condition characterized by an actual increase in the size and weight of the brain, due in part to a proliferative type of gliosis. Enlargement of the skull may be noted at birth, though most of the gross increase in size occurs later. The skull tends to be square rather than globular, and as in the hydrocephalic, the frontal prominences are pronounced. The greater circumference is at the level of the superciliary ridges, which are well marked. Pneumoencephalography may show the ventricular system to be enlarged only slightly.

Most cases are severely mentally defective. Headache, convulsions, and poor vision are common. The life-span is generally shortened except in those milder cases without severe epilepsy.

MICROCEPHALY According to clinical tradition, the term microcephaly is reserved for cases with an adult head circumference of 42 cm. (17 in.) or less. The corresponding criterion for children is 13 in. at 6 months; 14 in. at one year; and 15 in. at two years.

"True" or primary microcephaly presents a characteristic clinical picture and is considered to be transmitted as a single recessive gene. In this type of microcephaly, the face is not as reduced in size as the head, so that a relatively normal nose and chin, and large ears contrast with the receding forehead and low vertex. The head is greatly diminished in width and vertical measurement, and to a lesser extent in length. The contrast between the small cranium and the relatively well-developed face is diagnostic. The scalp is sometimes loose and wrinkled longitudinally as though too big for the skull; the skull may be ridged with bony crests along the saggital, coronal, and, occasionally, the lambdoid sutures.

The primary microcephalic is invariably moderately to severely defective. There may be associated defects such as epilepsy, cataracts, microphthalmia, coloboma of the retina, and incomplete formation of the optic nerve. Microcephaly may also occur secondary to exogenous lesions due to prenatal infections such as rubella or toxoplasmosis, or to trauma such as fetal irradiation, neonatal asphyxia, or birth injury.

CEREBRAL PALSY The generic term "cerebral palsy" embraces a number of conditions that produce brain lesions affecting motor control. The etiology is often obscure but includes the hereditary ataxias, maternal rubella, birth injury, cerebral anoxia, kernicterus, encephalitis, and meningitis. The clinical picture is diverse. About 50 per cent of these patients have spasticity of one or more limbs (monoplegia, hemiplegia, or quadriplegia). Basal ganglia lesions produce rigidity, athetosis, and tremor. About a third of these children will be so severely impaired that only custodial care can be given. Another third will require the close cooperation of parents, physicians, therapists, and teachers in providing specialized training and education. These children are usually of average intelligence but have serious physical handicaps. The third group, minimally impaired, can attend regular schools.

Diagnostic Behavioral Foci in Mental Deficiency

Many of the conditions listed above produce markedly defective children with progressive cerebral pathology, leading to deterioration and death at an early age. These children are given custodial care. Perhaps it is the exposure to such cases in pediatric training that often gives the medical student the mistaken idea that most cases of mental deficiency are "hopeless." This is not the case. A broad spectrum of capabilities exists in these children, ranging from defects incompatible with life to educable children capable of social and vocational adequacy. Various rating scales have been devised to describe the intellectual, emotional, and social capabilities of the mentally defective.[13, 14]

It is clear, especially in psychiatry, that in any particular case we are faced with several diagnostic problems. Nowhere is this more true than in cases of mental deficiency. The medical-neurological status of the individual is one diagnostic problem; the clinical psychological evaluation of intellectual and personality factors represents another. How these evaluations can be meaningfully related to each other so as to lead to still another diagnostic formulation is a third problem. Relating different diagnostic formulations (for example, medical-neurological, clinical-psychological, psychiatric) to each other is not merely a task of summating information. Unless these different diagnostic formulations can be integrated in a way so as to provide a basis for planning and management, we have little cause for satisfaction. For example, the neurological findings should illuminate the development and behavior of the child so that they give direction to what one might do in the here-and-now to effect better utilization of potential. To the clinician operating in other areas, such comments may represent glimpses of the obvious. Unfortunately, however, these commonplaces are rarely reflected in case studies of mentally defective children. Generally, such studies contain the unadorned diagnostic formulations of the different specialists, with little attempt to interrelate them or to plan a course of action.

It is not enough to proceed as if the child was the sole focus of the diagnostic effort. Frequently this has the effect of blinding one not only to the need for a clinical assessment of the effects of the child on the family, but also to the degree of help one can render to the family. Even if it is true, as it is in some cases, that there is little one can do for the child, it would still seem to be an obligation of the clinician to work with those members of the family who can utilize such help. Almost without exception the mentally deficient patient has a marked effect on the lives of the members of his family as individuals and as a social group. And these effects are usually negative: high levels of unhappiness and personal discontent, derogatory self-attitudes, social withdrawal, interference with vocational efficiency, and the like. Our diagnostic interest, then, should not be merely in terms of consequences for the child but also in terms of what can be done to enable the members of the family to live more satisfying and productive lives. To accomplish such aims—to utilize our clinical skills for the benefit of the afflicted and nonafflicted members of the family—requires adherence to the highest standards of diagnosis and treatment formulation.

Psychosis and Mental Deficiency

The relationship between psychosis and subnormal functioning has received a fair amount of attention over the years. A review of the problem and the literature has been presented elsewhere.[22] We will summarize briefly some of the known relationships between psychosis and subnormal functioning: (1) Psychosis is found at all levels of subnormal functioning. Even in the case of mentally subnormal patients with very low I.Q.'s, marked and dramatic psychoticlike changes in behavior have been noted. In some instances the behavior seemingly is episodic; in others, it is followed by deterioration. (2) Psychosis occurs in cases with no discernible brain pathology as well as in those with marked pathology. (3) Virtually every major psychotic symptom that has been described in the nondefective patient has also been noted in many defective cases. There appears to be little justification for the generalization that when psychosis occurs in a mentally defective patient it is less "complex" than when found in the nondefective individual. There is also little support for the equally sweeping generalization that psychosis or psychoticlike behavior in the defective individual tends to be of short duration. (4) As a result of work in the past twenty years on childhood schizophrenia, there is little doubt that many children who were committed to an institution for the mentally defective were in fact misdiagnosed and misplaced. Kanner's now-classic descriptions of the autistic child provided further evidence that there are many institutionalized patients in whom personality or affective rather than intellectual maldevelopment is the primary factor. (5) The schizophrenic type of reaction is the most frequently found psychosis among the mentally defective. (6) The incidence of mental illness among the mentally deficient appears to be much higher than in the general population.

It has been argued by some that the undisputed fact that psychotic, particularly schizophrenic-like, symptomatology is frequently observed in the lower grades of mental defect is no basis for assuming that we are dealing with the same condition as when these symptoms are observed in the intellectually normal person, or even the high-grade mental defect. According to this argument the schizophrenic symptomatology—particularly some of the bizarre and repetitive motor phenomena—is a more-or-less direct reflection of the organic pathologies so many of these cases have. Although organic pathology certainly cannot be considered a fortuitous factor, there has been no convincing demonstration of the nature of the relation between organic pathology and the behavioral symptoms; nor does the organic pathology seem capable of explaining either the episodic or the chronic nature of the motor and emotional symptomatology. It is our opinion that the state of our present knowledge is such that we cannot rule out the possibility that psychological factors play a role in the psychoticlike behavior of many severely defective individuals.

The Mentally Retarded

The mentally retarded have at different times been called "subcultural," "familial," "garden-variety," or "environmentally deprived," labels that were meant to reflect the fact that intellectual retardation is most frequently found in the lowest social classes. It represents the largest grouping in the institutional population and in special classes in the public schools. There is no evidence of any associated central nervous system pathology.[19]

The clearest demonstration of the relation of mental retardation to sociocultural variables has been made by E. Ginzberg and D. W. Bray[10] in their analysis of 716,000 World War II draftees rejected because of presumed mental deficiency. Clearly, this is a staggering national problem. On the basis of their detailed analysis, Ginzberg and Bray concluded: "The regional patterning of the rejections indicates that the screening assessed primarily the individual's educational background." The rejection rate varied from 97 per thousand in the Southeast to 10 per thousand in the Far West. Omitting the Negro registrants, the rates were 52 per thousand in the Southeast and nine per thousand in the Far West. The fact that these regions differ strikingly in expenditures for educational facilities tempts one to the conclusion that the rejection rates are *caused* by differences in educational opportunities. In a broad sociological frame of reference such a conclusion has meaning, although even in such a frame of reference it is dangerous to use correlational data to suggest causation. The two areas differ in many respects other than quantity and quality of educational resources; and it is possible that we are dealing with two different populations, people who differ culturally in some important respects. Other factors include differences in attitude toward education, in the kind and extent of personal rewards available through education, in how these groups conceive of "success" and "achievement." The relationship between educational opportunity and educational (and intellectual) attainment or level is complex; the quantity and quality of educational resources may be symptomatic of a cultural constellation that is primary in the sense that it gives rise both to the educational resources and to the attitudes toward education.

The term mental retardation indicates in a very general way something about the environment in which the individual exists, but it does not represent an individual diagnosis. Why is *this* child from *this* subculture intellectually and academically retarded, while other children from *this* subculture are not? The same question many times can be asked as between siblings. In other words, knowing that a child comes from a social class background that differs markedly from our own (and that of teachers in our schools), and knowing in addition that this background is in some general way related to poor test and school performance, hardly constitutes an individual diagnosis, let alone a basis for formulating a treatment or management program. Just as one cannot understand a juvenile delinquent by simply pointing to broad background factors, one explains little by pointing to an "impoverished" background as the cause of mental retardation.

The fruitfulness of research that takes seriously the possibilities of the relationships between sociocultural factors on the one hand, and intellectual and organic factors on the other, is exemplified by the studies of B. Pasamanick and his colleagues.[14,15,20,21] This program of research has given strong support to the hypothesis that sociocultural variables are intimately related to a variety of intellectual and organic difficulties. Prematurity, complications of pregnancy, intellectual subnormality, and neuropsychiatric disorders were all found to be related to socioeconomic stratification. On the basis of his various researches, Pasamanick[20] concludes: "If our findings and hypotheses have any validity we can estimate, admittedly quite crudely, that approximately 5–10 per cent of organically defective individuals fall into the hereditary category, and the remainder are largely prenatally damaged with a greater percentage functioning in the lower ranges. Accepting an IQ cutting point of 75, we can further expect that twice as many more will be retarded as defective, presumably on a sociocultural basis, with almost all in the upper ranges. However, it is obvious that the continuum of causality extends upwards into the normal range, affecting fewer individuals as it proceeds. The continuum of social retardation extends downwards so that the two overlap and indeed, since the two are often present in the same individual, become indistinguishable."

Although there is little doubt that there is a relationship between sociocultural variables and intellectual level and development, details of this relationship remain unclear. An outstanding beginning to this problem has been made by E. Zigler *et al.* in their research on social deprivation.[29] Of particular significance is Zigler's[30] conclusion that the behavior and performance of the subnormal individual are shaped by, and respond to, the environment in much the same way as the normal individual of the same mental age. Pasamanick's epidemiological studies and Zigler's experimental approach are of major significance to the clinical psychiatrist.

Constitutional factors (that is, "innate" capacity, frustration tolerance) may be important in retardation as well as the parent–child relationship. Lower-class preschool children are apt to be less supervised, to have less "training" and less intellectual stimulation than middle-class children. For example, middle-class parents are more apt to name objects, to guide in the selection and execution of solutions along lines of known effectiveness, to provide toys and experiences that stimulate curiosity and interest, to answer questions, and to be interested in and respect their child's developing intellectual capacities. In studies of adopted children born to lower-class mothers, H. M. Skeels and I. Harms[23] found that these children, whose real mothers often had borderline I.Q.'s, themselves, developed I.Q.'s averaging well in the normal range in middle-class homes, and those adopted into superior homes had correspondingly superior I.Q.'s. The child from a lower-class family enters school with a severe handicap in terms of intellectual and motor skills required for successful performance.

Emotionally disturbed children may also present with intellectual retardation. Disturbances in the parent–child interaction (that is, perfectionistic parents who demand superior achievement as the price for love) can produce learning difficulties and a disturbed family situation (parental strife) that can be reflected in inattentiveness, and behavior problems in school. Teachers who are insensitive to these factors can magnify the problem. Longitudinal studies of children reared in orphanages also reveal intellectual deficits related to stimulus deprivation.

Treatment

It is well-known that an emotionally stable child, in a supportive environment, with an I.Q. of 40 can learn a simple job, whereas an emotionally disturbed child with an I.Q. of 70 may be untrainable. The I.Q. defines individual capabilities within broad limits, so that treatment measures are aimed at permitting the child to develop optimally.

Of importance to the mental defective is the correction of physical defects or the adoption of specialized training techniques to permit maximum utilization of remaining skills. Examples would be orthopedic procedures in cerebral palsy, special reading and writing devices, and speech therapy. A group of children, dubbed "pseudofeebleminded," with sensory defects (that is, deaf or blind) or emotional blocking of learning may appear to be subnormal. The lack of specialized learning techniques permits the attendant social isolation to retard potential development. There is a great need for systematic research in education techniques for the subnormal individual.

Emotional factors within the child (feelings of inferiority, isolation, insecurity, frustration) as well as in the family (feelings of rejection, shame, overprotection) are an essential concern of any treatment program. Hopefully, the family can provide the stable, structured, supportive environment the defective child requires. Counseling and psychotherapeutic services for child and family are an important part of the total program. Setting realistic treatment goals is essential for the development of confidence and self-esteem in the child.

In recent years institutions for the care of the subnormal child have become active treatment, training, and research centers. The A.A.M.D. has published a set of standards[1] involving philosophy, practices, goals, and staffing for such institutions. Federal grants have stimulated the growth of community clinics providing specialized diagnostic and treatment services for the subnormal.

Genetic counseling, improved prenatal care and obstetrical practices, control of infectious disease, and research into the etiology and pathogenesis of the various syndromes may all contribute to prevention of mental deficiency. George L. Wadsworth[27] has outlined the present status and future needs of programs for the subnormal.

Excerpts from a case are given below. It is hoped that this material may give the reader, unacquainted with this area, a taste of some of the problems frequently met. More, it should indicate the significance of the need to recognize and cope with these problems early, in order to maximize the possibility that the potentialities of the individual can be utilized to compensate for certain deficits.

The patient, an eighteen-year-old girl, was brought to the outpatient clinic in order to determine eligibility for hospital admission. Since birth the left side of her body had been paralyzed. She was living with her parents and an older brother. The brother indicated that the patient had been overprotected all her life and had not been given an opportunity to learn tasks which were within her reach and from which she could derive satisfaction. The brother stated that she was alone most of the day and had become increasingly unstable. The family, who appeared affluent, seemed attached to the patient and looked upon hospitalization as a means for her to develop feelings and habits of independence that would make her happier when she returned home. She had attended school for three years, and subsequent private tutoring had not been successful. An EEG revealed "a mild degree of diffuse cerebral damage more on the right than on the left and with a definite focus in the right parietal region."

The patient, very neatly dressed, was a dark-haired and dark-complexioned young woman, with circles under her eyes. Her left hand appeared stiff, with some of the fingers clenched and the others extended rigidly. She seemed unable to engage in any activity that involved the coordination of both hands and usually prearranged the fingers of her left hand in a position to enable them to be of some aid. She was able to move her left arm quite well, although not as freely as her right. Hand tremors were observed. She was able to print letters with long bold strokes. Her left foot was stiff and dragged a bit. There was a defect in visual following movements.

During psychological testing she seemed very fearful, frequently rubbed her eyes, and exclaimed excitedly, "I'm too nervous to talk. Look how I'm shaking." Although she became more relaxed as testing progressed, she was prone to anticipate and become upset by failure. She seemed fearful of having her inadequacies exposed and tried to disguise them by offering vague, general answers to questions. She had great difficulty in understanding directions; how much of this was due to a mental defect and how much to the anxiety aroused by her feelings of inadequacy was difficult to estimate. In conversational speech, as well as in response to the vocabulary list, this girl's enunciation and use of words were excellent, in marked contrast to over-all test inadequacy. When responding to questions about her activities and family relationships, the coherence, fluency and "insightfulness" of her replies were atypical for mental defectives. Verbalized feelings of inadequacy usually were followed by statements about her strong desire to learn to do something useful, so that she would not be so dependent on her family. Her tendency to self-derogation was so strong that any achievement on her part was viewed as insignificant and consequently not a source of encouragement.

To interpret the intelligence quotients earned on the tests according to usual psychometric classifications would be to neglect important aspects of the patient's behavior. Though technically the results suggested mental deficiency, her facility with and correct use of language would not be expected in a defective individual. Her mental functioning was uneven. This irregularity was due to brain pathology combined with emotional instability. How much of her social incompetence was due to the brain defect and how much to overprotection was difficult to estimate. The problem was to decide whether admission to the training school was warranted. To expect institutionalization to reduce anxiety and instil independence in a girl who had been overprotected all her life did not seem reasonable. To compensate even to a small degree for the privations that the girl had experienced all her life by being so handicapped would take a great deal of individual attention. And to expect a woman whose only security had been the affection of her family to become more stable in alien surroundings was illogical. In terms of the family's purposes, then, institutionalization was not recommended.

It was felt that learning some tasks was essential for the patient's well-being, and a plan that could utilize community resources was recommended. It was suggested that she be enrolled in the training program of the workshop of the Society for Crippled Children in her city. When this possibility for training was advanced, the brother pointed out that this still would not solve the problem of her being left alone most of the time. The possibility of a companion was discussed; the brother indicated that the family had tried to get one, but that those who applied for the job were unsatisfactory.

The patient was first enrolled in the workshop. It was the opinion of the staff that she could be taught to go to and from home, increase use of her left hand, and learn some skills that would occupy her when she was alone. Although she gained considerably in self-confidence as a result of the workshop program, she was unable to learn to go from her home to the workshop. Since it was not possible to get a companion for her, and since she was still alone a good part of the time, the workshop recommended that she be admitted to the training school. This recommendation was carried out. Because of this girl's experience of overprotection and the traumatic shock of her separation from her family, it was arranged that she be seen each day by a psychologist on a psychotherapeutic basis. An initial problem was her inability to go from her cottage to the psychologist's office, a distance somewhat less than a quarter of a mile, without getting lost. At first she refused to go, saying that she would get lost. On the first few trips she was accompanied by the psychologist, who attempted to point out cues that she might use as bearings. Being accompanied by the psychologist reduced the patient's apprehension, increased her desire to come to the office, and made it easier for her to attempt the trip herself. The first few times she came alone she was told that the psychologist would be watching from his office in order to see where she might make a mistake, and to make sure that she did not get lost. After a few trials she was able to come to the office without difficulty. She also learned to go to other parts of the institution. For the first few weeks the interviews were largely taken up with her attitudes toward the other girls in her cottage. She was surprised at how rough they were and the coarse language they used, and she was afraid that they might not like her and would pick on her. Her adjustment to the other girls was complicated by their jealousy of the fine clothes she had and the attention and affection her family demonstrated by visiting frequently. She constantly reiterated that the girls "are not my type." The interviews seemed to give her an opportunity to unburden her feelings, to feel that despite separation from her family there was someone interested in her and to anticipate and reduce the apprehension that would arise with each new situation.

She then was enrolled in the occupational therapy and continuation school programs. Because of her intense desire to read, and in light of a severe visual defect, special reading techniques were employed. An apparatus was devised, which allowed only one line at a time to be exposed, thus correcting her tendency to wander all over the page. She was also instructed to spell each word to herself, then to spell it aloud, and then to attempt to pronounce it. She was aided by the teacher, who began with words the patient already knew. Within a period of two years, she was able to read and comprehend on about the fifth-grade level, although for optimal results it was necessary for the teacher to observe her directly, because even with the mechanical aid there was a noticeable tendency for her visual gaze to shift unexpectedly to other parts of the page. The patient, who had never been able to write words before, was taught to write a legible and coherent letter. At this point, the patient was returned to her family home. The parents asked for and received guidance in managing her daily activities, and the community workshop provided further training experience.

It is important to note that in this case a significant degree of improvement (in spatial orientation and reading) was achieved—a degree of improvement that had notably positive effects not only for the patient but for those responsible for her in the institution. The intriguing question this case allows us to raise is to what extent the course of this patient's development would have been different if early in her life a treatment program had been formulated with the aim of helping her compensate for her *specific* neurological defects.

This problem was first brought into sharp focus for the writer by the case of a man in his late twenties who was committed to an institution for mental defectives. Physically, this man was virtually totally handicapped, an appalling combination of spasticity and athetosis. However, he was surprisingly bright. He would sit in front of a checkerboard; each square of the board contained a letter of the alphabet in sequence. The patient would answer questions by running his finger slowly over the letters, beginning with the letter A. Although his body was in continuous motion, when his finger came to the letter at which he wanted to stop, his movements intensified markedly. In this way he was able to spell out answers to a number of questions.

How and by whom was such a severely handicapped patient reached and taught? We do not know; the patient had been entirely cared for by his mother whose death precipitated the commitment. The father had died a number of years previously. We can assume that the mother was responsible for his rearing, but unfortunately the details of his development are lost to us. Despite the lack of specific information, however, a case of this kind does seem to justify the hypothesis that if (early) diagnostic formulations are of a kind that lead to treatment programs aimed specifically at compensation for known defects, the development of many of these children might be significantly advanced.

The psychiatrist is concerned with the relationship between actual and potential performance, that is, the degree of discrepancy between what an individual does and what he potentially can do. Since a major problem in the field of mental subnormality involves the relationships between observed behavior and performance on the one hand, and potentialities for change and development on the other, it is clear that this should be an area of interest to the psychiatrist. Study of mental subnormality can contribute to the development of a more comprehensive view of human personality and development. For example, within the past few decades there has developed an interest in "social psychiatry," reflecting the impact of the viewpoints and findings of anthropologists, sociologists, social psychologists, and other social scientists. It was not until psychiatrists began to look at these findings that their possible significance for psychiatric theory and practice became apparent. Until that time, the psychiatrist could see no reason why the behavior of a so-called primitive group, for example, the lower social classes, so markedly different in so many ways from the patients with whom he came into contact, should be of any special interest to him *as a psychiatrist.* Although one cannot say to what extent psychiatric theory and practice will be changed by these relatively recent developments, it is safe to say that their impact will be considerable.

It is no great exaggeration to say that psychiatry now stands in the same relation to the field of mental subnormality as it earlier did to the study of "primitive" cultures. To the extent that this gulf continues unbridged, psychiatry is losing an opportunity of testing its theories and practices about human behavior—robbing itself of the opportunity of being changed by virtue of new experiences.

NOTES

1. American Association on Mental Deficiency Steering Committee on Standards for Residential Institutions, B. Pasamanick, chairman, "Standards for State Residential Institutions for the Mentally Retarded," *American Journal of Mental Deficiency*, 68 (1963–64).

2. C. E. Bender, "Mongolism: A Comprehensive Review," *Archives of Pediatrics,* 73 (1956), 391.
3. B. Blatt, "Towards a More Acceptable Terminology in Mental Retardation," *The Training School Bulletin,* 58 (1961), 47.
4. G. N. Cantor, "A Critique of Garfield and Wittson's Reaction to the Revised Manual on Terminology and Classification," *American Journal of Mental Deficiency,* 64 (1960), 954.
5. Bronson Crothers and Richmond S. Paine, *The Natural History of Cerebral Palsy* (Cambridge: Harvard University Press, 1959).
6. Eric Denhoff and Isabel Robinault, *Cerebral Palsy and Related Disorders* (New York: McGraw-Hill, 1960).
7. A. Foelling, "Über Ausscheidung von Phenylbrenztraubensäure im Harn als Stoffwechselanomalie in Verbindung mit Imbecillität," *Hoppe-Seylers Z. physiol. Chem.,* 227 (1934), 169.
8. S. L. Garfield and C. Wittson, "Comments on Dr. Cantor's Remarks," *American Journal of Mental Deficiency,* 64 (1960), 957.
9. S. L. Garfield and C. Wittson, "Some Reactions to the Revised 'Manual on Terminology and Classification in Mental Retardation,'" *American Journal of Mental Deficiency,* 64 (1960), 951.
10. Eli Ginzberg and D. W. Bray, *The Uneducated* (New York: Columbia University Press, 1953).
11. H. Harris, "Metabolic Defects and Mental Retardation," in Lawrence C. Kolb, Richard L. Masland, and R. E. Cooke, eds., *Mental Retardation* (Baltimore: Williams & Wilkins, 1962).
12. R. Heber, "A Manual on Terminology and Classification in Mental Retardation," *American Journal of Mental Deficiency,* Monograph Supplement, 64 (1959), No. 2.
13. Leo Kanner, *A Miniature Textbook of Feeble-Mindedness* (Child Care Monographs; New York: Child Care Publications, 1949), No. 1.
14. H. Knobloch and B. Pasamanick, "Prematurity and Development," *British Journal of Obstetrics and Gynaecology,* 66 (1959), 729.
15. H. Knobloch and B. Pasamanick, "Environmental Factors Affecting Human Development before and after Birth," *Pediatrics,* 26 (1960), 210.
16. Lawrence C. Kolb, Richard L. Masland, and R. E. Cooke, eds., *Mental Retardation* (Baltimore: Williams & Wilkins, 1962).
17. J. Lejeune and R. Turpin, "Somatic Chromosomes in Mongolism," in Lawrence C. Kolb, Richard L. Masland, and R. E. Cooke, eds., *Mental Retardation* (Baltimore: Williams & Wilkins, 1962).
18. J. Lejeune, M. Gautier, and R. Turpin, "Les Chromosomes humains en culture de tissue," *C. R. Acad. Sci. (Paris),* 248 (1959), 602.
19. Richard L. Masland, "The Prevention of Mental Retardation," *Journal of Diseases of Children,* 1 (1958), 95.
20. B. Pasamanick, "Research on the Influence of Sociocultural Variables upon Organic Factors in Mental Retardation," in *Approaches to Research in*

Mental Retardation (American Association of Mental Deficiency Conference, May 1–3, 1959).

21. B. Pasamanick and H. Knobloch, "Complications of Pregnancy and Neuropsychiatric Disorder," *British Journal of Obstetrics and Gynaecology*, 66 (1959), 753.
22. Seymour B. Sarason, *Psychological Problems in Mental Deficiency, 3d ed.* (New York: Harper, 1959).
23. H. M. Skeels and I. Harms, "Children with Interior Social Histories: Their Mental Development in Adoptive Homes," *Journal of Genetic Psychology*, 71 (1948), 283.
24. W. Sloane and J. W. Birch, "A Rationale for Degrees of Retardation," *American Journal of Mental Deficiency*, 60 (1955–1956), 258.
25. Arthur G. Steinberg, ed., *Medical Genetics* (New York: Grune & Stratton, 1961).
26. The Training School, "Conference on Diagnosis in Mental Retardation," *Training School Bulletin*, Vineland, N. J., 1958.
27. George L. Wadsworth, "Today's Plan, Tomorrow's Promise" (Presidential Address, 88 Annual Convention, American Association on Mental Deficiency, 1964) *American Journal of Mental Deficiency*, 69 (July 1964), 4.
28. World Health Organization, "The Mentally Subnormal Child," (*World Health Organization Technical Report Series*, No. 75 [1954]),
29. E. Zigler, "Rigidity in the Feebleminded," in E. Philip Trapp and Philip Himmelstein, eds., *Research Readings on the Exceptional Child* (New York: Appleton-Century-Crofts, 1962).
30. E. Zigler, "Social Reinforcement, Environmental Conditions and the Child," *American Journal of Orthopsychiatry*, 33 (July 1963), 614–623.

CHAPTER TWENTY

Behavior Disorders in Childhood and Adolescence

Seymour L. Lustman

Contemporary Concerns

Youthfulness characterizes not only the subject matter of child psychiatry, but the profession itself. Although its historical antecedents are distant, the life-span of child psychiatry proper is most correctly dated from the turn of the century. However few, they have been vigorous years of intellectual ferment and accelerated professional growth; years which have been witness to the emergence of child psychiatry as a clearly demarcated and well-differentiated subspecialty of psychiatry. At the same time, it remains a unique subspecialty whose foundation is broader than medicine alone, and which can be understood only in terms of its historical antecedents.

Since our interest is not primarily historical, no attempt will be made to trace the diverse and remote origins of interest in the child. The primary sources of child psychiatry are more proximate and limited. Beyond religions, we must turn to that enterprise which has always shouldered a major responsibility for children—education. Jean Jacques Rousseau, J. H. Pestalozzi, F. Froebel, and J. Dewey, among others, made efforts to probe the nature of the child and childhood as part of their philosophical concerns with education. These were profound attempts going beyond pure pedagogy, since the educational process and the life of the thoughtful educator was confounded by the problems of special needs. Simply stated, in addition to pedagogic techniques, the chief problem became how to recognize and separate those children who could not utilize the usual educational methods from the masses who could. The issues of why they were different and what could be done about it remained in the background.

Education, in turning to psychological testing, stimulated the development of the intelligence test and the broader area of psychometrics (Binet, Terman, Rorschach). Of greater import than the search for normative standards against which to evaluate deviation, this represented the acknowledgment of pathology and underlined the existence of individual differences. The unique problems presented by the necessity to house, care for, and train the so-called feeble-minded child became more prominent.

Researches in further differentiation of this group and more effective training methods (H. H. Goddard) followed. A shift from a purely custodial perspective was demanded. In great measure this was motivated by social action around the needs of dependent children. Enlightened laymen as well as diverse professions had to cope anew with the institutionalization, care, training and placement of the orphan, the physically handicapped, and the mentally defective child. Children's aid societies and foster-home placement programs evolved. The next major impetus came from concerns with delinquency (Healy) and the hope of preventing crime through clinics.

The culmination of this multifaceted approach was the continued elaboration of specialized children's services, which was to result in the establishment of a widespread child-guidance movement (Beers). This was and continued to be a multidisciplinary venture with contributions from psychiatry, social work, psychology, and pediatrics. For the most part, these early clinics functioned as diagnostic units, and care continued to be environmental—primarily custodial, educational, and manipulative. The further development of psychotherapeutic methods, treatment-centered clinics, and in-patient services were modifications brought about by the impact of Sigmund Freud. However, the multidisciplinary heritage remains the hallmark of child psychiatry with areas of contiguous interest and responsibility demanding cooperation with child analysis, education, social work, pediatrics, psychiatry, and the law.

Psychoanalytic theory had the most profound impact on research and practice. It presented a genetic theory of great direct and heuristic influence, which spotlighted childhood as the crucial formative years. It developed an invaluable technique for the understanding and treatment of the child via his play. Apart from its method and content, the formal contribution that will concern us most, for the moment, is the emphasis on a developmental approach to psychological forces in man.

Developmental Concepts

In spite of the aforementioned multidisciplinary characteristics and its official relationship to general psychiatry, child psychiatry remains a unique discipline with its own distinctive problems, techniques, and training requirements. In view of the degree of specialization, one may well question the advantages that accrue from the study of the child to any save those who intend to spend their professional careers immersed in clinical work with children.

The crucial value to the psychiatrist lies in the utility of a well-articulated developmental theory with its central concept of genetic and epigenetic continuity. The clinical psychiatrist must account for the influence of the past on the present, and both on the future. These can be formulated as the clinical questions of how did this patient come to be the person he is, and have the disturbance he manifests, and how can he be helped?

All theories, ranging from the psychoanalytic theory through dynamic theories to learning theories have within them developmental concepts to try to answer these two questions and, in varying degrees, relate the second to the first. Thus, one major advantage that accrues from the study of the child is the sense of genetic continuity it affords. This applies not only to the understanding of the individual case but has particularly important theoretical and practical implications for the rapidly expanding areas of family psychiatry and social psychiatry with their crucial concepts of preventive psychiatry (see Chapter 24). In this sense, to the degree that it focuses on child development, child psychiatry may be conceived of as one of the foundations of general psychiatry.

Why is the concept of development so central? Primarily because, in addition to the study of species-specific developmental changes shared by all, it provides the most productive and useful framework with which to study individuality. The major developmental facts of individuality faced daily by psychiatrists are not only the individual's function as related to peer group norms but also a hierarchy of levels of organization that exist within each single individual, which makes him capable of a vast range of thought, feeling, and overt behavior. This hierarchical structuring of levels of integration makes it possible for the same individual to function with varying degrees of maturity or primitiveness reflective of internal states of such organization.

It is within a developmental framework that one can best conceptualize the ebb and flow of regressive and progressive shifts that so characterize human behavior and interaction. These shifts are most dramatically apparent in fluctuating psychotic states where the mature and the archaic stand in bold contrast.[48]

It is also vividly demonstrated by the observation of all teachers and parents, that when a four-year-old child is under great stress such as in the death of a parent, or hospitalization, or a severe trauma of other sorts, his current level of organization will "regress" and earlier, previously given up activities such as biting, sucking, or enuresis will reappear, heralding function on another and lower level of organization. Speech, thought, and action will also show such regression. The ebb and flow of regression and progression are particularly characteristic of the psychotherapeutic interaction, which again demonstrates fluctuating developmental levels. This has particular pertinence to the study of all creative endeavor wherein the creative person, as Ernst Kris[38] has suggested, must have the ability to regress in the service of the ego.

One other major concept, common to both biological and psychological development, states that *variability is the essence of development.*[32, 61, 62] Although development is normative and sequential, the expression of individual differences within the norms are unlimited. The clinical implications of these two crucial concepts—developmental hierarchy and variability—form the backbone of a developmental, clinical psychiatry.

A theoretical conceptualization useful for child psychiatry and psychiatry in general may be stated as follows: structural growth and maturation of equipmental factors (gene determined, but which in itself involves organization and differentiation) precedes psychological development. As formulated by Heinz Hartmann,[33] the human infant is born adapted to an average expectable environment before processes of adaptation begin. Erik H. Erikson[17] describes this as follows: "His inborn and more or less coordinated ability to take in by mouth meets the breast's and the mother's and the society's more or less coordinated ability and intention to feed him and welcome him—'mutuality.' "

From Hartmann's "undifferentiated phase," equipment, motivation, and experience interact in an infinitely complex and inextricable fashion. When so considered, the number of possible personality permutations are astronomical, but in keeping with clinical data. Nevertheless, development progresses through a relatively orderly and normative sequential course, which can be phenomenologically and theoretically delineated into phases, each with phase-specific skills, conflicts, and crises; and each with phase-specific socially determined tasks and institutions designed to meet needs.[17] To this developmental complex, Erikson has recently added the historic moment.

Viewed in this dimension, pathological development represents deviations from normative development. The ultimate resultant is a unique person—very different from, yet very much like all other persons—whose functions are differentiated, articulated, and organized, and whose functioning is controlled by an internalized hierarchy of levels of integration. This can best be understood in terms of the antecedent maturation and development that created and organized the hierarchy.

Communication

There is, perhaps, no more striking demonstration of differing developmental levels than that afforded by the study of communication between adult and child. If we consider two major aspects of communication that primarily concern psychiatry as motivation and means, examination of the adult patient vis-à-vis the psychiatrist and the child patient vis-à-vis the psychiatrist reveals dramatic and characteristic differences.

The developmental differences make for profound contrasts in modes of patient–psychiatrist interaction and are so great that the departures from the adult techniques bear examination. In the usual out-patient setting, the psychiatrist anticipates a patient in pain, coming at least partially on his own determination, and seeking relief and help. This is the characteristic clinical motivation that sets the clinical situation apart. One regularly depends on it to overcome the original strangeness of the clinical interview. One continues to rely on it (among other factors) for sustaining the regularity and the depth of both diagnostic study and psychotherapy. The usual (but not universal) circumstance of the child as a patient is that he experiences little pain from his symptomatology, is rarely (if ever) self-referred, and is brought to the psychiatrist by the family, which does experience the pain. He is infrequently motivated to tell his problems and is most often in the psychiatrist's office against his will. Even the anxiety, suspicion, uncertainty, and fear he may share with an adult patient are experienced by the child on different and more absolute levels.

Yet the major difficulty has more to do with the anticipation on the part of the psychiatrist that the child will primarily use verbal language for communication. With the adult, although varying degrees of mutual awareness of nonverbal communication exist, that is, expressive movements, atmosphere, and the like, both psychiatrist and adult depend primarily on verbal means of communication. These usually occur on appropriate levels of mutually understood and adapted levels of abstraction.

The wish that the child express his problems in speech was one of the major stumbling blocks to the development of child psychiatry. The historical literature of early efforts to establish child psychiatry abounds with statements to the effect that the treatment of the child by the physician was impossible because of the lack of language development and the resulting difficulty in understanding and making oneself understood. If speech and verbal exploration of the child's problems remain the wish and expectation of the psychiatrist, frustration and disappointment is inevitable.

Returning to matters of motivation and delineation of problems, one very essential means of overcoming these obstacles is the inclusion of the family in the diagnostic and treatment framework. Although there are differences of opinion about this, and this need alters as the child approaches adolescence, it is generally felt to be a quite natural way of functioning. This is true of the parent *and* the child, who both anticipate that the parent will tell the psychiatrist about the problems. Until the onset of adolescence, this usually represents no violence to confidentiality for the child, since it is in accord with his experience to date. It is quite usual for most child psychiatrists—even when the parents are in treatment themselves or are being seen by social workers—to have regular contact with the parents, which extends even to involved teachers and other important figures in the child's life. The involvement and support of these key people has a beneficial effect on the young child in the sense of its being a direct expression of the importance of the psychiatrist in his life.

The major problem of communication with the child himself bears closer scrutiny. Remaining cognizant of demonstrable increasing verbal ability with increasing age, it still may be stated that, in general, the child simply does not have either the vocabulary or the conceptualizing and abstracting ability to describe and explore his inner states and his problems with reality. This is true even if one assumes that he has the desire to impart this information. The language and the underlying thinking processes of the child are unique to childhood and mitigate against such communication. They are strikingly different from those of the adult, even though glimpses of this earlier mode of functioning may be apparent in all adults. Jean Piaget[47] has schematized the language and thought of the child as "egocentric" and not socially oriented. They are characterized by rules of logic that are peculiar to the child, with unique concepts of precausality, concreteness, an animistic quality, syncretism, and a need for justification at any price. This applies to both understanding and expression. For example, a four-year-old child, when asked to describe her recent surgery, said, "A man stuck me with a needle and then I disappeared."

Such egocentrism in language and thought is ". . . obedient to the self's good pleasure and not to the dictates of impersonal logic . . ." and logical communications with others. The immaturity of language, thought, and modes of behavior was conceptualized by Freud[27] as the *primary process* (see Chapter 3). In general, this process can be characterized as being under the sway of peremptory demands of inner needs that tolerate no control and demand immediate gratification. Speech, thought, and motor behavior demonstrate a lack of time sense, a confusing, illogical sequence of events in which contradictory opposites appear side by side, in which there is representation by analogy or allusion, where parts stand for wholes and wholes for parts, and nonverbal means of communication are primary. The Freudian concepts of displacement and condensation, so prominent in the dream, are quite apparent in the child's speech, thought, and motor behavior.

All of this is not to say that language is not available to the child, since we are not speaking of the mute child, who is a particular case. It is, rather, to emphasize the fact that his stage of development is such that notable alterations in technique must be used. The situation could be described somewhat as follows: the child psychiatrist is in the anomalous situation of trying to understand and treat a child who not only may not want to be there but who is not even able to tell (in words) of his troubles. One cannot expect the child to equal the developmental maturity of the adult. It thus becomes vital for the adult to adapt himself to the level of development of the child, and to the means of communication used by the child. He must do this in order to understand and to make himself understood. To effect this, he must create a situation and an environmental atmosphere in which the child is free to communicate in his own developmentally specific manner.

The major aspects of communication come about only through an intensive study of the play of the child, which yields the clues and techniques for understanding him. It was not until the development of psychoanalysis and the very creative development of the use of play for this purpose by Melanie Klein and Anna Freud (it should be noted that there are major differences in both technique and theoretical orientation between the two), that order could be introduced into the communicative relationship with children. Prior to the development of psychoanalysis, the major theories put forth to explain the child's play precluded its use as communication. For the most part, these theories were teleological, stating that the play of the child prepared him for the function of adulthood, and they were couched in energic terms, that is, stating that such play permitted the discharge of "the excessive energies so peculiar to children."

Current psychoanalytic theory about play is derived from the work of Sigmund Freud,[26] Anna Freud and her followers,[21, 22] Robert Waelder,[59] Kris,[38] and Lili Peller.[46] This theory accepts K. Bühler's concept of "functional pleasure," which states that there is pleasure for the child in the movement and the game itself. However, the usefulness of play to the psychiatrist lies in its being a mode of communication. Play is the natural behavior of the child, in which the ever-present mechanism of displacement makes it the repository and arena for his problems. Empirical observations show that anxiety-producing events passively experienced by the child appear in his play.

Whereas in actuality the event tends to be overwhelming, in play both internal and external experiences are broken up into smaller, more manageable segments. These segments are then repetitiously played out, permitting the child to gain a degree of mastery over the attendant anxiety. Thus, the psychiatrist can see in the play the anxiety-producing situation and the struggle for mastery. The impact of both external events and internal forces upon the child can be understood if one realizes that the child transforms a passively experienced event into play, wherein he is the active member. As an example of this, one need only think of the young child filling and drilling clay teeth following a visit in which he was a dental patient. Through play, wish-fulfilment becomes apparent, and is made all the more palpable by a leave of absence from the constraints of reality and conscience. This makes accessible to the psychiatrist the child's fantasies about himself and the significant others.

In passing, we may note that play interviews require a playroom stocked with an appropriate range of play materials and a psychiatrist who responds to play and playing in an appropriate manner. This role of participant-observer imposes unique strains on the psychiatrist: he must play freely and creatively as a subjective participant, while remaining an objective observer. He must be able to regress, yet retain control over the seductiveness of such regression in himself. Play interviews demand a true regression in the service of the ego,[38] and for the child psychiatrist presupposes that he be in contact with his own childhood.[5]

Psychopathology of Childhood

Prior to considering psychopathological development of children, it is best to review several basic premises about human infancy and childhood. First among these premises is the conceptualization of the epigenetic, sequential, normal development of the human being, which merges both genetic and equipmental endowment with environmental forces. Of primary import is the uniquely prolonged helplessness of the human infant, which accentuates the dependency upon a nurturing person—usually the mother. With increasing age, the personality and character of the child becomes increasingly delineated and stable so that one can speak of a structuralization or an internalization of structures into the psychic apparatus of the child.

In a practical sense, this means that the human infant and his genetic equipment molds and is molded continually via an extremely sensitive interrelationship between himself and his mother, father, family, and subsequently extended social environment. Any disturbance or tension reflected in these relationships may be manifested by a transient response on the part of the child. The transient quality of this response implies, first, that enduring structuralization has not yet occurred in the development of the child; second, that it is reversible if the underlying situational stress is corrected. Such transient symptomatology is referred to as the "Adjustment Reactions of Infancy and Childhood."

As a rule, the younger the child, the more fleeting and transient are the disturbances. As the child grows and matures, and if the disturbance continues over a prolonged period of time, there is every likelihood that this will progress beyond a reactive response to the point where it can be spoken of as an internalized problem within the child, in the form of a neurotic disorder or a character disorder.

In the evaluation of children, the psychiatrist must, therefore, retain as a crucial element of his professional skill a thorough knowledge of normal development. Within this framework, he can then use his clinical skills and judgment in the diagnostic workup of the child and his or her family. This necessitates appropriate interviews with the child, and in addition, with the parents. It may also be essential, with the permission of the parents and the child, to interview other persons crucial to the referral, such as teachers, if it is a school or learning problem. Beyond this, the psychiatrist may use other professional contributions such as those stemming from pediatric evaluation, and other paramedical services as they are required.

Prior to any further discussion of pathology in the child, one must note one particular circumstance, which stems from the fact that the child is always brought to the psychiatrist by the family. The mere fact that the child is brought to a psychiatrist for consultation does not necessarily indicate illness in the child. There are times when an essentially normal youngster is brought for evaluation. Study may reveal this to be the only way the mother or father or family can present themselves to a psychiatrist for help with their own problems. This happens frequently enough to have been generally labeled as using the child as a "ticket of admission." As such, it represents yet another cogent reason for routinely seeing parents.

It is thus not infrequent that one finds a child coping quite successfully with the situational stresses, but with a mother speaking more and more about her own concerns—if given the opportunity. As an example of this, I think of a young mother who brought her perfectly placid youngster in for consultation because of her concern about his lack of playmates. She subsequently entered into treatment herself because of her own phobic behavior, which prevented her from taking the child outside to play.

Organic Brain Disease

The child is subject to the entire gamut of organic brain disease. This ranges from birth injury of varying degrees of severity, to cerebral palsy, traumatic injuries, infectious diseases, metabolic disorders, exogenous poisons, and the like. The manifestations of such disturbances are quite broad. In large part they are dictated by the nature of the injury and extent of it, the developmental level achieved prior to the injury, the potential for continued development, and the psychological reaction to such injury on the part of the individual child and parents.[14, 23]

Because of the complexity of these interacting variables, it is sometimes quite difficult to make the differential diagnosis between certain forms of psychological conduct disorders and brain damage. This is particularly true in a large number of children with so-called minimal brain damage. It is necessary to distinguish those behavioral manifestations due to specific brain damage from those that represent underlying personality characteristics and psychological adaptation to the disorder. In making such differentiations (both prognostically and in terms of treatment and management plans), it is helpful to note that in spite of the complexity of the total organism, brain damage itself produces some very consistent and distinctive features.

Whatever the etiological factor, diffuse brain damage characteristically produces deficits in the level of awareness and in certain intellectual functions. One may note fluctuations in levels of consciousness; impairment in orientation, learning ability, memory, abstract thinking, motor skills; and decreased ability to concentrate and maintain attention.

Some of these features may be present in conduct disorders without demonstrable brain damage, particularly impulse disorders. However, the defects in attention and intellectual function are consistent enough to constitute fairly reliable diagnostic criteria. Temporal lobe damage may produce more specific manifestations of depersonalization, hallucinations, aphasia, intense anxiety, and rage reactions. The latter may be of the "catastrophic reaction" type in the sense that they are not usually provoked or not in keeping with the degree of provocation, have an episodic characteristic, and have a sudden beginning and ending. A sound knowledge of localizing neurological signs and seizure-states is of great help to the psychiatrist.

These conditions will not be reviewed more extensively here because they are always interdisciplinary concerns, involving pediatrics, neurology, psychiatry, psychology, social work, and education. In this area, the psychiatrist will find psychological evaluation particularly helpful, since a number of available tests are particularly sensitive to intellectual deficits based on organic brain disease.

Treatment of the brain-damaged child is never exclusively a matter of psychotherapy. This can be quite helpful, but the total care of the child demands a well-thought-out, integrated interdisciplinary management plan. Utilization of special training, rehabilitation, and educational facilities is crucial to these children and their families. Such facilities as cerebral palsy centers, vocational rehabilitation centers, special problem classes, and individual tutoring unfortunately are not available in every community. Yet every attempt must be made to bring such benefits to the child. One great service the psychiatrist can render is therapeutic counseling to the parents of such children. This contact should never be ignored, nor should its direct aid to the child and his family be minimized.

Adjustment Reactions of Infancy and Early Childhood

For the purpose of this discussion, we will limit ourselves primarily to those psychiatric disorders in which clear-cut brain damage is not a component. When one is dealing with the so-called adjustment reactions, or reactive responses, it is to be expected that those developmental processes and tasks that are at the moment in the ascendancy will primarily reflect the distress. The more advanced developmental processes and tasks, which have not yet achieved a degree of autonomous functioning, may be given up via regression for previously abandoned forms of behavior, or may themselves become involved in conflict. For example, in a four-year-old, one may find a reappearance of enuresis or thumb-sucking, or a developing function such as speech may become the locus of the conflict via stammering. The psychiatrist must always establish whether current behavioral manifestations are in fact regressions or if they represent, rather, fixations beyond which the child has not progressed. The prognostic implications are quite different and more guarded in the latter case.

In the very young infant, the most crucial interaction with the mother takes place around the feeding experience. This is never a simple matter of food ingestion alone. From the very beginning this complex relationship is intensely invested with important feelings. It is quite likely that for the infant this is at first experienced in terms of increasing or decreasing tension states, which very quickly evolve into more complicated feelings. At the outset this is even more complicated for the mother who experiences more convoluted qualities of pleasure or displeasure, here considered as both shifts in tension states and hedonic tone.

Although the over-all atmosphere is created by mother and child, it is the psychological state of the mother that will contribute the most to the affective tone of this experience. The infant contributes by virtue of such factors as his state of health, restlessness, hunger, communicative quality of crying, sucking vigor, nutritional response, and degree of satiation experienced and communicated. The maternal contribution may often be a response to some of the characteristics in the child. For example, variations in feeding and sucking needs may be quite disagreeable to the young mother who may respond to this as repulsive gluttony; or an insatiable infant may exaggerate feelings of maternal inadequacy in an insecure and uncertain woman. Such maternal feelings are then "fed back" into the relationship in gross or subtle ways.

Disturbances between the mother–child pair very readily reflect themselves in eating difficulties. The recognition that feeding problems in the infant may be an expression of the psychological distress of the mother has a long history. Generations ago, wise pediatricians considered the way a newborn infant ate as a barometer of the emotional climate within the home. The increasing professional awareness of this knowledge is particularly apparent around the evolution of concepts of breast-feeding. It is now felt that if the mother cannot be very comfortable and impart loving tenderness in such a situation, then breast-feeding does not afford the child the "ideal nourishment"—here used in the broadest sense of the word.

Feeding disturbances may range from colic to the fairly common pediatric diagnosis of "failure to thrive." In the latter, the complaint is usually that the child is apathetic, does not feed well, nor gain weight, and may perhaps even be losing weight. It is very frequent that such infants, when admitted to the hospital and placed in the care of a nurse especially selected for her warm, affectionate interest, quickly regain their spontaneity and responsivity, and do very well. If they are returned to an unchanged home, they may relapse to the same apathetic state.

Other reactive disturbances may also manifest themselves in the form of hyperexcitability, irritability, and such adjustment reactions as sleep disturbances. Again, in evaluating such young infants, one must always attempt an evaluation of equipmental factors in the child, in view of the fact that recent research so clearly indicates the extensive individual differences that exist in terms of congenital endowment.[7,28,41,51] As in feeding problems, such factors in themselves may be major components in disrupting the harmonious mother–child relationships. For example, the child who is hyperexcitable or is motorically hyperactive by virtue of endowment may be quite distressing to the mother who is unable to cope with this.[52] The conscious and unconscious parental anticipations about the sex, appearance, and behavior of the infant are also components of such reactions. Of basic import are the relationship between the two parents and the meaning to them of the pregnancy, the birth, and the child, since these set the "climate" into which the child is introduced.[10]

Particularly pertinent to these reactions of the infant is a group of conditions summarized under the term "affect deprivations." Interest in this area first arose from the reconstruction of the childhood of delinquent adolescents. This was corroborated by the study of the institutionalized infant, either in hospital or in orphan asylum. It has been amply demonstrated that the growing infant requires a great deal of stimulus nourishment on the part of the care-taking person. Ideally, this stimulation should occur within an atmosphere of love, tenderness, and trust. If such stimulation is absent because of the absence of the parent or the parent's inability, the child inevitably reacts with some distortion of rate or direction of development. This can be quite transient and reversible, as in the instance of the child who is very briefly hospitalized and then returned to his parents. However, prolonged deprivation, either in terms of prolonged hospitalization, institutional placement, or inability of the mother to accept a maternal role within the home can be productive of a long-lasting developmental retardation and serious personality disorders. There is reason to postulate that the nurturing person acts as an organizer for many psychic functions (in a way analogous to the organizer in embryology) and that children so deprived during crucial developmental periods are subsequently unable to completely develop the areas of function involved. Such "affect-deprived" children, even though subsequently placed in normal homes, seem never to develop intellectually and emotionally to the degree that their home-reared peer group does.[9, 49, 58]

Observation of such children reveals the severe extent to which the child is capable of manifesting a depressive reaction. Such depressive states differ from those of the adult and, at least until adolescence, do not have the same quality as the depressive psychoses of the adult. They seem more reactive in nature and seem to be directly related to the loss of the love-object and later to the threat of loss of love. They can be quite overwhelming and lead to apathy as seen in "mirasmus" of infancy, or in any loss of the significant adults in later childhood. The prolonged dependency of the human child leads to clear depressive reactions when such dependency is unfulfilled. This can occur through loss of the parent as in death or prolonged separation, or it may be brought about by a severe depression in one of the parents. Here, there is an identification element in addition to the unavailability of parental care. Such an early and prolonged depressive personality structure has important developmental significance for later phenomena such as accident proneness in childhood, suicide, and the depressive psychoses of adult life.

Adjustment Reactions of Later Childhood

The phase-specific developmental tasks of childhood include the functions of eating, sleeping, bladder and bowel training, cleanliness, motility, separation from the mother, school and learning, and intellectual development among others. Thus the adjustment reactions of childhood, reflecting the deviations of phase-specific development, manifest themselves in the form of thumb-sucking, nail-biting, enuresis, constipation, fecal soiling, excessive clinging, inability to sleep, and the like.

Failure of bowel and bladder training represent the most frequently involved of these normal developmental tasks. Although the range of individual differences is great, the average child achieves bowel control between the ages of two and two-and-one-half years, and control of his bladder perhaps six months to one year later. Encopresis and enuresis are most profitably thought of as symptoms rather than disease entities since they do not lend themselves readily to any classificatory schema and can appear as encapsulated phenomena in essentially normal children or may be present in any of the more serious forms of childhood psychopathology. Both symptoms have physiological and psychological significance and may be caused by organic factors such as congenital anomalies, factors of local disease such as localized infections, or any degree of complex emotional stress. However, because of the psychological importance of the body zones involved, the inevitable parental–child interaction around the symptom, and the social consequences, one may always anticipate some degree of emotional reaction in even those instances where the etiological factors are obviously organic.

Although a local disease process, or an aganglionic segment of the colon may give rise to encopresis, the most frequent situation is one of psychological stress as an outgrowth of the toilet-training phase. Normally this is characteristically an intense parent–child interaction wherein obstinacy and rebellion are the usual childhood temperamental concomitant reactions. The successfully trained child emerges with a greater sense of autonomy and mastery. In the case of encopresis, a mixture of infantile sexual pleasure and rebellion and revenge against the parents coexist. If the condition persists into the school-age period, its meaning and consequences become even more complicated by virtue of its extended social significance, which is usually along the dimension of teasing and ostracism from the peer group.

Enuresis differs somewhat in that it is primarily nocturnal and is more easily made a family secret. Although there are no adequate incidence figures available, it is variously estimated that 10 to 15 per cent of children suffer from enuresis. As with the encopretic child, in addition to psychological factors, one must consider congenital factors and factors due to local disease conditions in one's differential diagnosis. In spite of the fact that organically caused symptoms are comparatively rare, they are frequent enough to warrant carefully thought-out physical evaluation. Such workups must be carefully considered and considerately carried out, since the effects of such procedures as cystoscopy and proctoscopy are not inconsequential to the child. Among the emotional conflicts that have been implicated in the symptom of enuresis, the most frequent are hostility with revenge components, castration fears, sexual confusion, identification problems, and characterological problems. Here again, as with all developmental processes, judgments must be made concerning the regressive or the fixated quality of the symptom, particularly since the prognostic implications are more reserved in the later instance.

It is usual to distinguish a group of disturbances called *conduct disorders*, where the manifestations of the child's reactions are focused around behavior itself, in the home, school, or community. This behavior can range all the way from helplessness to provocative and predelinquent behavior and may progress to delinquent and sociopathic behavior. It is sometimes quite difficult to differentiate whether this is an adjustment reaction or the early indications of more profound disorders such as psychosis, or severe psychopathy.

Another usual division in classification is that of *neurotic traits*, which include tics, peculiar habits, spasms, somnambulism, stammering, hyperactivity, and the like. As in the conduct disorder, more serious conditions frequently have such symptomatology as a part of an early pattern. At times, prolonged observation of the child as he continues to develop is necessary to differentiate reactive traits from those which may herald the onset of severe disturbance.

Psychoneurotic and Character Disorders

Solidification and consolidation into individually characteristic structure is the essence of development. As this process continues, it is quite possible for the child to internalize what was at one time a reactive response into a core of a neurosis. This is more common with the older child. Thus, one will find among older children true phobias, obsessive and compulsive neuroses with full-blown rituals and ceremonials, anxiety reactions, dissociative reactions, and conversion reactions.[29, 37, 53] Neuroses in children appear to be less common than conduct disorders, and phobias represent the most frequent type. The neuroses become increasingly more prevalent in older age groups. As the child grows into preadolescence and adolescence, the form of the neurosis approaches more nearly that of the adult but continues to be marked by the dramatic characteristics of adolescence. This may represent a particular problem for the assessment of hysterias in adolescence since many of them are incorrectly diagnosed as schizophrenics.[13]

Hysteria in early childhood is an infrequent diagnosis. A survey of children admitted to a New York hospital over a fifteen-year period revealed only twenty-seven cases out of 51,311 admissions.[53] These were almost exclusively females. However, this does not represent a true incidence figure, since many of these cases are treated in pediatricians' offices and in outpatient psychiatric facilities. As pointed out by I. Kaufman,[37] hysteria has historical importance for the development of dynamic psychiatry and remains the prototype of the relatively treatable psychoneurotic disorder.

Throughout late childhood the neurosis becomes refractory to the kinds of manipulative efforts which might have been effective earlier. At this stage, even profound changes in the parents will not, in and of themselves, affect the neurosis. Whereas in a younger child one could conceivably modify the child's situation by treating only the adults, extensive treatment of the child now becomes imperative. This may or may not include the adult, although it is most frequent that their participation must be enlisted.

It is equally true of character disorders that one can trace the development of character traits that are at first consonant with the wishes and demands of the parents and can, in an early stage, be altered through impact on such parental longings and expectations. Yet as the child grows and develops, these facets become internalized into a quite unique character structure, which is then no longer amenable to impact from changed parental attitudes.[42] One frequently sees this enduring quality where behavior of a characterological sort is highly prized in the very young child and then found to be distressing to the parent as the child grows older. For example, some parents will respond with delight to the evidences of masculinity in a young girl, or femininity in a boy—in terms of their own needs. As adolescence approaches, however, they may find this sexual confusion quite distressing. By this time masculine or feminine traits have been consolidated into the character structure of the child in a much more enduring form.

Case Illustration

A fourteen-year-old girl was brought to the psychiatrist because her family feared she was developing into a homosexual. Study of the family revealed that they had longed for a boy during this pregnancy and had been barely able to cope with the disappointment of their mutually shared anticipations. Their combined reluctance to accept the child as a girl was apparent in the boy's nickname she was given, as well as the masculine athletic behavior that was encouraged and rewarded. As she grew older, this familial attitude was unchanged but subtly channeled into the form of intellectual competition with her peer group. The situation reached explosive proportions for both the parents and the child at the onset of menarche. The child was unable to accept this "affront of femininity" and continued to deny her femininity by increasing her masculine strivings. The unhappy parental attempts at this point to force the child to take dancing lessons and to "behave like a young lady" became an increasing source of friction within the home. The child was confused, depressed, and incapable of comprehending what she experienced as a bewildering loss.

School Phobia

This is being considered separately in view of its frequency and the difficulty it presents in treatment. It may be quite true that a child's refusal to go to school represents a true phobic response displaced to the school. However, this is not the usual case. A major developmental task for the young child is separating himself from his mother. This separation demands a stage of development that presupposes a basic trust in the constancy of the maternal object in the sense that the child must have arrived at a stage of development where "out of sight" does not mean "out of existence." Equally pertinent to our problem is the fact that this also demands a willingness on the part of the parent to accomplish the separation. It is quite usual that even though there have been preliminary short-term separations, the focus of any problem in this sphere comes to the fore around the child entering school.

It is usually found that the school phobia is a misnomer in the sense that the child is not truly phobic, but is, rather, in a state of anxiety around separating from the parent. The vast majority of problems of this sort are in reality separation anxiety.

Clinical Illustration

A five-year-old boy was brought to psychiatric care for his inability to attend school. The mother very touchingly described her attempts to put the boy on the school bus as follows: she would carry the increasingly agitated child in her arms down the long hill from their house to the school bus stop. As they neared the bus, he would cry and scream, until at the very door of the bus she would give up and take him home.

As treatment changed this pattern and the boy was able to go off to school on his own, the mother described that morning after morning as she stood in the window and watched her child go happily into the school bus, she would break into uncontrollable tears.

It has been empirically demonstrated that the longer a child is permitted to stay out of school, the more entrenched becomes the symptom and the more difficult the problem of returning the child to school. Many communities have set up emergency types of treatment for this specific problem, in which every attempt is made to return the child to school immediately and simultaneous attempts are made to deal with the separation anxiety of *both* the mother and the child.[60]

Psychosis

The now-classic description of infantile autism by Leo Kanner[35] in 1934, gave impetus to a tremendous amount of research on this condition. The high incidence of this disorder and the kinds of global care and construction of special facilities needed for its treatment makes it a matter of extreme practical import. But more than that, it has great theoretical import because it is the first known psychotic state in man, and its possible relationships to schizophrenia have not yet been worked out. The classic infantile autism of Kanner shows an autistic aloneness from the very start of life, characterized by the absence of any of the usual kinds of relating of young infants to parents and by a seemingly complete indifference to the presence of the adult. Other features of this disease are a failure to develop speech or a failure to use language for the purpose of communication. These children manifest an obsessive preservation of sameness characterized by repetitive activities in which the child may become addicted to such activities as spinning, turning on or off light switches, or flushing toilets. Although many of these children have been classified as mentally defective, it is important to note that they do relate to inanimate objects with fascination and may develop great skills in fine motor movements. It is generally felt that these children demonstrate "good cognitive potentialities."

Extensive research by Kanner, [35,36] L. Eisenberg,[15] H. Potter, Lauretta A. Bender,[3] Margaret Mahler,[43, 44] William Goldfarb,[30] and others indicates quite clearly that the complexities of this problem warrant its being considered as a collection of different etiologically determined diseases having very similar symptomatological manifestations.[48]

Clinical Illustration

A boy of five was brought for initial consultation because his school could not accept his behavior. The history taken from his parents reveals that from early infancy he was considered an incredibly "good" child. He never cried, never fussed, and was content to be alone in his crib for as long as the parents would permit. They then noted that he seemed oblivious to them and nonresponsive. Their first concern was for his hearing. He was evaluated by the family physician and referred to pediatric examination for possible deafness. Subsequent examination ruled this out, and careful neurological examinations were completed to rule out the possibility of brain damage. His behavior became more bizarre, with hand clapping, twirling, jumping and bouncing, and peculiar posturing. The family was unable to toilet-train the child or teach him any verbal communication. Yet he seemed very bright—almost gifted in certain ways. For example, he developed highly skilled fine motor coordination in playing endlessly with small toys and subsequently developed phenomenal skill in ball throwing and catching. He never developed speech and subsequently had to be institutionalized in a special school, where he was able to achieve a good institutional adjustment.

A great deal of current research is focused on diagnostic procedures, prognostic evaluations, and treatment of these children. Infantile autism, or childhood schizophrenia, is the most severe disorder of childhood, and represents the most distressing burden for those responsible for the child's care and management. Greater familiarity with the problem has resulted in a marked increase in appropriate diagnoses and increasing demands for specialized treatment, focusing on in-patient, day center and out-patient facilities. To date, researchers have implicated parental etiological factors, inborn constitutional factors, factors of brain damage, maturational lag, and factors of familial interaction. Infantile autism and the area of mental deficiency represent two of the most vigorously pursued research areas in child psychiatry. This has been spurred by the genetic and biochemical progress of research in phenylketonuria, a disease of inborn metabolism of phenylalanine. This condition, now very easily detected by a simple urine test and readily controlled by appropriate diet, until recently routinely progressed to oligophrenia.

Adolescence

There is no developmental phase more flamboyantly stressful to both children and parents than adolescence. The momentous biological and psychological changes are so great in this transition from childhood to young adulthood that the lines between normal and pathological are never more blurred or indistinct.

The question of what is normal and abnormal in adolescence can only be answered from the point of view of the developmental tasks of the period. As emphasized by Erikson,[18] the tasks of adolescence are ". . . . to maintain the most important ego defenses against the vastly growing intensity of impulses (now invested in a matured genital apparatus and a powerful muscle system); to learn to consolidate the most important conflict-free achievements in line with work opportunity, and to resynthesize all childhood identifications in some unique way, and yet in concordance with the rules offered by some wider section of society. . . . This means that the young person finds himself exposed to a combination of inner and outer experiences which demand his simultaneous commitments to physical intimacy, to decisive occupational choice, to energetic competition, and to psychosocial self-definition."

To Anna Freud[24] disharmony is the basic fact of adolescence. Turbulence and tumultuous upheavals are inevitable and predictable. They represent the external indications of internal adjustments and, even if they take a pathological direction, they represent also a potentially useful way of regaining mental stability. To Anna Freud, a steady equilibrium during the adolescent process in itself is abnormal. One cannot improve on her classic description:

> I take it that it is normal for an adolescent to behave, for a considerable length of time, in an inconsistent and unpredictable manner; to fight his impulses and to accept them; to ward them off successfully and to be overrun by

them; to love his parents and to hate them; to revolt against them and to be dependent on them; to be deeply ashamed to acknowledge his mother before others and unexpectedly, to desire heart to heart talks with her; to thrive on imitation of an identification with others while searching unceasingly for his own identity; to be more idealistic, artistic, generous and unselfish than he will ever be again, but also the opposite: self-centered, egotistic, calculating. Such fluctuations between extreme opposites will be deemed highly abnormal at any other time of life. At this time they may signify no more than that an adult structure of personality takes a long time to emerge, that the ego of the individual in question does not cease to experiment and is in no hurry to close down on possibilities. If the temporary solutions seem abnormal to the onlooker, they are less so, nevertheless, than the hasty decisions made in other cases of one sided suppression, or revolt, or flight, or withdrawal, or regression, or asceticism, which are responsible for the truly pathological developments.

The psychopathology of adolescence can be approached from many frameworks. Cross-cultural anthropological and sociological studies have focused on the sexual mores of different societies, the study of value-judgments of different adolescent cultures, heroes and leadership, and the social mobility via athletic competition, beauty, intelligence, and so forth.[11] Clinically, however, the psychiatrist is usually faced with the behavioral manifestations of attempts on the part of the adolescent to establish for himself independence and a sense of his own identity. Erikson's[18] concepts of identity crisis, identity diffusion, negative identity, and psychological moratorium have great clinical usefulness. The adolescent seems always to ask, "Who am I and what can I become?"

Case Illustration

A sixteen-year-old son of a physician felt caught in the struggle of trying to find for himself what he wanted to become as opposed to his father's confused demands that he follow his professional footsteps. At the same time that he struggled with this as an unclear problem, he did know all of the things his parents did not want him to become. Their particular concern had taken the form of opposing his interest in music by allying it with "doped up jazz musicians." The uncertain internal confusion of what he could be was opposed by the stability of what he was not to be. He therefore began to experiment with his father's own drugs, which he pilfered, and focused more and more on a "negative identity," becoming a drug-addicted jazz musician.

Both psychiatrists and educators are becoming increasingly aware of the necessity for some adolescents to take a so-called moratorium before making lifelong occupational choices. It is becoming increasingly frequent for adolescents to drop out of college for one or two years, and, after having taken this moratorium, either through work, travel, or military service, to then return to college with a much clearer internal image of what it is they want. To some, the moratorium seems available only via very destructive acting out, which forces them out of the intolerable adolescent crisis into psychiatric treatment or institutionalization.

CASE ILLUSTRATION

An eighteen-year-old college freshman, beset by the confusions of homosexual versus heterosexual longings, professional choice, and great difficulties with competitive strivings as particularly manifested around collegiate intellectual activity, sought psychiatric treatment. Once in treatment, his first major decision was to drop out of school temporarily, using his treatment as the moratorium. This served to remove him from the intolerable pressure to make decisions while in the midst of a confused adolescent turmoil.

Anna Freud has pointed out that adolescent solutions may be classified as defenses against the dependency longings and defenses against increased impulses. The dependency upon one's parents can be resolved by avoiding adolescence and remaining forever a child. This may also be resolved by an abrupt detachment and flight from the parents. This usually is followed by very intense relationships with substitutes who are chosen for their dissimilarity to the original parents. The attachments can be to leaders who are idealized, as in youth movements, or in homosexual or heterosexual friendships, or group formations (gangs).

Anna Freud has particularly pointed out the danger to the adolescent who is unable to displace onto a broader circle than the family and who continues to act out within the family. Denial, reaction formation, may lead to more intolerable hostility and aggressiveness, which by means of projection may ultimately result in quite paranoid behavior. It is also quite possible for this hostility to be turned inward in the form of intense depression and even suicidal attempts.

The most severe result of the adolescent crisis is that of a psychotic break. It is frequently very difficult to determine whether this represents an unusually severe adolescent turmoil, or transient psychotic episode, as opposed to the ominous onset of a more chronic schizophrenic state. Recent research[60] has indicated, for example, that the issue of school phobia as manifested in adolescence is quite different from that manifested in the younger age group. Here it is no longer so much a matter of separation anxiety: instead one does find a large number of schizophrenic reactions in this group.

In summary, although one must remain ever-watchful for pathological development in the adolescent period, this must remain within the framework of adolescence as a normally tumultuous and turbulent period in which the child struggles to resynthesize and maintain his mental equilibrium. It remains particularly important during this evaluation process to remain cognizant of the needs of parents. Anna Freud, in speaking of the normal complexities of adolescence, states: "While an adolescent remains inconsistent and unpredictable in his behavior, he may suffer but does not seem to me to be in need of treatment. I think that he should be given time and scope to work out his own solutions. Rather, it may be his parents who need help and guidance so as to be able to bear with him. There are few situations in life which are more difficult to cope with than an adolescent son or daughter during the attempt to liberate themselves."

Juvenile Delinquency

It is impossible to speak of adolescence without some discussion of juvenile delinquency. It is common that the child may find himself in conflict with the law during the period of adolescent crisis. This is not always delinquency.

Juvenile delinquency is a legal term, not a psychiatric diagnosis. Nor is it exclusively a psychiatric problem. It is nonetheless an area in which psychiatry can make valuable contributions, and one for which psychiatry shares responsibility, along with social sciences such as sociology and anthropology, the law and law-enforcement agencies, and other community agencies.

It has been estimated that more than a half-million children are labeled as juvenile delinquents each year.[20] As Stuart M. Finch points out in his excellent review, this category is so broad that no person or discipline has studied the whole range. Each profession tends to focus only on its own definitions and samples. The highly charged quality of the area is apparent from the stance of professionals ranging from the demand for harsh punitive measures for the offender to the other extreme of blaming society for the plight of the delinquent.

Theories of etiology are abundant and tend to fall into two groups: those that stress individual pathology and those that focus on society and minimize individual pathology. Differences in training and approach make it difficult even to arrive at a common definition. However, in view of the fact that it is a legal term, one useful definition suggested[39] is ". . . behavior by nonadults which violates specific legal norms or the norms of a particular societal institution with sufficient frequency and/or seriousness so as to provide firm basis for legal action against the behaving individual or group . . ."

Sociologically oriented researchers point out that statistical incidence figures are only gross estimates, but the data reveal juvenile delinquency occurs in every country. Rates are highest in industrialized countries. It increases during periods of prosperity and decreases during periods of depression. It increases during periods of war. The ratio of boys to girls has remained at a rather constant four to five boys to one girl. Boys are often arrested for car-stealing, vandalism, or aggressive-destructive behavior; girls are primarily arrested for sexual misconduct and running away from home.

The lower socioeconomic levels contribute the highest ratio and, in keeping with this, arrests of Negro children are disproportionately high. However, there is every reason to believe this is not related to true incidence but is a function of such factors as the response to middle-class Caucasian children by both law-enforcing agencies and parents, which is the tendency to "bail them out."

The sociologists A. Cohen and J. Short[9] postulate three subcultures of delinquency. One is the "criminal" group in which children are relatively integrated into a criminal society in which they progress by means of criminal behavior. They abide by codes and ethics and develop status positions in the group.

The "conflict" subculture occurs around social disorganization with its many attendant frustrations. This, the largest group, tends to promote violent, irrational, and aggressive acting out. It is the problem of tension areas in segregation-desegregation disputes. The third subculture consists of "retreatists." They are characterized by adolescent drug addiction and withdrawal.

The psychiatrist tends to study the individual and focus on the common characteristic of acting-out behavior. The most usual diagnostic category used is that of the antisocial character disorder. It is usual to label latency children as predelinquent and adolescents as delinquents.

The most frequent psychiatric approach to the problem is to study such children within a psychodynamic framework to search for the etiological factors involved in the individual pathology. This has yielded a somewhat bewildering array of "causes" and conditions that manifest delinquent behavior. Delinquent behavior has been found to occur in neurotic, brain-damaged, schizophrenic, and other psychotic children, although the largest and most refractory group remains the character disorder. By such an individual approach it has not been possible to offer individual treatment to more than a small proportion of juvenile delinquents.

Starting with the work of Healy, the history of much of American child psychiatry is related to this problem. In a general developmental and etiological way, it has been related to the problem of maternal deprivation, frequent foster home placements, and for many has focused on the so-called affectless child. John Bowlby[6] characterized these children as having superficial relationships, as being exasperatingly inaccessible to help, having a curious lack of emotional response to situations where it would be expected, characterized by pointless deceit and evasion, lack of concentration in school, and a history of truancy and stealing that started quite early and became chronic. Many other workers have focused on the superego defect in these children and the manner in which this is transmitted by parents.

Treatment efforts are numerous and as yet bear the brunt of interprofessional confusion. The psychiatrist may recognize the "cry for help" of the neurotic child who can think of no other way of getting help.[1, 40] The methods of August Aichorn are still applicable to many of the character disorders. In working with the individual child, many modifications of psychotherapeutic technique are advised.

A major hurdle in treatment is to command the attention of the nonmotivated delinquent. One research approach has been for a worker (usually from social service) to "join" a group of delinquents. This is quite dangerous since it calls for participation in delinquent acts as a precondition for effective communication with the group. Another method suggested is to buy the time of the delinquent as a participant in a research project.[57] The more classical psychotherapeutic techniques have been effective primarily with neurotic delinquents. Intriguing as some of these techniques are, they are insufficient in the face of the overwhelming numbers and general inaccessibility of these youngsters.

The obvious needs are clear; the solutions elusive. It calls for more sophisticated research based on more adequate interprofessional communication. This is particularly true of treatment methods. One recent attempt has been the development of residential treatment centers. Others are therapeutic camping as practiced by the state of California and the University of Michigan, Boy's Clubs in underpriveleged areas and Fresh Air Camps. In addition, all must focus, as informed citizens, on those aspects of society which seem so directly to either cause or enhance delinquent behavior—such as slums, segregation, and educational deprivation, to name but a few.

Treatment

The forms of treatment available for work with the behavior disorders of children and adolescents include such organic therapies as psychosurgery, shock therapy, and pharmacologic agents. They also include such techniques as manipulation of environment or placement outside the home; educational techniques such as counseling with the parents; rehabilitation and retraining techniques as with the brain-damaged and mentally defective child; and psychotherapy, ranging from supportive relationship therapy and expressive cathartic techniques to child psychoanalysis.[1,3,21,22,26,40,45,55]

It is most usual to find various combinations of treatment techniques employed in the care of children. In general, there is a great reluctance to use such techniques as psychosurgery and shock therapy with children. However, shock has been used in treatment of childhood schizophrenia with rather confusing reports of results. Drug therapy, including sedatives, anticonvulsants, and tranquilizers is extensively used. This is particularly true of pediatric care of behavior disorders and treatment by general practitioners. The increasing incidence of side-effects such as extrapyramidal signs, has been noted and suggests widespread and indiscriminate use of drugs by physicians. Although psychopharmacological agents are used extensively by many child psychiatrists, they are usually used in conjunction with other forms of therapeutic intervention.

Adequately controlled research of drug effectiveness in children is unusually difficult. Few adequately conducted studies have been reported in the literature. Some of these suggest that the neurophysiologically less mature child responds differently than the adult. Another factor is the degree of psychological development attained. For example, although drug therapy has been reported to induce remissions in adult schizophrenics, it has been demonstrated as having no impact on the underlying process in autism or juvenile schizophrenia. The same state of affairs applies to the efficacy of shock therapy.

The few studies reported seem to indicate that the effectiveness or ineffectiveness of drugs is directly related to the contribution of psychological forces,[4] such as the relationship of the child to the care-taking adults and his peers. The most consistent use of drug therapy in child psychiatry is for the management of hyperactive, excitable, impulse-ridden children. In this group, prochlorperazine and meprobamate demonstrated no significant therapeutic benefit. On the other hand, dextro-amphetamine produced a marked reduction in symptomatic disturbed behavior. Prolonged use of this drug, however, resulted in marked weight loss.[15] In one study of eighty out-patient children, placebo demonstrated the same effectiveness as prochlorperazine, meprobamate, and perphenazine.[12] Benadryl and other antihistamines also are of some use in control of impulsive behavior. Sedatives are not generally used, since they either tend to make the child too drowsy or produce excitement in the hyperactive child. The most effective use of drugs in children's disorders has been the incalculable benefits to the group of seizure-states.

Increasing concern with training and care for the very seriously disturbed child has stimulated the development of in-patient facilities, day-care programs, and halfway house facilities, in addition to the more traditional out-patient clinics.[2] Collaborative treatment for the autistic child,[10, 00, 10, 11] and concern with the sensory-deprived child have become matters of increasing importance. In this regard, the recent publication by E. B. Omwake and A. J. Solnit[45] delineates a very poignant contribution from education to treatment of a blind child.

Yet it remains true that the majority of children are treated on an out-patient basis either in clinics or in private practice. Thus, the character of psychotherapy has been markedly affected by the patterning of the psychotherapeutic practices of the usual child psychiatry clinic. This is the orthopsychiatric team approach of psychologist, psychiatrist, and social worker. At first the definition of function within this team was quite clearly delineated, but in some settings there is now a great deal of overlap.

In view of the child's involvement with his parents and the impact of the omnipresent mutual stimulation, the usual practice is to take the entire family into treatment insofar as the family permits this. The most usual arrangement is for the mother and the child to be in simultaneous treatment with separate therapists. Increasing efforts are now made to include the father and other family members in such treatment efforts. Increasing concern with the familial interactions of pathological families has brought with it much experimentation in treatment methods. Group therapy with parents of disturbed children has long been part of the psychotherapeutic armamentarium. This has been extended to group psychotherapy with individual families, each family including one group leader, or simultaneous individual treatment of family members by the same psychotherapist. The choice of any of these techniques depends on the severity of the illness, the availability of the family, and the skills of the psychiatrist.

The typical arrangement remains that of the child psychiatrist treating the child, while a colleague, either from psychiatry, psychology, or social work does psychotherapy, counseling, or casework with the parent or parents.

The treatment of the child himself is accomplished via the techniques of play therapy. This takes into account the problems of communication as outlined above. It necessitates the structure of an adequately stocked playroom, which includes in it a wide variety of play materials that particularly lend themselves to the expression of conflicts. These include puppets, doll families, clay, guns, painting materials, and so forth. Through the medium of such play, the psychiatrist can understand the displacement into the play of the child's conflicts and can help the child to come to a conscious understanding of his problems.

Although interpretations are frequently made in the play, it remains very important that the psychiatrist conceptualize and verbalize the problems for the child in language the child understands. The therapeutic importance of this lies in the fact that thought is one of the most important developmental ways of controlling and directing impulses. Thus, every time the psychiatrist is able to identify in words the feeling states and complexities of relationships to the child, he gives him the adequate tools of thought with which he can make the appropriate abstractions and conceptualizations of himself and his relationships to others. For example, the child's understanding of "funny feeling" can be enlarged to this as his expression of the internal state of anxiety and the circumstances that arouse it and the ways he has of dealing with it. In this sense, psychotherapy with children—and particularly child psychoanalysis—can be thought of as aiding crucial developmental processes and are thus educational in the broadest sense of the word.

Play therapy, with or without the modifications listed above, has been most effective with those psychiatric problems of childhood which are amenable to psychotherapy. It has not contributed as much to the treatment of psychotic conditions, brain damage, and mental deficiency. The care, rehabilitation, and treatment of these disorders require newer techniques, which are constantly evolving out of clinical research centers. It appears quite likely that cooperation within multidisciplinary groups will become more important. It is further conceivable that new disciplines may emerge that will aid child psychiatry as it develops new modes of meeting and fulfilling its responsibility for the mental health of children.

NOTES

1. August Aichorn, *Wayward Youth* (New York: Viking Press, 1935).
2. Herschel Alt, *Residential Treatment for the Disturbed Child* (New York: International Universities Press, 1960).
3. Lauretta Bender, "Twenty Years of Clinical Research on Schizophrenic Children," in Gerald Caplan, ed., *Emotional Problems of Early Childhood* (New York: Basic Books, 1955).
4. M. Boatman and I. Berlin, "Some Implications of Incidental Experience with Psychopharmacological Drugs in a Children's Psychotherapeutic Program," *Journal of the American Academy of Child Psychiatry*, 1 (1962), 431–443.
5. Berta Bornstein, "Emotional Barriers in the Understanding and Treatment of Young Children," *American Journal of Orthopsychiatry*, 18 (1948), 691–97.
6. John Bowlby, *Maternal Care and Mental Health* (Monograph No. 2; Geneva: World Health Organization, 1951).
7. W. H. Bridger and Morton F. Reiser, "Psychophysiological Studies of the Neonate," *Psychosomatic Medicine*, 21 (1959), 265.
8. Stella Chess, *An Introduction to Child Psychiatry* (New York: Grune & Stratton, 1959).
9. A. Cohen and J. Short, "Research in Delinquent Sub-Cultures," *Journal of Social Issues*, 140 (1955), 20–37.
10. R. W. Coleman, Ernst Kris, and S. Provence, "The Study of Variations of Early Parental Attitudes," *The Psychoanalytic Study of the Child*, 8 (1953), 20–47.
11. James S. Coleman, *The Adolescent Society* (New York: Macmillan, 1961).
12. L. Cytryn, A. Gilbert, and L. Eisenberg, "The Effectiveness of Tranquilizing Drugs Plus Supportive Psychotherapy in Treating Behavior Disorders of Children: A Double-Blind Study of Eighty Out-Patients," *American Journal of Orthopsychiatry*, 30 (1960), 113–27.
13. L. Dawes, "The Psychoanalysis of a Case of 'Grand Hysteria of Charcot' in a Girl of Fifteen," *Nervous Child*, 10 (1953), 272–305.
14. L. Eisenberg, "Psychiatric Implications of Brain Damage in Children," *Psychiatric Quarterly*, 31 (January 1957), 72–92.
15. L. Eisenberg, R. Lachman, P. Molling, A. Lockner, J. Mizella, and A. Connors, "A Psychopharmacologic Experiment in a Training School for Delinquent Boys," *American Journal of Orthopsychiatry*, 30 (1963), 431–47.
16. R. Ekstein, K. Bryant, and S. Friedman, "Childhood Schizophrenia and Allied Conditions," in Leopold Bellak, ed., *Schizophrenia* (New York: Logos Press, 1958).

17. Erik H. Erikson, *Childhood and Society* (New York: Norton, 1950).
18. Erik H. Erikson, "The Problem of Ego-Identity," *Journal of the American Psychoanalytic Association*, 4 (1956), 56–121.
19. Sibylle K. Escalona, "The Study of Individual Differences and the Problem of State," *Journal of the American Academy of Child Psychiatry*, 1 (1962), 11–37.
20. Stuart M. Finch, "The Psychiatrist and Juvenile Delinquency," *Journal of the American Academy of Child Psychiatry*, 1 (1962), 619–36.
21. Anna Freud, *Introduction to Techniques of Child Analysis* (Nervous and Mental Disease Monograph Series No. 48; New York: Nervous and Mental Disease Publishing Company, 1928).
22. Anna Freud, *The Ego and Mechanisms of Defence* (New York: International Universities Press, 1946).
23. Anna Freud, "The Role of Bodily Illness in the Mental Life of Children," *The Psychoanalytic Study of the Child*, 7 (1952), 69–81.
24. Anna Freud, "Adolescence," *The Psychoanalytic Study of the Child*, 13 (1958), 255–78.
25. Anna Freud, *The Psychoanalytic Treatment of Children* (New York: International Universities Press, 1959).
26. Sigmund Freud, "The Analysis of a Phobia in a Five-Year-Old Boy" [1909], in *Collected Papers* (New York: Basic Books, 1959), Vol. III, pp. 149–295.
27. Sigmund Freud, "Formulations Regarding the Two Principles in Mental Functioning" [1911], *Collected Papers* (New York: Basic Books, 1959), Vol. IV, pp. 13–21.
28. Margaret E. Fries and Paul J. Woolf, "Some Hypotheses on the Role of Congenital Activity Type in Personality Development," *The Psychoanalytic Study of the Child*, 8 (1953), 48–62.
29. Margaret W. Gerard, "Enuresis: A Study in Etiology," *American Journal of Orthopsychiatry*, 9 (1939), 48.
30. William Goldfarb, *Childhood Schizophrenia* (Cambridge: Harvard University Press, 1962).
31. Group for the Advancement of Psychiatry, "The Diagnostic Process in Child Psychiatry," *The Group for the Advancement of Psychiatry Report* (August 1957), No. 38.
32. V. Hamburger, "The Concept of Development in Biology," in D. Harris, ed., *The Concept of Development* (Minneapolis: University of Minnesota Press, 1957).
33. Heinz Hartmann, *Ego Psychology and Processes of Adaptation* (New York: International Universities Press, 1960).
34. Heinz Hartmann and Ernst Kris, "The Genetic Approach in Psychoanalysis," *The Psychoanalytic Study of the Child*, 1 (1945), 11–30.
35. Leo Kanner, "Autistic Disturbances of Affective Contact," *Nervous Child*, 1 (1943), 217–50.
36. Leo Kanner, "Early Infantile Autism," *American Journal of Psychiatry*, 108 (1951), 23–26.

37. I. Kaufman, "Conversion Hysteria in Latency," *Journal of the American Academy of Child Psychiatry*, 1 (1962), 385–96.
38. Ernst Kris, *Psychoanalytic Exploration in Art* (New York: International Universities Press, 1952).
39. W. Kvoraceuis and B. Miller, *Delinquent Behavior; Culture and Individual* (Washington, D. C.: National Education Association, 1959).
40. Sandor Lorand and Henry Schneer, eds., *Adolescents* (New York: Paul B. Hoeber, 1961).
41. Seymour L. Lustman, "Rudiment of the Ego," *The Psychoanalytic Study of the Child*, 11 (1956), 89–98.
42. Seymour L. Lustman, "Defense, Symptom and Character," *The Psychoanalytic Study of the Child*, 17 (1962), 216–44.
43. Margaret Mahler, "On Child Psychosis and Schizophrenia," *The Psychoanalytic Study of the Child*, 7 (1952), 286–305.
44. Margaret Mahler, Manuel Furer, and Calvin F. Settlage, "Severe Emotional Disturbances in Childhood: Psychosis," in Silvano Arieti, ed., *The American Handbook of Psychiatry* (New York: Basic Books, 1959), Vol. I, pp. 816–840.
45. Eveline B. Omwake and A. J. Solnit, "It Isn't Fair: The Treatment of a Blind Child," *The Psychoanalytic Study of the Child*, 16 (1961), 352–404.
46. Lili Peller, "Libidinal Phases, Ego Development and Play," *The Psychoanalytic Study of the Child*, 9 (1954), 178–98.
47. Jean Piaget, *The Language and Thought of the Child* (London: Routledge and Kegan Paul Ltd., 1932).
48. William Pious, "A Provisional Hypothesis about the Nature of Schizophrenic Behavior," in Arthur Burton, ed., *Psychotherapy of the Psychoses* (New York. Basic Books, 1961).
49. S. Provence and Samuel Ritvo, "Effects of Deprivation on Institutionalized Infants," *The Psychoanalytic Study of the Child*, 16 (1961), 189–205.
50. David Rapaport and M. M. Gill, "The Points of View and Assumptions of Meta-Psychology," *International Journal of Psycho-Analysis*, 40 (1959), 189–205.
51. J. B. Richmond and Seymour L. Lustman, "Autonomic Function in the Neonate," *Psychosomatic Medicine*, 17 (1955), 269–75.
52. Samuel Ritvo and A. J. Solnit, "Influences of Early Mother–Child Interaction on Indentification Processes," *The Psychoanalytic Study of the Child*, 13, (1958), 64–91.
53. E. Robbins and P. O'Neal, "Clinical Features of Hysteria in Children," *Nervous Child*, 10 (1953), 246–71.
54. J. D. Salinger, *Catcher in the Rye* (New York: Little, Brown, 1945).
55. Milton J. E. Senn, "Changing Concepts of Child Care: A Historical Review," in *Society and Medicine*, New York Academy of Medicine, No. XVII (New York: International Universities Press, 1955).
56. Milton J. E. Senn, "Relationship of Pediatrics and Psychiatry," *American Journal of Diseases of Children*, 71 (1946), 537–49.

57. C. Slack, "Experimenter–Subject Psychotherapy," *Mental Hygiene*, 44 (1960), 238–56.
58. René Spitz and Katherine Wolf, "Anaclitic Depression," *The Psychoanalytic Study of the Child*, 2 (1946), 313–42.
59. Robert Waelder, "The Psychoanalytic Theory of Play," *Psychoanalytic Quarterly*, 1 (1933), 208–24.
60. S. Waldfogel, J. C. Coolidge, and P. B. Hahn, "The Development, Meaning and Management of School Phobia," *American Journal of Orthopsychiatry*, 27 (1957), 754–80.
61. Paul Weiss, *Principles of Development* (New York: Holt, 1939).
62. Paul Weiss, *Self-Differentiation of the Basic Patterns of Co-ordination*, Comparative Psychology Monograph, Vol. 17 (1941), No. 4.
63. Heinz Werner, *Comparative Psychology of Mental Development* (New York: International Universities Press, 1957).
64. World Health Organization, Geneva [1956], *Discussions on Child Development* (New York: International Universities Press, 1960).

CHAPTER TWENTY-ONE

Behavior Disorders in Old Age

Old Age and Senility

Prejudice, ignorance, and lack of empathy pervade our comprehension of the aged. Whatever determines the attitude that those undoubtedly near death are already half-dead, we cannot afford to be uninterested in aging and the aged. The increase in life-span alone has directed medical, social, and legal attention to this rapidly growing "minority group." Much of our specialized knowledge of the aged derives from a skewed sample of persons who have come to psychiatric and medical attention in hospitals and nursing homes; 96 per cent of old people reside in the community, unstudied by specialists. The student should be advised of this source of traditional knowledge; there are, however, growing research efforts to disentangle organic and psychological factors of the aging process and also to differentiate the common diseases of the aged from normal aging.[20] A scientific approach to the old has begun to replace traditional attitudes of awed reverence, which perhaps inhibited research in the field. Some behavior disorders found in old age are psychologically determined reactions; others are accompanied by pathological alterations of the brain parenchyma and its vascular system. The biological definition of aging has not yet been specified adequately; it is a process of multiple changes, which do not necessarily occur in an interrelated or synchronous manner. Although aging is not at this juncture a reversible process, factors contributing to disorders of aging may well be treatable, and growing insight into psychodynamic and social factors should allow a more confident statement about normal ranges of age-specific behavior change.

From the available data, it appears that aging presents a condition that, of itself, brings relatively few impairments of psychological function. On the other hand, it is a state in which vulnerability to some effects of biological and psychosocial stress is enhanced.[32] Thus, the pathological changes in cognitive function, memory, attention, and interest, and the regressive personality changes that constitute senile behavior ought to be—if possible—differentiated from behavior in normal aging. Disorders of old age range from relatively mild maladjustment, without brain disease, to very severe disorders leading rapidly to devastating deterioration and death. The severe behavior disorders with deterioration, the so-called senile psychoses, are usually accompanied by cerebral changes.

The Scope of the Problem

Populations of aged persons have increased all over the world. This increase has been both relative and absolute. In 1900, the total population of the United States was 75,000,000 with 4 per cent, or about 3,000, over 65 years of age. In 1960, the population was about 180,000,000 with 7 per cent, or 14,400,000, over 65. Similar changes are taking place in most industrialized countries. As the number of children has also increased very rapidly, this poses a serious problem; the ever-increasing number of children and old people have to be supported by a proportionally ever-smaller group of productive middle-aged people. In an article on arteriosclerosis, W. Dock remarks that persons best fitted to survive are those whose parents leave a nice nest egg after the children reach maturity and then obligingly disappear.[10]

The bulk of problems attendant on the expanding population is far beyond the tasks and scopes of psychiatry. Yet the psychiatric problem in itself is quite formidable. In a reasonably accurate survey carried out in Sweden, a country of 7,000,000, it was determined that 9,000 persons suffer from severe senile mental disorders;[37] applying this rate to the United States would put the number of such patients at approximately 250,000. Figures based on the research of E. M. Gruenberg, J. H. Cummings *et al.* are even higher.[17] These investigators found, in six census tracts in a random population of about 1,600 persons over 65 in Syracuse, New York, that 100 were "certifiable," that is, unable to take care of themselves or dangerous to themselves or others; by extrapolation, this would mean that in the United States roughly 1,000,000 would fall into the "certifiable" category. One must keep in mind not only that experts may disagree on criteria for illness but that criteria of helplessness and potential danger are by no means the same in urban and rural settings and among the different social strata; the problem of old age is particularly acute in urban communities. It is also clear from Gruenberg's data that only a small proportion of aged psychiatric patients are in mental hospitals; most are found in nursing homes or with their own families. Ironically, those in mental hospitals are not always mentally ill; they are sent there because there is no other place for them to go.

In the New Haven study, it was found that only approximately 10 per cent of the total psychiatric patient population under treatment were labeled as senile or arteriosclerotic behavior disorders.[18] In the state of New York, senile patients constitute 15 per cent of all mental hospital admissions, and this figure is on the rise.[27] This increase does not reflect the "medicated survival of the unfit" but rather the tendency, particularly in urban areas, to send senile members of the family to institutions. The three-generation family unit, particularly in the urban middle class, is gradually disappearing. William Malamud has remarked that with progress in the treatment of cardiovascular, degenerative, and neoplastic diseases, the problem of behavior disorders of old age will become an even greater challenge.[26]

Problems of Classification

In most older textbooks, two major classes of behavior disorders of old age, the senile and arteriosclerotic, are stressed. The senile disorders are subdivided according to symptoms into: (1) simple dementia; (2) delirious and confused types; (3) paranoid states; (4) depressed and agitated types; and (5) presbyophrenic types. Disorders due to the so-called presenile diseases of middle age are listed separately. Whether senile and arteriosclerotic cases should be put into one or two broad epidemiological classes cannot be answered categorically; essentially it depends upon the aims of such studies.

Recently, M. Roth has proposed a new classification of mental disorders occurring in old age.[31] He proposes a division into: (1) affective psychoses; (2) senile psychoses; (3) arteriosclerotic psychoses; (4) delirious states; and (5) late paraphrenia. Although no classification of disease limited to an age period is completely satisfactory, Roth's proposal is a distinct advance. It recognizes the important fact that the majority of disorders of old age are not characterized merely by profound and progressive deterioration. In a future classification of severe behavior disorders of the aged, one might divide the population into those with minimal, moderate, and severe intellectual deficit and state in addition whether the patients show affective, paraphrenic, or delirious symptoms. It is also essential to add a neurotic and sociopathic group, because many aged patients show merely their lifelong neurotic behavior or an aggravation of such traits. Most of all, to be effective, any classification must take into account the many gradual transitions from the normal aged to senility, from no cerebral disease to known and accountable cerebral pathology.

The Aged Person

The typical, or expected, behavior of old persons is not known with any precision. Erik H. Erikson noted that the life-crisis of old age was centered about a sense of integrity versus disgust and despair.[12] S. Perlin and A. S. Butler point to the "life review" as an intrinsic normal feature of aging, ranging from nostalgic reminiscence and story-telling to "broken records" of bitter regret.[28] Creative outcomes of such reviews are apparent in the valuable judgments and perspectives found in the memoirs of such men as Galileo Galilei, Johann Wolfgang von Goethe, Benjamin Franklin, Winston Churchill, Albert Schweitzer, and others. Such persons generally show an appetite for the life they live, whatever their age.

From the seventh decade of life on, a certain deficit is unmistakable, just as certain physical characteristics, such as a decrease in muscular power and speed, in acuity of sight and hearing, and the presence of certain cardiovascular changes are the rule. Nevertheless, the performance of aged persons can be outstanding, and investigators of old age have found that many old people are vigorous, alert, candid, and deeply involved in everyday living. Recent studies showed that cognitive performance in a well-adjusted group of aged living in the community compared favorably with young people, although some slowing in reaction time and processes requiring speed was evident. The factor of speed as well as cognitive functions were sensitive to the presence of stresses such as minimal disease states, including arteriosclerosis. Thus, the rigidity or lack of interest in new learning associated with aging may prove not to be a direct consequence of aging.[4]

Nevertheless, the *vulnerability* to impairment of mental function in the aged, the possibility for periodicity in excellence of performance, and the physical and sensorimotor deficits of aging provide, with the changing life situation, a changed set of circumstances and factors, which frequently lead to consequential limitations of over-all function. In varying degrees, old persons are aware of any failing performance or shifts of status and usually are quite defensive about it. Fear of death, loneliness, uselessness, and changes of body image and self-concept are encountered. Among the changing social relationships they face, is the decimation of their ranks of friends. Contact with children and younger colleagues, as well as peers, must be patterned in some gratifying way. Some, knowing life is short, show vigor in working out solutions to change; pre-existing personality traits may be adapted to meet changes or may interfere with adjustment. Many try to compensate for deficits by counterphobic maneuvers and at times endanger themselves thereby. Again, some tend to avoid new situations and give the impression of being conservative as well as rigid. They usually report some memory deficit, particularly for recent events, and are inclined to dwell on the remote past. When forced into new or puzzling situations or tasks requiring abstraction, they respond with anxiety, irritation, and withdrawal.

Many elderly persons become somewhat egocentric and possessive and show a preoccupation with their poor health. All these traits can be explained as responses to threats and losses. The existence of such a threatening reality is often denied. In general, it is not just behavioral deficit but new stresses in old age that generate troubles for the solution of which society turns to psychiatry.

The Aged Neurotic and Sociopath

Transition from the normal to the neurotic aged person is gradual; in this group, as at other age levels, it is not possible to draw a clear line of demarcation. In spite of their clinical significance, neuroses of old age are largely ignored in the literature.[8] In all likelihood, it is not a lack of "cortical reserve" that causes previously compensated neuroses to recur but rather such psychosocial events as the loss of persons or possessions, the presence of injuries and illnesses, or the decrease in status and independence. The aged patient responds according to previously acquired patterns and may become quarrelsome, complaining, negativistic, apathetic, or agitated. Exaggerations of complaints about physical discomfort, headaches, constipation, lack of appetite, and insomnia become very prominent. Irritability is a very notable trait in neurotic aged; antisocial behavior may be transient; often it is no more than a response to provocative and highly disturbing experiences, and extremes of behavior usually disappear with the removal of stress. The clinical impression is that many lifelong paranoid personalities and sociopaths do not improve in old age but get worse. Paranoid schizophrenics, on the other hand, reportedly improve. Perlin and Butler have pointed out that some personality traits (for example, obsessiveness or schizoid traits) are adaptively used to adjust to the relative isolation that too often characterizes the life situation of the aged.[28] Old age indeed provides a natural laboratory in which the general issue of the role of previous behavior patterns in new contexts can be studied. Butler has remarked, with no little justification, that few psychiatrists are familiar with the nature of the aging experience and the detailed problems of this process.

The following brief account of an elderly patient exemplifies a not uncommon pattern of neurotic behavior in the aged.

> A seventy-nine-year-old woman became increasingly hypochondriacal in her old age. She had always feared illness, liked to dwell on her ailments, and enjoyed being taken care of by doctors and by her family. There were many instances of histrionic behavior, such as dramatic outbursts of anger, of conversion symptoms such as losing her voice, and of brief amnesic episodes. After her husband had several illnesses and operations, her own behavior deteriorated. She felt she was not needed and neglected and that everyone in the family wanted her to die. She had to be reassured incessantly that she was loved and needed. Her excessively demanding behavior only provoked and irritated her family; to such irritation she responded with more dependent demands, complaints, and anger. She developed numerous symptoms: pains in the bladder, constant headaches, generalized itching, and "twitching of the nerves." She consulted more than one physician and received huge supplies of tranquilizing drugs, which potentiated each other and produced only increased forgetfulness, confusion, and apathy alternating with irritability. The patient improved markedly after a new physician took over, eliminated the excessive medication, and discussed with her in a simple way the obvious reasons for her demanding and histrionic behavior.

Severe Behavior Disorders in Old Age

SIMPLE DETERIORATION One might ask what is "simple" about a condition in which the patient becomes incapacitated and utterly helpless and dependent. The word simple implies that such deterioration is not markedly complicated by paranoid, manic, or depressive symptoms. The intellectual deficit is presumably the result of cerebral changes. The syndrome of senile dementia may develop slowly or rapidly. As old people are rarely in responsible occupational positions, their deficiencies usually are revealed at home and in social situations. Nonetheless, failure on the job, and subsequent forced retirement may be a calamitous experience. Often, the patient's deterioration, as when contracts and wills are involved, becomes a legal issue. At the beginning, forgetfulness, failures (particularly in novel situations), a certain lack of judgment, or silliness in opinion and conversation may be noticeable. Performance of abstract tasks in tests is impaired. Items of practical knowledge are retained longer than theoretical or abstract knowledge; in severe cases, however, practical judgment is usually defective at a fairly early stage. As deterioration progresses, the patient becomes unable to carry out even very simple tasks; he requires constant supervision, which may be difficult to provide at home even under favorable circumstances. If difficulties of recall are prominent, memory for the remote past relatively intact, and the patient confabulates to cover up or deny his deficit, we speak of *presbyophrenia*. This syndrome is similar to the one described by S. S. Korsakoff, although, of course, without the toxic polyneuropathy (see Chapter 21). It is very doubtful if it is a real disease entity. Actually, we are unable to determine why some senile patients develop one type of deficit instead of another. The presbyophrenic reaction is closely related to the confused and delirious reactions.

All patients with simple deterioration also develop striking emotional changes. Catastrophic anxiety reactions occur. Some patients are in a constant and restless state of agitation. The most common behavior is depression and apathy; this is probably the characteristic mood, particularly in those who are restricted to the lifeless atmosphere of back wards. A small minority becomes hostile and aggressive; generally, these disturbances subside under proper management since the paranoid ideas usually are not fixed. Most senile temper tantrums are responses to provocations. Suspicion and mild paranoid reactions related to the current situation are common. Many of these patients, lacking in ability to test reality, realize dimly that they are unwanted and develop paranoid delusions that others are stealing their belongings and their food, or that murderers are hiding nearby. Not infrequently these patients, particularly women, think that persons in their surroundings are sexually interested in them and that sexual proposals are being made. If sexual misdemeanors occur, they are usually of an infantile nature, exhibitionistic or voyeuristic, or involve the seduction of children to sexual play.

PARANOID REACTIONS These are diagnosed when paranoid traits reach a high intensity and systematization. Such reactions, which can occur with and without significant deterioration in old age, were described by Emil Kraepelin.[22] Most of the above-mentioned, mildly paranoid patients in this age-bracket, if well treated, are not difficult to manage if attention is paid to their stresses. It should be remembered that even slight losses of hearing and (to a lesser extent) of vision may contribute to the development of paranoid reactions in old people. Confidently presented and followed through, simple and practical maneuvers aimed at the specific perceptual deficit (for example, training in lip reading or providing hearing aids) may be helpful.

AFFECTIVE DISORDERS Depressive reactions in old age, often with minimal intellectual deficit, are frequent, and old persons are particularly apt to react to threats, losses, and frustrations with dejection and apathy. Superficially, this may resemble deterioration; in reality, it is usually the profound resignation and indignation of a deeply wounded person who feels unloved, unwanted, and abandoned. Irritability and irascibility similarly express struggles toward self-esteem. Guilt over lifelong failures and sins may be prominent although not necessarily overtly expressed. The severity and duration of depressive reactions vary greatly, ranging from mild, fleeting reactions to severe, lasting, and recurring depressions. A small number of depressions in old age are recurrences of manic-depressive disorders. True manic states in the senile are rare. The nearest to it are silly euphoric reactions and a tendency to tell inappropriate or inane jokes. When provoked, such patients can, at times, become quite agitated and destructive. It must be kept in mind that the statistical likelihood of suicide in old age is high; even mildly depressed patients in this age group frequently make suicidal attempts or show self-destructive behavior, which may be tantamount to suicide.

DELIRIOUS AND CONFUSED REACTIONS Even a slight cerebral deficit very markedly increases the chance of disorientation and confusion. Confused states are common in patients with cerebral arteriosclerosis and in those who suffer from convulsive seizures. Confused states are frequently seen at night or when patients change environments or undergo operations with general anesthesia. In the days when patients had to be restrained and blindfolded, ophthalmic surgery invariably provoked delirious reactions in old persons, which quickly subsided on return of sight and the accustomed environment. Arnold Pick described an interesting syndrome, apperceptive blindness of the senile, in which arteriosclerotic patients with occipital lesions without peripheral visual impairment do not fix their gaze on objects or pay attention to visual cues in their surroundings.[29]

Clinical Symptoms of the Presenile Diseases

The rather heterogeneous group of presenile diseases is characterized mostly by intellectual deterioration and personality disintegration closely resembling severe senile changes, but the onset occurs in the forties and fifties. The best-known types are the diseases described by Pick[29] and A. Alzheimer;[1] they are quite rare; not more than a few hundred cases have been described in the total literature. T. Sjögren thinks that Pick's disease is an independent disease entity but suggests that Alzheimer's disease is a variation of a senile deterioration.[34] Once an organic process is diagnosed and differentiated from treatable disorders, the distinction between Pick's and Alzheimer's diseases (or the even rarer syndromes described as Jacob-Kreutzfeld's disease, Binswanger's disease, and other diffuse demyelinizing encephalopathies) has little practical significance. An interest in picayune and often erroneous differentiation of these many syndromes was seemingly a favorite indoor sport of an older generation of psychiatrists. Nevertheless, for research to advance, the detection of organic dysfunction and identification of regular differences are required, and the contemporary disinterest in differentiation may be too radical.

ALZHEIMER'S DISEASE Clinically, one can distinguish four stages in this disorder. Onset is in the fourth or fifth decade of life; Armando Ferraro thinks that earlier, so-called juvenile forms, do not constitute true Alzheimer's disease.[15] The *first stage* is not essentially different from ordinary senile deterioration, although it is usually quite severe and progresses rapidly; memory deficits are quite marked, and patients tend to be agitated. The *second stage* is characterized by aphasias, agnosias, and apraxias; although temporal and parietal syndromes may be recognized, the most frequent disturbance is semantic aphasia with general deterioration. Convulsive seizures are not frequent. During the *third stage*, extrapyramidal signs become important; patients become rigid; tremors accompanied by athetoid and ballistic movements appear. The rigidity may lead to an inability to stand and walk. Such rigidity is by no means pathognomic; it occurs in many diseases of the basal ganglia and also in certain forms of arteriosclerosis.[5] During the *fourth stage*, the patient becomes incontinent, marasmic, and utterly helpless. He develops decubital ulcers and cachexia, which quickly lead to death. Few patients live beyond four or five years from the onset of the illness. R. G. Feldman, K. A. Chandler, and co-workers made a longitudinal study of a family with Alzheimer's disease.[13] In reading the full report of this unusual study, we are impressed with the fact that early symptoms may persist for a period of time and may masquerade as behavior disorders of various types. Examining relatives who were not yet symptomatic but "suspect," Feldman *et al.*, found early signs that did not consist solely of affective and memory changes; they observed mild paraphasia, denial, and various neurotic and sociopathic behavior patterns, which were viewed as attempts to cope with the effects of early subliminal changes. Abnormal EEG response to hyperventilation was seen in the "suspect" group.

PICK'S DISEASE Notwithstanding a number of published reports and textbook statements to the contrary, the authors believe that the clinical course of the disease, especially by the time the patient arrives for a diagnosis, is quite similar to that of Alzheimer's disease and rarely can be differentiated in the living patient. It also begins in the fourth or fifth decade of life; females are more frequently afflicted than men. There is good evidence that it is transmitted by an autosomal dominant gene.[34] The four stages are very similar to those of Alzheimer's; as frontal lobes are involved quite frequently, changes of incentive and of ethical behavior are more prominent. Patients become careless, sloppy, and dirty, or tactless and crude, and they may commit acts that are not compatible with previous moral values. Extrapyramidal symptoms may be less marked than in Alzheimer's illness; the terminal stages are identical.

Thus diagnoses of both Alzheimer's and Pick's diseases are based on: (1) occurrence of rapidly progressing intractable deterioration of intellect and personality, usually before senium; (2) aphasia, agnosia, and apraxia; and (3) extrapyramidal and basal ganglia symptoms. Essentially, diagnosis of these diseases is made by exclusion; other organic reactions, such as brain tumors, syphilis of the central nervous system, postencephalitic reactions, and a number of degenerative diseases, must be ruled out. The EEG findings are quite unspecific. Diffuse or regional cortical atrophy and dilation of the ventricular system may be demonstrated by air encephalography. The pathological anatomical findings of Alzheimer's and Pick's diseases will be discussed in the section on etiology.

Behavior Disorders with Arteriosclerotic Brain Disease

Cerebral arteriosclerosis and cerebral senile changes may occur separately or as mixed forms. To attribute a given behavior disorder in old age to vascular or parenchymatous change is often difficult; yet the differential diagnosis may be important because vascular impairment is amenable to therapy. Arteriosclerotic brain disease is not always accompanied by general arteriosclerosis; cerebral arteriosclerosis is frequently associated with hypertension, and it may be preferable to speak of vascular brain disease.

As many persons over sixty years of age have a certain degree of general and cerebral arteriosclerosis, the clinical diagnosis of cerebral arteriosclerosis or vascular brain disease is justified only if the changes are quite clear and massive. The diagnosis should be based on demonstrable evidence of pathology of the cerebral vessels, such as cerebral accidents and vascular retinopathy; it should not be based simply on peripheral arteriosclerosis and hypertension. We must be reasonably sure that the so-called general psychiatric symptoms—irritability, mild depression and apathy—are caused by vascular brain disease. Deterioration is usually slight. There is a certain insight into these changes and there are subjective complaints of failure of memory; objective tests often do not reveal deficit. Headaches and dizziness are frequent symptoms. All these symptoms are of an intermittent character, as one would expect in a vascular disease. The diagnosis is quite unspecific and can be made only if other organic causes for cerebral deficit are excluded. E. Eduardo Krapf felt that hypertension produced characteristic psychiatric syndromes such as transient twilight states.[23] N. S. Apter, Ward C. Halstead, and R. F. Heimburger describe, in mild hypertensive brain disease, a syndrome of repressed hostility; dependency; reduction of the need for perfection; mild judgmental defects; insomnia; loss of energy; and anxiety.[2] Severe cases of hypertensive encephalopathy with renal insufficiency present a more definite syndrome, usually with organic deficit and delirious and confused episodes. Persistent high systolic and diastolic blood pressure, renal impairment, and severe retinopathy are ominous signs. Cerebral hemorrhage, embolism, and thrombosis are the concern of the neurologist; even postictal confusions are rarely treated by the psychiatrist alone. However, he should have some knowledge of the differential diagnosis of hemorrhage, embolism, and thrombosis, the course of these diseases, and the most important specific syndromes of vascular occlusion.

The following case illustrates a typical depression associated with arteriosclerotic brain disease in a patient who improved in the hospital but relapsed after he was exposed again to the stresses of family life.

A seventy-five-year-old civil engineer was admitted to the hospital because, after being seriously depressed for about two months, he had tried to harm himself by banging his head and also had made a more serious attempt by self-strangulation. The depression began when his son left to seek employment in another state. Shortly after this, the patient took a job as janitor of a local school, although he had not worked for nine years previously. It was not clear why he decided to work again, but the family did not fully accept his explanation that he was bored and tired of inactivity. It soon became obvious that he was not up to this job, even when he was assisted in some of his chores by relatives. It was difficult for him to understand instructions; when he felt exasperated by them he retched, was anorectic, and said he felt ill. He constantly demanded attention and exasperated his family, first by threats of suicide and later by swallowing his wrist watch, rubber tubing, neckties, clothespins, and toothpaste tubes. He asked his family not to watch but help him to finish his wretched life and injured himself by banging his head. Once he tried to stuff his head in a fishbowl; another time he tried to stick himself with a pin. Escaping surveillance, he was found at the beach with wet hands and wet feet, but also made a dangerous suicidal attempt of strangling himself with a rope. This happened after the older son returned for a visit but stayed with his father for only one hour. The family physician found that the patient had high blood pressure and an irregular heart rate. He made the diagnosis of arteriosclerosis and advised hospitalization.

The patient's father had been a mining engineer who traveled a great deal. Both parents were said to be outgoing, well-adjusted people who died in their eighties. There was no mental illness in the family. The patient left school at fifteen, became a plumber and later a contractor. A skilful craftsman, he had little business sense and was forced into bankruptcy twice. He married a rather sickly girl when he was twenty-two. They had two sons and one daughter, who has frequent spells of sadness. The patient was particularly attached to the older son. After thirty years his wife died, and he remarried, a widow with two children, seemingly quite content with the new family.

Physical examination showed an obese man with artificial upper and lower dentures, marked arcus senilis, relatively normal vision and hearing, and moderate emphysema. The left cardiac border was slightly enlarged to percussion; blood pressure was 140/90. He had marked tortuosity of the retinal and peripheral arteries, varicose veins, and a small hydrocele. The ECG showed auricular fibrillation and left shift of the axis. Neurological examination and associated laboratory and X-ray findings were not remarkable. The EEG revealed 6/sec. frequency dominant in all leads with occasional 2/sec. waves, a pattern consistent with arteriosclerosis.

During most of the stay on the ward, the patient was tense, anxious, and depressed. The impression was of dullness, although on clinical testing there was relatively little deterioration. He was oriented but had no insight into his depressive mood or his continued histrionic and dangerous attempts at self-injury. On one occasion he burned himself quite severely by pressing his foot against a radiator.

After a week, when the staff had established a friendly contact, this behavior stopped; he began to sleep well and required no daytime medication. He was discharged in the care of his daughter but soon relapsed into his old behavior pattern and was committed to another institution for continuous care.

Multifactorial Etiology

Until the fifties, the problem of the etiology of behavior disorders of old age was considered to be quite simple: a few relatively well-defined entities, all with profound deterioration, all caused by definite neuropathological changes. It is now known that the clinical entities are by no means clearly defined, but show infinite shadings; we also know that clinical and neuropathological findings are not well correlated.[32] We now must assume that both organic and psychosocial factors determine senile behavior; neuropathological changes alone cannot be considered as essential in the pathogenesis of senile behavior. Parenchymatous and vascular brain disease in old age without a behavior disorder and senile behavior without marked brain disease can be observed. Thus, "pathways" to senile behavior disorders, as with other behavior disorders, require careful assessment to determine their relative weight in any individual case.

NEUROPATHOLOGICAL FINDINGS What constitutes the essence of aging of the central nervous system is unknown. In their exemplary monograph on human aging, James E. Birren, Robert N. Butler *et al.* mention the reduction of cerebral blood flow, decrease of oxygenation, and a change in the utilization of glucose by neural tissue as important biological factors that produce cortical damage and behavioral impairment.[39] In the absence of neuronal changes and vascular disease, which leads to cerebral vascular insufficiency and hypoxia, EEG changes are minimal; a slight trend to a shift to lower frequencies of the alpha range (8–14 C.P.S.) is noted. We know more about senile brain changes than about changes characteristic for normal aging. When atrophy is present, it is usually general; the total weight of the brain is reduced. Sulci are wide, gyri narrow; the ventricles are enlarged. Dura and leptomeninges are thickened; chronic subdural hematoma is frequently seen, particularly in neglected patients. There is a definite reduction in the number of cells, particularly in the third cortical layer. Cells may show the neurofibrillary changes described by Alzheimer, as well as senile plaques consisting of small areas of degenerated tissue with debris from necrotic cells, hyaline, and amyloid substances, and proliferated glia. In most senile brains, varying degrees of arteriosclerotic changes are present.

Neuropathological changes in *Alzheimer's disease* are essentially the same as in senile brains, but more severe. The atrophy is more marked and involves mostly the parietal, temporal, and occipital lobes without any definite demarcation. Neurofibrillary cell changes, which are invariably present in Alzheimer's disease, are, however, not pathognomic. In *Pick's disease,* there is a more circumscribed atrophy, particularly of the frontal lobes. Ferraro stresses the presence of certain swollen ganglion cells and argyrophilic inclusions, which are characteristic but not specific.[14]

In *arteriosclerotic brain disease,* large blood vessels lose their elasticity, appear convoluted, and show knotty projections. The intima contains yellow lipid deposits and areas of hyaline degeneration and calcification. In smaller vessels, the intima shows proliferation and also atherosclerotic changes, which produce occlusions and narrow the lumen and, secondarily, cellular damage. In *hypertensive brain disease,* there is thickening of all three layers of the vessels. In smaller vessels, a differentiation of arteriosclerotic and hypertensive disease is not possible. If occlusion of a vessel occurs, the supplied parenchymatous area degenerates and becomes necrotic. Size of the vessels, speed of occlusion, and presence or absence of hemorrhage determine the neuropathological picture. If small areas are affected, there may be only neuronal degeneration and glial proliferation. This will also occur on the periphery of large lesions; the center of large lesions becomes necrotic and eventually liquefied. Advanced cases may show a great many such areas, with various degrees and stages of degeneration.

GENETIC-CONSTITUTIONAL FACTORS Heredity plays a role in the development of senile disorders, although the extent of its influence is not clear. Senile disorders are more frequent in those families whose antecedents suffered from such disorders. Franz Kallmann found that, in dizygotic twin pairs, 8 per cent of the twins showed concordance in the development of severe senile disorders; in monozygotes the concordance was 43 per cent.[19] In Pick's disease, heredity plays a definite and important role. Heredity seems also to be etiologically significant in vascular brain disease. Certain ethnic groups, for example, East European Jews, are reported to be more afflicted by arteriosclerosis than other groups. The important problem of the role of diet in general, and of lipids in particular, in the etiology of arteriosclerosis is still an open question.

The Precipitating Role of Diseases and Accidents

One of the most important findings in the Syracuse study of senile and arteriosclerotic behavior disorders was the significant role of diseases and accidents as precipitating events.[17] James L. Titchener and his co-workers found that operations, anesthesia, and even hospitalization may precipitate severe behavior disorders in the aged.[35] Diseases and accidents thus must be seen as threats, generating catastrophic anxiety, against which the aged patient cannot defend himself. They also offer a variety of secondary gains to the vulnerable aged person; to a certain extent, this accounts for the frequent hypochondriacal attitudes.

PSYCHOSOCIAL FACTORS These operate for all aged persons, and their impact depends on the adaptive use the patient can make of his prior patterns and the presence of cerebral changes, of the "reserve" he can muster to cope with deficits, as well as the factor of enhanced vulnerability to stress.[33] Not only diseases and injuries but any kind of threat may precipitate a delirious state, agitation, or deep apathy. A new environment or situation the senile aged person is unable to master can be especially threatening. With his intellectual deficit and impairment, the patient has obvious difficulties in solving problems; quite naturally, he tends to withdraw to a fixed routine that avoids such challenges and stresses, in which case retirement may be helpful. For the normal aged, social patterns such as retirement at a fixed age may specifically evoke problems. Some of the problems that confront the retired normal person are focused on loss of status, which undercuts self-esteem and prepares the ground for depression and apathy. Psychological and real losses of persons, ideals, and worldly goods may increase the depression and produce anxiety and anger in the lonely and frustrated old person.[3] Loss of autonomy, especially in control over funds, is particularly important. We have known older persons, promised lifelong care by their children, who are nonetheless aggravatingly conservative with their money; their children forget that, at seventy-five, their parent may see himself with fifteen or twenty, as well as with but a few years, ahead. The prospect of helplessness is terrifying for many, and the indignity of having nothing of one's own independently to manage and dispose may lead to regressed behavior. Persons with high anxiety, unsatisfactory relationships, and previous incapacity to solve problems of living are more likely to develop behavior disorders than are stable and effective persons with good relationships. In particular, it is the lonely elderly person, the widowed, the unmarried, and the divorced who are vulnerable to the stresses of old age. E. W. Busse and his co-workers found that a high percentage of his severely disturbed seniles were considered poor parents by their children.[6] Some anxiously clinging and dependent persons, however, may adapt well to the personnel in institutions, and old age may offer advantages to some. The lack of economic competition may put the old person under less stress if he is not threatened by lack of subsistence. Some older persons can achieve a perspective that reduces neurotic guilt; diminished sex drive may play a role here. Regression to pregenital activity, if present, may or may not produce severe conflict, and generally there may be some "atrophy of the superego," which helps to alleviate certain conflicts. Some cultures, notably in the Far East, are more permissive than ours and provide opportunities for play, recreation, and regression to infantile pleasures for old persons. The Western world, however, does not exhibit such accepting attitudes; this difference may explain the reports of a lower frequency of senile disorders in the cultures of the Far East and in many primitive societies.

Diagnosis

To make a diagnosis that is not just a storage label but a concise summary of findings that points to appropriate therapeutic action, the following questions should be answered: (1) Is the patient intellectually deteriorated? To what extent? Clinical examination and psychological tests will help to answer these questions. (2) What is the type of the disorder and how severe is it? Is the patient depressed or agitated? Paranoid? Confused and delirious? Is his behavior essentially a continuation, exaggeration, or rearrangement of lifelong neurotic or sociopathic traits? A thorough history and examination will furnish the necessary data and will also establish the patient's role in his family and community. (3) Is the patient's behavioral difficulty complicated or caused by organic illness or injuries? Does he suffer from vascular brain disease, which can be treated? Are there sensory and perceptual impairments (often amenable to repair and/or rehabilitation)? This will determine whether other medical specialists can help. (4) To what extent is the patient's abnormal behavior a response to interpersonal difficulties in his family, occupation, or community? Most of the milder and more transitory maladjustments of the aged can be explained on this basis. (5) How does the patient's suffering affect other persons in his family or natural environment? To what degree does he depend on social and medical care? To what degree can persons in his environment be realistically expected to cope with his difficulties? Is the patient dangerous to himself? To others? Fortunately, aggressive and sexual crimes by senile persons are rare, but considerable harm may come from their defective judgment; hostile impulses of which the patient may be utterly unaware, of course, may play a role when senile persons set fires, drop babies, cause traffic accidents, or injure themselves. A consideration of the points listed above leads to a more practical and pragmatic diagnostic view than does overconcern with rare and refined diagnoses, which can hardly be proven, even by histopathological findings.

Course and Prognosis

Although the probability of senile cerebral changes and of some limitation in behavior increases with age, the degree of these neuropathological changes and their correlations with behavior disorders are extremely variable. In very severe cases, the patient may not live longer than two years. Roth found that the chances of survival are lowest in senile and presenile deterioration; next are the patients with cerebral arteriosclerosis.[31] Patients with depressions have a good prognosis for life and recovery; paranoid patients do not recover but live on. In considering the course of a senile disorder, one must recall that it is incorrect to assume that senile cerebral changes produce permanent changes in behavior. Just as in vascular brain disease, disorders may be very transient and seem, generally speaking, to depend more on behavioral and environmental, than on neuropathological, processes. Extensive and massive brain damage, of course, will produce permanent defects.

Therapy and Rehabilitation

There are few psychiatric problems where the old saw, "Cure few, relieve many, and comfort all," is more true than in senile disorders. A mere decrease in suffering is a realistic goal, but a great many old patients with behavior disorders can be rehabilitated and helped to live a reasonably happy and even productive life.

WHO SHOULD TREAT THE AGED PATIENTS? Perhaps one should ask: who wants to treat the aged patient with behavior disorders? Most psychiatrists have found little gratification in treating or taking care of the aged—undoubtedly a result of their training—but the situation is changing, and we have begun to realize that aged and senile patients can, in fact, be treated. The consensus seems to be, however, that priority for treatment should be with the disorders of younger age groups and that senile patients can be helped very effectively by general practitioners, psychiatrically trained community nurses and social workers. Certain specific problems, as re-education of aphasic patients, require very specific skills and enormous amounts of time and are entirely in the hands of specially trained speech therapists. In any case, there is an increasingly strong feeling in the psychiatric profession that psychiatrists can and must play a stronger and more vigorous role in the treatment of the aged mentally ill.

WHERE TO TREAT? Hospitalization of the aged patient is invariably a stressful event. It is also well known that the rate of hospitalization of "older" age patients has increased, that they are often sent to mental hospitals where they may not belong, and that there is an appalling shortage of adequate facilities for aged psychiatric patients. Nonadmission to a hospital may be even more stressful for the aged patient and his family than admission. However, we have become more conscious of the fact that intrafamilial adjustments are often possible and may prevent hospitalization. We also know that, when an aged patient enters a hospital, he often leaves the community forever. In Connecticut, and in other states, many patients over the years have been committed to state mental hospitals because there was nowhere else they could go. When, in 1950, Governor Chester Bowles asked that these patients be transferred to nursing homes and general hospitals, the hospitals and homes refused to admit them because they had once been committed to mental hospitals and were thus "insane." Today, many senile patients are cared for in nursing homes. The great majority of these nursing homes, in the United States, are privately owned and run for profit, and they very often provide something less than ideal care and treatment. The concept of an entirely new institution, day centers in the community, is being developed. In these senior citizen centers which are in live contact with the community, old persons, including many mildly disturbed persons, may find proper recreation, social contact, and a new content for life.

PSYCHOTHERAPY Psychotherapy may help the aged mental patient a great deal, but the shortage of psychiatric manpower limits its use. Alvin Goldfarb gives an eloquent description of goals and techniques in his particular approach to the psychotherapy of the elderly patient.[16] Obviously, there is less emphasis on insight and the kind of self-realization dynamic psychiatrists try to achieve with younger patients. The aims, rather, are a decrease of anxiety and hostility and an increase of security, comfort and, particularly, self-esteem. This is achieved primarily by establishing an accepting and trusting relationship. Elderly patients are quite likely to enter such a relationship because of their need to affiliate. Abram Kardiner pointed to the reversal of the child–parent relationship in the old.[21] If this shift is made possible by reducing its inherent threats, therapists may be able to help aged patients greatly. The psychotherapeutic contacts may be short but frequent and continuing, if necessary, indefinitely. Some vigorous old people seek and achieve insight with special problems and respond to the shortness of life with high motivation to live well. Very few analysts have attempted to work with aged and terminal patients, although the work of Kurt Eissler[11] and of A. D. Weisman and T. P. Hackett with dying patients has been both therapeutically rewarding and theoretically provocative. Not to withdraw from the dying patient is of the utmost importance. In psychotherapy with aged persons, there are special problems of countertransference: the general dread of illness and death and the therapist's attitudes to a dependent and failing parental figure. This countertransference may lead to unrealistic attitudes such as hostility, undue resignation, and withdrawal or overoptimistic denial.

REHABILITATION The importance of working with the families of these patients has been stressed by many. Without good understanding of the family constellation, little can be done for most patients. Of course, a large proportion of aged mental patients has no families; this lonely group poses some of the most difficult therapeutic problems. To be gainfully employed is often of central importance for the elderly person, but modern competitive societies have made this difficult save in rare instances. Rehabilitation by trained occupational counselors has shown that occupational involvement of aged persons, even with considerable physical and psychological handicaps, is often possible and therapeutically valuable. If the old person's abilities are not overtaxed, this kind of intervention may effectively complement individual and group psychotherapy.

ORGANIC THERAPIES All aged patients require general medical care, including careful attention to proper nutrition, which old people are apt to neglect. There are no specific organic therapies for senile and presenile diseases. In arteriosclerotic patients, the rather intricate somatic therapy depends on the nature of the vascular pathology; usually, such therapy is the concern of internists and neurologists. In the senile behavior disorders, there are certain organic treatments psychiatrists may judiciously use. In seriously depressed patients, electric convulsive therapy may be the treatment of choice, but the use of the method is limited in view of the complications of fractures and temporary deterioration in the aged patient. Rather fewer than more shocks should be given, since muscular relaxants in convulsive therapy, even in the hands of an experienced anesthesiologist, are not without danger in the aged patient. In our experience, electric shock treatment is not effective in rapidly deteriorating patients. In agitated senile patients, tranquilizing drugs (the phenothiazines, chlordiazepoxide, and meprobamate) have been used widely but with moderate success.[30] Dependency on drugs and particularly on narcotics often is used as a hostile and dependent link to the physician; this must be monitored, and dosages that unduly relax and confuse the patient should be avoided, since they may reinforce fears of failing with age. The senile patient is apt to suffer more from idiosyncratic reactions and from side-effects such as hypotension and episodes of delirium than younger patients, and, in general, drug application in senile patients requires special caution. The antidepressants like imipramine have been of value in depressed patients.[7]

The problem of caring for an ever-increasing number of aged persons has intensified interest in preventive measures. As Paul V. Lemkau put it, the functional atrophy of the personality should be reduced to a minimum.[25] Clearly this will require gerontological research as well as major social and legislative measures designed to protect elderly people from the threats of poverty and crippling illness, enabling them to live with some gratification. Lawrence S. Kubie expressed the imaginative idea that someday medical science will help man to live forever.[24] We find the prospect of fulfilling this age-old dream somewhat appalling! But undoubtedly psychiatrists can help the aged patient to live better and to die with a minimum of misery.

NOTES

1. Alois Alzheimer, "Über eine eigenartige Erkrankung der Hirnrnide," *Allg. Z. Psychiat.*, 64 (1907), 146.
2. Nathan S. Apter, Ward C. Halstead, and R. F. Heimburger, "Impaired Cerebral Functions in Essential Hypertension," *American Journal of Psychiatry*, 107 (1951), 808.
3. James E. Birren, Robert N. Butler, S. Greenhouse, L. Sokoloff, and M. Yarrow, eds., *Human Aging, A Biological and Behavioral Study* (Bethesda, Md.: U. S. Public Health Service Publications, 1963), No. 986.
4. Jack Botwinick and James E. Birren, "Mental Abilities and Psychomotor Responses in Healthy Aged Men," in James E. Birren and Robert N. Butler, eds., *Human Aging, a Biological and Behavioral Study* (Bethesda, Md.: U. S. Public Health Service Publications, 1963), No. 986.
5. Walter L. Bruetsch and C. L. Williams, "Arteriosclerotic Muscular Rigidity with Special Reference to Gait Disturbances," *American Journal of Psychiatry*, 111 (1954), 332.
6. Ewald W. Busse, R. H. Barnes, A. J. Silverman, M. Thaler, and L. L. Frost, "Studies of the Processes of Aging X. The Strengths and Weaknesses of Psychic Functioning in the Aged," *American Journal of Psychiatry*, 111 (1955), 896.
7. D. Ewen Cameron, "The Use of Tofranil in the Aged," *Canadian Psychiatric Association Journal*, 4 (1959), Special Suppl. S160.
8. Norman Cameron, "Neuroses of Later Maturity" in Oscar J. Kaplan, ed., *Mental Disorders in Later Life* (2nd ed., Stanford: Stanford University Press, 1956).
9. Darab K. Dastur, M. Lane, O. Hansen, S. Kety, R. Butler, Seymour Perlin, and L. Sokoloff "Effects of Aging on Cerebral Circulation and Metabolism in Man," in James E. Birren, Robert N. Butler, S. Greenhouse, L. Sokoloff, and M. Yarrow, eds., *Human Aging, A Biological and Behavioral Study*, (Bethesda, Md.: U. S. Public Health Service Publications, 1963), No. 986.
10. W. Dock, "Arteriosclerosis," in T. R. Harrison, ed., *Principles of Internal Medicine* (New York: McGraw-Hill, 1958).
11. Kurt Eissler, *The Psychiatrist and the Dying Patient* (New York: International Universities Press, 1955).

12. Erik H. Erikson, "Selected Papers," *Identity and the Life Cycle, Psychological Issues*, Vol. I, No. 1, (New York: International Universities Press, 1959).
13. Robert G. Feldman, K. A. Chandler, L. L. Levy, and G. H. Glaser, "Familial Alzheimer's Disease," *Neurology*, 13 (1963), 811.
14. Armando Ferraro, "Senile Psychoses"; "Presenile Psychoses"; "Psychoses with Cerebral Arteriosclerosis," in Silvano Arieti, ed., *American Handbook of Psychiatry* (New York: Basic Books, 1959), Vol. II, pp. 1021, 1046, 1078.
15. Armando Ferraro, R. Hernandes, and G. A. Jervis, "Alzheimer's Disease," *Psychiatric Quarterly*, 15 (1941), 3.
16. Alvin Goldfarb, "Minor Maladjustments in the Aged," in Silvano Arieti, ed., *American Handbook of Psychiatry* (New York: Basic Books, 1959), Vol. I, p. 378.
17. Ernest M. Gruenberg and J. H. Cummings, "A Mental Health Survey of Older People," *Psychiatric Quarterly Supplement* (1959).
18. August B. Hollingshead and Fredrick C. Redlich, *Social Class and Mental Illness* (New York: John Wiley, 1958).
19. Franz Kallmann, *Heredity in Health and Mental Disorder; Principles of Psychiatric Genetics in the Light of Comparative Twin Studies* (New York: Norton, 1953).
20. Oscar J. Kaplan, ed., *Mental Disorders in Later Life* (Stanford: Stanford University Press, 1956).
21. Abram Kardiner, "Psychological Factors in Old Age," in *Mental Hygiene in Old Age* (New York: Family Service Association of America, 1937).
22. Emil Kraepelin, *Clinical Psychiatry; A Textbook for Students and Physicians*. Abstracted and Adapted by A. Ross Diefendorf from the 7th German edition of *Lehrbuch der Psychiatrie* (New York: Macmillan, 1923).
23. E. Eduardo Krapf, Über zerebrale Störungen bei Hypertonikern," *Verh. dtsch. Ges. Kreisl-Forsch*, 5 (1932), 131.
24. Lawrence S. Kubie, "A Fortieth Reunion in 2156, a Salute from Harvard 1916," *Harvard Alumni Bulletin* (Sept. 29, 1956).
25. Paul V. Lemkau, "The Mental Hygiene of Aging," *Public Health Reports*, 167 (1952), 237.
26. William Malamud, "Presidential Address," *Mental Hospitals*, 11 (1960), 5.
27. Benjamin Malzberg, "The Expectation of Psychoses with Cerebral Arteriosclerosis in New York State, 1920, 1930, 1940," *Psychiatric Quarterly*, 19 (1945), 122.
28. Seymour Perlin and R. N. Butler, "Psychiatric Aspects of Adaptation to the Aging Experience," in James E. Birren and Robert N. Butler, eds., *Human Aging, a Biological and Behavioral Study* (Bethesda, Md.: U. S. Public Health Service Publications, 1963), No. 986.
29. Arnold Pick, *Zur Symptomatologie des atrophischen Hinterhauptlappens* (Berlin: Karger, 1908).
30. Benjamin Pollack, "The Addition of Chlorpromazine to the Treatment Pro-

gram for Emotional and Behavior Disorders in the Aging," *Geriatrics*, 11 (1956), 253.

31. Martin Roth, "The Natural History of Mental Disorder in Old Age," *Journal of Mental Science*, 101 (1955), 281.
32. David Rothschild, "Pathologic Changes in Senile Psychoses and Their Psychobiologic Significance," *American Journal of Psychiatry*, 93 (1937), 757.
33. David Rothschild, "Senile Psychoses and Psychoses with Cerebral Arteriosclerosis," in O. J. Kaplan, ed., *Mental Disease in Later Life* (Stanford: Stanford University Press, 1956).
34. Tomsten Sjögren, H. Sjögren, and A. G. H. Lindgren, "Morbus Alzheimer and Morbus Pick," *Acta Psychiatric Scandinavia*, 82 (1952), Supplement.
35. James L. Titchener, Israel Zwerling, Louis Gottschalk, and Maurice Levine, "Psychological Reactions of the Aged to Surgery," *Archives of Neurology and Psychiatry*, 79 (1958), 63.
36. Avery D. Weisman and T. P. Hackett, "Predilection to Death: Death and Dying as a Psychiatric Problem," *Psychosomatic Medicine*, 23 (1961), 232.
37. World Health Organization, Expert Committee on Mental Health, *Mental Health Problems of Aging and the Aged* (Geneva: World Health Organization Technical Report Series, 1959), No. 171.

CHAPTER TWENTY-TWO

The Drug Addictions

◆ The Expert Committee of the United Nations speaks of drug addiction as a state of periodic or chronic intoxication, detrimental to the individual and to society, produced by the repeated consumption of a natural or synthetic drug.[38] V. H. Vogel, H. Isbell, and K. W. Chapman define addiction as a state in which a person has lost the power of self-control with reference to a drug and abuses the drug to such an extent that he or society is harmed.[33] A. Wikler put it this way: "Drug addiction exists when the behavior of an individual is determined to a considerable extent by the use of chemical agents which are harmful to himself, society or both."[36] The term "addiction" is commonly applied to many of life's habits, which cannot be considered addictions in terms of such definitions as these; it is loosely used, for example, when one speaks of an addiction to food (most obese people are "food addicts") and to work. Excessive smoking, according to current medical knowledge a more dangerous habit than excessive drinking, is not a true addiction. Since abuse of alcohol is the subject of a separate chapter, this chapter deals only with addictions to the opiates, stimulants, and the barbiturates.

In order fully to understand what follows, several terms pertaining to addiction should be made clear. *Physical dependence* refers to physiological changes after prolonged drug use, which are, so far, not sufficiently grasped. Although this dependence is thought (more by empathy than proof) to "create" a motive for "repetition of the drug," it is more precisely understood by observations of the withdrawal effects. If certain drugs that produce physical dependence are suddenly withdrawn, the *abstinence syndrome* develops. *Tolerance*, a characteristic that is also not well understood, refers to the need for increased doses of certain drugs in order to produce the effect originally achieved by smaller doses. Tolerance is operationally defined as a decrement of effect contingent upon dosage schedule. *Habituation*, or *psychological dependence*, refers to the craving for the drug and to the individual's drug-seeking behavior. Although avoidance of abstinence (or seeking partial abstinence to justify further drug use) and the cycle of increasing dosage represented by physiological dependence and tolerance are important, they cannot account for addiction, since many tolerant or dependent individuals can stop taking the drug when there is no longer medical reason for administration. Further, and more than is generally appreciated, many users will carefully restrict drug intake for fear of the consequences of tolerance. Thus, psychiatrists are most concerned with psychological dependence and are inclined to consider it the essential feature of addiction. It is also important to keep in mind that *excessive use of drugs* is not synonymous with addiction.

The Modern Addiction Problem

Addiction-producing drugs have been used since the dawn of history. The gods of old Indian scriptures drank soma; the Greek gods, ambrosia. The Aztecs ate peyote and the Incas, cola. The intoxicating effect of opium and derivatives of the hemp plant were known in the ancient world. A worldwide drug problem in the modern sense, however, did not exist before the chemical extraction of active alkaloids and the industrial revolution, which permitted large-scale production and merchandising of addictive drugs and also created a more avid consumer. Norman E. Zinberg and David C. Lewis, reviewing the history of narcotic usage in the United States,[39] note that the invention of the hypodermic needle in 1843 facilitated the widespread "soldier's illness" (narcotic addiction) of the Civil War, but the meaning and mechanism of addiction was not recognized until the turn of the century; indeed, heroin (and Demerol, fifty years later) was thought to be a cure for morphine addiction. Habituation, tolerance, and dependence were not identified and distinguished until the turn of the century; and the Harrison Narcotic Act of 1914 focused on policing and taxing rather than on treatment measures. Public clinics were established after World War I, but poor planning, excessive dosages, and relapses led to sensationalism and violent attack in the public press, and court rulings and American Medical Association opinion, for a time, put a halt both to individual and dispensary treatment of the addict. The therapist, today, though less restricted, is usually still dependent on hospital care of his addicted patient. The federal hospitals at Lexington and Fort Worth, pioneering in research and treatment, nevertheless are aware of readdictions of up to 90 per cent of patients. The 1962 White House Conference noted the failure of restrictive legislation to control individual addiction and the dismal results of compulsory confinement in federal hospitals. This has led to renewed interest in clinic treatment which is supervised and controlled in the community.

Incidence and Prevalence

There are no reliable figures on the incidence and prevalence of drug addiction. The United States Bureau of Narcotics reports that there are 50,000 adult addicts and 10,000 juvenile addicts in the United States, but many experts consider these estimates far too low. Sampling studies of juvenile street-corner gangs suggest much higher rates. Whether addiction in the United States is increasing or decreasing is uncertain. Very little is known about incidence and prevalence in other countries. For the United Kingdom, Marie Nyswander quotes from British reports the absurd figure of 400.[29] In some Asiatic countries there is, according to general impression, a large number of addicts. However, it is also felt that these addictions are not so serious as Western addictions; intake is perhaps better controlled by the Oriental addict in an environment with a more benign response to the habit. Attitudes toward addiction, particularly in the United States, are severe, moralistic, and punitive. In the United States, before the Harrison Drug Act was passed in 1914, female addicts outnumbered men. Women consumed tonics and vegetable nostrums that contained opiates. The teen-age addict and the use of opiates by the urban poor and disadvantaged are relatively modern phenomena. At present, there are four times as many male addicts as women. Addiction occurs for the most part in metropolitan areas. Published statistical data have derived largely from studies of addicts of the lower classes who came to the attention of police and health agencies. In the United States, there has been a steady increase in the number of Negro addicts. In the health professions, the number of addicts is high; it is estimated that in Germany (and probably elsewhere) one per cent of physicians are addicts.[9]

General Remarks about the Nature and Causes of Addiction

Western literature has stressed the pathological and dismal aspects of the effects of prolonged intake of addiction-producing drugs, exaggerating the evil consequences and minimizing beneficial effects, such as relief of pain and insomnia and decrease of anxiety and tension. For some persons, existence without the beneficial effects of these drugs would be very difficult or impossible. Of course, the effects of such drugs are not lasting. In either extensive or nondiscriminate use, drugs encroach on those motivations and means by which skill in coping with nondrug reality is maintained; difficulties may be compounded because of tolerance. The practical rather than moral issue is, then, the difficulty many (but not all) users have in controlling their intake of such drugs and integrating their use into a satisfactory life pattern. The negative effects, such as increased suffering in hangover and abstinence, the inducement to an unrealistic orientation, and the deleterious effects on the organism when tolerance increases, are strong reasons to consider these drugs as dangerous, if not deadly, weapons, which are apt to produce more harm than good. The harm, however, is greatly increased through unreasonable and punitive social attitudes and legal sanctions.

In discussing drug effects, one must focus on three parameters and correlate such data: the drug, the patient, and the sociocultural context in which the drug is given and taken. Through advances in cell chemistry, behavioral pharmacology, and physiology our chances of gaining fundamental knowledge about the mechanisms and the effects of addictive properties of drugs have greatly increased. As yet, however, no biological explanation of physical dependence and tolerance exists.

The Personalities of Addicts

Sigmund Freud mentioned intoxication, together with ecstasy, neurosis, psychosis, and humor, as major mechanisms of coping with internal and external dangers and stresses[12] and alluded to the similarities between neurosis and addiction. The relief from tension, the avoidance of reality and the regression induced by drugs and, most critically, the temptation (or compulsion) to repeat these experiences in the presence of conflict and the substitution of drug for alternative action—all this constitutes in essence much of what a neurotic symptom achieves. Sandor Rado stressed that drugs, self-administered magical substances, dispel reality and its pain and enable patients to indulge in megalomanic narcissism.[31] Edward Glover emphasized the poor interpersonal relationships of addicts; objects, that is, drugs, and not persons, supply gratification.[15] Erich Lindemann and L. D. Clarke stress the role the addictive drugs play in providing a compensatory ego integration.[24] Alfred Gross and other psychoanalysts stressed the tendency of drugs to produce regression and facilitate a return to primary processes.[61] Robert P. Knight held that addicts as infants are conditioned to expect relief from discomfort by taking something into their mouths; if comfort is not obtained, they react with chronic disappointment and rage.[21] He also pointed to the low self-esteem addicts have in connection with their inferiority feelings and passive needs. Based on his work with alcoholics, John W. Higgins found the orality thesis of addiction too restrictive and suggests that many apparent uniformities in personality are secondary; addicts defend, not just against unacceptable oral needs, but also against other instinctual needs.[18] He stressed the defensive as well as the gratifying function of the drugs. Thus, a picture emerges of addicts as generally impulsive personalities who have remained infantile or have regressed to infantile patterns of living. They are unable to bear pain, tension, anxiety, guilt and grief; they are easily frustrated and discouraged and are unable to delay gratification of their needs. They do not attempt to solve problems by facing them squarely or by seeking to change reality when this is possible. Drugs, it would seem, provide them with a temporary means of avoiding internal stress.

It is questionable, then, whether one can speak meaningfully of an addictive personality beyond the tautological statement that such a person, for one or another reason, has the compulsion to take drugs. At present, we are inclined to believe that addicts are a heterogeneous lot. The clinical impression is that there are some differences among addicts in terms of the drugs to which they are addicted. This is not difficult to understand because there appear to be definite, though not easily defined, differences in the needs that are gratified with the help of specific drugs.[6] Morphinists seem for the most part to want to obtain peace, freedom from tension and anxiety; cocaine and marihuana users attempt to lower inhibitions; and amphetamine addicts wish to reduce their drives. Such general statements, of course, should not be swallowed whole; they must be variously qualified, for example, by the observation that many addicts take more than one drug, and most addicts take what is available. Although the method by which a drug is incorporated does not serve to differentiate groups of addicts, the rituals of smoking, swallowing, or injecting cannot be without psychological meaning. It is easy to make glib interpretations of the meanings of these methods, but the fact is we know little about them.

It is our feeling that investigators exploring personalities of drug addicts have not differentiated sufficiently between the personalities of addicts before and after they became users. Most descriptions of personality types of addicts are based on syndromes encountered after addiction is well established. The clinical syndromes vary greatly, depending on whether one observes a population under ambulatory therapy or in a hospital or prison. The percentage of antisocial personalities in penal institutions obviously is much greater than in a sample of unapprehended addicts. R. H. Felix examined institutionalized addicts and divided them into conventional diagnostic types; he also warned of the limitations and dangers of this kind of classification.[11] He emphasizes that addicts should not be viewed as creatures apart; certainly this is very important in treating the addict. A small number of addicts, between three and four per cent of the patients, was considered normal or well integrated before addiction; these were patients who suffered from severe pain and used drugs only to relieve the pain. The majority of patients were sociopaths of various types; neurotic addicts were in the minority.[37] Based on experiences with addicts in outpatient settings, there is good reason to believe that "normal" and neurotic addicts are by no means rare. D. L. Gerard and C. Kornetsky found that half of the patients of the hospital in Lexington were incipient schizophrenics but made no claim for a representative sample.[14] Some schizophrenics may take drugs defensively, and some persons may try to avoid psychotic disintegration by taking drugs. There are, however, toxic psychoses produced by cocaine and amphetamine, and there is evidence for more enduring cerebral damage occurring after the chronic abuse of bromides. Some psychotic states are produced by withdrawal, particularly of barbiturates. In general, however, toxic and organic psychoses due to drug abuse are not common.

Zinberg and Lewis proposed a classification of drug addiction (particularly opiate addicts) that is of greater practical value to physicians than the conventional psychiatric classifications.[39] They distinguished five groups, as follows: (1) Pseudo addicts act as if they habitually use drugs; such persons belong to social groups who admire drug usage. (2) Demanding patients request drugs, often on pseudomedical grounds, from their frequently harassed physicians, without really wanting them; essentially, these patients are overinvolved with their emotions and crave attention and support. (3) There are patients who use drugs regularly but do not develop tolerance or withdrawal symptoms. (4) Patients who suffer from severe pain may be convinced they need drugs; they have overt physical symptoms (for example, severe headaches), but pain dominates the picture, and the physician finds relentless demands for increased relief by drugs. (5) The last group consists of true addicts. The above classification represents groups commonly encountered in medical practice rather than in special social situations, such as juvenile gangs. Whether a significant number of true drug addicts is delinquent—and why they become delinquent—are even more involved questions, which will be considered in the following section.

Sociocultural Factors

The family structure and relationships of addicts show no distinctly recognizable patterns. Whether addicts come from broken homes seems less important than the fact that, according to most case studies, fathers of male addicts are weak or irresponsible and the mothers are dominant, seductive, and inconsistent. When the child is later addicted, parents have frequently been known to procure relatively harmless drugs or proffer money for their purchase. Such a general pattern may facilitate the development of a passive, impulsive, deviant male who, under certain sociocultural conditions, may become an addict. In addicts of both sexes, confusion about the sexual role and fixation at an infantile level of sexuality have been stressed as predisposing factors. Why some persons become addicts and why others develop different "solutions" to their problems is, at bottom, still unknown.

The generally disapproving and punitive attitude to addiction in Western society has already been mentioned. Degree of disapproval is related to the kind of drug; Western society is relatively tolerant of alcohol addiction, less so of persons addicted (or habituated) to barbiturates and amphetamines and marihuana, and least tolerant of addicts to cocaine and the morphine group. In some countries of the Far East, opium addiction is no more frowned upon than excessive drinking; however, nowhere is addiction approved. Different attitudes to different drugs, such as relative acceptance of the use of alcohol and, to a lesser degree, of sedatives, and the militant disapproval of the use of certain alkaloids, cannot be rationally accounted for nor explained by the different noxious effects of these drugs. Attitudes differ as a function of ethnicity, religion, and social class, and this accounts for some differences in addictive habits.

In the United States, most morphine and cocaine addicts have been dealt with as criminals. According to Supreme Court rulings, addiction per se is not a crime, but illegal possession of narcotics is. Since the Narcotics Control Act of 1956, punishment in the United States for possession of addictive drugs without licensed prescription is a two-to-five year penitentiary term; for illicit sale, five to ten years; and for selling drugs to a minor, the death sentence may be legally invoked. The attitudes reflected by such statutes, needless to say, are unwarranted and interfere with therapeutic and rehabilitative goals. This, however, is not to say that a stern but realistic approach to the individual addict and to the general problem of addiction is unwarranted.

Isidor Chein[5] and John A. Clausen[6] have pointed to certain social characteristics of drug addicts. Adult opiate addicts, in contrast to cocaine addicts, are lone users; juvenile opiate addicts of the lower classes are usually found to be members of gangs. These addictive gangs have a strong group solidarity, although the individual addict is a rather passive person with weak interpersonal ties. Addictive members are often not delinquent until they develop what Wikler calls purposive abstinence symptoms, or the need to obtain the drug at any cost.[36] In these street-corner societies, the absence of social controls and the lack of identification with strong, masculine, socially integrated figures are usually striking. Although the deep reasons for the genesis of addiction of the total gang or individual user often remain obscure, seduction and initiation by group members seem more important than the influence of peddlers. The magical power of "turning someone on" has a sexual overtone; the fact that sexual experience is less interesting than drug effects indicates the extent to which the drugs involve a regression to pregenital experience.

The fact that in some middle-class addicts (who were not medically initiated) petty crimes, theft and fraud, sexual misbehavior, and prostitution are not infrequent tends to bolster the stereotype of the criminal addict. There is, however, no solid evidence that addiction is linked in a causal way to a disposition to criminal activities. To be sure, there is a relation between crime and addiction, but this is explained in part by the milieu from which most current drug addicts come: the slum. It is not certain whether members of juvenile gangs who take drugs are more inclined to commit criminal acts than those who are not addicts. From the study of gangs, we have learned that social factors breed crime and also addiction, but crime does not always precede addiction, nor does addiction necessarily lead to crime unless specific incentives exist. The most important incentive to crime by addicts is the insatiable need to procure drugs by any means and at any price; this drives the addict to stealing, "hooking," and pimping, and, most of all, to dope-peddling. The complex problem of addiction and criminality still awaits careful study. One psychological factor to be considered is the powerful motive of "hustling"; many addicts seem to value the search for illicit drugs and even prefer this highly absorbing chase to assured medical sources of supply.

In summary, then, statements about the etiology of addiction must be guarded and quite unspecific. Just as descriptions of addicts are vague and general (or, even worse, false stereotypes, such as the lower-class derelict addict), we must remember that the etiology of addiction, beyond all doubt, involves multiple determinants. Constitutional factors, such as certain biochemical deficiencies, have been assumed to exist and will be considered in some detail in connection with alcoholism; so far, however, no solid evidence for such assumptions has been found. It does appear that the confirmed addict responds differently to a number of drugs affecting mood than does the normal subject. The alleged carelessness with which physicians prescribe those drugs is much overstressed. In general, physicians are less apt to be overpermissive or careless in their prescription of drugs than to be caught in the dilemma of when to prescribe and when not. The focus of this troublesome issue is our inability to assess realistically the therapeutic and dangerous consequences of drugs, which is due not only to a lack of empirical and theoretical available knowledge but also to the emotionally charged atmosphere surrounding the prescription of addictive drugs.

Diagnosis

To arrive at a satisfactory diagnostic formulation, we must obtain, in addition to a medical anamnesis and examination and a good psychiatric history, answers to specific questions. How was the addict introduced to drugs? What does he take and how much? It should be remembered that many addicts take more than one drug and give false information about dosage lest their supply be cut off. What reinforced the habit? Wikler has shown, clinically and experimentally, that such reinforcement is of great significance.[35] What needs do the drugs gratify? What is the patient's basic personality? Did definite personality changes occur following the onset of addiction? Is there any evidence of intellectual deterioration, psychosis, or asocial behavior? Finally, it is important to assess the patient's motivation for treatment, on which the chances for therapeutic success largely depend. No evaluation of addiction is possible without appreciation of the reinforcing power of the sociocultural setting. What is there in the social setting that promotes or inhibits addiction in this patient? Are the sanctions against the sale and consumption of drugs reasonable or adequate, or do they promote further social disorganization and crime? The weekend consumer of marihuana, the lone morphinist, the youthful heroin addict in a street-corner gang, and the addicted dope peddler with many convictions in court can be properly diagnosed only if the social milieu in which the addiction developed is carefully considered. Knowledge of the psychosocial forces shaping addiction is of central importance in designing proper steps for prevention, treatment, and rehabilitation.

General Principles of Treatment and Prevention

The following broad statements about the treatment and prevention of addiction apply to all forms of addiction; specific treatment problems are taken up in the sections dealing with individual drugs. Treatment of addiction presents us with some of the most difficult and complex problems of psychiatric therapy. To keep an addict only temporarily off drugs and help him assume his social and occupational responsibilities is of itself an achievement. We distinguish between (1) treatment of the basic personality of the addict; (2) treatment of the addiction proper; and (3) treatment of the consequences of addiction, such as physical illnesses, psychoses, and various forms of asocial and antisocial behavior.

It is difficult to treat any patient who is required to give up pleasure. The essence of addiction lies in the irresistible and insatiable need for gratification and the low tolerance of pain, frustration, tension, and anxiety. And there is an additional difficulty: addicts seek not only pleasure but also punishment—or the security, attention, authoritative structure, and contrition entailed in punishment. Through evoking and experiencing punishment, deeper conflicts and aggressions may be expressed and atoned for; such conflicts are also contained and limited by an external authority willing to exercise the responsibility the patient avoids. Society and its experts are only too ready to punish the addict overtly and covertly.

Expert therapists of addicts know that motivation for treatment is all-important. Results of treatment of patients in most penal institutions, where therapy is mandatory, are dismally poor even though many of these patients are first offenders and hence not necessarily irrevocably confirmed addicts. Patients who want treatment and are not sentenced to it fare much better. A very important task for the therapist is to reinforce the patient's motivation for treatment, but in a system that threatens incarceration and that is experienced by patients as hostile and humiliating, such motivation rarely can be maintained. Sustained motivation and acceptance of responsibility for his part in the work is not easy for the addict. The therapist should appreciate the ease with which drug addicts exploit a supportive agency, in part testing the trustworthiness of the therapist; addicts are easily discouraged by failures and setbacks, guiltily avoiding available help. To an extent difficult to believe, the world of the addict can revolve around securing his supply of drug, and his capacity to disguise this interest can easily mislead the therapist focusing on "proper" therapeutic topics rather than the realities of the patient's life. There is some promise in the approach of *Synanon,* a new "self-help group" modeled to some extent on Alcoholics Anonymous, to which the addict may turn.

All experts agree that psychotherapy of an addict is extremely difficult, usually taxing to the limit the devotion and skill of a therapist. The inevitable relapses of the patient are provocative and discouraging. To treat addicts requires almost inexhaustible patience and devotion on the part of the therapist, who must steer a very narrow course between a sympathetic, tolerant understanding and a realistic sternness with the ability to set limits. Usually, failures are explained by the patient's inability to relate and by his extreme dependence. A lack of "ego strength" usually excludes the use of classical analysis, although a few patients have been treated successfully by this method.

The general dictum, to treat addicts in institutions, is questionable. Only certain addicts with physical dependence during withdrawal need to be treated in institutions. Withdrawal, however, is only part of the treatment, usually the easiest part, even if the patients find it most difficult. In some addictions, hospitalization may be very short, or even unnecessary. Psychiatrists have gradually become more aware of the importance of social approaches, such as group therapy and attempts to alter the milieu in which addictions originate and become reinforced. Many addicts relapse because the social approaches to rehabilitation are neglected, and, in fact, these approaches are realistically very difficult to arrange without extensive group and community help.[32]

In general, neither society nor the expert has dealt very successfully with the problem of preventing addiction; relatively little has been achieved, and millions remain addicted to drugs. Although some progress in the control of drug addiction has been made in many countries, it is difficult to evaluate the efficiency of these controls. The most incisive measure of control consists of supervision and regulation of production of addictive chemical substances. It is said that opium smoking has been virtually eradicated in the People's Republic of China through control of drug production and traffic as well as through public health education. At present, however, in spite of controlling measures, more addictive drugs are produced than are required by medical needs. Physicians, who are often unjustly accused of "soft" attitudes, have always favored effective legal measures to control production and sale of addictive drugs and have accepted and supported strict licensing procedures which specify the persons who may dispense such drugs, but such cooperative efforts are not sufficient. The illegal production and smuggling of drugs, powered by deep psychological and social motives, continue in many countries. We contend that one approach which is primarily punitive will not solve the problem. Punitive social attitudes are exemplified by severe sanctions and also by the strict quasi-legal prohibition against the administration of drugs to patients with abstinence syndromes outside of certain institutions. These punitive approaches discourage treatment, drive patients into the underworld, and remove them from the medical purview. Most of all, it is highly doubtful that these approaches, embodied in the United States in the Harrison Drug Act of 1914, are efficient. The Harrison Act requires licensure of drug dispensers and establishes their strict supervision. Self-administration of drugs, even under the supervision of a physician, is unlawful. Any infraction of the Harrison Act is considered a crime and punished according to the criminal code. Critics point to other countries, notably Great Britain, which without such severe legislation have fared better than the United States by keeping certain addicts on a maintenance dosage when cure is not possible. Progressive physicians and lawyers certainly do not wish to let dope peddlers pursue their trade freely but would like to see more effective measures introduced. Organized underworld activities related to illicit trade in drugs should, of course, be dealt with rigorously, but there is no reason for a sweeping punitive approach. Realistically, we believe—as the elder Lawrence C. Kolb, a veteran fighter for progressive legislation believes—that although the outlook for the immediate future is not bright, eventual changes for the better are inevitable.[22] These changes will entail a pragmatic approach to the problem of appropriate therapeutic goals; it is important to treat even if we cannot completely cure. If so, a realistic start with the current problem can be made; some addicts may have to be maintained, but eventually some of these will be cured. With the diminution of punitive attitudes and the legal rather than illicit dispensing of drugs, a start toward cure and then toward prevention can be made.

Addiction to Opiates

The juice of the opium poppy, *papaver somniferum*, contains a number of alkaloids; the most important ones with addictive properties are morphine and codeine, also pantopon and dilaudid. Synthetic morphine derivatives used by addicts are heroin, meperidine, methadone, and levosphan. The effects of the morphine group are, in part, species-specific. Morphine, the protoype of these alkaloids, is a cortical depressant but also has excitatory properties. Wikler's studies showed excitatory and inhibitory effects at most levels of the neuraxis;[36] some workers speculate that the addictive properties of the drug are related to the need to overcome depressant effects. It has only slight inhibitory effects on the reticular activating system, although it produces some drowsiness in man. Morphine produces nausea, vomiting, and constriction of pupils. It has a strongly depressant effect on respiration; in acute morphine poisoning, death is the result of respiratory paralysis. Neurophysiological studies have not "explained" its analgesic action, but a number of studies have made clear the role of fear and anticipation in pain. The effects of both lobotomy and morphine, which lead to a perception of pain but an indifference to it, and the influence of set and situation on the analgesic effects, indicate the critical role of psychological factors in drug effect. It has been noted that lobotomized persons are not addictable; if this is really so, the neurophysiological and neurobehavioral basis for addiction could be more concisely approached in controlled observations.

The main effect of morphine is its singular capacity to reduce pain without marked alterations of consciousness or marked changes in perception; it may produce a certain euphoria in some subjects. Morphine and related drugs decrease hunger and sex drive and possibly fatigue, as well as the need to be active. In his theory of addiction, Wikler stresses the capacity of morphine to reduce primary drives.[34] Many potential addicts do not experience euphoria and often report some malaise; they simply take the drug to avoid abstinence symptoms, but a reduction of tension and anxiety, which the drug produces, certainly seems very important to the addict. Some subjects become passive and sleepy; they "nod." Others become overactive and boisterous; they "drive." When the drug is intravenously injected, some subjects experience an abdominal "thrill" comparable to orgasm. Chronic drug users often develop a curiously ambivalent attitude toward morphine and other drugs, which they express by calling the drug "dirt" or "crap." Wikler also notes an augmentation of a tendency, under varying environmental conditions, to respond with reaction patterns most stable for the subject. Previously "neurotic" animals responded with neurotic behavior, whereas there were decreased signs of such behavior in those drugged animals with freshly induced experimental neurosis. Some persons can continue their work schedule under the drug; others retreat.

Physical dependence, or tolerance, has been observed both in man and animals. Although a lethal dose for a normal person is about 100 mgm., Wikler reports that in addicts 750 mgm. have been given without harm. The nature of both the physical dependence and of tolerance, which are associated but separable phenomena, is obscure. Recent experiments show a change in the response of brain norepinephrine to tolerance dosage schedules; whether this is primary or secondary to the decrement in excitatory effects is not known.[26] Neural as well as biochemical and behavioral factors are probably involved. J. Cochin and C. Kornetsky have found tolerance to morphine effects persisting for a year following termination of drug, a strange but interesting instance of a behavioral or biological "drug memory."[7]

It is difficult to induce habituation in animals; and there is, intriguingly, wide variability in the degree to which experimental animals will seek drugs under conditions of stress or discomfort. They do become tolerant and apparently dependent when morphine is injected, and when the animal "controls" the input of a drug by self-injection; but it is doubtful whether such studies will provide a precise behavioral model for human addiction. Such approaches, combined with studies of neurophysiologic and chemical structures, may, however, begin to clarify the relevant biological mechanisms. Wikler speaks of physiological or nonpurposive abstinence and purposive abstinence in man; the latter refers to the attempts of the patient to obtain the drug, often at any cost and to heighten the effects of a lower dose.[36] There are notable exceptions: some patients have no need to increase the dose and carefully regulate their intake.

If the drug is withheld from a true addict, abstinence symptoms appear. In the mild abstinence syndrome, symptoms resemble a common cold or an allergic reaction, with sore throat, rhinorrhea, lacrimation, sweating, and slightly elevated temperature. The patient appears ill in the more severe cases and also suffers from nausea and diarrhea; occasionally spontaneous ejaculation occurs, and shock and convulsions may be seen. A drop in blood eosinphils has been noted, indicating activation of the pituitary-adrenal system; a few fatalities have been recorded. In a few cases, psychological symptoms are severe and intolerable; they include insomnia, hallucinations, and delirious symptoms. Occasionally, acute abstinence symptoms last from forty-eight to seventy-two hours. A dramatic precipitation of abstinence symptoms may be produced when n-allylnormorphine is administered to a morphine-tolerant patient. A potent antagonist of morphine, it is the drug of choice in the treatment of morphine poisoning. Given to nontolerant individuals, the drug produces effects similar to opiates, with the possible additional symptom of hallucinations. The administration of n-allylnormorphine in doses of 3 to 5 mg. can constitute a diagnostic test to determine whether the patient is tolerant and undergoing a true abstinence syndrome.

Older persons, particularly those who suffer pain, and the addicts in the medical and nursing professions tend to take morphine and synthetic drugs, particularly meperidine. Codeine addiction is rare, possibly because it provides little euphoria; there does not appear to be dependence. Heroin, referred to as "horse," the drug of juvenile gangs, provides the greatest "kick," especially when taken intravenously; as in morphine, however, the euphoric effects can be maintained only with ever-increasing doses. Its potency permits peddlers to "cut" the product, and contaminants can cause adventitious serious reactions. In contrast to the countries of the Far East and South East Asia, where opium is smoked, heroin, morphine, and related synthetic drugs are injected subcutaneously or intravenously by Western addicts. Infection of the injected sites, even in physicians, is common. Nelson Algren's novel, *Man with the Golden Arm*, and William Burroughs' book, *Naked Lunch*, provide vivid descriptions of the argot, experiences, fantasies, and life patterns of contemporary heroin addicts.

Addiction to opiates may develop rapidly—within a week. Patients with chronic pain who become addicted, however, rarely derive any orgastic experience from morphine or related synthetic drugs. The physical symptoms of habitual use of opiates are relatively mild. They consist of a diminution of appetite, loss of weight, and a decrease of sexual drive and potency. There may be, through the analgesic effect of morphine, a masking of acute and dangerous illness. More serious is a certain withdrawal from reality and social responsibility; life begins to revolve solely around the question of how to obtain the panacea in ever-increasing doses. To think of all opiate addicts as destitute persons is incorrect; if healthy and well off, they may be indistinguishable from any other person of similar social status. The popular stereotype of the addict as a lazy, deceitful, depraved person who indulges in vice and has only one desire, to seduce others to his miserable way of life, is a far cry from the truth. But all too frequently this is the accusation made by moralistic persecutors, and it is one of the unfortunate consequences of a social system that makes an outcast of the lower-class addict. On the whole, morphine addicts, though not intrinsically criminal, do not make good citizens. Some addicts live a well-regulated life or conduct a business successfully, but this degree of social integration is not too commonly seen even in countries where the attitude toward abuse of opiates is reasonable.

TREATMENT All opiate addicts should be treated, with the sole exception of those with severe, terminal, painful diseases. Even in such cases a judicious attempt to reduce doses and make the patient more independent of a drug that is losing its effectiveness is often indicated. Addicts may be kept off drugs for considerable periods of time, even if no complete and lasting cure takes place. Nyswander feels, and this is also our strong impression, that when treatment occurs under voluntary auspices, the results can be much more favorable.[29]

Expert consensus is that withdrawal must be carried out in hospitals under skilled and close supervision. It is unfortunately but nonetheless true that one cannot avoid the role of a detective in searching for hidden drugs, because desperate addicts can be fantastically resourceful if they are not motivated to cooperate with their therapists. Three methods of withdrawal have been practiced: sudden withdrawal, slow withdrawal, and the substitution for opiates by other drugs that produce less severe abstinence syndromes. In the United States, sudden withdrawal is considered inhuman and dangerous and is not frequently practiced. Prior to treatment, patients must be given a thorough physical examination, which helps determine the risk and need of treatment. Recommendations are to begin with the full dose patients claim they need, but not to exceed 120 mgm., in four divided doses. After the patient has been stabilized in such a fashion, rapid substitution of methadone for morphine, combined with reduction of morphine, is initiated. Usually, 3 mgm. of morphine is replaced by 1 mg. of methadone, which produces a less severe abstinence syndrome. Patients are rapidly withdrawn in three to seven days. Recently, the use of phenothiazines for the alleviation of withdrawal symptoms has been recommended,[13] but their use has not been adopted generally. Withdrawal symptoms vary not only with the dose but also with the individual patient; they seem less severe in the voluntary and cooperative patient. During withdrawal, the physician must be alert to the occurrence and therapy of severe and dangerous abstinence symptoms such as vasomotor shock and convulsive seizures, especially after Demerol. Fortunately, preconvulsive tremors can be monitored and promptly treated by administration of the addicting drug. The most difficult task is not withdrawal but psychotherapy and rehabilitation of the patient. Although Nyswander is fairly optimistic about the chances of permanent or long-lasting cure of patients in competent psychotherapy, most psychotherapists have been reluctant, if not unwilling, to take these difficult patients into treatment.[28] The most difficult part of treatment is the phase in which the patient who has been withdrawn and, hopefully, has received psychotherapy is rehabilitated in his community through the combined efforts of psychotherapists and social workers. Undoubtedly, rapport and responsiveness to the cultural realities of the patient is important. If doctors are "authorities" to whom the patient cannot relate and toward whom fear rather than trust is engendered, treatment will be less successful than it could be.

Cocaine Addiction

Cocaine, the oldest local anesthetic, has an excitatory action on the central nervous system; its ability to relieve fatigue is attributed to "cortical excitation." It produces hyperthermia, potentiates the sympathetic nervous system reaction to epinephrine, and dilates the pupils. In acute cocaine poisoning, patients usually become restless, excited, and develop delirious reactions. They complain of headache, nausea, and abdominal pains; temperature is elevated and vomiting is frequent. Convulsions occur, and in terminal cases Cheyne Stokes respirations are followed by respiratory arrest. Lethal doses are 1–2 gm. Treatment of acute cocaine poisoning consists of administration of quick-acting barbiturates.

Pure cocaine addiction is relatively rare. In a strict sense, cocaine is not an addictive drug because there is no physical dependence or tolerance.[25] It is usually sniffed as a powder; more rarely it is chewed; the average dose is 0.5 gm. When it is sniffed for a prolonged period of time, it usually produces perforating ulcers in the nasal septum. The drug is rarely taken alone; most cocaine addicts also take opiates; and taking a combination of heroin and cocaine, the so-called *speedball,* is common. Cocaine is sometimes called the martini of the addictive drugs because cocaine users are more gregarious than morphine addicts; it purportedly was once a favorite of bohemians and the denizens of the underworld. South American Indians have been known to chew the leaves of *erythroxylus coca,* which contain caffeine and cocaine and have a mild alerting and euphoric effect; this widely spread habit cannot be equated with cocaine addiction in industrialized countries.

The habituating properties of cocaine are seemingly related to the sexual excitation and the feeling of power it produces. Perceptions become vivid; the drug creates a feeling of indefatigability and creativity. When taken over longer periods of time, it produces visual, auditory, and particularly tactile hallucinations. Cocaine addicts frequently develop paranoid and megalomanic delusions and aggressive behavior. In this stage, they may be dangerous, especially when driven to impulsive acts by terrifying hallucinations. Withdrawal from cocaine can be abrupt because no abstinence symptoms occur. Psychotherapy and rehabilitation of cocaine addicts, who are invariably severely disturbed or antisocial personalities, are notably difficult.

Marihuana Addiction

Indian hemp, or *cannabis indica,* also known as hashish and marihuana, has been known as a euphoriant in Asia and Africa for hundreds of years. The drug is obtained from the flowers of the plant which is easily grown in tropical and in temperate climates. As it may be cultivated inconspicuously at home, its production can hardly be controlled. On the other hand, it can be said that marihuana effects and marihuana addiction per se are relatively harmless. The chief danger lies in the fact that juvenile drug users are first seduced to marihuana and then proceed to heroin. Marihuana is eaten, drunk, or smoked, largely varying with local customs. In Western metropolitan centers, the "weed" is mostly smoked, generally in groups. It is a drug used by the fringe of the entertainment world, particularly some jazz musicians, who claim to derive from it an increased sense of rhythm and timing; C. K. Aldrich demonstrated that the improvement of rhythm and timing is only subjective.[1] The effects of marihuana are similar to certain effects of alcohol; it produces reddening of the conjunctivae, photophobia, and mild rhinorrhea, tachycardia and rise in blood pressure. There may also be some dizziness, but no serious central nervous effects except hyperreflexia and slight incoordination are occasionally noted. In higher doses, it produces nausea and somnolence; however, no serious acute toxic effects are known. When the drug is taken, most habitual users experience an elevation of mood and excitability followed by lassitude. J. Moreau[27] and, a hundred years later, Karl Beringer[4] noted in classical reports the occurrence of symptomatic psychoses. S. Allentuck and Karl M. Bowman reported that 9 of 77 had mild symptomatic psychoses.[2] There are no known lasting serious effects of the drug, no alterations of mentation or personality. There is, of course, the general inclination to withdraw and escape from reality, which is characteristic of most addicts. There is no evidence of physical dependence or tolerance. In general marihuana addicts are often in need of psychotherapy and social rehabilitation.

Amphetamine Addiction

E. Guttman was the first investigator to report abuses of amphetamine.[17] Since the 1940's, a number of articles and an important monograph have appeared on addiction to amphetamines.[8, 20] This sympathicomimetic drug has effects similar to those of ephedrine. It constricts peripheral blood vessels; stimulates the heart and elevates blood pressure; relaxes the bronchial and intestinal muscles; decreases appetite, probably by a direct hypothalamic action; and has been widely used as a drug in the treatment of obesity. To psychiatrists, the alerting and exciting effects are of particular interest;

the amphetamines have been utilized in combating and preventing fatigue and also in the treatment of narcolepsy.[30] Psychological effects vary but, in general, it produces a feeling of mild euphoria, increased confidence and mental powers, and decreased fatigue. Actually, there is no good evidence that mental powers are increased (unless, for example, they have been decreased by sleep deprivation); apart from a slight increase in motor performance, no enhancement of behavior seems to occur without a prior decrement. Its effect on sexual function is not entirely clear, but it seems to increase sex drive while retarding orgasm and to weaken defenses and inhibitions.[3] Psychiatrists have used it in combination with other drugs, especially amobarbital, in the treatment of depression. The euphoria amphetamine produces in some persons is usually accompanied by a disagreeable feeling of tension, anxiety, and prolonged insomnia; this is probably a reason that amphetamine addiction is not frequent. There is no physical dependence, although doses that can be absorbed without side-effects vary greatly. Normal doses are 5 to 30 mgm. per day by mouth in adults, but as much as 1500 mgm. has been taken. The ordinary sources are benzedrine inhalers and amphetamine tablets, which are taken orally. Amphetamine addiction occurs frequently among inmates of penitentiaries and also in juvenile gangs. In Japan after World War II, mass addiction in adolescents and a virtual epidemic of psychoses were observed. Chronic high dosage of amphetamine produces acute symptomatic psychoses with lively visual or auditory hallucinations and paranoid delusions. The patients usually are restless, excited, irritable, and inclined to be assaultive. What is most striking is the difficulty in differentiating these from schizophrenic psychoses. The symptoms may persist for some months after withdrawal. A toxic picture is not necessarily seen. We have known some patients who have recovered from the acute psychosis, yet report on inquiry that they still believe their old delusions but prefer to ignore them. A characteristic feature of early onset of these psychoses is an extraordinary sensitivity to reflected images from surfaces; patients are distracted by minutiae and endow them with meaning. As the psychosis developed in one patient, the reflection of the sun on a car became, over a few days, a plot to confuse the city with visions of naked women. He had been overworking for four months, was sleep-deprived, and had forged prescriptions for 60–100 mg. amphetamine daily, together with barbiturates and meprobamate. Treatment of amphetamine addiction consists of sudden withdrawal and the painstaking efforts of individual and group psychotherapy, family and milieu therapy, and rehabilitation, which are essential in the treatment of all addictions.

Barbiturate Addiction

Barbiturates produce true addiction with the characteristics of physical dependence, habituation, and tolerance, although tolerance is relatively slight compared to that seen with opiates. It is a widespread and medically dangerous form of addiction in industrialized countries and more damaging than opiates. Curiously enough, in the United States, where there is vehement reaction to other addictions, the production and sale of barbiturates is not as strictly controlled as that of other addictive drugs. There is a vast overproduction of barbiturates.[38] Although no reliable estimates of the number of barbiturate addicts exist, it can be assumed that it is second only to alcohol addiction and much higher than addiction to all other drugs combined.

For psychiatrists, barbiturates have been important drugs, which are used as hypnotics, sedatives, anticonvulsants, and also as agents to produce narcoanalysis. Although, in subhypnotic dosage or under particular motivational circumstances, a facilitory effect on psychomotor function can be seen in man and animals, the drugs are used clinically for their depressive effect, which varies from mild sedation to deep coma and death through respiratory paralysis. As margins of safety are small and deaths from barbiturate poisoning are relatively frequent, psychiatrists must be familiar with the symptoms of acute poisoning through accidental or deliberate overdose. When barbiturates produce a confusional state, a small additional amount taken without any (conscious) suicidal intent may lead to serious complications and death. Symptoms consist of deep sleep that progresses to coma; respiration becomes stertorous, then shallow; in the dangerous phase, the patient becomes cyanotic; the blood pressure sinks and pupils dilate. Urine formation is decreased. The diagnosis is confirmed by chemical examination of blood, urine, and the contents of the stomach. Treatment consists of removal of the drug by gastric lavage with a solution of sodium permanganate, 1:5000, and treatment with analeptics, artificial respiration, and oxygen. Preventive measures against hypostatic pneumonia and care to avoid regurgitation are important; tracheotomy may be advisable. Plasma dialysis with artificial kidneys has been employed to rid the organism of drug. Direct antagonists, although under development, are not as yet specific. Patients with severe damage to their central nervous systems may remain under dialysis in prolonged coma for weeks and months or, in less severe cases, develop delirious and dysmnesic psychoses.

Addiction to barbiturates is frequently the result of medical prescription. The barbiturate addict, in certain respects, resembles the alcohol addict; barbiturate and alcohol addiction often go together. In most barbiturate addicts, doses are gradually increased. Addicts take these drugs primarily to fight insomnia and to obtain sedation and reduction of tension. In a significant number of patients, the drug supplies a temporary kick. The role of personality variables determining such reactions have been demonstrated; some addicts respond with euphoria, whereas a normal population does not. Neurological signs after chronic use of high doses may be seen; these consist of cerebellar disturbance of coordination, tremor, and optokinetic nystagmus. Other symptoms are dyspepsia and toxic skin rashes. Behavioral changes after prolonged use of barbiturates are a certain sluggishness, emotional lability, and irritability. There is definite evidence of the occurrence of symptomatic psychoses and also, in some cases, of an organic deterioration.[19]

Withdrawal symptoms may be very serious and consist of convulsions and delirium, psychosis and, in milder cases, insomnia, nausea, vomiting, abdominal cramps, and severe anxiety and restlessness. Usually, withdrawal symptoms last from a few days to weeks. These symptoms make it necessary to hospitalize barbiturate addicts and withdraw them gradually. Psychotherapy and rehabilitation present difficulties similar to those in other addictions. Kornetsky described the psychological effects of experimental barbiturate intoxication and withdrawal.[23] From Rorschach tests, he could infer that persons with constricted personalities and poor resources to cope with stress tended to produce psychotic symptoms within a few days following withdrawal. Giving doses of .6–.8 gm. of secobarbital daily for 38–58 days, the Lexington group found 79 per cent of the subjects had seizures and 69 per cent transient psychoses on high dosage, but only 10 per cent showed such symptoms in the moderate-dosage group. Obviously, withdrawal symptoms are dependent upon dosage schedule as well as personality.[19]

Barbiturate and Amphetamine Addiction in a Middle-Class Woman

A fifty-three year old single woman was admitted to the psychiatric service because she had been taking high doses of barbiturates—probably between 0.5 and 1 gm. of amytal and about 50 mgm. of benzedrine per day. She had been an addict for some twenty years. Before admission, she lived with her married brother, who wanted to help her but found it increasingly difficult to cope with the patient's drug habits, her tendency to lie about in the apartment in a nightgown or in the nude, and to say embarrassing things to family and friends. When she was moved into an apartment of her own, the situation became worse and admission to a psychiatric hospital was the only solution.

The patient is the illegitimate child of an erratic mother and a wealthy man, who willed a large amount of money in trust to her. After the patient's birth, her mother married an actor, by whom she had two children. The family had to move around the country a good deal, and the household was never stable. The patient's formal education was sporadic and incomplete, with no vocational preparation. For short periods of time she was farmed out to various relatives. She was described as a moody, unhappy, and lonely child who often shut herself up in her room for days. When she was twenty-two, the mother divorced her husband; she asked the patient to testify falsely that the husband had tried to seduce his stepdaughter when she was a teen-ager. Years later, when she wrote to her stepfather, he proposed marriage. The patient's mother married again, a wealthy man, but continued to pay little attention to her daughter, who lived an irregular and erratic life in a Southern California artists' colony. She there shared an apartment with two other women, with whom she constantly quarreled. Always promiscuous, the patient had sexual relations with many soldiers from a nearby military installation because she believed in "free love." It was at this time that she became addicted. Barbiturates were first medically prescribed for insomnia; she took benzedrine on the advice of a soldier-friend so as not to become groggy during her alcoholic binges. At first, the drug made her anxious and tense; she later has felt depressed without it. She still uses barbiturates when she wants to sleep and benzedrine in the daytime, but occasionally combines them.

She became attached to one young soldier and tried to shoot herself when he left her. After this, she was hospitalized in a private psychiatric hospital and received a series of shock treatments. Two years later, the patient almost died after taking an overdose of barbiturates and was hospitalized in a general hospital at that time. She fell in love with a medical student fifteen years younger and married him; after six weeks of violent quarrels and beatings, the marriage was annulled because both partners were intoxicated when they got married.

On admission to the psychiatric service, the patient was rambling, circumstantial, incoherent, and forgetful. She was only partially oriented to time and person. Her mood was euphoric; she seemed intellectually deteriorated on clinical examination. Psychological testing at that time was impossible. She was markedly undernourished and had edematous lower extremities. The blood pressure was 180/100; during hospitalization it reached normal limits. The initial diagnosis was drug psychosis and malnutrition. Barbiturates were withdrawn within two weeks, benzedrine within three days. A progressive clearing of mental function followed, but the patient became more overtly depressed. When she was tested psychologically during the fourth week, there was no evidence of any organic deficit. She related well to the therapist and developed some insight into her difficulties. She gradually overcame her seclusiveness and took a maternal interest in a young schizophrenic girl. She was discharged after five months into the custody of her half-brother. In a follow-up inquiry one year later, she was still off drugs and seemed to get along reasonably well.

Other Addiction-Producing Drugs

Other drugs that occasionally produce addiction are *paraldehyde, chloral hydrate,* and *ether.* Usually, they are taken by chronic and derelict alcoholics and barbiturate addicts. Abuse of bromides today is only of historical interest. Addictions to more recent arrivals on the drug market, such as *glutethimide* (Doriden), *methyprylon* (Noludar), *ethinamate* (Valmid), *ethylchlorynol* (Placidyl); have been reported to occur in some users. Doriden, in daily doses above 2.5 gm., may produce intoxication, and doses of 10–20 gm. in nontolerant persons may be lethal. Autonomic signs, convulsions, hallucinations, and delirium are seen on withdrawal, with an onset as late as six days following cessation of drug. Similar syndromes have been seen with Nodular (lethal dose 6 gm. or more) and Placidyl. These "safe" hypnotic drugs appear not only to intoxicate and probably induce tolerance and dependence, but also to potentiate alcohol effects. Addictions, tolerance and abstinence syndromes are similar to those produced by barbiturates. Tolerance and withdrawal symptoms on high doses—above 1600 mg. daily

—have occasionally been reported with *meprobamate;* six of 25 schizophrenic patients on 2400 gm. daily for nine months developed convulsions on withdrawal. EEG abnormalities and even death have been related to sudden withdrawal (from 10 gm. to 1.6 gm.) of this drug.[10] *Chlordiazepoxide,* although useful in treating alcoholism (including delirium tremens), has habituating and addicting properties. While doses of 200 mg. can be given in a six-hour period, and while it may have anticonvulsant effects, withdrawal after 300 mg. daily produces abstinence symptoms, and intoxication coma may be seen after 300 mg. daily. Abrupt withdrawal may lead to convulsions as late as four to eight days later. So far, no addiction to major tranquilizers and antidepressants has been reported. There is also no true addiction to the common psychotomimetics (see Chapter 10), but habituation and cult formation around these drugs is clear; further, their effects on reality orientation and judgment when taken in certain settings is yet to be assessed; these drugs, unwisely used, produce disorganized and socially undesirable behavior and may have consequences requiring control.

NOTES

1. C. Knight Aldrich, "The Effects of a Synthetic Marihuana-like Compound on Musical Talent as Measured by the Reaction Test," *Public Health Reports,* 59 (1944), 431.
2. Samuel Allentuck and Karl M. Bowman, "The Psychiatric Aspects of Marihuana Intoxication," *American Journal of Psychiatry,* 99 (1942), 248.
3. D. S. Bell and W. H. Trethowan, "Amphetamine Addiction and Disturbed Sexuality," *Archives of General Psychiatry,* 4 (1961), 74.
4. Karl Beringer, "Zur Klinik des Haschischrausches," *Nervenarzt.,* 5 (1932), 337.
5. Isidor Chein, Donald L. Gerard, Robert S. Lee, and Eva Rosenfeld, *The Road to H* (New York: Basic Books, 1964).
6. John A. Clausen, "Social Patterns, Personality and Adolescent Drug Use," in Alexander H. Leighton, John A. Clausen, and Robert N. Wilson, eds., *Explorations in Social Psychiatry* (New York: Basic Books, 1957).
7. Joseph Cochin and C. Kornetsky, "Development and Loss of Tolerance to Morphine in the Rat after Single and Multiple Injections," *Journal of Pharmacology and Experimental Therapeutics,* 145 (1964), 1.
8. Philip H. Connell, *Amphetamine Psychoses,* Maudsley Monograph, No. 5 (London: Chapman and Hall, 1958).
9. Helmuth Ehrhardt, "Drug Addiction in the Medical and Allied Professions in Germany" (U. N. Bulletin on Narcotics, 11 [1959]), 18.
10. Carl F. Essig, "Addiction to Nonbarbiturate Sedative and Tranquilizing Drugs," *Clinical Pharmacology and Therapeutics,* 5 (1964), 334.

11. Robert H. Felix, "An Appraisal of the Personality Types of the Addict," *American Journal of Psychiatry*, 100 (1944), 462.
12. Sigmund Freud, "Humour" [1927], *Standard Edition* (London: Hogarth Press, 1961), Vol. XXI.
13. Charles E. Friedgood and C. B. Ripstein, "Use of Chlorpromazine in the Withdrawal of Addicting Drugs," *New England Journal of Medicine*, 252 (1955), 230.
14. Donald L. Gerard and Conan Kornetsky, "A Social and Psychiatric Study of Adolescent Opiate Addicts," *Psychiatry Quarterly*, 28 (1954), 113.
15. Edward Glover, "On Aetiology of Drug-Addiction," *International Journal of Psycho-Analysis*, 13 (July 1932), 298.
16. Alfred Gross, "The Psychic Effects of Toxic and Toxoid Substances," *International Journal of Psycho-Analysis*, 16 (1935), 425.
17. Erich Guttman, "Discussion of Benzedrine; Uses and Abuses" *Proceedings of the Royal Society of Medicine*, 32 (1939), 388.
18. John W. Higgins, "Psychodynamics in the Excessive Drinking of Alcohol," *Archives of Neurology and Psychiatry*, 69 (1953), 713.
19. Harris Isbell and H. F. Fraser, "Addiction to Analgesics and Barbiturates," *Pharmacological Reviews*, 2 (1950), 355.
20. Peter H. Knapp, "Amphetamine and Addiction," *Journal of Nervous and Mental Disease*, 115 (1952), 406.
21. Robert P. Knight, "The Psychodynamics of Chronic Alcoholism," *Journal of Nervous and Mental Disease*, 86 (1937), 538.
22. Lawrence Kolb, *Drug Addiction* (Springfield: Charles C Thomas, 1962).
23. Conan H. Kornetsky, "Psychological Effects of Chronic Barbiturate Intoxication," *Archives of Neurology and Psychiatry*, 65 (1951), 557.
24. Erich Lindemann and L. D. Clarke, "Modifications in Ego Structure and Personality Reactions under the Influence of the Effects of Drugs," *American Journal of Psychiatry*, 108 (1952), 561.
25. Hans W. Maier, *Der Kokainismus* (Leipzig: Georg Thieme-Verlag, 1926).
26. Everett W. Maynert and Gerda I. Klingman, "Tolerance to Morphine, I. Effects on Catecholamines in the Brain and Adrenal Glands," *Journal of Pharmacology and Experimental Therapeutics*, 135 (1962), 285.
27. Jacques Joseph Moreau, *Du Hashisch et de l'alienation mentale* (Paris: Fortin, Mason, 1845).
28. Marie Nyswander, *The Drug Addict as a Patient* (New York: Grune & Stratton, 1956).
29. Marie Nyswander, "Drug Addictions," in Silvano Arieti, ed., *American Handbook of Psychiatry* (New York: Basic Books, 1959), Vol. I., pp. 614–623.
30. Myron Prinzmetal and W. Bloomberg, "The Use of Benzedrine for the Treatment of Narcolepsy," *Journal of the American Medical Association*, 105 (1935), 2051.

31. Sandor Rado, "The Psychoanalysis of Pharmacothymia (Drug Addiction)," *Psychoanalytic Quarterly*, 2 (1933), 1.
32. *Rehabilitation of Drug Addicts*, Mental Health Monograph No. 3 (Bethesda: National Institute of Mental Health, 1963; U. S. Public Health Service Pub. No. 1013).
33. Victor H. Vogel, H. Isbell, and K. W. Chapman, "Present Status of Narcotic Addiction," *Journal of the American Medical Association*, 138 (1948), 1019.
34. Abraham Wikler, "Mechanisms of Action of Drugs That Modify Personality Function," *American Journal of Psychiatry*, 108 (1952), 590.
35. Abraham Wikler, "A Psychodynamic Study of a Patient during Experimental Self-regulated Re-addiction to Morphine," *Psychiatric Quarterly*, 26 (1952), 270.
36. Abraham Wikler, "Drug Addiction," in A. B. Baker, ed., *Clinical Neurology* (New York: Paul B. Hoeber, 1955).
37. Charles Winnick, "Maturing Out of Narcotic Addiction," *Bulletin on Narcotics*, 14 (1962), 1.
38. World Health Organization, Expert Committee on Drugs Liable to Produce Addiction, "Report of the Second Session," Technical Report Series No. 21 (Geneva: World Health Organization, 1950).
39. Norman E. Zinberg and David C. Lewis, "Narcotic Usage," *New England Journal of Medicine*, 270 (1964), 989.

CHAPTER TWENTY-THREE

Alcoholism

The Nature of Alcoholism

Ethyl alcohol is the most important chemical substance associated with intoxication and addiction; excessive and uncontrolled drinking produces more serious psychosocial and physical consequences than any of the previously mentioned drugs. Man has used alcohol from the Stone Age to the present, but abuse of alcohol became a serious problem only after the spread of industrialization in the eighteenth century. Alcoholism, according to Mark Keller, is a chronic behavioral disorder manifested by repeated drinking of alcoholic beverages in excess of the dietary and social uses of the community, and to an extent that interferes with the drinker's health or his social or economic functioning.[19] E. M. Jellinek's definition is even more generic and deliberately broad: alcoholism refers to any use of an alcoholic beverage that causes any damage to the individual or society.[16] Such definitions are not entirely useful since they do not highlight certain "gray" areas; for example, the use of alcohol in an addictive way is frequently observed, but the patient can still function apparently well. Loss of control does not occur in some addictions; in others, it is subtle and graded and often difficult to detect. In the literature on alcoholism, many terms are used with dismaying vagueness. Impairment, usually of a temporary nature—getting drunk—is called alcoholic intoxication and referred to in bad medical vernacular as acute alcoholism. The vague term, excessive drinking, refers both to an isolated occasion and to the ingrained behavioral patterns and drinking habits of alcoholics. Jellinek speaks of alcoholism as a disease—in the sense that psychiatrists speak of mental diseases. We see it, as Keller does, as a behavior disorder; either term puts us in a position to apply a scientific, enlightened, and objective approach to alcohol addiction rather than to contend with moralistic points of view in contrast to some of psychiatry's great leaders—August Forel, Emil Kraepelin, Eugen Bleuler—who were prominent in the temperance and abstinence movements. The trend today is less toward premature action based on condemnation of drinking and more toward impartial investigation of this complex problem.

Is alcoholism a true addiction? If we define addiction broadly as a psychological dependence on alcohol, it clearly is. A large number of, but not all, alcoholics also develop tolerance. A large proportion develops physical dependence and serious withdrawal states. That the drug does frequently produce physical dependence in the sense of withdrawal symptoms is clear both from clinical evidence and the experimental studies of H. Isbell and others;[15] drug addicts volunteered to consume large quantities of alcohol for weeks, and in the majority (but not all subjects) withdrawal produced hallucinosis and convulsions. J. H. Mendelson reported different findings in a group of volunteers.[25] Individuals vary in the level of blood alcohol required to produce intoxication, but many heavy drinkers show *acquired tolerance* (in terms of blood levels this apparently has an enzymatic basis,) [25] which permits large intake without marked neurobehavioral impairment; the sudden loss of this tolerance at some stage of a drinking career confronts the drinker with new consequences of his dependence on alcohol. Tolerance varies and does not correlate at all precisely with the occurrence or severity of withdrawal syndromes. Whereas tissue and metabolic mechanisms are undoubtedly active, their role in sustaining or compelling the likelihood of further drinking is not at all clear and probably varies, not only in individuals, but in various phases and stages of different patterns of drinking behavior.[25] Alcohol, as with most drugs, produces a sequence of altered neurobehavioral states in which psychological and situational factors, precipitating, and conditioning factors interact to produce the manifest behavioral patterns. Individuals may be *psychologically dependent,* since some persons compulsively resume drinking after a period of abstinence quite independently of any tolerance or withdrawal. Other individuals show an inability to abstain, but retain control over the amount of intake; others show loss of control—an inability to stop continued heavy drinking rather than a simple inability to abstain from moderate drinking. Again, the student must be alert to two series of determinants, organic and psychological. For many drinkers, the first drink is sufficient to induce, not drunkenness, but a mental state in which there is loss of focus on realistic necessities and inability to heed warning signs of danger. Too often the notion of *physiological dependence* is taken as a condition that "cannot be argued with"; such dependence, it is assumed, cannot be influenced by psychological means or conditioned by psychological events; and if psychological causes are found, the effects of the drug, alcohol, are too often ignored. In fact, physiological disturbances can sometimes best be treated expectantly; on other occasions, they require specific medical therapy. Similarly, the effects of alcohol can revise the "rules" by which psychological forces are usually expected to operate in therapy. Dogmatic and essentially unrealistic views of the exclusive role of one or another factor simply will not—practically speaking—work, if one wishes to treat alcoholics.

Psychiatrists deal with only certain segments of the problem of alcoholism, which concerns many other professions: the medical profession in general, biological and behavioral scientists, as well as administrators, legislators, and law-enforcing personnel. It is the psychiatrist's task to diagnose and treat behavior disorders and neuropsychiatric diseases of the individual alcoholic. It is also his task to contribute to a rational approach to the problem of alcoholism; this, so far, has been largely neglected.

Pharmacological Effects of Alcohol

Alcohol is a nutritive substance. It produces 7.1 calories per gm. and is dietetically and medically used for its food value. In large doses, alcohol increases the organism's vitamin requirements, perhaps because it represents an additional intake of calories. Alcoholic beverages may be sought as nourishment and for their taste (which is not so much the property of the alcohol but of so-called congeners), but its main attraction to the consumer lies in its intoxicating, sedating, and anesthetizing qualities. L. A. Greenberg defines an intoxicating beverage as one that may produce a state of abnormal behavior with blood alcohol concentration of 0.15 per cent or more; levels above 0.2 per cent correspond to moderate-to-severe intoxication, and blood alcohol levels of 0.5 per cent may be fatal.[11] A concentration of 0.15 per cent blood alcohol is established as a legal test for inebriation in many countries and states. Beer, according to Greenberg, is not an intoxicating beverage because the amounts that can be consumed without distress do not produce an intoxicating blood alcohol level. Although beer may not raise blood levels of alcohol to the extent that other products do, alcoholics should not drink beer because it does have a mental effect; it "pulls them" away from reality and facilitates the start of a bout of uncontrolled drinking.

Alcohol is mostly absorbed from the small intestine and distributed into all tissues. From 2 to 10 per cent is excreted through lungs, kidneys, and skin. The rest, depending on the magnitude of intake, is broken down, largely in the liver by a DPN (diphospho-pyridine nucleotide) dependent enzyme to acetaldehyde and by a DPN-dependent aldehyde dehydrogenase to acetate. Alcohol can enter the brain, which can oxidize and degrade it, but insufficient data exist on these central biochemical changes; energy metabolism has been implicated in the effects of alcohol, but the specificity of this is unclear. Alcohol is a central nervous system depressant with possibly slight excitatory effects on respiratory centers. Its so-called stimulating qualities are deemed to be the result of release of inhibition. In larger doses, it is a severe depressant of respiratory centers. Just how alcohol acts on ganglion cells and what precise neurochemical sequences produce intoxication are not definitely known. It raises the pain threshold in man; this action, in part, is due to a shift of concern and to euphoria.

After a brief period of neurological and psychological release, the depressing effects of alcohol on the central nervous system predominate. During early intoxication, patients show vascular dilation of the skin, with a flushed and sweaty face, increased pulse, and deepened and accelerated respiration. Gastric secretion is increased. Even in small doses, ataxia of the fine coordinated movements occurs. Central mechanisms regulating the various stages of sleep are affected by alcohol; there is an initial depression of fast (REM) sleep; with daily dosage, there is an "escape" and a great increase of fast sleep, which persists for a time following withdrawal of the drug.[43]

In ordinary drunkenness, often the excitation phase is followed by somnolence and sleep. Simple intoxication does not last longer than twelve hours, and symptoms of "hangover" may then ensue. With increasing intoxication, cerebellar ataxia with unsteadiness of gait and dysarthria appear. The waking EEG shows a decrease of frequency and an increase of amplitude, depending on the severity of intoxication. Alcohol poisoning is discussed in a later section.

Behavioral Effects of Alcohol

John A. Carpenter *et al.*, in the first study of the effects of alcohol on complex thought processes, showed that certain tasks involving "inductive reasoning" showed impairment with increasing doses; whereas over the same range of doses, the "deductive" tasks showed no change or even showed improvement.[7] It is thought that, for certain creative tasks, any impairment is offset by a decrease of intellectual inhibitions. Thus, under the influence of alcohol, some artists or writers may do better, not only subjectively but also objectively. This decrease in inhibition—the release effect of alcohol—is considered by A. Wikler and others the outstanding behavioral effect.[39] Wikler makes a good general point, even though the manifest behavior is far more variable; a great variety of drives may be selectively released in different alcoholics, whose personalities vary greatly. The release effect is held responsible both for the transient feeling of well-being and for the fact that the drinker is more apt to fulfill some of his inhibited and conflicted needs. Just what such frustrations are, depends on the basic personality pattern and the current situation, so that the effects of alcohol vary greatly. Often, the needs and conflicts brought to the surface have been hidden—In *vino veritas!* The reduction of conflict and the emergence of truth about hidden wishes is bought at the expense of a firm estimate of the demands of reality. Judgment, and particularly the ability and will to distinguish between wish and act, are impaired, and false estimations of limitations and underestimation of danger are common. The reduction of defenses and anxiety and the release from social and ethical inhibitions can lead to freer but also to unconventional, and occasionally, antisocial behavior. The timid man becomes courageous; an aggressive woman becomes more passive and feminine. Suspicion and fear may be relaxed, love shown more openly, and dependence expressed more freely.

Even the sedating function of alcohol seems to vary greatly. Some persons become sleepy; others are stimulated to prolonged aggressive harangues. The impact of moderate doses of alcohol on sexual behavior is also complex.

It increases sexual desire in the inhibited and may even help the performance of sexual intercourse through a decrease of anxiety. Alcohol is the favorite aphrodisiac of the newlywed. Nevertheless, there is reason to believe that, for the male, willingness to perform is greater than capacity, so that the drug does not in fact fulfill the wishes for a magical potency potion. Its retardation of ejaculation is well known, and potency disturbances in drunkenness are common. Most important is the general tendency for conscious and unconscious unacceptable sexual needs to be less upsetting. A man with strong but unconscious, inhibited homosexual needs, who usually feels tense and unhappy and avoids people, may relax sufficiently at a bar to enjoy at least superficial social contacts with men, which he otherwise has to deny himself. Alcohol, as we say colloquially, dissolves conscience, rarely a welcome, and more often a socially dangerous effect.

Alcohol adversely influences psychomotor performance and increases reaction time. Decrease in motor skills, reactivity, and judgment, as well as an overestimation of one's abilities and released aggressiveness, are responsible for traffic accidents in intoxicated drivers. K. Bjerver and L. Goldberg found a decrease of skills in simulated driving tests of 18 to 32 per cent at the low blood level of 0.04 per cent.[5] All other subjects in a simulated automobile driving test showed some impairment of function at blood alcohol concentrations of 0.05 per cent. Although, in the public mind, acute intoxication is often linked with criminal behavior, it is noteworthy that the behavioral release phenomena rarely are seriously antisocial. Only occasionally will an individual deliberately drink to bolster courage for a crime; this does occur in cases of aggressive and sexual crimes executed by groups, such as rape by a group or lynching. Details of normal, and particularly of antisocial, behavior during intoxication are often not recalled with accuracy. Hysterical drinkers, especially, are apt to repress antisocial details of their behavior, but usually in ordinary drunkenness the amnesia is more often wished for than truly attained. In general, for the average drinker, consciousness and memory in moderate degrees of intoxication are surprisingly intact.

"Blackouts," the memory deficits that occur during and following drinking, which are so characteristic for the alcoholic problem drinker and a warning sign of dangerous alcoholism, deserve far more study than they have received. Whether information is registered; and, if registered, "consolidated"; and, if consolidated, accessible for retrieval is not clear; effects on various neural and chemical systems are conceivably sufficient, directly to impair the normal requirements for memory functions in heavy drinkers.

Socioeconomic Aspects of Drinking and Alcoholism

S. Sariola aptly reviewed social and cultural aspects of drinking and alcoholism.[31] France is the largest consumer of alcoholic beverages; the average Frenchman drinks 17 liters of absolute alcohol per year, of which 78 per cent is imbibed as wine, mostly taken with meals. In the United States, 40 million men and 28 million women consume alcoholic beverages; 5.8 liters of alcohol are imbibed per person per year. Middle-aged persons are more likely to drink than persons under twenty or over fifty. Urban populations drink more than rural populations, with the exception of the wine-producing regions. It is generally believed that certain professionals, such as clergymen, teachers, and welfare workers, are more likely to be abstinent than others; creative artists, actors, musicians, journalists, salesmen, and housepainters have the reputation of drinking more than the average population. In the United States, there are more abstainers among Protestants than among Catholics, and least among Jews; in Moslem cultures, drinking is forbidden. Drinking habits in the social classes differ according to social pattern, kind of drink, and participation by the sexes. In the upper and lower classes, men and women drink; in the lower-middle class, women are more frequently abstinent. The cocktail parties of the "smart set" and the drinking of the unskilled laborer after a monotonous day of hard work are worlds apart. According to world-wide statistics, drinking in all cultures and classes seems to be increasing.[31] Greater affluence may be an explanatory factor.

It is important to remember that only a fraction of drinkers become alcoholics, although many more have serious problems associated with drinking. In the United States, about 47 million, or roughly 7 per cent of the drinking population, are estimated to be alcoholics. International statistics, which are not on very firm ground, suggest that alcoholism has the highest rate in the United States, with France second and Sweden third.[42] Alcoholism is low in certain cultures, such as in Moslem, Italian, and Chinese-American cultures; Italians are accustomed to drinking wine at mealtimes, but the alcoholism rate is low. In the United States, Protestants have the highest proportion of alcoholics; there are fewer alcoholics among Catholics, and Jews have the lowest rate of all. It is of interest that Orthodox Jews drink regularly from an early age but rarely become alcoholics. In all cultures, male alcoholics outnumber females, although an increase in female alcoholics has been noted in the past decade. The percentage of single, divorced, and widowed alcoholics is relatively high; and the majority of alcoholics is found in the middle-age range. Alcoholism is found in all classes; in certain subcultures, excessive drinking may become a prestige symbol.

It has been estimated that, in the United States, 2 to 4 per cent of manpower-hours are lost because of excessive drinking. The cost of the abuse of alcohol in the United States has been estimated at 779 million dollars per year. Alcoholism lowers life expectancy from 61.3 to 51.1 years. In working with a population of alcoholics, one is clinically impressed with the disappearance of patients due to fatal illness and suicide. Confirmed alcoholics are responsible for fewer traffic accidents than intoxicated nonalcoholics, perhaps because many have lost their drivers' licenses. The disruption of family life by alcoholism, with its disastrous effects on marriage and child-rearing, cannot, of course, be expressed in cold figures. In spite of such grim evidence of the psychosocial consequences of alcoholism, for some rare individuals excessive drinking and even chronic alcoholism may be a relatively benign solution, protecting them from crime, perversion, and insanity.

Classification of Alcoholism

It is obvious that medical descriptions of various forms of alcoholic behavior disorder are contingent on special viewpoints. We intervene when patients are brought to us and accordingly tend to describe what we most frequently encounter. This restricted viewpoint has been further confounded by a host of divergent theories but a paucity of longitudinal observations to specify and justify them. For a comprehensive understanding, a truly behavioral description of the various alcoholisms will have to be linked with both biological and psychosocial factors, which operate through time.[25] At one juncture, psychosocial factors may be predominantly important; at another, biological factors may play the central roles.

Types of Alcoholism

Based on a lifelong study, Jellinek proposes a division of alcoholism into several types.[16] Of all clinical classifications of alcoholism, it is the one that deserves to be taken most seriously. *Alpha Alcoholism* is characterized by excessive and inappropriate drinking without any loss of control or the inability to abstain. There are consequences of such drinking, for example, social and occupational difficulties and impairment of physical health, but in general there is no progression of the disorder. In *Beta Alcoholism,* physical diseases such as cirrhosis, gastritis, and neuritis occur. The nutritional habits of these patients are faulty. There is, however, no clear-cut evidence of psychological or physical dependence. The most important and serious type is *Gamma Alcoholism.* It corresponds to popular concepts of alcoholism and is characterized by a progressive course, physical dependence, often acquired tolerance, and, invariably, psychological dependence with an inability to control drinking.

Jellinek also described other types. *Delta Alcoholics,* encountered particularly in wine-drinking countries, develop tolerance and withdrawal symptoms. They appear unable to abstain but can control the quantity of alcohol ingested. The *Epsilon Alcoholic,* in the psychiatric literature, is often refered to as the dipsomaniac who goes on episodic long binges without apparent cause and may have long intervals of abstinence. Among the various patterns of drinking are spree-drinkers, the fiesta and convention drinker, and a number of drinking types, which differ according to ethnic and social status from Skid Row to Wall Street, and from Russia to Chile. The role of alcohol in overcoming inhibitions, isolation, withdrawal, and in promoting group identity, and the importance of psychosocial factors in reinforcing these patterns may differ among these types.

There are some special reactions related to alcohol intake which may be described as *complicated intoxication,* in contrast to simple intoxication.[4] One of the reactions is *alcohol intolerance,* characterized by an acute excitatory phase with clouding of consciousness similar in some aspects to neurological and behavioral manifestations of anesthesia produced by volatile anesthetics.[4] Unlike ether, however, alcohol produces progressive diffuse slowing of the EEG, which, in general, correlates with the extent of behavioral intoxication; blood levels of alcohol, especially in chronic intoxication, do not necessarily correlate with behavioral and EEG changes. This dissociation is not the case with volatile anesthetics. In general, intoxications produced by different agents are arrived at through different pathways and may show consequential differences at a number of points in the sequence of neurobehavioral events. Among persons who show signs and symptoms of acute intoxication after minimal quantities of alcohol are epileptics, mental deficients, patients with brain damage, hysterical personalities, and also some seemingly normal persons. Often, deviating from their normal standards, they quarrel, fight, and exhibit unacceptable sexual behavior with minimal intake of alcohol. Memory for such behavior is blurred, but complete amnesia is rare. *Pathological intoxication* is characterized by sudden severe excitation, clouding of consciousness, and an occurrence of typical intoxication with the addition of antisocial, aggressive, and sexual behavior for which the patient has a complete or almost complete amnesia; the episode is followed by sleep. The extent to which a cerebral disposition exists for the reaction is unclear. The uncommon patient who has commit-

Phases of Alcoholism

ted violent, aggressive crimes during such episodes is usually bland, timid, and constricted. The crimes may be understood as explosive eruptions of repressed drives that had been checked by lifelong characterological defenses and were discharged unexpectedly during intoxication. The existence of the syndrome is not universally recognized.

For the Gamma Alcoholic—the prototype of alcoholism—Jellinek distinguishes definite phases of development of the disorder. In the *prealcoholic symptomatic phase,* the patient drinks socially; but, as drinking reduces tension significantly, he starts drinking daily and excessively. He may have to increase his consumption in order to obtain relief. Members of Alcoholics Anonymous, given often to apt slogans, remark that one drink is too many and twenty drinks aren't enough. They describe the motive in this phase as drinking for courage and to avoid internal or external demands. In the *prodromal phase*, blackouts occur. It becomes obvious that the patient needs a drug rather than a beverage. He suffers not only physiological, but "psychological hangovers," characterized by depression, remorse, and guilt. Sneaking and gulping drinks are characteristic. Lies about drinking and, more crucially, a system of alibis to explain away the drinking, are commonplace. These patterns may proceed to drinking "eye-openers" in the morning and to missing work because of depression and hangover. In the *crucial phase*, there is a definite loss of control over drinking. Episodes of solitary drinking, of more-or-less uncontrolled binges, may occur; so-called benders, social decline, a constant hangover, "the shakes," a sequence of apologies, lies, and further drinking may herald this phase. The alcoholic has not only got into serious difficulties but also has suffered a marked loss of self-esteem. His life is organized to protect the liquor supply, and unreasonable, almost paranoid resentments and childish projection of blame, nameless anxieties, enhanced dependency, and reactive anger come to dominate behavior. Intellectual and ethical deterioration are apparent. The patient has slipped socially; he may proceed to drink anything he can get and associate with inferior companions. Acquired tolerance is marked and may be lost; metalcoholic disorders and behavior disorders may supervene. Usually it takes ten to twelve years for a Gamma Alcoholic to reach the last disastrous phase. In work, persons with drinking problems may be covered for long periods by alibis (the wife phoning in to report "absence due to a cold") or by loyalty of friends who do his work and do not report his ailment. Such pre-alcoholic behavior may occur for a long time until management is faced with a highly placed employee (or physicians with a trusted colleague) who is now obviously impaired and intrenched in his crucial phase. Similarly, daytime drinking—taking a nip or cocktails—among housewives is recognized as an increasingly common pre-alcoholic pattern, which may develop into other phases or may be hidden for years, since the consequences of drinking may be less apparently disrupting than in business.

Personality Patterns in Alcoholism

Is there a personality pattern which predisposes to alcoholism? Oskar M. Diethelm denied this, but many clinical investigators are inclined to the opposite view.[9] The question is much like the broader problem of whether an addictive personality exists. In our opinion, it is not possible to reduce the personality traits of alcoholics to one basic type. The general descriptive attributes of the personality of the alcohol addict include, according to Israel Zwerling and Milton Rosenbaum: (1) schizoid traits; (2) depressive traits; (3) dependent traits; (4) hostile and self-destructive impulses; and (5) sexual immaturity.[44] J. Levine mentioned the sexual immaturity of alcoholics; latent homosexual strivings are notable.[23] Karl Menninger found marked self-destructive tendencies.[26] When alcoholism was rarer in women than it is today, the psychopathology of alcoholic women was generally found to be more severe than that of alcoholic men. Ben Karpman, in extensive clinical studies, noted the existence of masculine strivings and identification in female alcoholics.[18] Many male alcoholics seem inclined to marry older, maternal women, and a group of female alcoholics tends to prefer younger, passive men whom they try to dominate. Our own clinical observations confirm that alcoholics, whether shy or gregarious, generally are inhibited and passive persons with a great yearning for love, recognition, and security. The infantile nature of their sexual, dependent, and aggressive needs often makes acceptable gratification difficult; they attempt, usually in vain, to overcome their frustrations and conflicts in alcohol.

Causes of Drinking

Many factors play a role in the etiology of alcoholism, and it is very difficult to disentangle the web of predisposing, precipitating, and contributing factors. Psychologists have viewed abnormal drinking as a form of learned behavior; psychoanalysts have pointed to unconscious, oral, and homosexual conflicts; sociologists and cultural anthopologists stress cultural pressures and prohibitions or the lack of such taboos; biologically oriented investigators point to constitutional and biochemical causes. The fact is, we cannot state with any precision or authority either for the individual patient or groups of patients why they develop into alcoholics, although we have considerable knowledge about the conditions under which such a development takes place. If it were not sufficiently clear from study of other disorders, behavior disorders associated with drugs make it evident that there are sequences through time in which multiple factors differentially operate. A biological factor—the drug—can create states in which there are reactions that in turn generate psychological responses; these may then lead to both biological and psychological consequences. The chief problem is not to confuse the effects of a drug, which generally produces a certain uniform pattern such as regression or orality, with predisposing causes.

Jorge Mardones, R. Onfray, and B. E. Onfray demonstrated that rats, maintained on a diet free of thermolabile elements of the Vitamin B complex increased their alcohol intake by self-selection.[24] When given vitamins, the animals decreased their alcohol consumption. Roger J. Williams, working on the general problem of biochemical individuality, confirmed and developed their findings further; he considered alcoholism a genetic, metabolic deficiency disease and was able to develop strains of rodents with differential preferences.[41] In his view, partial "genetic blocks" lead to a diminished potentiality for necessary biochemical responses and hence to an augmented requirement for the intake of nutritional substances—for example, alcohol. Williams, however, does not explain why such a genetic deficiency becomes clinically manifest at a certain time. His studies were based in part on preference tests; D. Lester and Greenberg found that vitamin-deficient rats did not choose alcohol if they were given a sugar solution as an alternative.[22] In general, it has not been possible to create alcohol addiction in animals, although behavioral effects of alcohol can be experimentally studied. Perhaps man, with his more complicated neural apparatus, his wide array of alternative mechanisms for adaptation, his dependence on symbolic systems for finely attuned and sustained performance, is more vulnerable than lower animals to the changes in experience and perception induced by drugs and hence psychologically predisposed to developing psychological dependence and addictive patterns of behavior. Rather than a prisoner of the drug, he is a prisoner of his heightened responsiveness to the drug.

In any event, the inordinately costly behavior generated by a presumed genetic mechanism in alcoholism is not easy to explain. Psychosocial factors would appear to us crucial to account for the behavioral pattern in alcoholism. As in other such problems, it is easier (although not necessarily more accurate) to view the biochemical fault as "taxing" the ease with which psychosocial factors could operate (for example, attempts to stop drinking) than to imagine biological factors generating anything as specific as sustained alcohol intake. Once such intake patterns are established, physiological dependence, of course, plays a much clearer (though not psychologically insurmountable) role in sustaining drinking behavior. Biological factors—sensitivity (not allergy, as Alcoholics Anonymous calls it) could also make the establishment of a drinking pattern more probable. The chief reinforcement in drinking, on which most drinkers and observers agree, is some form of relief of tension, whether this is achieved through specific pharmacological effects or a general psychological regression and shift of focus.

There is wide agreement that patterns of drinking behavior are not inherited but transmitted through culture and child-rearing practices. The alcoholic undoubtedly learns to reduce tension and shifts his field of perception and action by consuming alcohol in spite of the various punishments and taboos inherent in his environment. A learning approach is appealing, and there have been recent attempts to explain, in some detail, the sequence of events that lead to chronic alcoholism.[20] In animal experiments, alcohol appears to reduce conflict and to become a source of reinforcement facilitating the expression of basic drives. One thing is amply clear: alcohol is a reinforcement much more potent than the drastically punitive consequences; thus, alcoholics have to muster far more determination than is generally appreciated before this pattern will be given up. How such reinforcement works is not known. Does the alcoholic drink to become intoxicated, to experience relief, to avoid withdrawal, or to avoid consequences and demands? Does drinking induce a partial regression, and does this psychological state create its own secondary rewards?

The research literature has provided no solid evidence for any personality variable or set of variables predisposing to alcoholism. Broken homes occur frequently in the history of alcoholics, and disturbed relationships with one or both parents have been found. In families of alcoholics, occurrence of alcoholism is frequent, and identification with the alcoholic parent can undoubtedly play a role in generating alcoholism in children. The alcoholic man who remembers hating his father's treatment of the mother and his drunken violence toward the children, or the daughter of such a marriage who nurses her own alcoholic husband, are examples. We have already mentioned the unspecific family constellation of a weak and undisciplined father and a domineering and seductive mother in all types of addictions and in many other behavior disorders. Frequently, we have encountered not only the needs of a patient to be nursed but also his considerable aptitude in finding a mate whose integrity and nursing capacity grows as the patient becomes more of a problem. Yet, the very circumstances engendered by drinking would naturally foster such a pattern. We are also struck by the frequency with which we encounter histories of excessive intimacy of the alcoholic and his mother, in patients who had to care physically for a sick mother, for example. Nursing and being nursed are, then, focal patterns observed in some patients.

Although we must rely on conjectures about the early predisposing factors to excessive drinking, we are on firmer ground in studying precipitating stresses that produce drinking. With many patients, it is possible to pinpoint preconscious and unconscious rebellion against an ambivalently loved person, or anger over a real or imagined frustration, slight, or humiliation as precipitating stimuli. In some cases, patients escape from sexual temptation by drinking excessively, particularly if their desires are infantile or forbidden, mobilize too much aggression, or cast the patient in a passive role that he cannot accept. Intoxication reduces, at least temporarily, the anxiety and guilt these aggressive and sexual acts or desires generate.

There can be little question that sociocultural factors contribute to the etiology of chronic alcoholism. D. Horton, after analyzing drinking habits in primitive societies, concluded that excessive drinking is related to subsistence anxiety over hazards of living, failure of crops, and the like.[14] Robert F. Bales explained the moderation of such minorities as Jews and Chinese-Americans by their need to avoid scandal and persecution.[2] Religious taboos and feelings of superiority to drinking groups undoubtedly also enter into some of these cultural attitudes. Our current multifactorial approach to the problem of alcoholism is defensible even if it does not permit easy conclusions. The clinical psychiatrist must be satisfied with an approximate understanding of the many forces at work in the individual alcoholic patient. He must distinguish as clearly as possible between predisposing, precipitating, and contributory events that produce excessive drinking and, in some individuals, lead in lawful sequence to the different forms of chronic alcoholism.

General Principles of Treatment

Treatment of patients with alcohol problems can be divided into therapies of states of intoxication and withdrawal states and therapies of habitual excessive drinking. The former are largely medical; the latter, re-educational and rehabilitative. As to the individual patient, a combination of physical, psychological, and social measures is usually needed.[1] Note that this should put the psychiatrist into a very favorable position to assume responsibility for the therapy of these patients; in reality, however, psychiatrists have treated patients with alcohol problems only grudgingly and with undue pessimism. The psychotherapeutically oriented psychiatrist prefers a patient who is capable of gaining insight into his problems, or applying this insight, and of controlling his impulses. The alcoholic is not such a patient; typically, he is more motivated to drink than to abstain and is quite capable of provoking his therapist by his aggression, supersensitivity, clinging dependence, and, most of all, by his relapses. Yet, with these patients, one cannot engage in a power struggle or in moralistic preachments about drinking; the realistic support of a therapist who cannot be manipulated and calmly sets limits is required.

Although there have been many published reports that cite statistics on cure and improvement by various methods, the data are notably unreliable, and we have only a very rudimentary knowledge of the efficiency of different methods. The tentative consensus is that about one-fourth of chronic alcoholics can be greatly helped (and stay sober from two to four years);[6] another one-half can be helped to some degree. Only future work with carefully matched and controlled populations will provide more accurate data.

GOALS OF TREATMENT There are three levels of aspiration in the treatment of alcoholism: (1) The specific treatment of withdrawal states and alcohol poisoning, which will be discussed in the sections dealing with the nosological entities. (2) At the next level, a therapist attempts to help the patient stay sober without any explicit attempt to change his personality. (3) Finally, there is exploratory and clarifying psychotherapy to aid the patient with his neurotic problems. For many alcoholics, maintenance of sobriety is, for all practical purposes, the ultimate aim. A relationship with a professional person, a friend, an employer, such social groups as clubs, churches, and, most of all, Alcoholics Anonymous can be a major resource for the patient stopping drinking or maintaining sobriety. We know many therapists who enjoy a social drink and who have a moralistic—rather than realistic—vision of mental strength through therapy; they strive to help the patient to drink socially and to "analyze" any counterphobic tendencies against drinking, which, in fact, are realistic and helpful to one who has experienced the dangers of addiction. Any reasonable device the patient employs to stop drinking is useful, since the resumption of drinking exponentially increases the chance for a loss of painfully attained gains. One eighty-year-old former alcoholic told us why he did not take even one drink: "It might be okay, but I don't know; and I *do* know I can't afford to gamble." The regressive "pull" of the drug effect is not confined to an evening's fling; it engulfs and transforms the patient's total way of living. Recovered alcoholics don't just "stop" drinking. They describe themselves as stopping drinking each day "for today"; they take a "step at a time" in order not to intoxicate themselves with excessive ambition. For a few, something like a conversion—a total shift of attitude—appears to accompany a "decision" to abstain.

Thus, the knowledgeable therapist knows that there are more crucial problems to discuss than whether the patient theoretically can or cannot drink; this issue surely has been settled through ample demonstrations before the patient arrived for treatment. The therapist sees the patient as an individual in deep trouble, a person with deeply wounded pride. Alcoholic patients are easily hurt by slights (the therapist is three minutes late or changes a fixed appointment) and, with low frustration tolerance, give up easily. The schemes and dreams of the alcoholic, his "future plans," and his capacity for wishful fantasy cannot be underestimated, nor should his "resolutions" be solicited or regarded as realistic. A casually reported casual drink may signal that a consequential decision has once more been avoided. The therapist does not then condemn; nor is he lulled; he indicates, rather, curiosity and his awareness of a continuing problem. Tolerance of the poor morale, easy frustration, and defeat of these often gifted but infantile persons and, most of all, patience, are required. The habits of being accessible to help and of remembering that realistic control over drinking requires some humility and help must be continuously reinforced, whether by therapy, conditioning, group or chemical procedures.

Individual or group psychotherapy, in the narrow sense of the word, not only helps the patient to find ways to overcome drinking but may also serve as a means for working with the range of personal problems that arise. Harry M. Tiebout, treating alcoholics and studying the therapeutic process implicit in Alcoholics Anonymous, stresses the need for patients to "hit bottom" to be truly motivated; for a satisfactory therapeutic relationship, he feels the patient must undergo some "ego reduction" and surrender ominipotent and magical notions.[35] There are no specific methods particularly suited for the psychotherapy of alcoholics. Experiences with classical psychoanalysis have not been encouraging, and relatively few analysts are willing to treat chronic alcoholics. A supportive relationship, with attention to principal current conflicts and with attempts to restore the patient's low self-esteem, is more apt to succeed. It is not possible to set therapeutic goals at the beginning of treatment. Alcoholics, once their alcohol intake is stopped, are individuals with widely different problems. Only after therapist and patient have worked together for some time can decisions be made about the aims of therapy, and the treatment of neurotic problems is no different than in the nonalcoholic. But in terms of the problems engendered by addiction, there do seem to be characteristic attitudes to be worked through. If all goes well, the patient comes to realize how, under the mask of shyness, he domineers, pushes, but fears his own drives. The high demands and the dreams of glory of the alcoholic, as well as his infantile bossiness and imperviousness—all recognized as very much a part of the *inner* life of even the overtly shy alcoholic—can be modified as the patient learns he can get along without all the answers, without being always in control. Quite commonly, as the patient improves, he reasserts a notion that he can run his life according to his wishes, and this may lead to relapse.

GROUP THERAPIES As a rule, group therapy of alcoholics is superior to individual therapy. Many alcoholics, though inhibited, are gregarious, like to help their cosufferers, and are stimulated by shared experiences. For this reason, it is more advantageous to treat groups made up exclusively of alcoholics than mixed groups. For many therapists, groups of alcoholics are also more comfortable; some patients, at least, make progress, which mitigates the sharp disappointment felt by the individual therapist and patient after a relapse. As the number of therapists is small and the number of alcoholics great, group therapy is also a more economic approach. Yet relatively few mental health workers are trained to conduct such group therapy. The important group therapies are carried out not by professional workers but by alcoholics themselves.

The most significant endeavor of this type is the work of *Alcoholics Anonymous*. This self-help group of alcoholics was partly inspired by a religious sect, the Oxford Group. It is, as its founder, W. William, put it, on the middle ground between medicine and religion,[40] nonsectarian, but stressing reliance on an individually defined God as "a power greater than ourselves." It attempts to help the individual alcoholic and also promotes the acceptance by society of alcoholics as sick persons. The organization provides aid to alcoholics in the form of emergency service and continuous contact through individual and group relationships.[29] If an alcoholic who feels the urge to drink or has started on a binge calls for help, Alcoholics Anonymous can often offer direct personal contact. Older abstinent members come to the aid of new alcoholic members and provide opportunities for identification. In open and closed meetings, problems of drinkers are discussed in a rather permissive, informal fashion, which is much akin to the atmosphere of certain types of group psychotherapy; such meetings are definitely not prayer meetings, as some of our cloistered colleagues carelessly imagine. Alcoholics Anonymous, through its religious orientation, has been well accepted by denominational groups, especially Protestants; the movement is powerful in the United States and has also taken root in other countries.

FAMILY THERAPY AND REHABILITATION Relationships in the families of alcoholics are usually disturbed before the onset of drinking and are further aggravated by drinking; it is, therefore, imperative to estabish therapeutic contact with family members. Relatives of alcoholics may need help because of their own pathology; they invariably need guidance to become helpful to the patient. Without family therapy, chances for successful treatment of alcoholics are seriously diminished. In studying family relationships, specific conflicts and alliances can often be discovered, which upset the patient and add to his difficulties in keeping from drinking. Spouses often play such a role unconsciously; although they are overtly helpful and seriously concerned about the patient's fate, they give in, provide liquor, bail out their mates, and, without help, generally cannot refrain from neurotic involvements. Programs of rehabilitation of alcoholics are also carried out in industrial clinics.[27] Industry, business, and the armed forces have begun to realize that the serious problem of alcoholism in these organizations is best met by an active therapeutic approach.

Hospitalization of Alcoholic Patients

A person with simple intoxication may need a little friendliness and patience (not easy to get), perhaps a bed, and possibly aspirin, antacids, and nonalcoholic beverages for his hangover. The intoxicated alcoholic needs more than such assistance. Withdrawal states may become complicated psychiatric and medical problems requiring measures that can be supplied only in hospitals. The alcoholic also benefits from hospitalization because it removes him from the stresses of an environment that has produced the need to drink excessively. It permits him to establish positive relationships in a protective environment during a period of abstinence. It does not ensure, however, that the wish to stop drinking is truly enhanced. Prolonged hospitalization (beyond three to six months) is not indicated; patients experience it as punishment. Sooner or later, an alcoholic has to fight his problems in the arena of his everyday life.

BIOLOGICAL TREATMENT OF ALCOHOLISM Many alcoholic patients are generally undernourished and suffer from specific vitamin deficiencies. The therapist must determine whether patients are receiving a calorically adequate diet containing the necessary vitamins; in cases of deficiency, vitamins must be administered in adequate doses. There is no evidence that other specific diets remedying hypothetical metabolic deficiencies are of therapeutic value. Feeding alcoholics with proper care also has a psychological impact in this orally deprived group.

Many tense, anxious, and depressed chronic alcoholics who are not accessible to intensive psychotherapy are helped materially by such drugs as chlordiazepoxide, the different phenothiazines, and, to a lesser degree, by imipramine. For nighttime sedation, chloral hydrate is preferable to barbiturates with their strong addictive properties. Both physicians and alcoholics have begun to warn us about the addictive pattern of intake of these psychotropic drugs; many feel that any drug will be employed by the alcoholic for the same defensive and avoidance purposes as alcohol and that the best therapy is activity by the patient to stay sober and a minimum of pharmacological agents. There have been reports that one or two large doses of LSD-25 in a supportive and specially prepared environment can lead to a profound change of attitude about drinking (in what amounts to a conversion).[8] The drug enhances the urge to communicate for a few hours of its action and, because of the greater difficulty in maintaining secure controls, the need to rely on the surroundings for structure and support is facilitated if not compelled. Thus, LSD and related drugs are "cultogenic" drugs—binding groups together—and to date this factor of the need for environmental structuring through support and "explanations" has been overlooked in the enthusiastic reports of success. Seemingly the patient *needs* to agree and adopt "beliefs" in this setting, which, however, provides no checks in reality for mutually engendered enthusiasms. Adequate controlled studies of such treatment have not yet appeared.

CONDITIONING THERAPY WITH EMETICS Since 1912, conditioning procedures have been employed with apomorphine or emetine to produce nausea and aversion in alcoholics when they reach for a drink.[13] The technique consists of administering an emetic followed by the offer of the favorite drink. The administration of the emetic must be timed to ensure that nausea quickly follows the alcoholic euphoria. This treatment is administered daily to individual patients or groups until, after several weeks, the patients become nauseated when they merely see or smell alcohol; the treatment is then stopped. We see no evidence that such procedures are generally effective, although they may prove useful as adjuncts to a continuing therapy. The popularity of forcefully unpleasant conditioning therapies probably attests to the formidable problems and disappointments inherent in therapy of alcoholism. The temptation for the patient—to drink—is dramatically evident both to the physician and the patient (as hidden neurotic temptations are not); obviously, if in "one-trial" learning the alcoholic were to develop an aversion to drink, one could begin to work with other problems. We wonder if lack of marked success does not breed ever-new efforts at deconditioning with new drugs of equally little promise.

DISULFIRAM THERAPY J. Hald, E. Jacobsen, and V. Larsen discovered the intraorganismic incompatibility of alcohol and tetraethylthiuram disulfide (disulfiram, or Antabuse), a chemical used in the rubber industry.[12] When it is ingested simultaneously with alcohol, patients develop a characteristic reddening of face, neck, and conjunctiva, as well as headache, palpitations, and lowering of blood pressure with faintness, sweating, and nausea.[17] Vomiting, chest pain, and dyspnea are usually harmless. The biochemical process underlying these reactions involves an accumulation of acetaldehyde, because of a block of aldehyde dehydrogenases; there is also a block of the enzyme converting dopamine to norepinephrine. Jacobsen and Larsen developed their observations into a carefully worked out therapeutic procedure. After medical examination to exclude cardiac decompensation and severe liver disease, patients receive 0.5 gm. disulfiram by mouth for three days. On the fourth day, they receive a drink containing 10 cc. of alcohol. This gives the therapist and the patient an opportunity to observe the disulfiram-alcohol reaction. The ordinary maintenance dose of disulfiram varies between 0.15 gm. and 0.25 gm. and needs to be carefully supervised. Hugo Solms, who used this method extensively, does not consider it an aversion method but a crutch, which, together with psychosocial approaches, enables the patient to resist the temptation to drink.[34] It has been said that disulfiram acts as a chemical policeman. When the patient drinks, he not only feels most uncomfortable, but he also betrays his indiscretion to others by his red face. This treatment method, without any other attempt to educate or rehabilitate the drinker is, of course, entirely symptomatic. One difficulty is that of inducing the patient to take the drug regularly; this may be almost as difficult as keeping him from drinking. The method is not without danger; apart from cardiovascular complications, convulsions and toxic psychoses have been observed. At present, disulfiram therapy is still used extensively, particularly in Europe, but (like most therapies, even the good ones) with less enthusiasm than after the initial reports.

PREVENTIVE MEASURES The passage (in 1919) of legal prohibition of the production and sale of alcoholic beverages in the United States and its repeal (in 1933) after evident failure to solve the problem was an important step in stimulating the search for more rational rather than punitive approaches. Milder measures, such as high taxation and controls on time and place of sale, are now employed in part to discourage excessive drinking. More promising are educational measures and the establishment of community facilities for treatment, such as have been organized effectively in Czechoslovakia.[32] So far, most programs are recommended without the benefit of planned experiments. It is hoped that a more scientific approach to the problem will lead to better-designed preventive methods and to more effective social and legal implementations.

Physical Illness in Chronic Alcoholism

In a word, chronic alcoholics are a sick lot. Their physical health is significantly impaired, and their life expectancy is ten years below the average. There follows a brief resumé of the most important medical illnesses found in alcoholics; for a more detailed discussion, the reader is referred to textbooks of internal medicine and neurology.

Chronic alcoholics frequently suffer from acute and chronic gastritis. Gastric pain, nausea and vomiting, and anorexia are common symptoms, which, in turn, produce malnutrition, underweight, and a disposition to succumb to acute and chronic infections. Alcoholics rarely suffer from full-blown Vitamin B deficiencies, but mild syndromes are frequent. Half of the cases with Laennec's cirrhosis are chronic alcoholics.

Peripheral neuropathies (probably related to nutritional deficiencies) of one or several nerves with flaccid paralysis or weakness, absent deep tendon reflexes, anesthesias and hyperthesias, and paresthesias are found. The most frequent neuropathy involves the peroneal nerve, with a resulting dropfoot and steppage gait; neuropathies of the large nerves of the upper extremities are less frequent. Pressure lesions of the radial nerve, the so-called Saturday-night palsy, are common when alcoholics awake from binges. Treatment of alcoholic neuropathies consists of bed rest, splinting of foot- or wrist-drop, physical therapy and exercise, high caloric diet, and high doses of vitamins of the B complex.

Alcoholics who are not epileptics rarely develop convulsive seizures, even if there is considerable brain damage. The so-called rum fits are in all likelihood related to an abstinence syndrome. In some epileptics, seizures are produced by alcohol intake; the mechanism is probably less related to the direct effect of alcohol than to the temporary water retention produced by alcohol. In any case, epileptics must strictly refrain from drinking alcohol, especially distilled liquor.

Alcohol Poisoning

The difference between a heavy and a lethal dose of alcohol is small, and alcohol in high doses is a dangerous central nervous system poison. Symptoms of anesthesia appear rapidly and without warning. Shallow respiration; tachycardia; hypotension; pupillary dilation; sluggish tendon reflexes, which become weak and disappear; and pyramidal signs are observed; death is caused by paralysis of respiratory centers. In the differential diagnosis, diabetic and hepatic coma are considered; poisoning is based on alcohol odor of the breath and laboratory tests of stomach contents, blood alcohol level, and, when obtainable, the history of excessive alcohol intake. In patients with alcoholic coma, it is important not to overlook head injuries and respiratory diseases. Therapy consists of intravenous administration of analeptics; occasionally insulin, to aid carbohydrate metabolism, maintenance of respiration, and fluid balance; high doses of Vitamin B complex, and preventive measures against pneumonia. Dialysis has been employed in extreme instances.

Alcohol Withdrawal

After withdrawal of alcohol in severe alcoholics there is a continuum of symptoms, which range from mild to severe. In alcoholics, tremor, weakness, hyperhidrosis, hyperreflexia, gastrointestinal symptoms, and occasional elevation of temperature are observed for twenty-four to seventy-two hours following the end of a bout of heavy drinking. When convulsions occur, they are generally noted between twenty-four and forty-eight hours after withdrawal; the incidence in mild and severe withdrawal is fairly constant—about 10 per cent.[28] The most important withdrawal syndromes, delirium tremens and alcohol hallucination, are taken up in the next section. The drinking and eating patterns preceding withdrawal cannot as yet be directly related to the type of severity of the withdrawal reaction; hence, no true prevention of withdrawal reactions exists. In practice, we recommend that withdrawal in severe alcoholics be carried out under medical supervision with attention to nutrition, water and mineral metabolism, and proper sedation. It is recommended that such patients be given paraldehyde (15–40 cc. daily) or chlordiazepoxide (up to 200 mgm. daily) for several days. Prompt treatment of alcohol withdrawal prevents the development of the more serious syndromes.[36] For mild (but not severe) cases, phenothiazine treatment is quite effective; prolonged withdrawal states should not be treated with these drugs.[36]

Metalcoholic Psychoses

Of particular interest to the psychiatrist are certain brain diseases and severe behavior disorders that occur in alcoholic patients. They have been referred to as metalcoholic psychoses.[34] Some of them, such as delirium tremens and acute alcoholic hallucinosis, are highly specific withdrawal states; others, such as the dysmnesic syndromes, paranoid reactions, and intellectual deterioration, are unspecific sequelae of alcohol abuse.

Delirium Tremens

Delirium tremens is the most common of the metalcoholic diseases. John Romano has reviewed early contributions to the study of this disorder, which was named by Thomas Sutton in 1813 but astutely and accurately described before him.[30] The incidence of the disorder is difficult to determine, since, among other reasons, some of the symptoms lie on a continuum of responses to other, milder forms of alcohol withdrawal. In addition, treatment agencies differ in the readiness with which patients with varying degrees of withdrawal syndromes are admitted for treatment. There is no clear relation between duration or quantity of intake and incidence of delirium tremens, although it certainly occurs most frequently in heavy drinkers of long standing.

Although the typical delirium may appear to have an abrupt onset, there is usually evidence of prodromal symptoms. Some patients appear to attempt to counteract withdrawal syndromes by alcohol intake for a period of weeks prior to the occurrence of delirium. An increasing tremulousness—"the shakes"—and the appearance of illusions, insomnia, restlessness, watchfulness, fear and dread, accompanied by diminution of appetite and bouts of excessive perspiration may be noted. These symptoms also dominate the full-blown delirium, and many patients describe themselves as "now unable to come back to reality." George L. Engel and J. Romano[10], in contrast to M. Victor and R. D. Adams,[37] doubt that delirium tremens is a true delirium because the characteristic EEG changes are absent. With the full-blown syndrome, patients are invariably restless and disoriented for time and place. They appear oblivious to the environment for long periods, assuming they are in their customary settings; occupational hallucinations are common and may range from simple explanations concocted to answer the physician's questions to vivid and elaborated experiences. Visual, tactile, and, rarely, auditory hallucinations are encountered; micropsia or macropsia, optical illusions, hallucinations of small animals such as vermin occur, the latter frequently associated with altered sensation of the skin. There is a general tremor, which is noted both at rest and in motion. Even in the absence of infection, elevations of temperature are regularly observed, and pulse and respiration are accelerated. Due to sweating and tachypnea, patients can become dehydrated. Many suffer from polyneuritis, and about 10 per cent have convulsive seizures. Apart from the typical tremors, neurological examination is normal, and the EEG in most cases shows no pathological changes. Severe physical symptoms are generally denied by patients; some disregard even painful wounds and fractures. Mark Twain gave a very accurate and vivid description of delirium tremens in *Huckleberry Finn.*

There is considerable variation both in the intensity and course of the disease. The first episode may or may not lead to a full-blown syndrome. The typical delirium lasts from one to four days, although milder cases, punctuated by long lucid intervals, may be protracted for weeks. The delirium often ends with the so-called critical sleep. In some patients, a dysmnesic syndrome may follow delirium tremens. When sleep does not occur, patients continue to exhaust themselves; the temperature becomes elevated, the pulse rapid, and signs of vascular collapse appear. There is a mortality rate of 4 to 15 per cent, depending on treatment and population, and this has varied little since the turn of the century.

Douglas W. Thomas and Daniel X. Freedman[36] found that an assessment of severity of alcohol withdrawal could be reliably made by recording tremulousness, disorientation, hallucinations, fear, agitation, eating, and sleeping; most critical and differentiating were the pulse rate and temperature. Mild delirium was marked by diaphoresis; a pulse of 100–120/min., and a temperature of 99°–100° F. defined moderate delirium tremens in highly restless patients; in severe cases, the pulse was above 120/min. and temperature 100° F. or more. These signs, noted on admission, not only predicted severity but also occurred in medically uncomplicated fatal cases and appeared in every fatal case. *Pathological findings* are sparse; some authors report cortical and subcortical cell degeneration; others, only perivascular hemorrhages and exudates, particularly in the central gray and the basal ganglia.

Victor and Adams found in virtually all their cases that the outbreak of delirium tremens was preceded by abrupt cessation of drinking.[37] However, not all heavy drinkers who stop develop the syndrome,[25] and it is not known if predisposition exists. Further, the syndrome occurs in the presence of alcohol intake, and, even with treatment—which is suppressive, dampening rather than abolishing symptoms—the disorder to some extent follows a self-contained course. Withdrawal is a major but not sufficient causal factor.

The *therapy* of delirium tremens has changed relatively little over the years. The most important steps are still: adequate sedation with the aim of preventing exhaustion of the agitated or debilitated patient and of inducing sleep. Paraldehyde in high daily doses from 10 to 40 cc. may be given orally with nursing skill and patience; intramuscular or rectal administration may be occasionally necessary, but is not desirable. The drug has a high margin of safety and is definitely preferable to barbiturates, phenothiazines, and reserpine. Paraldehyde, it should be recalled, may produce sufficient ataxia to mask recovery from the delirium. Perhaps the best current therapy is immediate treatment with chloridiazepoxide, using intramuscular doses of 50–100 mg. i.m. followed by 50 mg. at intervals, up to 200 mg. daily. Although some patients must be restrained—if proper nursing care is not available—every attempt must be made to restrain as little as possible and for the shortest possible time. Prolonged restraint is definitely harmful; in animals such treatment clearly enhances stress and, in delirium of man, it may increase the heightened sympathetic response. Proper nursing and proper sedation can nearly always make restraint unnecessary; newly recovered patients can help to solicit the cooperation of sicker patients and to reduce their isolation and fear.

It is obvious that a high caloric diet is desirable; routinely, high doses of Vitamin B are given in most treatment centers. This is essential in patients with definite signs of Vitamin B deficiency; otherwise it is of no value. In the light of J. J. Smith's theory,[33] which assumes similar mechanisms in Addisonian crises and delirium tremens, ACTH and cortisone therapy have been recommended. As the theory has not been substantiated, such treatment is not based on a sound rationale. It is of great importance to prevent dehydration by supplying fluids by mouth, or, if necessary, by intravenous infusion. Elegant cocktails of glucose, insulin, ACTH, and the like are unwarranted. Some therapists recommend prophylactic medication with penicillin or broad-spectrum antibiotics to prevent pneumonia.

The following case contains features characteristic of severe delirium tremens.

A forty-five-year-old, white, married, Catholic truck driver was admitted to a state hospital for alcoholism and delirium tremens. This was his third admission. He had had a problem with excessive drinking of alcohol for fifteen years. Since his last admission ten months earlier, he had been drinking whisky heavily, though intermittently, and had eaten poorly. In the two days prior to admission, he developed tremors and sweating and had intermittent periods in which his attention was diverted by the sight of a small bird in a tree, the sound of tires on cement, and he found he had to pull himself forcefully back to the demands of the moment.

On admission, the patient alternated between belligerence and an ingratiating, friendly mood, in which he would expansively express fondness for everyone about him. His speech was slurred, and his breath bore the odor of alcohol. Physical examination revealed a wiry, moderately well-nourished man looking somewhat younger than his stated age, with a slight tremor in the upper extremities, a mild conjunctivitis, and mild glossitis and cheilosis. The pulse was 140 and regular; blood pressure was 170/100. The liver edge was palpable 3 cm. below the costal margin and was not tender; there were small external hemorrhoids, but no jaundice, spiders, gynecomastia, or other signs of hepatic involvement and venous congestion. Neurological examination revealed dilated pupils of 7½ mm., which responded sluggishly to light. The reflexes were all hypoactive, the achilles tendon reflexes could not be elicited. Gait was broad based and unsteady, Romberg's sign was positive, the patient falling to the right. Coordination was somewhat impaired. There was diminished sensation to pain, light touch, and vibratory sense in the legs and loss of position sense in the toes bilaterally.

The patient was placed on a regimen of 200 mg. daily of promazine and was put to bed, taking his medicine, vitamins, and fluids by mouth. Twelve hours following admission he began to sweat more profusely, seemed frightened, and appeared to be warding off hallucinations by closing his eyes and brushing invisible objects off the bed. He carried on conversations with various members of his family and his friends and appeared to both see them in his room and hear their voices. His mental state shifted frequently: at times, it was possible to break into the delirium, and the patient would answer some simple questions; at other times, he either ignored the interviewer or incorporated him into his hallucinations by identifying him as a particular friend; at still other times he showed insight into his state. He began to insist that he was at a bar, smoking a cigar, and certainly not lying in bed. He was suggestible; he could be induced to see an imaginary sign on the wall of the bar. He first insisted the sign was blurred and then contented himself by reading just the large print. Much of the time, he was in a truck, which was going to crash because he could not reach the brake pedals. He talked incessantly to his private acquaintances, imploring them for help, getting angry when they apparently would not respond, screaming: "How the hell do you expect me to do it—I can't reach the pedals." Family, friends, and employers seemed to appear and disappear as he would call to them, imploring aid.

The tremulousness and sweating continued, but the state of awareness shifted in cycles throughout the day. He alternated between a condition of complete involvement in his hallucinations to lucid intervals when he knew his name and knew that he was in the hospital and was hallucinating. In an intermediate state, he could be interrupted momentarily and could focus his attention on his surroundings and "return to reality," as he later put it. Alternatively, during a period of contact with the environment, a slight movement or faint noise would suddenly startle the patient and be interpreted in a hallucinatory context as some kind of threat.

This picture persisted, with the periods of hallucinosis increasing in length, especially at night, when the ward was quiet and (because of staffing problems) he was alone at intervals; his room, however, was kept well lighted. He refused all nourishment and appeared dehydrated; accordingly, parenteral fluids with vitamins and intravenous promazine were instituted late on the second day of the delirium. By the third day of the delirium, his temperature was 104, there were no lucid intervals, and his general condition seemed worse. He was noisy and resistant to nursing care, shouting "You're poisoning me—get away—what's that?—is that you Frank?—listen, tell Mary to bring the car over—why not? I want you to tell her—get that out of here, Frank!" It was necessary at this point to restrain the patient since he began to walk to Frank's house, dragging the intravenous equipment and the Foley catheter with him. He slept only in short naps, wakening suddenly, apparently disturbed by some slight noise. No specific infection was found. Liver function tests were normal. Because of the high specific gravity of the urine (in the presence of normal hematocritic findings), parenteral fluids were increased.

In the fourth day of the delirium, the patient appeared more alert for longer periods and was less tremulous; there was less sweating and the pulse was not so rapid. His naps seemed more restful. At night, however, he was noisy and uncooperative; the frightening hallucinations returned, evoking hallucinatory attempts to neutralize them. On the fifth day, the patient was greatly improved, with normal vital signs. He sat up in bed, took adequate oral nourishment, and was aware of his surroundings. He apologized to the staff for having "bothered" them, and hoped that he had not insulted anyone; this seemed to be his chief concern. The sensorium remained clear throughout the day. He slept through the night but complained in the morning of having had several terrible nightmares that awakened him. He would not disclose the content of these. His delirium seemed to be at an end. The liver remained enlarged, but laboratory tests continued to reveal no abnormalities in liver function. Vital signs remained within normal limits. The neurological examination returned to normal findings after two weeks of continued vitamin therapy, and he was discharged thirty days after admission, in accordance with hospital practice.

Alcohol Hallucinosis

Most psychiatrists consider alcohol hallucinosis—or hallucinatory insanity of drunkards, as Kraepelin called it—a separate disease. Some think it is closely related to delirium tremens; others, to schizophrenia. Patients with pure types of alcoholic hallucinosis suffer from auditory hallucinations, usually of a threatening nature, which produce great anxiety. Visual hallucinations and illusions usually are described as sinister; patients mistake persons for ghosts, devils, and evil figures; they see nightmarish, fantastic, and bizarre scenes of murder, cannibalism, gruesome sex acts, and scenes of judgment in which they are threatened with torture and execution. Very clearly, in these hallucinations and delusions there are strong self-incriminatory projections, as is the case in patients suffering from depressions. Patients with alcohol hallucinosis are oriented to time and space, in marked contrast to delirium tremens; there is only slight clouding or narrowing of consciousness. They show little restlessness and rarely have occupational deliria. The striking physical symptoms of delirium tremens are absent. In about one-fourth of the cases, however, according to G. Benedetti, the syndrome of alcohol hallucinosis is not so clear; delirium and hallucinatory symptoms occur together and blend into each other.[3] A combination with a dysmnesic syndrome is also occasionally seen.

The frequent occurrence of relatively mild forms of metalcoholic diseases has been noted by many investigators.[37] One form is characterized by tremulousness, mild disorientation, and insomnia; another, by fleeting hallucinations, nightmares, and severe anxiety. These syndromes usually clear up after a few days. Mixed forms of the milder syndromes are seen frequently.

Benedetti differentiates acute from chronic hallucinosis. Acute hallucinosis, which Victor and Adams describe as a separate syndrome,[37] is a relatively mild symptomatic psychosis with a duration from hours to days; the prognosis is relatively good. Of Benedetti's 123 cases, all but 23 recovered. The prognosis of chronic hallucinosis, however, is poor. Practically all patients deteriorate; half of them show symptoms that cannot be differentiated from those of deteriorated schizophrenia, and the remainder resemble organic deficit states. According to Benedetti, alcohol hallucinosis does not have the same genetic family pattern as schizophrenia; it would be interesting, in the light of new family research in schizophrenia, to examine the structure of families of patients with chronic alcohol hallucinosis.

Alcohol hallucinosis is treated very much like delirium tremens, with paraldehyde or chlordiazepoxide, diet and fluids, and the general therapeutic procedures recommended for acute symptomatic psychoses. If the patient is extremely frightened, the use of phenothiazines is permissible. Chronic and deteriorated hallucinoses are treated like deteriorated schizophrenias. Of course, complete abstinence at all times is mandatory.

THE DYSMNESIC SYNDROME The dysmnesic, or Korsakoff's syndrome,[21] occurs relatively frequently but not exclusively in chronic alcoholics. The symptoms—disturbance of recall of newly acquired mnemic material, disorientation in time and space, confabulation, and general intellectual deterioration—were described in Chapter 16. Alcoholics with Korsakoff's syndrome invariably suffer from peripheral neuropathies. The alcoholic dysmnesic syndrome has a grave prognosis. Although improvement with and without treatment has been observed, residual organic deficit states are common. The neuropathology of the syndrome consists of atrophic and degenerating cell changes, glial proliferation, and perivascular hemorrhages in thalamic and mesencephalic region. It is assumed that B_1 avitaminosis plays a role in the etiology of the alcoholic dysmnesic syndrome. Massive doses of Vitamin B complex for weeks and months, a high caloric diet, and general medical and nursing care, besides a slow program of retraining in a supportive hospital environment, are the recommended measures.

Alcoholic Encephalopathies

Hemorrhagic superior poliencephalitis, described by Carl Wernicke[38] in 1881, and named after him, has an acute onset with nausea, vomiting, and clouding of consciousness or develops more slowly from a delirious or a dysmnesic syndrome. Its symptoms are external ophthalmoplegias and also disturbances of the pupillary reactions to light and convergence; the pupils are usually small and unequal. There is usually a cerebellar form of ataxia; disturbances of coordination of intentional movements are rare. Most of these patients also suffer from peripheral polyneuropathies. The patients are apathetic, unresponsive, and suffer from a dysmnesic syndrome, which, at times, may be obscured by severe clouding of consciousness. Victor and Adams consider the syndrome described by Korsakoff to be identical to Wernicke's disease[37] and view Wernicke's disease as the most severe form of a Korsakoff syndrome. The majority of patients suffering from Wernickes' disease are chronic alcoholics with severe dietary deficiencies; the disease also occurs in persons with severe malnutrition, such as inmates of prison camps. The principal cause of Wernicke's disease is thiamin (B_1) deficiency, which produces a disturbance of the oxidation of pyruvic acid. Adams and Victor report a mortality rate of 16 per cent. Pathological findings are acute perivascular hemorrhages, necroses, and degeneration of nerve cell and fibers, and proliferative changes of astrocytes in the perivascular regions of thalamus and hypothalamus, the mamillary bodies, and the region adjacent to the sylvian aqueduct. The changes are not caused by cerebral inflammation. Therapy consists of thiamin administration (100 mgm. daily i.v.) and the general therapeutic measures mentioned in the treatment of the dysmnesic syndrome.

Nicotinic-acid deficiency encephalopathy, described by Joliffe and others, has been observed in chronic alcoholics[17] and also in febrile symptomatic psychoses. Many of these patients have typical pellagra symptoms, and all are undernourished. The symptoms are those of clouding of consciousness and delirium, increased sucking and grasping reflexes, cogwheel rigidity, and fleeting pyramidal signs. These patients improve after a high caloric, high vitamin diet and therapy with nicotinic acid, 500–1000 mg., or with nicotinamide, 100–200 mg., which should be continued for seven days.

A rare disease of the corpus callosum, known as *Marchiafava's Disease,* occurs after the chronic and cxcessive consumption of cheap red wine. The patients are deteriorated alcoholics, often showing aphasic, agnosic, and apractic symptoms. The degenerative changes are primarily in the corpus callosum; besides this pathology, there are multiple encephalomalacias of cortex and subcortex. Severe *cerebellar ataxia,* with degenerative changes in the cerebellum, has also been described in chronic alcoholics.

Alcoholic Paranoia

It is questionable whether a genuine syndrome of alcoholic paranoia exists; it is much more likely that patients labeled as "alcoholic paranoiacs" are schizophrenics and paranoid sociopaths who are addicted to alcohol. Many of them are deteriorated alcoholics. The cardinal symptom is pathological jealousy. Practically all alcoholic paranoiacs that have been described are men; the writers, however, have seen at least one female patient in whom delusions did not center around jealousy but around the fear that her family and, later, her professional colleagues, were trying to eliminate her. The typical patient might see not one but several men going in and out of his house, presumably to have intercourse with his wife; he may find suspicious spots on the bedsheets and on her underclothing and marked money which she has received. Alcoholic paranoiacs can be very brutal to their wives, examining their genitalia, beating and assaulting them; these patients usually have been impotent for some time but show much interest in the sexual activities of other men. Many are overtly homosexual or bisexual. At times, the jealousy may be directed against a daughter, with a strong, repressed, ambivalent affection for her lover or husband; this type of incestuous conflict is wonderfully portrayed in Arthur Miller's play, *A View from the Bridge.* There are also cases in which the patient fears that son and wife are plotting against him. Wives are often accused by patients of perversions with their own children or with house pets. Whether the paranoia is entirely delusional cannot always be easily demonstrated; at times, this becomes a job more for a detective than a psychiatrist. These patients seem to have, unconsciously, a tendency to choose unfaithful partners and do much to provoke their infidelity. In most cases of alcoholic paranoia, however, there is clinical evidence of pathological jealousy, and delusions of jealousy are quite obvious. The spate of accusations is usually fantastic; the patient is uncritical of the lack of proof. The projections of the patient can be easily discerned in his accusations. The prognosis in deteriorated patients is poor. Even when no deterioration is present, only the most skillful psychotherapists are able to work with these patients who, as other paranoid patients, are much inclined to act out their impulses. The tendency to view a majority of alcoholics as warding off schizophrenia by drink is not warranted; some alcoholics do have underlying schizophrenia, but this is not a rule.

Alcoholic Deterioration

The stereotyped public image of a chronic alcoholic is incorrect; it is more applicable to the deteriorated alcoholic. Only a few chronic alcoholics develop signs of organic deterioration. We have described the signs of such deterioration in Chapter 16. The deficit may be almost imperceptible in everyday life and, even in clinical examination, become evident only in careful psychological testing. Severe cases resemble general paretics, and this condition is described as *alcoholic pseudoparesis*. Emotional changes, such as rather severe depression or euphoria, or—in milder cases—emotional lability and irritability, are frequent. Aggressive, self-destructive, and infantile sexual behavior, which is characteristic for most organic deficit states, is strikingly manifest in deteriorated alcoholics and may present serious problems in clinical management. Pathological findings are unspecific and consist of cerebral atrophy, cerebellar degeneration, and chronic leptomeningitis. Psychiatric therapy of such patients follows the general outline of therapy with organic deficit states. As in all alcoholics, strict avoidance of drinking is of paramount importance.

NOTES

1. Selden D. Bacon, "Alcoholism," *Federal Probation*, 11 (1947), 24.
2. Robert F. Bales, "Cultural Differences in Rates of Alcoholism," *Quarterly Journal of Studies on Alcohol*, 6 (1946), 480.
3. Gaetano Benedetti, *Die Alkoholhalluzinosen* (Stuttgart: Thieme, 1952).
4. Hans Binder, "Über Alkoholische Rauschzustände," *Schweizer Archiv für Neurologie, Neurochirurgie und Psychiat.*, 35 (1935), 209.
5. K. Bjerver and L. Goldberg, "Effect on Alcohol Ingestion on Driving Ability," *Quarterly Journal of Studies on Alcohol*, 11 (1950), 1.
6. Karl M. Bowman and E. M. Jellinek, "Alcohol Addiction and Its Treatment," *Quarterly Journal of Studies on Alcohol*, 2 (1941), 98.
7. John A. Carpenter, Omar K. Moore, Charles R. Snyder, and Edith S. Lisansky, "Alcohol and Higher-Order Problem Solving," *Quarterly Journal of Studies on Alcohol*, 22 (1961), 183.
8. Nicholas Chwelos, D. B. Blewett, C. M. Smith, and A. Hoffer, "Use of d-Lysergic Acid Diethylamide in the Treatment of Alcoholism," *Quarterly Journal of Studies on Alcohol*, 20 (1959), 577.
9. Oskar M. Diethelm, ed., *Etiology of Chronic Alcoholism* (Springfield: Charles C Thomas, 1955).

10. George L. Engel and John Romano, "Delirium, a Syndrome of Cerebral Insufficiency," *Journal of Chronic Diseases*, 9 (1959), 260.
11. Leon A. Greenberg, "The Definition of an Intoxicating Beverage," *Quarterly Journal of Studies on Alcohol*, 16 (1955), 316.
12. Jens Hald, E. Jacobsen, and V. Larsen, "The Sensitizing Effect of Tetraethyl-Thiuramdisulfide (Antabuse) to Ethyl Alcohol," *Acta. Pharmacologica et Toxicologia Scandinavica*, 4 (1948), 285.
13. Francis E. Hare, *On Alcoholism* (London: Churchill, 1912).
14. Donald Horton, "The Functions of Alcohol in Primitive Societies," *Quarterly Journal of Studies on Alcohol*, 4 (1943), 199.
15. Harris Isbell, H. F. Fraser, A. Wikler, R. E. Belleville, and A. J. Eisenman, "An Experimental Study of the Etiology of 'Rum-Fits' and Delirium Tremens," *Quarterly Journal of Studies on Alcohol*, 16 (1955), 1–33.
16. E. M. Jellinek, *The Disease Concept of Alcoholism* (New Haven: Hillhouse Press, 1960).
17. Norman Jolliffe, Karl M. Bowman, L. A. Rosenbloom, and H. D. Fein, "Nicotinic Acid Deficiency Encephalopathy," *Journal of the American Medical Association*, 114 (1940), 307.
18. Ben Karpman, *The Alcoholic Woman* (Washington, D. C.: Lineacre, 1948).
19. Mark Keller, "The Definition of Alcoholism and the Estimation of Its Prevalence," in David J. Pittman and Charles R. Snyder, eds., *Society, Culture and Drinking Patterns* (New York: John Wiley, 1962).
20. Richard J. Kingham, "Alcoholism and the Reinforcement Theory of Learning," *Quarterly Journal of Studies on Alcohol*, 19 (1958), 320.
21. Syergei S. Korsakoff, "Über eine besondere Form psychischer Störung mit multipler Neuritis," *Archiv. Psychiat. Nervenkr.*, 21 (1890), 669.
22. David Lester and L. A. Greenberg, "Nutrition and the Etiology of Alcoholism," *Quarterly Journal of Studies on Alcohol*, 13 (1952), 553.
23. Jacob Levine, "The Sexual Adjustment of Alcoholics," *Quarterly Journal of Studies on Alcohol*, 16 (1955), 675.
24. Jorge Mardones, R. Onfray, and B. E. Onfray, "Influencia de una Substancia de la Levadura (Elementa del Complejo Vitamínico B) Sobre el Consumo de Alcohol en Hatas en Experimentos de Autoseleccíon," *Rev. Med. Aliment.*, Chile, 5 (1942), 148.
25. Jack H. Mendelson, ed., "Experimentally Induced Chronic Intoxication and Withdrawal in Alcoholics," *Quarterly Journal of Studies on Alcohol*, Supplement 2 (May 1964).
26. Karl Menninger, *Man against Himself* (New York: Basic Books, 1938).
27. Arnold Z. Pfeffer *et al.*, "A Treatment Program for the Alcoholic in Industry," *Journal of the American Medical Association*, 161 (1956), 827.
28. John W. Rhinehart, "Factors Determining 'Rum Fits,' " *American Journal of Psychiatry*, 118 (1961), 251.
29. Herbert S. Ripley and J. K. Jackson, "Therapeutic Factors in Alcoholics Anonymous," *American Journal of Psychiatry*, 116 (1959), 44.

30. John Romano, "Early Contributions to the Study of Delirium Tremens," *Annals of Medical History*, 3 (1941), 128.
31. Sakari Sariola, "Social Implications of Alcoholism," in Hans W. Gruhle, R. Jung, W. Mayer-Gross, and M. Müller, eds., *Psychiatrie der Gegenwart* (Berlin: Springer, 1960), Vol. II.
32. J. Skala, *The Problem of Alcoholism and the Organization of Treatment and Control of Alcoholics in Czechoslovakia* ("Studies in the Prevention of Alcoholism" [Geneva: 1957]).
33. James J. Smith, "The Endocrine Basis of Hormonal Therapy of Alcoholism," *New York State Journal of Medicine*, 50 (1950), 1704.
34. Hugo Solms, "Die Behandlung der akuten Alkoholvergiftung und der akuten und chronischen Formen des Alkoholismus," in H. W. Gruhle, R. Jung, W. Mayer-Gross, and M. Müller, eds., *Psychiatrie der Gegenwart* (Berlin: Springer, 1960), Vol. II.
35. Harry M. Tiebout, "Alcoholics Anonymous—An Experiment of Nature," *Quarterly Journal of Studies on Alcohol*, 22 (1961), 52.
36. Douglas W. Thomas and Daniel X. Freedman, "Treatment of the Alcohol Withdrawal Syndrome," *Journal of the American Medical Association*, 188 (1964), 316.
37. Maurice Victor and R. D. Adams, "The Effect of Alcohol on the Nervous System," *Association for Research in Nervous and Mental Diseases Proceedings*, 32 (1953), 526.
38. Carl Wernicke, *Lehrbuch der Gehirn-Krankheiten für Studierende und Ärzte* (Berlin: Fischer, 1881).
39. Abraham Wikler, "Mechanisms of Actions of Drugs that Modify Personality Function," *American Journal of Psychiatry*, 108 (1952), 590.
40. W. William, "The Society of Alcoholics Anonymous," *American Journal of Psychiatry*, 106 (1949), 370.
41. Roger J. Williams, *Nutrition and Alcoholism* (Norman, Oklahoma: University of Oklahoma Press, 1951).
42. World Health Organization, Expert Committee on Mental Health (Alcoholism), "Report on Second Session" (October 1951).
43. R. B. Yules, Daniel X. Freedman, and K. A. Chandler, *The Physiological Effect of Ethyl Alcohol on Man's Electroencephalographic Sleep Cycle* (Abstract, presented at Association for the Psychophysiological Study of Sleep [March 1965]).
44. Israel Zwerling and Milton Rosenbaum, "Alcoholic Addiction and Personality," in Silvano Arieti, ed., *The American Handbook of Psychiatry* (New York: Basic Books, 1959), Vol. I, pp. 623–644.

CHAPTER TWENTY-FOUR

Psychiatry and Law

Lawyers and Psychiatrists

Civil and criminal laws are created and administered by vast and complex organizations in which lawyers naturally play a decisive role. They are key persons in public administration and legislation, in courts and penal institutions, implementing the defined patterns of social control that are characteristic of a given society. Psychiatrists are called upon to apply their technical skills in a variety of legal situations. Their role in such situations is usually somewhat peripheral, not clearly defined, and not properly apprehended by the participants. Thomas S. Szasz has asserted, in several challenging articles, that by participating in legal work, psychiatrists step out of their central role as individual therapists, a role change he vigorously opposes.[29] We believe that, in this instance, Szasz defines the function of psychiatry too narrowly; the assistance some qualified psychiatrists may render in legal matters is desirable and necessary. What is crucial, of course, is that psychiatrists understand their role and limitations, and appreciate, as in all social psychiatry, the extent to which they have developed special competence.

Apart from the fact that lawyers and psychiatrists both deal with internal and external controls of human relationships, the two professions have very different traditions, philosophies, methods, and aims. Law is a normative discipline; psychiatry, in part at least, is a child of a technology based on the natural sciences. Natural sciences recognize the existence of infinite variation, such as transitional states between the healthy and the pathological. Law requires strict and formal definitions and, in general, is not inclined to recognize vague boundaries; a man is guilty or not guilty. Law is essentially a body of rules for human conduct that must be created and administered. Many psychiatrists mistake the formality of law for rigidity; to them, the nature of the law and the legal process is more fixed and absolute than the scientific system on which psychiatry is based; lawyers, however, usually do not think that law is fixed and rigid. Law is constantly changing, not only by new legislation, but also by the ongoing process of legal interpretation and jurisdiction; the latter is particularly true for common or judge-made law.

Physicians, including psychiatrists, pull their observations together in the form of a diagnosis of what they consider the trouble. The diagnostic process makes little sense to lawyers; as they see it, descriptive diagnosis is mere labeling, and dynamic diagnosis seems to involve a very loose process of thinking. In spite of such reservations (or perhaps because of them), diagnoses are often exploited by lawyers in ways that alienate psychiatrists. The fact is that psychiatrists, like all physicians, are usually quite efficient in the synthesis of data that is embodied in the diagnostic process. They tend, however, to be quite sensitive to criticism and challenge and suffer when subjected to questioning, examination, or arguments in adversary procedures. Argumentation is at the root of legal procedure, and to understand this should make it easier for the psychiatrist to submit to it. Lawyers are usually less than well trained in scientific observation and synthesis; they consider it essential to look at any problem from different angles and thrive on differences of opinion. Physicians usually try to work toward a therapeutic recommendation or rehabilitation—types of intervention that, until very recently, have been alien to the thinking of most lawyers.

Understandably, such differences in fundamental philosophy and method create difficulties. In Anglo-Saxon countries, where adversary procedures are the most highly developed, these difficulties have been most acute. More recently, some outstanding lawyers and judges, concerned with a more enlightened and realistic view of motivation and conduct, have expressed the opinion that help from psychiatry and the behavioral sciences is much needed in the courtroom. Psychiatric insights are pertinent in the area of crime and its prevention but are of even greater value in many areas of family law as Joseph Goldstein and Jay Katz convincingly state.[12] An active and participant interest in mental health legislation is in fact crucial for the psychiatrist; otherwise, he may find himself confronted by legislation that is not compatible with his professional standards, knowledge, and responsibility to patients. Some of the more important general problems in psychiatry and law will be considered in the following sections. For a comparison of forensic psychiatry in different countries, the reader is referred to G. Rylander's article.[26] Psychiatrists who assist in these problems must, of course, familiarize themselves with the specific laws of their country or state.

Hospitalizing of the Mentally Ill

To hospitalize the mentally ill, a variety of medical and legal procedures is used. Admissions to mental hospitals may be either involuntary or voluntary. In a publication on a model commitment act,[1] two types of involuntary hospitalization are mentioned: (1) Hospitalization without consent because of inability to decide or act due to confusion, delusion, or deterioration, which requires an agent in court, a relative, or friend to act for the patient. (2) Compulsory hospitalization of an individual who is dangerous to himself or others. Actually, few persons fall into the second category. Dangerous behavior disorders, contrary to public opinion, are rare. Most dangerous persons are not suffering from severe behavior disorders in the narrow sense of the word. Szasz has observed that the attribute "dangerous" usually means endangering persons of high power and status.[30] We feel that psychiatrists tend strongly to avoid involuntary hospitalizations of patients who might create certain difficulties through a variety of social pressures and manipulations; thus, it is unduly difficult to commit argumentative and paranoid patients or patients of high status and power. This was borne out by the case of the mad Ludwig of Bavaria,[2] and the hospitalization of Earl Long, a former governor of Louisiana. The suicide of James Forrestal, Secretary of the Navy, while under psychiatric observation in a naval hospital, was another distressing illustration of the fact that it is a complicated and ticklish business to carry out procedures imposing restraint for the safety of persons of high position. Similarly, professional colleagues in medicine are apt to receive special, and hence—all too often—inadequate, care, occasioned more by misapplied concern for the privileged patient's pride than an appreciation of his emotional predicament. In all these instances, internal pressure may obscure the physician's judgment, and the responses of concerned authorities may tend to restrict sound therapeutic approaches. Certainly, commitments in many cases are entirely rational acts; however, in some cases there is evidence that psychiatrists and other involved persons are motivated, in part, by counteraggression toward very provocative patients. Such aggressive and punitive tendencies require commitment procedures to be strictly regulated by law. In many countries and in many states of the United States patients are deprived of their civil rights when they are committed to an institution; this seems entirely unjustified in most cases. In many states it is obligatory that the patient be examined by two physicians of which one must be a psychiatrist; the examining physicians must not be related to the patient nor affiliated with the institution to which he is sent. The patient is examined to ascertain if he is drugged or physically ill and to determine the nature of his mental disorder. A judge then must order that the patient be admitted to, and detained in, an institution for the mentally ill for as long as he needs treatment and care. In some states, a jury decides that the patient needs such treatment and care. Poorly considered legal safeguards can become cumbersome, if not irrelevant. In general, psychiatrists object to legal procedures, such as the patient's appearing in court, service of notice, and the like, and favor an entirely informal admission to psychiatric hospitals. To protect the patient's rights, commitment must be a psychiatric as well as legal procedure and requires, in legislation and administration, the cooperation and deliberation of both professions. There is agreement that voluntary admission of patients with behavior disorders need not be different from admission procedures for general hospitalization. One important modification of the standard commitment is certification by a physician that the patient is in need of temporary observation or therapy (usually not exceeding fifteen to thirty days) for a behavior disorder; this permits the hospital superintendent to receive and hold such patients and allows agents of the court or police to transport patients to the institution. This procedure has the advantage of dispensing with formal commitment and has become widely used. It is a speedy and efficient measure and may be considered, next to voluntary admissions, the most humane and medically satisfactory procedure, particularly for the patient who otherwise cannot make arrangements for admission or who is unreasonbly opposed to hospitalization. With all patients, whether committed or voluntarily admitted, modern psychiatrists press for minimal restraint and coercion in transporting the patient to the hospital and upon admission. Unfortunately, in many locations transporting the patient to the hospital is still in the hands of medically untrained personnel. As police officers in many metropolitan areas become educated in mental health problems, the patient can more frequently be dealt with in a reasonably humane fashion.

For some time, voluntary admissions have been the rule in private hospitals. However, even voluntarily admitted patients are deprived to a degree of some aspects of their ordinary freedom. This does not simply imply that they must submit to a certain institutional discipline, which, of course, is also the case in general hospitals. It often does mean that they cannot leave immediately, even if they give due notice; often, signed but not legally binding agreements with the director of the hospital stipulate that they remain for a certain period of time. It also means that subtle (and sometimes not so subtle) pressures in the family and community are used to keep patients in the institution. Such rules are established in the interest of the patients, but it is undeniable that they are restrictive. Although voluntary patients are not formally deprived of their right to vote, to make contracts, and the like, in reality such rights often *are* curtailed, even though many hospitalized patients are as capable as many nonhospitalized persons to carry out these functions. In many instances, hospitalization is the best way to deal with a phase or an aspect of a behavior disorder, but it is not, per se, a meaningful index for severity of illness. In the great majority of mental institutions, there is still a striking deprivation of physical freedom, ranging from restriction to closed wards to grounds parole and carefully limited outside visits. Many mental hospitals censor all mail and closely supervise all activities. When control is built into a therapeutic milieu, with mutual exchange of observations for purposes of therapy, the meaning of such restrictions is quite different and differently motivated than the usual instance in which such measures are for the convenience of inadequately staffed institutions and the protection of the staff from ill-considered community pressures. The point is that, applied indiscriminately to all patients, such constraint becomes therapeutically harmful. No wonder that mental hospitals have been compared with concentration camps and jails! Szasz actually recommends that all institutions to which patients are sent by compulsion should be called jails.[28] We believe it would be just as erroneous to do this as to call our prisons hospitals.

The present shift away from commitment by legal procedures to voluntary admissions reflects a very important trend. It suggests, first, that we are progressing on a path from custodial segregation to active treatment in which patients are permitted and encouraged to participate voluntarily. It also sanctions a fundamental right of persons in democracies to live as they like, even if they choose to live eccentrically, as long as they do not seriously or dangerously disturb their communities. Interestingly, however, the behavioral sciences have not yet been able to evolve simple and operational definitions of eccentricity or of "dangerousness." [18] As therapeutic interventions increase in intensity and scope, we more frequently encounter the question of a person impulsively leaving treatment when there appears to be a good chance that he could further improve his status and diminish his self-destructive behavior. Without some element of restraint, such a person might not have received therapeutic help at all. Nonetheless, it is probably best, both for society and for therapy of the patient, that coercion be restricted to the minimum necessary for the protection of life.

The discharge of voluntary patients and also of most committed patients who are not criminal offenders takes place by arrangement between physicians of the institutions, families, and patients and usually presents no legal difficulties. In the New Haven study of social class and mental illness, it was shown that lower-class patients had a significantly poorer chance to be discharged (although the prognosis on discharge may, because of lessened social demand and role expectations, be better for lower- than for middle-class patients).[15] After a patient has been committed, the patient, family, or counsel may, under Anglo-Saxon law, petition for a writ of release. The writ of *habeas corpus*, protecting a person from being restrained illegally, is used relatively rarely. In the case of a psychiatric offender sent to a mental hospital by the court, a new court decision is required to permit the hospital authorities to discharge the patient. In this connection, controversies occasionally develop between courts and hospitals on the issue of whether the patient is dangerous.

Psychiatric Aspects of Contracts, Wills, and Torts

Mental incompetence means the inability to carry out certain legal acts; it usually implies inability to understand the nature or effect of a transaction. The test of incompetence, however, is not strictly defined; it depends on the condition that causes the incompetence and also on the nature of the act. There is usually little argument about extreme deterioration. In mild deterioration, on the other hand, the test of mental incompetence may be very difficult. Paranoid delusions are considered causes of mental incompetence only if they directly affect the legal transaction in question. The nature of the legal act must be considered: complex business transactions require a very different degree of mental competence from that required for a simple deed for a small amount of money.

In all types of contracts, a reasonably intact intelligence, alertness, and contact with reality is demanded. Serious intellectual deficit and gross incapacity to remember or to recall, as in the serious organic disorders, may void a contract. In the case of schizophrenics, only disturbances in reality-testing that specifically affect the understanding of the contract can legally void it. In the case of the typical emotional changes in manic-depressive psychoses, the test of mental incompetence may be even more difficult.

In the case of wills, courts must be satisfied that the testator realized he was engaged in drawing a will, that he knew the nature and extent of his property, and the natural recipients of his bequests. This should mean he was able to recognize and appreciate who his heirs were and, if they were unusual, such as a pet, that he did not, psychotically, identify the pet with persons, or misrecognize persons. Courts have recognized wills that have conformed to prevalent mores even when the testator was far from mentally competent and have considered them invalid when the wills were odd or antisocial. Tests of incompetence are quite different in cases where a person wills his property to his children or to an educational, religious, or charitable institution from those where the legacy goes to a woman of ill repute, a domestic animal, or a strongly disapproved cause, especially when such wills are challenged. Psychiatrists, as Szasz says, become involved beyond the limits of their professional competence when asked to testify in the highly complex "inheritance game." [31] Since opinions typically must be based on historical evidence without the benefit of a personal examination, participation in this game is never easy; when contradictory claims are made that the testator was psychotic, the difficulties become formidable. Manfred S. Guttmacher and Henry Weihofen recommend that in all cases of unusual wills that are likely to be contested, lawyers should try to enlist the services of a psychiatrist while the testator is alive to ascertain the presence or lack of mental competence.[13] Psychiatrists have to testify from time to time in an evaluation of a possible suicide, because many insurance contracts are voided if the insured party commits suicide within a certain period of time. Psychiatrists sometimes are also involved in cases where guardians are appointed because of mental incompetence; their role is essentially the same as in other cases of evaluation of mental incompetence.

Frequently, psychiatrists are asked to determine the consequences of a damaging action, not only after an accident, but also after a tort, and to establish what "emotional shock" a person has suffered. In general, it is recommended that whenever such testimony is required, a psychiatrist who is the patient's therapist should not be pressed into the role of a witness, jeopardizing his therapeutic role, which is difficult enough to sustain. It is important to keep in mind that psychiatric patients who inflict torts on others are legally responsible, with their estates for these torts, in contrast to criminal acts for which they may not be punishable.

Sterilization and Abortion

In states and countries with laws recommending compulsory sterilization, psychiatrists are asked to evaluate psychiatric criteria for such procedures. Sound psychiatric indications for sterilization are rare.[12] There are few mental diseases clearly transmitted by genes, and most patients with severe behavior disorders do not procreate; this leaves, then, only certain cases of mental subnormality as candidates for this radical step. Even in these rare cases, sterilization is often indicated more from a social than from a eugenic standpoint. It is essential that psychiatrists, in such evaluations, not confound expert judgment with value judgment. Most such cases can be handled as voluntary sterilizations. The brutal sterilization laws of National Socialist Germany, which were not based on scientific data, have been swept out of existence, and others should follow.

Sound psychiatric indications for abortion are also the exception.[12] Pregnancy and childbirth are rarely events that endanger the life of psychiatric patients or seriously complicate the course of their disorders. Schizophrenia, manic-depressive psychoses, and reactive depressions with the danger of suicide are controversial indications. Some psychiatrists will recommend abortion because they anticipate that the stress of rearing a child may be too severe for the mother and also may endanger the favorable development of the child. Some, like the authors, are willing to recommend abortion in cases when pregnancy followed rape; however, the recommendation of the psychiatrist in such cases of clearly undesirable pregnancy is often based on his social and ethical convictions rather than on medical or psychiatric findings.

We do not clearly know the harmful effects of abortion. Young women frequently feel robbed and deprived following abortions they actively sought. In part, the context in which the abortion takes place is quite important; the family pulls and antagonisms surrounding the procedure (and the occasion for it) should be assessed. In general, when a mature, multiparous woman requires an abortion for psychiatric reasons and the family is essentially supportive and consenting, the after-effects are usually not harmful.

Family Law

Psychiatrists are sometimes asked to testify as expert witnesses to the mental competence of one of the parties in a challenged marriage contract in order to permit an annulment. If the marriage was performed when one or both partners was intoxicated, this is considered grounds for annulment. A marriage may also be annulled if one or both of the partners did not understand the contract because they were psychotic or mentally deficient;

however, most courts have ruled that it requires very little intelligence to understand marriage contracts.[6] In some countries, for instance, in Switzerland, Finland, and Norway, psychotics are not permitted to marry.[26]

In many countries, divorce is permitted if one of the marriage partners is suffering from chronic, incurable psychosis. Psychiatrists occasionally have been used as expert witnesses in divorce suits to testify on mistreatment during marriage and its consequences. To our minds, however, there are far more constructive ways to use psychiatric skills than in such adversary procedures. With the recognition that a well-functioning family is the most important preventive measure against mental disorders, psychiatrists have begun to study family relations and to treat and counsel before problems become severe and chronic. Some family courts now use psychiatrists in cases of pending divorce and separation, in working with other problems of the intact and broken family, with unmarried mothers, and in cases of adoption and custody of children.[12]

Responsibility for Criminal Acts

In all civilized countries, criminal law is based on the concept of responsibility or accountability. In Anglo-Saxon countries, the term responsibility is widely used; on the European continent, accountability is preferred. Man is considered a criminal not because he has committed a certain act, which is specified in the criminal code, but because he is charged with the intent to have committed an act, which he, as a rational human being, should not have committed and for which he is held responsible or accountable. For over a hundred years, psychiatrists have been asked, under a variety of legal statutes, to assist lawyers to disentangle problems around such intent and, in particular, to assess the capacity of the accused to act intentionally. Hippocrates' diagnosis of paranoia was regarded by the Athenian courts as cause for exemption from legal sanction in all but capital cases. In Anglo-Saxon law, one of the first pronouncements about mentally ill criminals was made in the eighteenth century by Judge Robert Tracy, who referred to such a person as someone who: ". . . does not know what he is doing, no more than a wild beast." The "wild beast test" became, according to Judge D. L. Bazelon, the model for the famous M'Naghten rule.[3] In 1843, M'Naghten, a paranoid schizophrenic, fatally shot Edward Drummond, the secretary of Sir Robert Peel, the Prime Minister of England, his intended victim. Nine physicians testified that M'Naghten was insane. He was acquitted and sent to a mental hospital where he remained until his death. Public indignation over the acquittal forced the House of Lords to conduct an inquiry into the problem of the criminal insane. The M'Naghten rule states that to establish a defense on the grounds of insanity it must be proven that at the time of committing the act, the accused party was laboring under such a defect of reason from disease of the mind as not to know the nature and quality of the act or, if he did know it, he did not know that what he was doing was wrong. In over half of the states of the United States and in Great Britain, rightly or wrongly, this is still the dominant rule for judging criminal insanity. Outstanding jurists and psychiatrists have criticized the M'Naghten rule. Objections are that not all facts about criminal behavior can be expressed under the headings right or wrong. Some lawyers favor the M'Naghten rule because they simply assume that rational human beings are responsible for their acts, and that such rationality can be established by psychiatric examination.[14] They also maintain that the power of reason either exists or is absent. We disagree with these assumptions and believe that the principles based on the M'Naghten rule reflect an antiquated approach that compartmentalizes intelligence, volition, and affect; does not recognize the importance of drives and unconscious motivation; overestimates the importance of intellectual processes and their influence on behavior; and does not permit sufficient consideration of medical and psychosocial data to give the court a complete psychiatric appraisal of the accused. Nor does the rule give psychiatrists the opportunity to testify to the best of their knowledge; it forces them to answer questions of right and wrong, on which they are not qualified to answer as experts.[13] Criticisms of this kind had in fact been expressed by Isaac Ray, America's pioneer in forensic psychiatry, at the time when the M'Naghten decision was first pronounced by Lord Chief Justice Nicholas C. Tyndal. Ray, through his *Treatise on the Medical Jurisprudence of Insanity*, was instrumental in inducing the New Hampshire Supreme Court to adopt a rule recommending to the jury that the accused should be acquitted if his act was the result of mental illness.[24] Essentially, this rule is contained in the famous Durham decision: Durham was brought before the court for breaking and entering, and prior to that for embezzlement, passing bad checks, and car theft. He had been in mental hospitals several times with the diagnosis of psychosis with psychopathic personality. After the verdict, he was sent to a public mental hospital. In the Durham decision, it was said: "legal and moral traditions of the Western world require that those who of their own free will and with evil intent . . . commit acts which violate the law shall be criminally responsible for those acts . . . where such acts stem from mental disease or defects, moral blame shall not attach and hence there will be no criminal responsibility." [9] By this decision, the accused is not held criminally responsible if his unlawful act was the product of mental illness or defect. The Durham rule has been attacked on the grounds that mental illness cannot be defined and because it is difficult to prove that an act was or was not the product of an illness.[16] The Durham rule may not be completely satisfactory, but it is vastly superior to the M'Naghten rule. In clear-cut cases of severe behavior disorders, such as in the schizophrenias, affective behavior disorders, behavior disorders associated with organic brain disease, severe mental deficiencies, and also in some epileptic hysterical reactions, it is usually not difficult to demonstrate that an act was the result of mental illness. In most neuroses and sociopathies such proof is difficult or impossible at our present level of knowledge. Furthermore, it must be pointed out that "insane" persons commit rational as well as irrational acts and that "insanity" may be a temporary state, a fact that is recognized in some statutes.

Under the Durham rule, however, the psychiatrist testifies only in areas where he is experienced: on behavior disorder and its possible relation to the alleged act; the question of responsibility is quite properly left to the jury. The spirit of the Durham decision is similar to the laws of Scandinavian countries and many other European countries, which state that no person can be punished who has committed an offense under the influence of a psychosis or other profound mental disability. One important point in Danish, Norwegian, and Swedish law is the breadth of the concept of mental abnormality, which permits consideration not only of psychotic but of other abnormal offenders.

In many European countries, a legal differentiation is made between *full and diminished responsibility*; in English-speaking countries, with only rare exceptions, the concept of diminished responsibility has not become important. Even where applied, the concept has not remained unchallenged; in Germany, it was the subject of controversy from its inception.[33] Psychiatrists generally are opposed to a black-or-white concept of insanity and abnormality, nor do they favor the thesis that diminished responsibility automatically entails a reduction in punishment. In fourteen states of the United States and in the Armed Forces, the *irresistible impulse rule* has been adopted, following an opinion and decision in 1886 by Judge Henderson Somerville of the Supreme Court of Alabama. The psychiatrist F. Wertham and many jurists doubt that irresistible impulse is an important motivation for crime.[32] From a psychiatric viewpoint, the irresistible impulse may be more satisfactory than the M'Naghten rule, but less satisfactory than the Durham rule and the laws of many European countries, which permit psychiatrists to testify efficiently and flexibly as expert witnesses. The following case report illustrates the complex issue of accountability.

A successful and competent accountant was indicted because he had not filed income-tax returns for many years. It was learned that he used his accumulated wealth most sparingly; he kept his money in checking accounts, lived frugally, and behaved—like his dead father, a rather unscrupulous merchant—ungenerously to his demanding mother and to his associates. He had hardly any friends and expanded his resentment of his father to include all authority figures and particularly "Uncle Sam"; this latter, seemingly, was related to a disappointing personal experience in the Navy during World War II. He first failed to pay his income tax one year after he returned from military duty. On psychiatric examination, he seemed chronically depressed, at times almost suicidal. He was not only unable to enjoy himself but showed definite self-destructive and self-damaging trends in his everyday living. Two psychiatrists examined the accused on behalf of the defense; one diagnosed him as a neurotic behavior disorder with obsessive and depressive symptoms; the other diagnosed a schizophrenic psychosis. The man was sentenced to a brief prison term because the judge considered the accused responsible for his crime. The judge was cognizant of the neurotic motivation for the crime and undoubtedly considered such motivation in his lenient sentence, as well as in his efforts to aid in the man's rehabilitation. The sentence, in the judge's private opinion, was meant to be a deterrent for other tax-dodgers. And in terms of the man's rehabilitation after (and definitely not through) imprisonment, he was undoubtedly better off not to have been labeled a psychotic.

This case touches on a number of important questions. It shows how difficult it is to establish or to rule out the relationship between certain traumatic experiences resulting in a behavior disorder and a criminal act. Did certain events in the experience of the accused, such as his hostility toward his father and his mother or his alleged mistreatment in the Armed Forces, relate directly to his unwillingness to pay taxes? Was his criminal behavior unavoidable, or might he have decided to behave differently? One would have to know clearly why other persons with similar family constellations and experiences behave differently, pay their taxes willingly or grudgingly, or possibly reduce their income tax by sharp but not illegal techniques. Is the virtuous taxpayer really free to act as he wishes, or is he unable to keep himself from sharing his earnings with the Government? These, we submit, are most complicated psychological and ethical problems. All too often psychiatrists are expected, as expert witnesses, to answer such questions; and all too often they yield to pressures ranging from pity for the accused to a vain sense of omniscience and give scientifically untenable answers, discrediting themselves and their profession.

The Sentence and the Psychiatrist

In American and British courts, the insanity defense is used mostly in capital crimes because the successful consequence, indeterminate confinement to a mental hospital, is too grave for the defense to use lightly. In Continental courts, which recognize diminished accountability, psychiatric evaluation is neither limited to a major crime nor to a major psychosis, which, in the psychiatrist's opinion, is a decided advantage over Anglo-American procedure. What to do with the insane criminal or with the convicted abnormal offender is a complex and very difficult problem, which, in the opinion of progressive lawyers and psychiatrists, is far from a solution. Judge David Bazelon has remarked that our thinking on how to deal with felons in general is still very confused.[4] Society seems uncertain whether it wants to retaliate and punish, to rehabilitate, to protect society, or to deter from crime. In most cases, with the exception of "temporary insanity" that existed only at the time of the crime, the insane criminal is sent to a mental hospital for an undetermined and usually long period of time. In major or repeated crimes by insane persons, the probability of discharge is very slight; a court decision is necessary for such a discharge, and this is not easily obtained. Even when superintendents were authorized to discharge patients who were committed to psychiatric hospitals after felonies, their decisions have been challenged and at times reversed by the courts. Katz and Goldstein, in discussing this controversial issue, make the point that the function of determining dangerousness for purposes of release belongs, not alone to psychiatrists, but to the community and to judges as construers of legislative determinations.[18] In deciding whether a patient is dangerous, psychiatrists, as experts in diagnosis, prognosis, and treatment, merely advise judges and courts.

Insane criminals are sent for treatment to general mental hospitals or to special institutions for the insane, but there is no doubt that in most of these institutions or on wards with "maximum security" in general mental hospitals, little or no therapy goes on. This situation will only change if the public becomes sufficiently interested to provide the necessary funds for such therapy and if psychiatrists will not only talk about therapy of mentally disordered criminals but actually attempt to treat them.

How to deal with the habitual offender who is not insane is an even more vexing problem. Are habitual nonpsychotic offenders necessarily abnormal persons? Many psychiatrists unhesitatingly assert that habitual criminals are always abnormal and fall into the descriptive category of sociopaths. It has been urged that such persons be treated and rehabilitated. In practice, however, such treatment poses well-nigh insoluble difficulties. In many cases, we have neither the manpower nor the technical skills to treat the habitual offender. However, the occasional success is encouraging enough to stimulate further attempts, perhaps with group techniques. One pressing need is to sharpen our diagnostic tools, to be able to determine who can be treated and who ought to be segregated in order to protect society. In some countries, jurisdiction has dealt with habitual offenders by sentencing them to indefinite penalties, with or without provision for treatment. In other countries, the law permits preventive sentences, in our opinion a highly questionable practice. If no attempt at treatment is made for such offenders, of course, the sentence is tantamount to permanent segregation, which may be necessary in the case of some deviants, but which is unsatisfactory and unjust in many other cases. A definite trend toward rehabilitation, reeducation and treatment of habitual offenders in special clinics and hospitals, however, is noticeable.

No deviant person is dealt with more inappropriately than the sexual deviate.[10] In many countries, punishment of these unfortunates until recently has been very cruel; even now, in a number of states of the United States, any type of sexual activity except certain forms of intercourse between husband and wife may be punished. There are extraordinary differences in legislation about sexual behavior; in New York State homosexuality is a misdemeanor; but in Nevada and Michigan the offender, if convicted, is subject to life imprisonment. Only gradually are these harsh and irrelevant measures being modified and legislation introduced that provides psychiatric examination and treatment for the sexual offender. Courts increasingly have been inclined to recommend psychiatric therapy and place offenders on probation, unless the offender is a hopeless recidivist or endangers other persons, which may require segregation in mental hospitals. The Scandinavian countries and the Netherlands have, in general, been progressive in their sex legislation but, amazingly, have retained (though, fortunately, rarely applied) castration of recidivist dangerous criminals as a measure of punishment and prevention.[27]

Legislation about crimes committed in a state of alcoholic intoxication varies in different countries. In most countries where common law prevails, drunkenness is not a defense for a crime. In practice, however, sentences have been frequently reduced when crimes were committed during a state of serious intoxication. In some countries, for example, in Germany, Austria, and Norway, a man is not held accountable for a crime committed in a state of severe drunkenness unless he became drunk with the purpose of committing the crime. In Austria, an alcoholic who commits a crime can be punished only for his drunkenness. Offenders suffering from an alcoholic psychosis usually have been dealt with as other psychotic offenders. There has been considerable debate about the validity of the syndrome of pathological intoxication; some authors doubt the existence of the syndrome and do not consider it a proper legal defense.[21] Psychiatrists and courts of law have been concerned with the commitment of the habitual alcoholic and the alcoholic offender; commitment, however, is indicated only in a very small fraction of alcoholics.

Lawyers as well as laymen have often expressed concern that recognition of mental disorders in some criminals will have the effect of letting these persons off easily and will encourage crime. Experience in Scandinavian countries, where courts have collaborated closely with medical and psychiatric experts, allays this fear. Actually, it is by no means certain that severe punishment is an effective deterrent to crime. At present, many an unfortunate person pays dearly for one criminal act, while habitual criminals, regardless of punishment, remain unchanged, unrehabilitated. Altogether, this is a challenge that calls for much thought and effort, and psychiatrists are expected to make a significant contribution to these problems.

Psychiatrists as Expert Witnesses

An expert witness is a person with specific technical knowledge who is asked to testify on a subject of his competence. Unlike other witnesses, he is permitted not only to state facts but also to offer opinions, conclusions, and inferences. Psychiatrists qualify as such witnesses, and one would assume that they would play a most useful role as technical experts and consultants to courts of law. On the European Continent they have, in varying degrees, fulfilled such a role; in the United States and the United Kingdom, their function has remained, with rare exceptions, considerably more dubious. The most important reason for unsatisfactory performance is that an expert medical witness cannot function effectively under conditions of argument. Guttmacher and Weihofen have noted that, "The doctor who undertakes to go into court to testify as an expert witness must bear in mind that he is stepping squarely into the middle of a fight. A trial is not a scientific investigation. It is not a search for objective truth. It is . . . an adversary proceeding." [13] This state of affairs is particularly pronounced in Anglo-Saxon law, where psychiatrists are usually retained by opposing parties. This often yields an array of opposing statements, which at times have given the courts, juries, and the public the impression that there is no objective truth in psychiatry and that psychiatrists can be bought (or bribed) to say almost anything for a fee. Psycihatrists have asked for this verdict; many appearing in court have performed poorly and not helped courts. Courts, however, could consider that psychiatrists do not function optimally under existing conditions. In cross-examination, which often aims at undermining the expert rather than sharpening the psychiatric issues, little enlightenment can be expected. Lawyers are likely to ask expert witnesses for answers to questions that are based on hypothetical facts. Such a device is not designed to bring out the kind of judgment relevant to the specific person and problem in question, which the psychiatrist is trained to offer. Beyond that, in criminal law, tests for insanity like the M'Naghten rule or the irresistible impulse rule have the effect of putting psychiatric opinion in a strait-jacket. In arguing for the elimination of the battle of the experts, Guttmacher and Weihofen make a number of recommendations:[13] (1) Experts should be appointed by the court and existing clinical facilities utilized. Unfortunately, under existing conditions in American and British courts, the best-qualified psychiatrists have often been unavailable to function as expert witnesses. (2) There should be opportunity for consultation of experts of the opposing parties before the trial. (3) Psychiatric reports should be filed prior to trials, and a more judicious use of the hypothetical question should be made in the courts. B. L. Diamond feels the system of partisan experts is superior to the system of impartial witnesses, because it realistically recognizes the fallibility of expert witnesses and gives the court an opportunity to arrive at its own conclusions from opposing views.[8] We believe that this argument is not valid because a system that uses more than one court-appointed expert witness certainly does not preclude different points of view. What Diamond, in an otherwise admirably frank and lucid editorial, describes as a court-appointed psychiatrist is actually a psychiatrist working at a low salary and tight budget for the prosecution. An impartial system, of course, should not utilize underpaid and poorly trained experts identified with the prosecution, but the expert known as *amicus curiae,* who assists judge and jury. In our opinion, only such experts—well trained, less preoccupied with their omniscience, and secure enough in public status to admit deficiencies of their own knowledge—are really free to give a relatively unbiased opinion. In very few places in this country is careful psychiatric evaluation provided; in Baltimore, for example, it is common for the courts to make referrals to hospitals and clinics. In Massachusetts the Briggs laws, calling for psychiatric examination of major recidivist offenders, has virtually eliminated the battle of the experts and contributed to better jurisdiction.[23] In general, however, psychiatric help in United States courts is easily available for the wealthy accused and difficult to obtain for the poor, who cannot retain their own expert witnesses.

Privileged Communication

Psychiatrists, like all other physicians, are bound by the Hippocratic oath not to harm their patients under any conditions. To reveal what a patient has told his physician could be harmful to the patient; hence, physicians insist that what they have heard in confidence from their patients should not be revealed in courts, unless a patient of the expert witness specifically permits such revelation. In the states of Georgia and Connecticut, privileged communication between psychiatrist and patient is granted by statute.[11] In six other states, a statute protects the communication between psychologists and their clients. Lawyers, in general, are opposed to privileged communication, holding that it is often against the public interest and may obstruct justice. Psychiatrists maintain that if communication were not confidential and privileged, patients would be deterred from seeking treatment and would not trust their psychiatrists. In a famous decision in Illinois, where no statute of privileged communication exists, the privilege to withhold information was granted to Dr. Roy R. Grinker when he was asked to make statements about one of his patients in a divorce suit.[5] The court recognized that the close relationship of trust between psychotherapist and patient is unique, and the therapist was not required to report on communications made in confidence. It is interesting that the Illinois court ruled that the psychiatrist–patient relationship is closer and involves more intimate confidence than the general doctor–patient relationship. This privilege, of course, can be waived by the patient. There is no privileged communication in Connecticut if the patient is examined at the court's behest. A judge may also find it in the interst of justice to waive the privilege in civil proceedings, in which the patient introduced his mental condition as an element of claim or defense, or when a mental hospital communicates about a patient committed to the institution. Regardless of the law, psychiatrists at times may find themselves in very difficult and conflictful situations as to what to reveal about their patients, not only in courts but in prelegal and extralegal situations. The ultimate principle should not be silence at any cost, but what will best serve the patient's interest.

Reliability of Witnesses

From a psychiatrist's point of view, courts of law overestimate the power of the rational mind. The legal rules of evidence—a system of elaborate techniques designed to establish facts, rule out hearsay, and detect conscious falsification—do not take cognizance of the power of unconscious forces that falsify reports. Lawrence S. Kubie, in several articles on the fallacy of memory, forcefully pointed to the distortions of perception and recall that are the result of unconscious motivation.[19] Such distortions in statements of witnesses are particularly strong when powerful emotions play a role. This is often clearly illustrated in statements of child witnesses or in reports about emotionally arousing crimes, particularly crimes involving sex. Psychiatrists, who are keenly aware of the fallacy of memory and the power of unconscious motivations of the witness, have occasionally been asked to examine witnesses to determine their reliability. In at least one famous case, the Alger Hiss trial, a competent psychiatrist, Dr. Carl Binger, had been asked by the defense to observe the witness, Whittaker Chambers, to cast doubt on his character and veracity; Dr. Binger, by necessity, had to give his opinion without the benefit of a clinical examination. He himself pointed to the limitations of such a procedure but was nevertheless criticized by his colleagues, who objected to expert testimony without a clinical examination. Psychiatric evidence is in fact largely based on historical material, but psychiatric testimony without the opportunity of clinical examination, although possibly valid, is nevertheless the more precarious. This arises frequently in contested wills and in life-insurance claims. Examination of the patient permits feedback, the checking of hunches, the explanation of *prima facie* damaging data, the proper evaluation of matters of degree and emphasis—an array of judgments tailored to the person in question. This is the essence of clinical knowledge: the person in question, not a hypothetical question.

Two techniques have been introduced to test the veracity of witnesses: the so-called lie detection test and the investigation under hypnosis or narcoanalysis. These procedures are far from satisfactory. Lie detector tests rely on the recording of physiological reactions such as heart rate, blood pressure, respiration, and psychogalvanic skin response, which accompany any emotional states such as anger, anxiety, or tension.[17] It is assumed that these responses differ when a person tells the truth and when he lies. This assumption, generally speaking, is correct, but there is one telling qualification: it cannot distinguish the individual who is convinced he is telling the truth. There is clinical evidence that many patients and many accused persons have been consciously convinced they were telling the truth while, in reality, they were not. The psychological responses merely reflect the affect, and affects do not differ so long as the subject believes his statements. The lie detector will register as true the conviction of a deluded person who thinks he is King Solomon or the sincere assertions of a man who denies his guilt because he has repressed the memory of his criminal act. For this and other reasons (for example, technical problems of decoding artifacts in the record, in stabilizing electrodes, and in establishing a reliable protocol of questions), great caution in the interpretation of lie detection tests is warranted.

Narcoanalysis to ascertain the truth also has serious limitations: confessions may be fantasies, and persons with great ego strength are able to resist the probing under narcoanalysis.[7, 25] In any case, interpretation of the confession requires skills similar to those needed for interpretation of dreams, because the confession is the result of a compromise of instinctual and defensive forces. Hypnosis, likewise, can be used to only a limited extent, if only for the reason that relatively few persons can be hypnotized.

In recent years the phenomena of so-called false confessions have become of interest to courts and to political and military authorities. Striking false confessions were made by American prisoners of war in North Korea and in many reported trials held in police states. In all likelihood the persons who made the confessions were not only threatened and possibly tortured but were also guilt-ridden, masochistic, and depressed individuals. In their anxiety, they identified with the aggressors and confessed what was expected of them without being aware of these mechanisms, even sincerely believing in their confessions. The skillful techniques used to acquire such confessions and also to promote sweeping changes of attitudes and opinions have been described by Joost A. M. Meerloo[22] and by Robert J. Lifton.[20] Following is an example of a false confession by a depressed man:

> C., a philosopher and historian, was a brilliant and effective adversary of totalitarian ideology. A person of great moral strength, he inspired not only the few who knew him well but the many who read his publications. After the National Socialists occupied his native country, upon a visit he was found distraught, anxious, and gloomy. One week later he astonished his friends by confessing to them that he had defrauded taxes, reported friends to the Gestapo, and had exploited and betrayed people who worked for him. All this sounded incredible, but it took another week to realize that the man was in a serious depression, of which these false and fantastic self-accusations were an important feature. Shortly afterward, he was arrested; he repeated his "confessions" and later committed suicide.
>
> In this extreme case, the "confessions" were psychotic self-accusations, and it was easy to detect the nature of his self-flagellation. In the early stage of his disorder, however, this distinguished scholar would have made an ideal case for public trial from the point of view of National Socialist propaganda.

Future Tasks

We have discussed some of the divergent orientations of lawyers and psychiatrists. More than once, psychiatrists have told lawyers that all criminals are sick, that psychiatrists should advise judges about sentences, that sentences must be indeterminate, and that no criminal should be returned to society before he is cured. Lawyers, perhaps understandably, have been annoyed by these statements; worse, they have not taken psychiatric knowledge about behavior seriously. They feel that psychiatrists have little understanding of the legal process and see them as well-meaning but uninformed and impractical champions of the offender.[29] Yet there can be little doubt that the ways we deal with crime and the criminal are archaic.

Do all or most criminals suffer from behavior disorders? Does punishment prevent crime or change criminals? If it does not, what else should be done? Are current legal practices compatible with what we know about human behavior? These are crucial questions, which can be settled only by hard-headed research and not by sentimental generalizations. The spectrum of criminal behavior is as broad as the differences in the individuals who commit crimes, and the range of disordered behavior is equally wide. We are only at the very beginning of learning something about possible relationships between crime and behavior disorders. In any case, psychiatrists have strong and well-founded convictions that certain forms of deviant behavior, which are punishable by law in many countries, require treatment; among these are certain sexual deviations, impulsive acts like kleptomania and pyromania, and most antisocial behavior of children and adolescents. Punishment, and particularly harsh punishment, is not a cure for crimes nor even a very effective deterrent. Certainly, it does not deter the large proportion of habitual criminals who populate our prisons, nor does, ordinarily, the degrading prison atmosphere reform the individual who has committed a single crime. But would a different system work better? What should be the principles and techniques of such a system? We have virtually no relevant data on which to base recommendations. Yet psychiatrists need not be ashamed of their profound skepticism about current practice, even if lawyers accuse our profession of being tender-minded, soft-hearted, and starry-eyed. Friedrich Dürrenmatt called mercy the highest form of justice; if we psychiatrists err, it is better to err on the side of mercy. There is little doubt that joint efforts of lawyers, psychiatrists, and behavioral scientists can make an important contribution by bringing research to the legal process and to penal administration. If society expects more than punishment, deterrence, and detention of the dangerous person, if rehabilitation and treatment are goals, a broad program of research in this area must be developed and social reforms (the last recourse a society will entertain) considered. In many countries of the European Continent, particularly Sweden, Great Britain, and some states of the United States, new approaches are under way. A less punitive legal approach to homosexuality in Czechoslovakia is an example. So far, legal procedures have been beyond the scrutiny of the scientist; to bring the methods of laboratory and clinic into these areas of human endeavor may not be very comfortable or appealing to many lawyers, but it may eventually have revolutionary results. An investigation, not only of the criminal but also of witnesses, of the nature of the legal evidence and proof, of all types of legal arguments of counsel, and even of juries and judges, should be carried out as time goes on. It should be extended to the study of police methods, of jails and their possible differences from other closed institutions such as mental hospitals. Even more important than work in forensic psychiatry is the application of dynamic psychiatric thought to the field of family law; this has far-reaching implications for family relations, child-rearing and, ultimately, for a more effective control and even prevention of deviant behavior.

As an agency of social control, the law requires information from a variety of sources. An exposure to knowledge about the organization of behavior and motivations, as it has emerged from clinical and experimental experience, should be beneficial to future judges, advocates, prison administrators, and parole officers. The lawyer who understands something about, say, the pattern of extravagant behavior, poor judgment, but lucid capacity for argument of the mental patient is likely to counsel his client with better judgment than one attorney we know who proudly and successfully liberated his convincing client from the clutches of a hospital only to be shocked at the suicide that followed within a few days. The extremes of behavior disorder and the attendant patterns of behavior with which psychiatrists are acquainted should be familiar to legal and penal experts. Similarly, the knowledge we do have about aberrant behavior and the contributory roles of psychosocial factors can be conveyed to advantage in legal education. But neither lawyers, penologists, nor psychiatrists are yet able to counsel in the majority of cases what "should be done" on the basis of such knowledge. Such applications represent an uncharted area in which little expertise or experience can be claimed. Collaborative attempts to define and evaluate problems and to find solutions are needed.

NOTES

1. A Draft Act Governing Hospitalization of the Mentality Ill, *Public Health Service Publication*, (U. S. Federal Security Agency 1951), No. 51.
2. Leo Alexander, "The Commitment and Suicide of King Ludwig II of Bavaria," *American Journal of Psychiatry*, 111 (1954), 100.
3. David L. Bazelon, "The Awesome Decision, Adventures of the Mind," *The Saturday Evening Post* (1960).

4. David L. Bazelon, "The Dilemma of Punishment," Louis D. Brandeis Memorial Lecture, Brandeis University, Waltham, Massachusetts, March 14, 1960.
5. Binder v. Ruvell, Circuit Court, Cook County, Ill., 5262535, (1951).
6. Henry A. Davidson, *Forensic Psychiatry* (New York: Ronald Press, 1952).
7. George H. Dession and Lawrence Z. Freedman, "Drug-induced Revelation and Criminal Investigation," *Yale Law Journal*, 62 (1953), 315.
8. Bernard L. Diamond, "The Fallacy of the Impartial Expert," *Archives of Criminal Psychodynamics*, 3 (Spring, 1959), 221.
9. Durham v. United States, 214F 2d 862 (D. C. Cir., 1954).
10. Paul H. Gebhard, J. H. Gagnon, W. H. Pomeroy and C. V. Christianson, *Sex Offenders* (New York: Harper and Row, 1965).
11. Abraham S. Goldstein and J. Katz, "Psychiatrist–Patient Privilege," *American Journal of Psychiatry*, 118 (1962), 733.
12. Joseph Goldstein and J. Katz, *The Family and the Law* (New York: The Free Press, 1965).
13. Manfred S. Guttmacher and Henry Weihofen, *Psychiatry and the Law* (New York: Norton, 1952).
14. Jerome Hall, "Psychiatry and Criminal Responsibility," *Yale Law Journal*, 65 (1950), 761.
15. August B. Hollingshead and Fredrick C. Redlich, *Social Class and Mental Illness* (New York: John Wiley, 1958).
16. "Implementation and Clarification of the Durham Decision of Criminal Responsibility," *Columbia Law Review*, 58 (1958), 1253.
17. F. E. Inban, *Lie Detectors and Criminal Interaction* (Baltimore: Williams & Wilkins, 1953).
18. Jay Katz and Joseph Goldstein, "Dangerousness and Mental Illness," *Journal of Nervous and Mental Disease*, 131 (1960), 404.
19. Lawrence S. Kubie, "Implications for Legal Procedure of the Fallibility of Human Memory," *University of Pennsylvania Law Review*, 108 (1959), 59.
20. Robert J. Lifton, *Thought Reform and the Psychology of Totalism* (New York: Norton, 1961).
21. John M. MacDonald, *Psychiatry and the Criminal* (Springfield: Charles C Thomas, 1958).
22. Joost A. M. Meerloo, *The Rape of the Mind: The Psychology of Thought Control* (New York: World Publishing Co., 1956).
23. Winfred Overholser, "The Briggs Law of Massachusetts," *Journal of Criminal Law, Criminology and Police Science*, 25 (1935), 859.
24. Isaac Ray, *A Treatise on the Medical Jurisprudence of Insanity* (Boston: Little, Brown, 1838).
25. Fredrick C. Redlich, L. Ravitz, and G. H. Dession, "Narcoanalysis and Truth," *American Journal of Psychiatry*, 107 (1951), 586.
26. Gösta Rylander, "Forensic Psychiatry in Relation to Legislation in Different

Countries," in *Psychiatrie der Gegenwart, Forschung und Praxis,* herausgegehen, von H. W. Gruble (Berlin: Springer, 1960).

27. G. Stürüp, "The Scandinavian Experience," *Law and Contemporary Problems,* 25 (1960), 361.
28. Thomas S. Szasz, "Commitment of the Mentally Ill: 'Treatment' or Social Restraint?" *Journal of Nervous and Mental Disease,* 125 (1957), 293.
29. Thomas S. Szasz, "Psychiatry, Ethics and the Criminal Law," *Columbia Law Review,* 58 (1958), 183.
30. Thomas S. Szasz, "Some Observations on the Relationship between Psychiatry and the Law," *Archives of Neurology and Psychiatry,* 75 (1956), 297.
31. Thomas S. Szasz, "The Concept of Testamentary Capacity," *Journal of Nervous and Mental Disease,* 125 (1957), 474.
32. Fredric Wertham, *Dark Legend* (New York: Doubleday, 1949).
33. Karl Wilmanns, *Die sogenannte verminderte Zurechnungsfähigkeit* (Berlin: Springer, 1927).

CHAPTER TWENTY-FIVE

Psychiatry and the Practice of Medicine and Surgery

Psychiatry's Role in Comprehensive Medicine

The most important application of psychiatric principles, apart from psychiatric practice itself, is in general medical practice and in the different medical specialties. Of all medically trained personnel, the psychiatrist, together with experts in preventive medicine, public health and rehabilitation, is less apt than others to develop a picture of the patient as an isolated organism and more likely to see an individual as a member of a real community. He has much to contribute to medical practice, but he also has much to learn from nonpsychiatric patient populations.

A comprehensive medical orientation is increasingly essential for the following reasons: (1) The number of physicians per capita is on the wane in many countries; in the United States, for instance, medical schools have not been able to supply the needed number of physicians. The result is an inability to give as much time to patients as doctors did even a generation ago. Furthermore, the many complex procedures mandatory in current medical practice are also more time-consuming. (2) The family physician is disappearing. Family physicians were able to get acquainted with their patients and their families; many physicians knew their patients all their lives. The specialist rarely has such broad knowledge and interests. It is in the very nature of specialization to focus on specific topics and medical problems for which a high level of skill in diagnosis and treatment has become necessary. (3) The increasing importance of hospital and office practice has further removed physicians from their patients. It is rare today for physicians to see their patients' homes, to know how they live, and understand their relationships with their families. For all these reasons it is not surprising that in medical schools psychiatry has often become the advocate of a holistic or comprehensive medical orientation; frequently, medical specialists concerned with comprehensive patient care seek the collaboration of psychiatry.

Comprehensive medicine maintains that for proper diagnosis, treatment, and prevention, we must know more than biological facts: we must consider the psychosocial aspects of human existence, and this requires technical knowledge. In due time, departments of behavioral sciences will be an integral part of our medical schools, just as today we have departments of anatomy, physiology, and biochemistry. For the present, psychiatrists have set themselves the task of teaching the behavioral sciences relevant for medicine; only recently, psychologists and social scientists have also begun to play a role in this aspect of medical education. Such teaching can arouse resistance, criticism, and even ridicule; psychiatrists are belittled and reproached for teaching "bedside manners" of a medicine about which they know little. It is true that very few psychiatrists have retained enough medical knowledge to teach comprehensive medicine well; the task therefore seems to be done best in collaboration. Eventually, specialists outside of psychiatry will have less need for the psychiatrist in this endeavor. To a certain degree, this has happened in pediatrics, where comprehensive pediatrics has been taught effectively by pediatricians in a number of medical schools.

The Cultural Context of Medical Practice

Physicians are not sufficiently aware that the culture of a given society determines the type of medicine—scientific, magical, or admixtures—which is practiced. The modern practitioner must be cognizant not only of his own value system but also of that of his patients. He must know how and in what terms his patients value health and what they believe about methods of preserving health. The most important aspect of the relationship of culture to medicine is the fact that value systems and socioeconomic resources of a group, as well as of an individual, determine therapeutic interaction and its outcome to a significant degree. In many parts of the world sick people suffer and die not because of a lack of medical knowledge, but because no physicians, drugs, or hospitals are available. This happens, too, because those who are sick are sometimes unwilling or unable to cooperate with health authorities to make therapeutic measures effective. All too often treatment cannot take place because cooperation between the individual patient and physician is lacking. An example is the case of parents, members of the sect of Jehovah's Witnesses, who endangered the life of their child by not permitting physicians to administer a blood transfusion. A court order was obtained to permit this. Unfortunately, after the transfusion the child died, which to the parents was a clear expression of the Lord's wrath.

Family members can help or, in the most subtle and surprising ways, hinder a person from seeking and using help. Scientific medicine is a relatively new endeavor and far from being universally accepted. Powerful social institutions, such as certain religious organizations, still advocate magical practice and oppose scientific methods. Belief in magic and resistance to scientific medicine is widespread; to a certain degree it may be observed in virtually all patients. More important, the intentional and unintentional need for magic is present in many physicians who openly are adherents of scientific medicine: otherwise, one cannot explain the flourishing of short- and long-lived fads of successful quacks inside the medical profession and the popularity of useless and even dangerous drugs and patent medicines.

Patient–Physician Relationship

Three contributions from psychoanalysis and the behavioral sciences are particularly useful for understanding the patient–physician relationship: (1) the concept of the sick role and the physician's role; (2) the concept of the participant observer; and (3) the concepts of transference and countertransference.

Talcott Parsons defines the social role of a person as expected behavior; he speaks of the physician's role and the sick role.[19] The *physician's role* is well expressed by the rules embodied in the Hippocratic oath: physicians must help and not harm (*primum non nocere*) and must not derive other benefits than reasonable income from their practice. Compensation for medical services and medical responsibilities are set explicitly or implicitly by society. The physician is required to give first aid or any medical help if he is the only one who can do this. He expects the patients to exhibit their bodies and reveal any secrets of body or mind that are pertinent to their health. In medical matters, physicians are in a strongly authoritative role; but this does not justify any extension of this authority to other areas of living. Physicians should not gain any social, sexual, political, or other personal advantages from their relationships with patients. They should not derive power from their practice, although it is natural that successful practice enhances prestige.

The *sick role*, which we discussed before on several occasions, is a culturally accepted set of rules which defines how patients are expected to cooperate with physicians. The patient will follow the doctor's orders; he will not window-shop or bargain-hunt for medical services; he is excused from work but has the obligation of doing everything in his power to get well. Deviations from the sick role bring about sanctions from the physician and also from society. These sanctions are not legalized, although they are strongly enforced by the prevailing mores. One of the results of deviation from such expected behavior is termination of treatment or an alteration in medical care, which is usually to the detriment of the patient.

In general medicine, physicians usually consider themselves detached observers. In psychiatry, the *concept of the participant-observer*, first used by Harry Stack Sullivan, prevails.[29] To be completely detached is impossible for any scientific observer and from the standpoint of medical practice, usually undesirable. Any observation of scientific data, and particularly the observation of human relations, is based on a transaction between the observer and the observed person. The observer is, so to say, his own and most important instrument. Whatever happens to the observed person is bound to produce a reaction in the observer, and vice versa. The expert in human observation is keenly aware of his own reactions and will draw on them freely in his interpretation of the other person.

Many of the reactions of both patient and physician are determined by unconscious motivations. Two very important classes of such reactions, determined by unconscious motivation, are transference and countertransference. *Transference* refers to the fact that the patient carries over, or transfers, preconscious and unconscious reactions of the past to the doctor–patient relationship. Think, for example, of the unreasonably uncooperative and angry patient whose attitude is a carry-over from childhood when the patient was sick or in a situation in which he was frightened, angry, and frustrated because he did not receive attention from the mothering person. Essentially, transference involves unconscious sets or attitudes and is not primarily based on specific childhood trauma. To be sick and need help may mean that someone has to pay attention; the patient anticipates that, as with the demands of a whining child, his complaints will be resented—the doctor will help only grudgingly. The patient may equate sickness with badness and in some way be ashamed to approach the doctor. He may "be sure" the doctor is not interested in his insignificant troubles and, therefore, tends to ignore, or keep his distance from, the doctor. We cannot, of course, explain all uncooperative behavior in this fashion; however, we not infrequently find that the patient's lack of cooperation and his struggle against his doctor are beyond his conscious control and, in any case, should not be considered personal insults to the physician. Merely to realize this may be very helpful in one's daily work.

Countertransference in medical practice means the archaic emotional reaction to the patient which the physician carries over from his own earlier preprofessional experiences. The role of "doctor" may unconsciously mean the one who helps, who never fails; or the one who can fix things better than anyone; the powerful privileged one who helps and thereby is exempt from demands and from the danger of illness; the one who can peek, touch, and poke where others may not—as in the doctor game of childhood. The consequences of transference and countertransference responses may be far reaching and can account for a great many problems and perplexities of medical work. Many mistakes and misunderstandings and many iatrogenic illnesses are the result of undetected and unfavorable transference and countertransference reactions. Transference and countertransference is not easily discerned by the physician untrained in psychodynamics. However, if physicians are aware of strong preconscious emotions in their patients and in themselves, this of itself is a real achievement.

Among the most important emotional reactions of patients are: anxiety, hostility, suspicion, passivity and dependence, seductiveness, and self-destructiveness. Of course, pure types of such reactions do not exist, and in actual practice we encounter complex mixtures; fusions of anxiety and hostility and of passivity and hostility are perhaps the most common. The seductive patient, even if he flatters his physician, often turns out to be basically angry and destructive. To all reactions, the physician will respond consciously and unconsciously. Where he is desired, honored, loved, flattered, needed, and seduced by an attractive patient, he can react by basking in glory, by wrestling with sexual temptation, by aloof withdrawal or, hopefully, by wise comprehension. He must refrain from encouraging these distractions and from toying with them, since these are potentially explosive emotions for anyone. The physician may be anxious, overdetached, particularly toward emotional problems of the patients, constantly angry, guilt-ridden over not doing enough for his patients, or too dependent on their gratitude. If his competence is questioned, he may doubt his proven abilities or unnecessarily retaliate. He may be aware of his feelings or, more often, unaware of them and assume that he is tired or that his work is unfulfilling.

Psychosocial Factors in Medical Practice

Awareness of cultural context, social role, and the conscious and unconscious aspects of the patient–physician relationship will add to the physician's grasp of the patient's medical problems. Good physicians have always been interested in the total patient and not merely in one of his diseased organs. A patient is neither a guinea pig nor a laboratory specimen, even if most medical schools impart a kind of corpse- and rat-orientation in the preclinical years. A holistic view, in our opinion, does not imply a reduction of all the patient's problems into one diagnosis. To the contrary, we believe it is preferable to make separately a biological and a psychosocial diagnosis; only a consideration of both kinds of data will permit a truly effective therapy.

The innumerable problems about which physicians are consulted can be divided into three classes. (1) Medical problems constitute the first group; physicians are adequately trained to handle biological aspects of these problems but not to uncover and appreciate the role of psychosocial factors in all illness. These tend to intrude at any number of points in the course of events. It is our conviction that these factors influence not only the so-called psychosomatic diseases and certain endocrine and metabolic diseases but all illnesses, although relatively few hard data are currently available to support this view. (2) Physicians are consulted about a variety of nonmedical problems; openly or covertly, patients bring problems of which physicians have no explicit knowledge. Some physicians are seduced into responding to pleas for nonmedical advice out of a feeling of kindness or omnipotence and omniscience. Such responses are, of course, not justified and are often detrimental to both patient and physician. (3) Patients also offer borderline problems, which may superficially involve medical considerations. The help of a physician is typically solicited in the absence of a more competent specialist or because of the patient's need to think of his difficulties as medical. Into this group fall many problems of living, some of them normal and some neurotic. The former include the universal crises in the various stages of life, during infancy, childhood, puberty, adolescence, menopause and old age, and the unavoidable difficulties that at times beset every marriage and family. To help patients with such "minor" problems is a "major" task. In general, medical educators are not yet fully aware that neither intuition, common sense, nor amateur skill is enough to prepare physicians for such a task; some technical knowledge is required. According to a verbal communication by H. E. Payson, 25 per cent of all problems encountered in the medical dispensary of a community and teaching hospital are medical problems; 15 per cent are nonmedical problems; and the remainder comprises a mixture.[20]

The Acute and the Chronic Sick Role in Medicine

In acute and severe illnesses, the roles of physicians and patients are clearly defined. The physician is in the role of the technically competent and authoritative helper. Here the stereotype is that of a person who saves life or limb, helps anyone who needs him regardless of color, creed, or status, and makes any sacrifice to achieve this goal. The greater the danger, the greater the physician's prestige. Franz Werfel in *The Man Who Conquered Death* said that the specialties closest to death—surgery and medicine—enjoy the greatest prestige. In contrast, the stereotype of the patient is of one who is helpless, suffers from pain, dysfunction, and feels endangered. He is dependent and temporarily in a childlike role but masters his anxieties like a brave boy. Physicians have been portrayed in the role of a heroic helper in popular fiction, theater, and media of mass communication. And the fact is that some of the finest and most rewarding work is done under circumstances that approximate this culturally defined pattern. In a relationship between a helpless, suffering patient and a truly competent physician, all moves as well as can be expected, and the situation offers relatively few psychosocial problems. The patient believes in his doctor, rewards him by paying directly or indirectly for his service, by honoring him, and, most of all, by getting well. If the patient does not get well, even if he dies, the physician will not be blamed if he has done what is possible. Medical and surgical work with patients in the "acute sick role" is in these terms most gratifying.

Physicians feel decidedly uneasy about the "chronic sick role" in contrast to the "acute sick role." Dependency is a psychological problem in all illnesses,[1] but in chronic illness it reaches major proportions. Often it is difficult to decide what to do with such a patient who does not get better, especially if the patient is bitter, hostile, and uncooperative, as is so often the case with people chronically ill. Physicians, in turn, react to these emotions with hostility and withdrawal, which may make the situation worse. Most physicians feel uncomfortable with maladjusted, infantile, dependent, and passive chronic patients who make too many demands with which the physician is not trained to cope.

Yet practitioners of medicine must reckon with the psychosocial consequences of chronic diseases, which have become medicine's greatest challenge. A very large number of chronic diseases, malformations, and defects result in lasting occupational, social, and sexual impairment. They produce severe secondary stresses, which cannot be mastered and which threaten the patient's existence. This is evident not only in chronic cardiac and pulmonary diseases, which endanger the patient's life, but also in many less threatening types of infirmity. The unattractiveness of a patient's chronic eczema or the devaluation of a sterile woman (in many cultures) may be experienced as deep psychological injuries, which tend to isolate the patient and drive him into more hopeless invalidism. All too frequently, instead of helping these patients, we increase their stresses by irrational, and, at times, even by rational, methods of treatment. Until recently, many patients with tuberculosis suffered as much from the isolating and regressive effects of traditional institutional therapy as from the disease itself. Similarly, many patients with coronary disease have unnecessarily been made lifelong cardiac invalids. In many parts of the world, patients with leprosy are still excluded from a normal and dignified life. The management of many chronic neurological diseases, such as multiple sclerosis, promotes invalidism, particularly in the lower-class patient. We have already mentioned how stressful the existence of an endocrine cripple can be. Thus, the chronic sick role into which the patient is cast by society and his physicians may be more harmful than the chronic illness.

Only a combined biological and psychosocial diagnostic and therapeutic approach can offer promise to such patients. This comprehensive approach is embodied in the important efforts of rehabilitation, medicine's newest major division.[26] Many patients with severe chronic disabilities, with aphasias, spinal cord injuries, disfigurations, and deafness and blindness have been returned to a fair degree of happiness, usefulness, and satisfaction through the efforts of teams of physicians, physical and occupational therapists, psychologists, social workers, and educators. Not infrequently all these skills combine in a single person—the general practitioner.

Psychosocial Problems in Medical and Surgical Specialties

Surgical specialties have been notably resistant to a psychological point of view. One plausible explanation which surgeons offer is the mere fact that their serious and highly technical responsibilities do not permit them to dwell on what many consider frills of clinical practice. Yet an increasing number of surgeons believes that this view is erroneous and has become convinced that many surgical failures occur not because of technical incompetence but because of a lack of appreciation of the patients' psychosocial problems.

Operations may be necessary, highly skillful procedures, sanctioned by elaborate legal and ethical codes. Although they are certainly not assaults, the patient's preconscious perception of an operation may be precisely that. In children, senile patients, and patients of primitive cultures, the dread of surgery is not suppressed or repressed; there is some degree of fear in all patients nevertheless, even in those whose intelligence and ego strength permit them to accept the inevitable. As anxiety and hostility not only unnecessarily increase suffering but also are disturbing factors in the management of surgical patients, proper steps should be taken to reduce such anxiety. Irving L. Janis has studied this problem both clinically and experimentally in patients undergoing surgical operations.[12] He recommends more careful information and preparation of patients for these procedures; patients should have a chance to vent their apprehensions and doubts; if this is not the case, Janis found that it may have a definite influence on the postoperative course; patients are apt to become uncooperative, depressed, overdependent, and hostile.[31] The irrational notion that operations are killing, mutilating, or castrating procedures is much more common than we think.[8] This is particularly true with respect to operations of the genitourinary tract, in ophthalmic and neurosurgery, in amputations, and in most operations that leave severe physiological or cosmetic defects.

Psychological preparation for surgery should come in steps, and patients should have a chance to absorb it. Incidents as the eye operation of an elderly patient who was completely unprepared for what was going to happen until the surgeon jabbed a needle with novocain into the patient's eye socket and said, cheerfully, "Here we go," surely can be avoided. The postoperative course of this particular patient was stormy—not necessarily because of this incident—and his anxiety and resentment considerable. Today, many experienced surgeons believe that a smoother postoperative course follows when patients are psychologically prepared for their operations.

One procedure often dreaded by patients is general anesthesia; it is clearly a fear of never waking up from the anesthesia. Spinal anesthesia can also be anxiety-producing. A number of anesthesiologists have realized the importance of a careful explanation and personal (rather than routine) reassurance, which takes some of the specific anxieties of the patient into account. Doctors should not talk about the patient until he is deeply anesthetized; we recall a postoperative psychosis in a woman who was panicked by what she overheard (correctly) before and misheard during the first stage of anesthesia. Care should be taken to give patients appropriate information, not only before the operation, but after it as well. Actually, most psychological and physiological complications develop in periods which for most surgeons are much less interesting than the operation itself; surgeons are apt to lose the war after they have won their battles. Reassurance and explanations, of themselves, are not the critical features of psychological management: merely telling someone something is *not* equivalent to two people participating. The opportunity for patients simply to express to a receptive and understanding physician their attitudes and sentiments concerning their situation, symptoms, and therapy is of much greater importance. For the patient, this means there is something he can do, he can reach the surgeon and be heard when there is need; and this securing of a pathway to relief is the crucial bond.

The problem of needless surgery, although severely dealt with in good hospitals, is a taboo subject. We believe that bad judgment, incompetence, and fads, and not greed, account for most cases of unneeded surgery. Psychologically, the most important cases are those in which a masochistic and self-destructive patient is able to provoke an unsuspecting and occasionally punitive surgeon into an unnecessary procedure. In our observation, self-destructive and self-punitive patients are apt to have more complications than others; not infrequently one operation necessitates another and may lead to what has been called surgical addiction. From a certain point on, the patient manages the surgeon. Lest it appear that we are trying to saddle the patient with the responsibility for unnecessary surgery, it should be clearly stated that the surgeon is responsible for such mismanagement. Usually, however, this is not because he is bent on performing unnecessary operations but because he fails to understand that he is being manipulated by a patient who blindly wants change and relief and at bottom is moving toward self-destruction. Once the vicious cycle is started, it is extremely difficult to stop; both skillful psychotherapy and a cooperative surgeon are needed to demonstrate to the patient that he is self-punitive and acts against his own interest. Karl Menninger has shown convincingly that many so-called surgical addicts are self-destructive persons.[18] An occupational hazard of all medicine and surgery is the tendency of the doctor to allow patients to elevate him to a godlike role. If this is compatible with the doctor's needs, he often finds himself searching for even the most unlikely explanations or unnecessary surgical procedures in order to maintain the role and continue to be needed. A reliable and freely communicating doctor–patient relationship is the surest safeguard.

Surgical subspecialties: Other specialties in which psychosocial factors are of considerable importance are ophthalmology and otolaryngology. In both specialties, medical approaches are gradually becoming as important as surgical interventions, and rehabilitation is becoming especially significant. Otolaryngologists have become interested in the psychological impact of a partial or complete loss of hearing, and ophthalmologists are concerned with the effects of congenital and acquired blindness on the personality of the visually handicapped patient. Impairment or loss of vision or hearing produces overt and covert anxieties, an inevitable degree of social isolation, and severe handicaps in learning, which are sometimes consciously or unconsciously interpreted as deserved or undeserved punishment. These anxieties mobilize powerful defense mechanisms. The prevalent defense in patients with impaired vision and blindness is denial, often resulting in bland, hysterical behavior in the seemingly well-adjusted patient. Recognition of the patient's responses to sensory loss has greatly helped in the re-education and rehabilitation of such patients.[16, 27] In severe cases, a high degree of autism is not infrequent. In patients who are hard of hearing or deaf, one is impressed with projective mechanisms, which manifest themselves as suspicion and paranoid attitudes. Urologists and proctologists also work in "touchy" areas, which makes an appreciation of the patient's concern and anxieties particularly important. It is obvious that neurosurgeons, who operate on the "organ of behavior," must have more than a casual knowledge of psychosocial factors in behavior.

Psychological Factors in Gynecology and Obstetrics

In the chapter on Psychosomatic Diseases, we have discussed the impact of psychological factors on certain gynecological diseases, on infertility, and on habitual abortion. Beyond the expert handling of these diseases, the gynecologist is often expected to guide his patients in their sexual problems and to help them in the crises of life that may arise during menarche and menopause. Psychological factors in normal pregnancy and delivery are even of greater significance for the practitioners of the specialty and those general practitioners who do obstetrical work.

To isolate those psychological factors which impinge on *pregnancy and childbirth* is, however, another matter. It is very difficult to predict which physically healthy women will go through pregnancy with a feeling of serenity, which will take it in stride, and which will suffer from such complications as morning sickness, salivation, and heartburn, which are considered to be, at least in part, of psychogenic origin; pica, or unusual appetite, is solely psychogenic. Some neurotic women actually feel free from anxiety and other neurotic symptoms during pregnancy; it seems that the pregnancy gives them a feeling of security, integrity, and worth. During pregnancy, women enjoy certain advantages: in general they can satisfy their needs for dependence and succor more readily; during the latter part of pregnancy, frigid women can escape from sexual relations, and this may lessen neurotic anxieties and conflicts. Other women are plagued by panicky fears of being mutilated or killed during delivery and remain in a state of agony for many months before the dreaded labor begins. The conscious rejection of the infant found in many unwed mothers is not related to a difficult or complicated pregnancy. Unconscious rejection of the child and the mother's fear of being mutilated are the most important psychogenic causes of complications.[7] Grete Bibring felt that identification of the pregnant woman with her own mother is decisive for the quality of the experience of pregnancy.[4]

Long before the days of psychosomatic medicine it was known that *lactation* is to a large degree a function of the mother's desire to nurse her child. There are authentic reports of the cessation of lactation after stress, and there are also observations of the continuation of the flow of milk after the separation of the child from the mother against her wishes. Therese F. Benedek considers the desire to nurse the child as a true instinct;[3] any interference of the symbiotic relationship of the mother and infant will reflect itself in a disturbance of this instinctual activity. Modern obstetrics and pediatrics believe that any arrangement that facilitates closeness between mother and child is desirable. Edith Jackson, a psychoanalyst and pediatrician, pioneered the so-called "rooming-in" program, which permits the mother to keep the baby in her hospital room, in contrast with the customary arrangement of isolating infants in separate units. Another, possibly even more important, method has become known as "natural childbirth" or "childbirth without fear." Although childbirth is invariably accompanied by some pain and fear, the new trend is notably constructive. It views pregnancy and delivery not as pathological but as physiological processes. The method, in essence, uses persuasive and clarifying statements to reinforce the mother's wish to have a child and to dispel her fears of pregnancy and labor. Contemporary techniques, which originated with Grantly Dick Read[21] in Great Britain and I. Z. Zvelovski[32] in Russia, were developed by H. Thoms[30] and C. Lee Buxton[5] in the United States. In France, Leon Chertok has attempted to understand the subtle mechanisms of the method, which, based on a better grasp of the psychological aspects of pregnancy, permit a significant reduction of anxiety.[6] This aspect is more fundamental than the ritual addition of relaxing exercises that Read recommended.

The Importance of a "Psychological Attitude" in Pediatric Practice

In no medical specialty is psychological knowledge more important than in pediatrics. J. B. Richmond reports that over 50 per cent of the contemporary pediatrician's time is spent with well children and their families.[23] For a pediatrician, the work with a family is almost as important as the work with his child patients. In this capacity, he must deal with normal and abnormal children, normal and abnormal families. In his role as pediatrician, he is an important adviser upon many problems of child-rearing, ranging from infant feeding to sexual instruction and the choice of schools. He must serve as a consultant to parents but at the same time not make them too dependent. He is often called upon to advise on child health and welfare in his community. His emphasis must be equally on disease and normal growth. Pediatricians are often consulted about problems of adoption, and this requires especially sensitive judgment and knowledge. Pediatricians share with child psychiatrists the treatment of many behavior problems in children.[28] Although psychiatrists usually take care of the more severe cases, there is no clear demarcation between the two professions, especially if the pediatrician has an orientation to psychological problems. The allotment of cases depends more on the availability of child psychiatrists and on the interest and aptitude of pediatricians to handle serious behavior problems than on membership in professional societies.

In severe and dangerous illnesses pediatricians have the additional task of dealing with the child's parents, and this is usually a greater challenge than dealing with families of adult patients. In the face of medical and emotional crises, parents are apt to feel very anxious, guilty, and inept; they look to the support of their pediatrician.

Some Psychological Problems in Dental Practice

There is a growing awareness of the significance of psychological factors in the practice of dentistry. As Alex H. Kaplan remarked, dentists work in one of the psychologically most important regions of the body.[13] Anxiety over oral manipulations is prone to be high, and dentists, in order to do their work properly, must be competent to deal with anxiety as well as able to alleviate physical pain. There have been assertions in the literature that certain common dental diseases such as caries and periodontal diseases are in part the result of emotional attitudes that alter salivary flow and the chemical milieu of the mouth. Thumb-sucking and bruxism may contribute to some cases of malocclusion. In severe abnormalities of the oral cavity, such as different forms of cleft palate, which are accompanied by serious impairment of speech, behavioral consequences are inevitable and striking. They require the very skillful teamwork of oral surgeons, otolaryngologists, speech therapists, teachers, and mental health workers.

Neurotic and Psychotic Patients in General Practice

The question is sometimes asked whether general practitioners and medical specialists should treat neurotics. The answer is very clear: it is unavoidable! The supply of fully trained medical and nonmedical psychotherapists now available does not begin to meet the need; thus the general practitioner perforce treats large numbers of neurotic patients. Many practitioners feel uncomfortable with neurotics; they discourage or neglect them and chase them away by overt or covert methods; of course, this can hardly be considered good practice. It is understood that general practitioners and medical specialists have neither the time nor the skill for intensive long-term psychotherapy; fortunately, such therapy is neither necessary nor desirable in many cases. Rather simple techniques of relating to the patient are often sufficient. The severely neurotic patient belongs in the hands of a psychiatrist; the milder case, however, can be helped by the family physician. He may not be cured (the term *cure* is applicable to few neurotics), but he may be seen through many crises of living.

Nonpsychiatric physicians usually tend to refer psychotic patients to a psychiatrist or to the nearest mental hospital with all possible speed. Neither such haste nor fear is justified in a great many cases. Unquestionably, the severely disturbed person should have the benefit of psychiatric therapy, yet many psychotics who, for various reasons, are neither in active psychiatric treatment nor in mental hospitals could and should be carried by general practitioners. As we have stated repeatedly, there are very few patients with psychiatric disorders who are dangerous. The small list of dangerous patients includes some paranoids, schizophrenics, patients with suicidal depression and very rarely epileptics. Even among the agitated, it is at times amazing how much a little kindness, freedom from fear, and the judicious use of a tranquilizing drug can do to restore the patient's equilibrium. An important and frequent problem is posed by patients who are physically ill and also suffer from a behavior disorder, which may or may not be directly connected with their physical illnesses.

Psychotic patients with physical illness rarely receive good medical care; most physicians, surgeons, and nurses have a regrettable, often unchecked tendency to avoid such patients. This probably explains, more than lack of funds and facilities, why physically ill patients in so many psychiatric institutions and in general hospitals get inferior medical and surgical treatment. These remarks also apply to the severe mental deficiencies. There is a curious resistance in most physicians to admit that a behavior disorder and a somatic illness can coexist. Presumably this is the result not only of the physician's training in parsimonious diagnosis but also of his aversion to deviant behavior in his patients. As a rule, physicians do not like anxious, hypochondriacal, or obsessive patients who dwell on their illness or deny it; they are suspicious of unconscious exaggeration and dramatization in hysterical patients and are enraged by malingerers. They seem actually to prefer passive patients, although these patients may create even more difficulties than outwardly aggressive and critical patients. Most of all, they dislike self-destructive patients who frustrate their efforts by not getting well. Yet general practitioners and nonpsychiatric specialists are charged with helping their patients, whether or not they suffer from a behavior disorder. In this connection it should be remembered that unnecessary, repetitive, and prolonged examinations can often reinforce in patients the conviction that they are ill and thus produce iatrogenic neuroses.

Psychotherapeutic Medicine

Every good physician has used one or another type of psychotherapy in his practice; he may use it intuitively or with clear awareness. In the following sections are briefly discussed some of the psychological therapies and attitudes that apply to all medical practice. Considered under separate headings, this implies a splitting of therapeutic activities into discrete elements, which of course is not the case. Although common sense is indispensable, these methods also involve a certain technical skill, which, within certain limits, can be learned.

INFORMATION To ensure the cooperation of patients, physicians are expected to provide information about the medical and surgical diseases they are treating; this, of course, will vary as a function of the patient's age, intelligence, emotional and social status, and the nature of the illness. To give this information effectively is an art; unfortunately, little effort has been made to teach it systematically. Providing information should not be equated with simply dumping information upon the hapless patient, nor with confessions concerning the physician's problems and burdens. Even when one physician, an expert, gives information to another in consultation, clarification is involved; one supplies what needs to be known to plan, to cope, and to act. The best guide for giving information is to listen, to learn what is wanted, and to anticipate the irrational fears that accompany illness in anyone. The doctor should also appreciate the patient's reticence to disclose these fears and, more importantly, to ask questions about medication or disease, which spring from unstated theories about disease.

In the recent past, there has been a tendency among physicians to be more open toward patients. We believe this trend is a consequence of rapid and publicized developments in scientific medicine and the rejection of a mystical and magical role in medicine. There is a growing conviction among laymen that they are entitled to know about the findings of modern scientific medicine from books, lectures and, most of all, from their doctors. Until recently, physicians larded their conversation with Latin phrases in the presence of their patients; in a way, this protected the patients from being hurt by words they might easily have misunderstood or misinterpreted. Studies of grand rounds clearly show that patients are easily hurt by words that are misunderstood or emotionally loaded;[14] it is equally important to understand the patient's language, which, of course, is quite different from professional language.[22]

Medical information is usually misunderstood for emotional and not for semantic or intellectual reasons. Anxiety is at the root of defensive maneuvers, which lead to gross misinterpretations of what is perceived, experienced, and understood by patients. Dangers may be grossly exaggerated or illness denied. This capacity for defensive maneuvers means that information that is threatening may be mitigated to avoid excessive anxiety; this is an important facet of the problem of imparting information in cases of severe and dangerous illness. One school of thought holds that threatening information should never be given; the opposite recommends being absolutely truthful. In practice, most physicians steer a course between these two extremes and adjust information given in terms of its content and their evaluation of the recipient. Often, however, these variations relate more closely to what the physician can tolerate than on the needs of the patient and his family. To put it simply, we recommend that physicians be both truthful and sensitive. Oliver Wendell Holmes once said that the patient is not necessarily entitled to the whole truth any more than he is entitled to all of the medicine in the doctor's saddlebag.[11] Patients and relatives can handle the truth if they are properly supported and understand that the physician will see them through pain, agony, and danger as well as possible.

One of the major tasks of a physician is to help his patients face approaching death.[9] The central factor in this always difficult situation is the physician's own anxiety: his realization that his power and his knowledge are limited, but also his own tendency to escape from the responsibility, to abandon the patient, or to reassure him with thinly disguised lies. Personally, the writers have found that in the case of approaching death as well as in the case of severe and dangerous illness, it is best to be honest. Honesty does not mean sadism (or deliberately hurting with the "truth"), nor forcing the patient to admit he has heard right; the extent of information and the manner in which the patients' relatives should be informed will, of course, vary greatly. It is wise to remember that the human being's capacity for denial and repression, and also the clouding of consciousness, help us to buffer the shock of the unbearable.[25] There are no special techniques for this ultimate task, although many have been tried, from hypnosis and drugs to psychoanalysis. It is best to be straightforward, as optimistic as one can realistically be, and, most of all, to stick to one's patient and not abandon him. One patient, a dentist, insisted that he was improving, that he was psychosomatically ill and not saddled with carcinoma; nevertheless he planned meticulously for his wife and children while, to the end, he continued to chide his physician for not agreeing that his progress was good. His attachment to his doctor was deep, and it was obvious that he appreciated the chance to deny and to blame the physician for being "gloomy." Honesty and realism should govern not only the information that is imparted to the dangerously ill patient but also that given to his family. Usually, it only complicates matters when patients are given different information from their relatives. However, the writers know of one case in which the patient was told in secrecy that he was hopelessly ill with cancer but was asked to keep it to himself and not to let his family know; the family was also told and asked not to let the patient know. Amazingly, they all behaved well, which, of course, was the physician's wish. When physicians are dealing with patients who are devoutly religious, close cooperation with the clergy can be helpful.

Advice

Even in medical matters, where physicians proudly feel that they tread on firm ground, their advice is not always strictly rational; it often betrays not only ignorance but also the need for assuming omniscient and omnipotent roles. The long history of fads and strange cures bears witness to this. Often advice is too vague and casual. Think of the patient, after a near-fatal coronary episode, who was told no more than to "take it easy"; then imagine going about the day's activities wondering *how easy* to take it: should one reach for one's hat, bend to tie one's shoes, get angry with a colleague, wrestle with the elevator door, walk a block or three blocks, hike, bend, grunt, reach, and argue vigorously or without heat? Such a patient is rarely advised about sexual intercourse and rarely given a chance to ask questions or ventilate his experiences. Some physicians impose unnecessary restrictions for too long a time on many chronic patients, such as those having coronary thrombosis or tuberculosis. One of the invidious forms of restriction is the rest cure, which—at long last—is in disrepute in Western medicine and psychiatry. Rest has its place after severe physical and emotional exhaustion, but prolonged rest cures have no sound physiological and psychological rationale; they only make patients passive and dependent. Such practices as these derive from a lack of definite knowledge and experience and also reflect the irrational needs both of patients and doctors, which make patients behave like little children and induce physicians to regress to the role of the magical healer.

In nonmedical matters, physicians have no authoritative opinion, but they are often pressed into authoritative roles by their patients or goaded by their own needs for status and power, which make them oblivious to their limitations. There also arise borderline situations, when medical facts are important but not the sole determinants of the issue: a physician may be consulted about a change of job or a change of location partly for health reasons. In case of doubt, it is generally better not to advise; the tendency to check one's own inclinations toward omnipotence is a sounder attitude than its obverse. More, such an attitude is in keeping with the decline of the authoritarian and avuncular position of the physician in Western society. For these reasons, physicians are today less likely to recommend marriage for hysterical girls or pregnancy for frustrated brides without knowing relevant details, which might justify such counsel. On the other hand, many are still apt to recommend unnecessary and expensive diagnostic procedures. As far as general problems of living are concerned, physicians can learn from good psychiatrists who are parsimonious with advice, not only because they are aware of their ignorance, but also because they feel it is desirable to let patients make their own decisions whenever possible.

It is unwise to tell patients to carry out activities that are not in keeping with the mores of the particular culture or subculture; for example, to advise a youngster to masturbate or go to a prostitute. It is also usually unsound to encourage a patient to be aggressive or passive or to vent his emotions. All this is an abuse of medical authority; it often backfires because it increases the patient's conflicts instead of reducing them. In any case, it is usually less effective then helping the patient make his own decisions or work through his problems, which are the result of a dilemma for which there is no general solution. Although advice should be dispensed in very sparing doses, physicians must be willing to help patients reach new adjustments that are needed following illnesses, accidents, and operations. A completely nondirective attitude may be startling and threatening to patients. To be nondirective does not mean to be nonsupportive; on the contrary, what is required is support, interest, inquiry, an occasional opinion, a clarifying statement, with advice limited to clearly defined areas of medical care. After this spate of advice to use advice most sparingly, we should also remind the physician to be aware of the resources of his own community; a good doctor must have a feeling for his community, its assets and liabilities, its welfare organizations, clubs, churches, schools, and recreational facilities, in addition to its hospitals and clinics. He should know how to collaborate with the social worker and how to use the services of the community nurse. Finally, he should always remember that patients have families and jobs and that here is where the bulk of loving, hating, and living is carried on. The close ties patients have to spouses who are objectively obnoxious must be respected; bitter complaints do not automatically represent a call for legal aid. Without such knowledge, the physician's therapy will remain restricted and his ingenuity and efforts to aid rehabilitation will often fail.

REASSURANCE AND SUGGESTION To reassure anxious and depressed patients is one of the oldest and most important of psychological techniques. Reassurance is not taught in any systematic way and, in general, the art of reassurance is not used too well. Some physicians and some psychiatrists advocate the use of certain pet phrases of reassurance. One experienced physician told his patients to repeat to themselves t. i. d.: "Easy does it." However, such mechanical approaches have little merit. It is more important to realize that reassurance and suggestion require a definite relationship between physician and patient. The physician must be in a position of authority; the patient must have trust, although complete trust is rare and too often not realistic. The person who suggests or reassures is a person with the power of magic; the verbal and behavioral messages of this powerful physician are accepted by the patient and reduce his anxiety. In very anxious and infantile patients, the need for reassurance will be particularly great. Behavioral suggestion and reassurance are usually greater than verbal suggestion and reassurance; for instance, when a physician stops a certain medication, it has a more powerful reassuring effect on the patient than mere words that the patient is getting better. Although reassurance and suggestion can have a magical quality, they must not stray too far from reality. Once reassurances fail, the likelihood for further reassurance and suggestion is also sharply diminished. It is our impression that lower-class patients have a greater need for reassurance and suggestion and that the better-educated patients of the upper classes more frequently demand realistic information. But all patients need to have the assurance that comes with confidence. At bottom, the wish to be cared for, to be cured, is a universally powerful motive, and this wish is transferred to the person in whose temporary care we put ourselves.

Hypnosis, which recently has come again into vogue in medical circles, is one specific and very important method of suggestion. Professional and unprofessional hypnotists are conducting widely attended courses and demonstrations, which are more than a little reminiscent of the old medicine show. They teach eager doctors how to use hypnosis in treating any kind of psychological difficulty, somatic disease, or pain. The range of patients and of problems in general practice that can be treated by hypnosis is quite limited. Most of the conditions hypnotists claim they can help are better treated by other somatic or psychological means. We believe it is wise for general practitioners and nonpsychiatric specialists to consult psychiatrists about the indications for hypnosis in a particular problem. Hypnosis is a therapeutic technique that has definite limitations and is also not without dangers; general practitioners should be aware of this.

Some patients virtually force a doctor to say things they want to hear; such reassurance, of course, cannot be effective. We have learned it is better to reassure by assigning the patient a more active role; the physician provides some correct medical information and recognizes the patient's feelings, but the patient has to do "the worry work," as Janis put it.[12] Instead of saying, in the case of a slow recovery, "You will be perfectly all right a month from now" (unless this is certain), it is better to say, "You are getting better, but it is slow, and you seem to be worried." This approach is more characteristic for the newer psychotherapeutic attitude, which will be discussed in the next section.

Psychotherapy in General Medical Practice

Will a universal psychotherapy for general practitioners evolve? Probably not; nevertheless certain trends are emerging, from which we can sketch, not a system of psychotherapy, but a simple, flexible, and widely applicable approach for the nonpsychiatric practitioner. It is shaped to a certain extent by techniques developed by C. Rogers, J. Coleman, and H. Kaiser and particularly adapted for the use of general practitioners by Hans K. Knöpfel[15] and Michael Balint.[2] The approach proposed here is based on five principles: (1) proper listening to the patient; (2) sensitive response by the therapist; (3) acceptance of the patient; (4) a relationship of trust; and (5) help toward psychological growth. In dealing with both organic medical and psychological problems, listening attentively and carefully, not only to content but also to the subtleties and manners of speech and nonverbal expressions, such as mimicry and gestures, is the most basic requirement. The therapist also must be aware of his own reactions, as was mentioned earlier in discussing the participant–observer relationship. In stressing the ability to listen well, it should be mentioned that most of us talk too much and about matters that we grasp only poorly. Listening provides the therapist with the cues he needs for responses. His responses must be sensitive and selective; there are some matters in which the therapist will show greater interest than others, which he bypasses or does not even notice. The therapist's responses will reinforce in the patient a trend to talk about these very things and not others. A sensitive response will focus on matters that are important for the patient and will help him to solve problems and grow psychologically. A relaxed, casual, and very mild form of banter may be an optimal stance. Any compulsive or extreme form of humor, particularly humor that is at the expense of the patient, must be avoided. The proper responses will produce a feeling of being understood in the patient. Such understanding, coupled with a friendly acceptance and the absence of punitive or ulterior motives, is, for most persons and for most patients, a rare if not unique experience; it has a liberating effect, which may permit the patient to come out of a depressed, anxious, sullen, or hostile isolation, and it will help to increase his self-esteem. Ultimately such a procedure will enable the patient to grow psychologically and to actualize himself. The therapist, in this process, is a mere catalyst: he provides the opportunity; the patient does the job. Significant changes may occur after only one encounter or over a period of years, and sometimes never. There is nothing miraculous in such an approach, which in fact is more an art than a technique; it calls for sensitivity and interest in human beings and must be learned not from books but in the context of the experience itself.

At times, the question arises whether medical and surgical specialists and general practitioners should attempt to use the so-called deeper techniques, such as the interpretation of dreams, of symbolic acts, or of transference and resistance. We advise against this; these techniques are complex and little will be gained from them unless they are competently, comfortably, and securely used by an expert. The reader's attention is directed to a distinction, which E. Bibring taught, between clarification of conscious and preconscious material and interpretation of unconscious material. The physician who is not analytically trained should stick to clarification.

PSYCHOSOCIAL ASPECTS OF DRUG THERAPY One of the great and unique duties and privileges of the physician is to prescribe drugs. This right endows the physician with great power and puts him in a position of singular trust. It is in part this privilege that endows the physician with power and status in the eyes of patient and society. Even with the rise of a scientific medicine, many diseases for which no known therapy exists are treated by "magic" today.[8] To make this clear: magic does not mean that supernatural forces cause or cure an illness; it means only the assumption of supernatural forces in the minds of the public and occasionally also unconsciously or consciously in the minds of physicians. Mark H. Hollender stated that there is a personal ingredient in every prescription.[10] There is also a bit of magic in most medications and therapeutic procedures. This is one reason why people so readily believe in "miracle" drugs and why many are afraid of drugs because they may be devilish potions and poisons. The "personal ingredient" is also the reason for double-blind studies in evaluating drugs. This ingredient is, however, elusive because the interlocking of individual somatic and interpersonal factors in every case is very complex.

Because patients are anxious about medication, they usually demand precise information on how drugs should be taken and increasingly more information about how drugs work. If the physician supplies this information it may diminish fears but does not always dispel them; the deep anxieties remain. Patients refuse to take drugs, do not carry out procedures, endanger themselves, and irritate physicians who are sensitive to such lack of cooperation. This behavior is variously rooted in anxiety or often in deep self-destructive tendencies of the patient, as well as in a desire to manipulate the environment, particularly evident in children and dependent persons. Self-destructive behavior is clearly seen in diabetics who have become comatose because of dietary indiscretions and faulty application of their insulin therapy.[24] Hollender pointed out that an important consideration in prescribing medicine is the physician's clear and honest awareness of the person for whom the medication is given;[10] is it for the patient, for the family, for the physician, or for a social organization? In pediatric practice, we find, for instance, that much medication is really given for the parent and not for the child. In psychiatric practice, we see the wholesale application of tranquilizing drugs for the benefit of the institution, that is, physicians, nurses, and administrators, and not always solely for the patient's sake. A similar consideration applies in general practice, where tranquilizers are given quite often indiscriminately; this abuse is particularly evident in pediatric practice when tranquilizers are all too readily prescribed—for the parents' sake. In such cases, drugs are not used for medical but for manipulative psychosocial reasons. Clear-thinking physicians must be aware of this and should not blur the distinction between biological and psychosocial uses of drugs.

Placebos are given for psychological reasons and often as a part of the give-and-take patients expect in the medical transaction. Whether relatively inactive drugs, or drugs with a dubious positive effect, should be given depends on the physician's judgment. In some cases it is wise to explain the placebo effect; in others it is not. There is reason to believe that virtually all medical procedures, including all psychotherapies, contain a suggestive effect. Certainly, a good deal of physiotherapy, hydrotherapy, sojourns in health resorts, and the like are successful because of this. Often it is the disguise, the medical coating, that permits the patient to accept a gratifying procedure without shame or guilt. A dependent but consciously proud adult man may need and be able to accept some tender loving care only in the form of medication, baths, and massage; a frustrated but puritanical patient may be able to accept attention to his oral needs only in the form of a prescribed diet and not otherwise. To prescribe such therapy requires discriminating clinical experience and wisdom; it cannot be done wholesale.

PSYCHOSOCIAL FACTORS IN HOSPITALIZATION Modern hospitals have become magnificent structures, veritable palaces of disease, with equipment reflecting the tremendous technical progress of our century. Unhappily, these advances have not been matched by an improvement in the psychosocial atmosphere of the modern hospital. In large hospitals particularly, psychosocial aspects of patient care are badly neglected. The patient characteristically is thrust into a huge impersonal machine where very little attention is paid to his personal needs, his anxiety, his regression, and often not even to his comfort. From the medical standpoint, the patient becomes a case: from the administrative view he becomes a social security or insurance number. He is dealt with by very impersonal medical, administrative, nursing, and technical task forces, which often have little communication with each other. In this environment, the patient's feelings of anxiety, guilt, shame, dependence, and resentment are enhanced rather than extinguished. He is subjected to repetitive examinations and taxing, incomprehensible procedures; he is apt to be underinformed, not only about his illness, but also about the rationale and the results of the many procedures to which he is subjected. He may wait idly for long periods of time or be suddenly told about a change of contemplated program without any explanation. Nurses will wake him up at unusual hours in the morning and sometimes shake him out of his sleep at night to give him a sedative. Because most hospitals are understaffed, he may call in vain for nurses when he badly needs help. Although orally deprived and without much appetite on account of his illness and inactivity, he may be served food which is the unappetizing product of diet kitchens. Visiting hours are inflexible and restricted, particularly on the public wards. This is annoying for everybody but definitely noxious for children and aged patients, who are more apt to react adversely to sensory deprivation and unfamiliar environments. Such experiences in American hospitals, held to be outstanding, are not uncommon. What is more, many of these hospitals, apart from their advanced technical aspects, are not only highly uncomfortable, anxiety-producing, and irritating environments but are also not conducive to good medicine. As physicians have the ultimate responsibility for the patient's care and treatment, it is their obligation to be aware of such conditions and to take active steps to improve them. Administrative actions affect the patient at every step of his hospitalization from admission to release, and physicians should not surrender to bureaucratic experts and accountants those decisions which so profoundly affect the welfare of sick persons. There is, ironically, one good feature about the atmosphere of such hospitals; they do not reinforce the patient's desire to stay any longer than absolutely necessary.

It does not require the insights of depth psychology to recognize such mismanagement of the ill in our hospitals; nor is it too difficult to see how these mistakes can be remedied. Nursing routines do not have to involve such flagrant disregard of personal comfort. Visiting hours can be arranged for the convenience of the patient. It is possible to make arrangements on pediatric wards so that parents can stay with their children; British hospitals have pioneered such programs. Information need not be haphazard, confusing, and alarming. If several physicians are involved in the care of the patient, one physician must assume the ultimate responsibility for the decisions and also for keeping the patient informed. If a junior physician is working with a patient, his senior colleague should function as a consultant and avoid giving the patient the impression that his doctor is inexperienced and unable to make decisions. A patient being admitted or discharged for aftercare need not be treated as if he were arriving at an austere bank for a loan; surely it is possible to prepare patients for procedures and inform them in terms of their needs and capabilities. All this can make for reduction in anxiety, confusion, and in regressive behavior.

A comprehensive medical approach in hospitals, clinics, and offices will lead not only to better medical practice but also to greater satisfaction and enjoyment on the part of the physician. There are serious obstacles to the achievement of this goal. Perhaps the most important is the physician's feeling either that he knows all about human beings anyhow—"it's all common sense"—or that this art cannot be learned; neither proposition is true! The second difficulty arises because many physicians are so overworked and harassed by their consuming duties and emergencies that it is difficult for them to be able to enter into a more relaxed relationship with their patients. They suffer from what communication experts call an overload in input. The third obstacle is an extreme in attitudes: emotional overinvolvement or intellectual overdetachment. Good professional work is difficult with either attitude. What is needed is compassionate understanding of the patient, his situation in life, and his illness.

NOTES

1. C. Knight Aldrich, *Psychiatry for the Family Physician* (New York: McGraw-Hill, 1955).
2. Michael Balint and Enid Balint, *Psychotherapeutic Techniques in Medicine* (Springfield: Charles C Thomas, 1962).
3. Therese F. Benedek, "Sexual Functions in Women and Their Disturbance," in Silvano Arieti, ed., *The American Handbook of Psychiatry* (New York: Basic Books, 1959), Vol. I, p. 727.

4. Grete Bibring, "Some Considerations of the Psychological Processes in Pregnancy," *Psychoanalytic Study of the Child*, 14 (1959), 113.
5. C. Lee Buxton, *A Study of Psychophysical Methods for Relief of Childbirth Pain* (Philadelphia: Saunders, 1962).
6. Leon Chertok, *Les Méthodes Psychosomatiques d'Accouchement sans Douleur* (Paris: Expansion Scientifique française, 1957).
7. Helene Deutsch, *The Psychology of Women: Motherhood* (New York: Grune & Stratton, 1944), Vol. II.
8. René Dubos, *Mirage of Health* (New York: Harper, 1959).
9. Kurt R. Eissler, *The Psychiatrist and the Dying Patient* (New York: International Universities Press, 1955).
10. Mark H. Hollender, ed., *The Psychology of Medical Practice* (Philadelphia: Saunders, 1958).
11. Oliver Wendell Holmes, quoted in F. Lapham, *Disease and the Man* (New York: Oxford University Press, 1937).
12. Irving L. Janis, *Psychological Stress* (New York: John Wiley, 1958).
13. Alex H. Kaplan, "Psychological Factors in the Practice of Dentistry," *Journal of the American Dental Association*, 57 (1958), 835.
14. M. Ralph Kaufmann, A. N. Franzblau, and David Kairys, "The Emotional Impact of Ward Rounds," *Journal of the Mt. Sinai Hospital*, 23 (1956), 782.
15. Hans K. Knöpfel, *Einfache Psychotherapie für den Hausarzt* (Stuttgart: H. Huber, 1962).
16. Edna S. Levine, *The Psychology of Deafness* (New York: Columbia University Press, 1960).
17. Erich Lindemann, "Observations on Psychiatric Sequelae to Surgical Operation in Women," *American Journal of Psychiatry*, 98 (1941), 132.
18. Karl A. Menninger, "Polysurgery and Polysurgic Addiction," *Psychoanalytic Quarterly*, 3 (1934), 173.
19. Talcott Parsons, *The Social System* (Glencoe, Ill.: The Free Press, 1951).
20. Henry E. Payson, unpublished material.
21. Grantly Dick Read, *Childbirth without Fear* (New York: Harper, 1944).
22. Fredrick C. Redlich, "The Patient's Language," *Yale Journal of Biology and Medicine*, 17 (1945), 427.
23. Jules B. Richmond, "The Pediatric Patient in Health," in H. M. Hollender, ed., *The Psychology of Medical Practice* (Philadelphia: Saunders, 1958).
24. Harold Rosen and T. Lidz, "Emotional Factors in the Precipitation of Recurrent Diabetic Acidosis," *Psychosomatic Medicine*, 11 (1949), 211.
25. Albert Rothenberg, "Psychological Problems in Terminal Cancer Management," *Cancer*, 14 (1961), 1063.
26. Howard Rusk, *Rehabilitation in Medicine* (St. Louis: Mosby, 1958).
27. Theodore F. Schlaegel and Millard Hoyt, *Psychosomatic Ophthalmology* (Baltimore: Williams & Wilkins, 1957).

28. Milton J. E. Senn, "Relationship of Pediatrics and Psychiatry," *American Journal of Diseases of Children*, 71 (1946), 537.
29. Harry Stack Sullivan, *The Psychiatric Interview* (New York: Norton, 1954).
30. Herbert Thoms, *Training for Childbirth* (New York: McGraw-Hill, 1950).
31. James L. Titchener and Maurice Levine, *Surgery as a Human Experience* (New York: Oxford University Press, 1960).
32. I. Z. Velovski, K. I. Platanov, V. A. Plotitcher, and E. A. Chugom, *Painless Childbirth through Psychoprophylaxis* (Moscow: Foreign Languages Publishing House, 1960).

CHAPTER TWENTY-SIX

Psychiatry and Society

Social Psychiatry

Early scientific developments in modern psychiatry were centered around problems of cerebral pathology; then followed an intense interest in the individual psychological history of life experiences. Only recently has an emphasis on social roles and transactions been added in this evolution. It is recognized today that behavior disorders occur in a social system within a particular culture at a given time of the history of mankind. "Psychohistorians," the newest breed of theoreticians, bridging the behavioral sciences and humanities, are applying clinical methods and concepts to historical exploration and also view behavior disorders in the light of history. For that matter, we view our total professional activities as transactions that depend on the historically determined values of the social system in which they occur; they are either reinforced or inhibited by them.

We define social psychiatry as the study of the impact of the social environment on the etiology and treatment of abnormal behavior. In this sense, social psychiatry is no more a clinical subspecialty than its counterpart, biological psychiatry; rather, it is an approach to a fundamental dimension of behavior, to a parameter of theoretical and practical interest. We distinguish social psychiatry, as Viola M. Bernard does, from community psychiatry,[7] which involves the practical approach of utilizing community resources in helping patients as well as the community where such patients live. Social psychiatry is also defined as a branch of psychiatry that is concerned with organizations rather than individuals.[15]

Those who look at social psychiatry as a subspecialty are inclined to divide it into further "subspecialties," such as family psychiatry, cross-cultural psychiatry, group dynamics, and what not. The boundaries between these segmental endeavors and interests are fuzzy, and social psychiatry itself, viewed as a special branch of psychiatry, cannot be sharply delineated from epidemiology, administrative psychiatry, preventive psychiatry, and so forth. All these subheadings may designate interests of a so-called social psychiatrist but make little sense if they become rigidly defined sections in a scheme of classification.

In the framework of social psychiatry, interaction between the psychiatric profession and social scientists, social psychologists, sociologists, cultural anthropologists, economists, political scientists, ecologists, and epidemiologists has been facilitated. Social scientists have become familiar with the publications of Sigmund Freud about mass psychology[23] and culture[22, 26] and the contributions by Harry Stack Sullivan[74] and Abram Kardiner.[40] Psychiatrists became acquainted with important theoretical concepts by social scientists which we mentioned earlier: Émile Durkheim's *anomie,*[16] Erich Fromm's *alienation,*[28] David Riesman's *directedness,*[66] Erik H. Erikson's *ego identity,*[17] and the highly useful concept of *social role,* for which we are particularly indebted to Talcott Parsons.[60] These are not constructs describing an unconnected environment, but rather are concepts that link individual and environment. What constitutes culture stress for an individual (such as deprivation and isolation, or precipitous and conflictful culture change) can be understood only in terms of that person's response and background; the individual interprets environmental phenomena and endows them with meaning; the critical social-psychological concept of alienation, for instance, means both estrangement from one's environment and from one's inner world.

Social psychiatry uses methods of the social sciences and of clinical psychiatry. Rarely will social scientists have the clinical dynamic sensitivity of the seasoned practitioner of psychiatry, nor will psychiatrists be trained in the rigorous methods of the social sciences exploring large and small groups and value systems. Some of the best work in the field has been the result of collaborative efforts. Social scientists have discovered deviant behavior to be a rich and important area of investigation. Psychiatrists have found it useful to explore the role of social systems and culture in the etiology of psychiatric disorders and treatment. Throughout this book we have mentioned the psychiatric investigations of the family, the impact of social class on etiology and treatment, and cross-cultural studies comparing phenomenology and dynamics of behavior disorders as well as different methods of intervention ranging from witchcraft to the more rational methods of modern psychiatry.

In studying social factors, psychiatrists encountered some old and some new social problems that have plagued mankind: poverty, migration, cultural exclusion. The scientific publications about these problems have largely come from political and social scientists, but psychiatrists have begun to make contributions of their own. The adverse effect of *poverty* on mental health is obvious. It has been demonstrated in individual case studies in epidemiological research and in surveys of psychiatric therapies that are available to the poor.[37, 67] Large-scale *migrations* in our time, as the result of war, political and racial persecution, economic depression, and population explosions have uprooted and upset millions of people. Migration from rural into urban areas has created vexing problems. H. B. M. Murphy studied psychiatric aspects of such migrations.[57] Confusion, anxiety, and depression in migrants are typical consequences. A few psychiatrists have explored racial bias and are inclined to view such prejudices as infantile forms of behavior. They can be interpreted in part at least as the result of unconscious anxieties and aggressions.[50] They are particularly apt to occur in authoritarian personalities.[2] The marginal and excluded person becomes not only the target of irrational fears and projections of hostile impulses but may acquire psychopathological traits; for example, depressive, aggressive, or furtive and deceitful traits, which reinforce the discriminatory behavior of the "superior" group.[41] Such explorations obviously are relevant for problems of segregation and integration. Psychiatrists have not only concerned themselves with such overwhelming social and political problems but also have applied their clinical concepts and methods to other "extratherapeutic" areas. In this chapter, we will briefly review such applications to the problems of marriage, education, occupation, esthetics, and religion. We will conclude with a discussion of community psychiatry.

Psychiatry and Marriage

It is generally agreed that sound methods of child-rearing would be fundamental for the prevention of many behavior disorders. Proper child-rearing presupposes stable, healthy, and mature parents who have established the framework of a good marriage. The problem, then, is how to help young married people to achieve this before they have children or when their children are young. Obviously the goal, if realistic, must be rather modest. In any case, this point of view emphasizes the importance of preparation for marriage and the maintenance of good marriages, in the sense of an environment that can facilitate the mutual and individual development of individuals of different generations. One pressing need for marriage counseling, commonly cited in alarm, is the high rate of family disorganization. This appears to be real enough, although how novel it is to our times requires careful scrutiny. Lawrence S. Kubie, for example, cites data showing that as marital disruptions by death have declined, divorce has, to a lesser extent, increased; a higher percentage of families, in fact, were holding together in 1940 than in 1890.[43] Longevity, he states, has exposed the fact that the human race has never been mature enough for enduring marriages.

Divorce is apt to entail stressful isolation of the divorced, but, obviously, broken homes not only affect the wives and husbands but also have serious implications for children, and even for other members of the family, friends, and the larger community, which relies (perhaps unjustly) on the expectation that recognized social units, such as a family, will be stable. This, of course, does not mean that separation and divorce should be prevented at all costs, because there can be little doubt that sustained strife can have equal or worse effects on all involved than actual separation and divorce. Psychiatrists do well not to have any fixed and rigid views on the matters of divorce and separation; they must, however, respect the views of their patients. It would be helpful if one could make knowledgeable predictions about the psychosocial consequences of separation and divorce for both parents and children; such knowledge does not exist yet, but it is possible to help parents and children through the crises of separation and divorce.[13]

That marriage has a crucial function both socially and psychologically is obvious; it is not only one way in which an adult may chose to live but, for most people, also represents the bridge by which earlier strivings of childhood are creatively translated into meaningful fulfillments. Of course, it is precisely these hidden earlier strivings, partially determining the choice of marital partners, which provide the neurotic potential in marital life. As these strivings depend in part upon events in the parents' union, one might say that marriages are significantly shaped by the fate of marriages of antecedents.[14] In Western culture, marriages are supposed to be unions of partners who have a romantic love relationship and must be happy with each other; this is markedly different from other cultures wherein the main emphasis is placed on the socioeconomic and procreative aspects of marriage.[56] In such cultures, marriages are prearranged mainly by parents or elders; marriages are supposed to function, but there is less accent on personal happiness. Happiness is not a goal in itself but merely the result of a job well done. Undoubtedly, many marital difficulties are linked to the culturally exaggerated notion of happiness and also the unrealistic attitudes that are a function of romantic love. However, it would be erroneous to say that romantic love relationships are entirely responsible for bad choices and incompatible living and that prearranged marriages are superior. Neither social pattern has a monopoly on misery or solutions to the unconscious conflicts; unconscious anxiety, guilt, and hostility underlie many, though not all, marital and familial difficulties. Specific problems and solutions may vary with the culture, but the unfortunate consequences of marital problems have not as yet been shown to have been avoided by any "advanced" civilization.

One cause of contemporary marital stress is the shifting roles of husband and wife. In Western society, the role of the wife has become very complex and is no longer confined to activities of homemaking and child-rearing. These new identities, often not fixed and rather diffuse in themselves, may contribute heavily to the particular instances of marital maladjustment we are likely to encounter. As the roles of husband and wife vary greatly and are undergoing rapid changes in the different social classes and also in various cultures and ethnic groups, social factors must be considered by the clinician in his assessment of the situation.

Marriage counseling, since time immemorial, has been in the hands of the clergy. Ministers have been aided in this task by the wisdom of common sense which, as Allan Gregg once remarked, is the gift of God and not the result of a technical education. Most premarital counseling is still carried out in a haphazard and unprofessional manner. There have been feeble efforts in secondary schools and colleges to inform the young adult about the problems of marriage. Only very recently psychologists, psychiatric social workers, and psychiatrists have become active in the marriage field. At present, psychiatric interest still centers around family dynamics in various mental disorders rather than in marriage itself. However, the observation of families in the current family therapies should yield a better knowledge of the communicative techniques by which families carry out their complex mutual and individual functions.

Psychiatrists are expected to fulfill two practical functions concerning marriage: counseling before marriage and counseling and psychotherapy in marital difficulties. Psychiatrists have been consulted for some time about problems of psychiatric genetics, which are, however, of concern only in rare cases when one of the partners suffers from a severe, genetically determined illness. Psychiatrists as well as physicians in general have also the opportunity to advise young people before their marriages on sexual matters, for example, techniques of sexual intercourse and contraceptive problems, and help the newlywed by dispelling the ignorance and anxieties surrounding these topics. This requires a thorough knowledge of sexual functions and an open mind about sexual matters, which, unfortunately, not all physicians and psychiatrists possess.[48] We tend to assume that the medical student is aware of methods of intercourse, psychological problems about them, and skills that can enhance mutually satisfactory relationships, although the fact is that the medical curriculum does not offer such material, and that there is a paucity of relevant research,[52, 53] while myth and parable abound. The reasonable approach is that mutual responsibility obtains; both parties seek satisfaction, and it is not only imperfect technique that impairs attainment of this but also a host of attitudes, inhibitions, and childish wishes that make a satisfying adaptation difficult. It is always preferable to explain and counsel in terms of individual needs rather than mechanically to refer to the pamphlets and books that have been written on the subject, although some of them are informative and helpful. Where books on techniques are consulted, the benefit to the reader probably derives in part from the willingness and interest to investigate, which can, in itself, give impetus to a shift of values and behavior. Although no truly good marriage is thinkable without satisfactory sexual relations, there is growing consensus that sexual disturbances are not always in the foreground of marital difficulties; marital troubles may be expressed in complete or partial impotence, frigidity, sexual deviations, and particularly, extramarital relations or promiscuity. Often these symptoms are only surface phenomena of deeper disturbances, usually indicating fear or hostility on the part of one or both marital partners.

Psychiatrists are often expected, through consultation or brief psychotherapy, to dispel doubts about impending marriage—a difficult if not impossible task! Occasionally, they are consulted by parents of young people with a request to interfere with marriages, which the parents consider undesirable; this is usually neither an easy nor an appealing task and in most cases psychiatrists rightly do not accept the assignment, although we have seen some instances in which they were helpful to all parties involved. One cheerful note is that persons with behavior disorders can have relatively good marriages if they complement each other in fulfillment of needs.

Most frequently, psychiatrists are asked to function as repairmen in marriages that are in serious trouble. Unhappily, motivation to seek help is generated all too often when it is too late and too difficult. Whether the more superficial instrument of counseling or more intensive psychotherapies are used, it is advantageous when both spouses are in treatment.[33] Some psychiatrists treat both spouses, separately or together; most psychiatrists prefer to work with one person and arrange for the other to be treated by another mental health worker. Under the impact of favorable reports from family psychotherapists, joint sessions of the couples have been more in vogue. The rationale for these various approaches, often providing therapists with very lively displays of marital tragedy or comedy, has not been satisfactorily confirmed, but they seem promising as practical procedures. Essentially, the therapeutic task has been to show how partners antagonize each other by subtle provocation, destructive and self-destructive maneuvers, instead of fulfilling mutual needs. One thinks of Arthur Schopenhauer's freezing porcupines, who would like to huddle together for warmth but repel each other with their quills as they move closer. As in all intensive psychotherapy, the uncovering of unconscious infantile needs and demands or goals that cannot be fulfilled, or the discovery and tactful and relevant demonstration of attitudes that are automatic and unmodified, is the task of the psychotherapist in treating marital difficulties. Another task is to demonstrate the occasions and tactics by which the marital couple annoy and frustrate each other.

Psychiatric Therapy in Schools

Psychiatry, based on psychoanalytic as well as learning theories, has had a definite effect on the practices of child-rearing and education. Results are the widespread use of new child-rearing techniques, such as demand feeding, modern toilet training, and more realistic attitudes toward reward and punishment, with emphasis on positive motivation rather than on deterrent methods. In general, we see today a more loving and more realistic attitude toward children in large parts of the world. In such different countries as the United States and the Union of Soviet Socialist Republics, a very strong interest in emotional and mental growth and development has sprung up; yet in many countries with population explosions the neglect of children is appalling. Problems of overpopulation and its consequences are among the most serious ones facing modern man and demand very determined efforts in research and social action. Hopefully, psychiatrists will play a role in such efforts.

The modern gospel of child-rearing has been effectively stated by educators, psychoanalysts, and enlightened pediatricians, such as Anna Freud, Jules Richmond, Milton Senn, and Benjamin Spock. Just what the effects of these new techniques on mental health will be cannot be predicted, but experts are inclined to believe that their effects will be beneficial, measurable objectively, and possibly very far-reaching.

The impact of psychiatry on the school system is less marked than the impact of child psychiatry on early child-rearing. Psychologists play a more prominent role in educational settings, and where individual treatment is carried out, it is limited to a few urban or expensive private schools. Educators and psychiatrists often have rather divergent views on learning and personality difficulties. There is controversy over the importance of mental health in schools. Many teachers consider the accent on mental health as an unrealistic and pampering approach. Psychiatrists, however, feel that many academic failures are essentially emotional crises and that it is possible to help such students by psychotherapy and counseling. As in so many applied fields, both specialists—psychiatrists and educators—have much to learn from each other. Some educators have undertaken provocative and new approaches to the total education of the normal child,[58] and psychiatrists should be interested in what a good teacher does and knows about children and parents and be ready to apply skills these persons have developed in their concrete situations of action. What is not desired is to convert skillful teachers into bad therapists or to provide educators with an exotic vocabulary for commentary about children while ignoring any implementation of behavioral techniques and principles that could practically help children. Research is clearly required in this area, since child-rearing and education are functions crucial for all cultures and most vulnerable to prejudice and passion.

As one would expect, the impact of psychiatry has been greatest in special institutions that deal with children with serious emotional, intellectual, and social problems. Psychiatrists and dynamic psychologists, such as the late August Aichorn[3] in Austria and his students, particularly Fritz Redl[62] and Bruno Bettelheim[8] in the United States, have developed pioneering approaches and progressive institutions. The psychosocial impact of the environment of such institutions has resulted in amazing changes in children who previously had been considered inaccessible by ordinary educational methods. In turn, these institutions have influenced the environments of hospitals, aiding the development of therapeutic communities.[39] The modern concept of student government was successfully developed in some of these progressive schools long before patient government was introduced into mental hospitals.

The functions of the psychiatrist in the regular schools include diagnostic workup, individual and group therapy of students, consultation with teachers and, hopefully, a certain influence on school policies and programs in order to promote better mental health. A school psychiatrist should be thoroughly familiar with the school environment and oriented to assess the impact of this environment on the student. Problems that school psychiatrists encounter embrace the ordinary scope of psychiatric difficulties in childhood and adolescence; in addition, there are special disciplinary and academic problems. One such is underachievement, or poor academic performance not explained by lack of intellectual endowment, physical handicaps, or organic reading difficulties. In some cases, underachievement is caused by a rebellious and overcompetitive or, also, a very passive attitude produced by emotional conflict in home or school;[72] the causes of underachievement however often remain obscure.[35]

As there is such a scarcity of psychiatrists in our schools, it has been found expedient to use them primarily as consultants to mental health workers in schools and to teachers rather than as therapists. For the most part, treatment—often cautiously called counseling—is carried out by school social workers, school psychologists, and specially trained teachers. Even the ordinary teacher who is helped to tolerate a difficult child is in a position to help him academically and personally. Acquisition of skills can be of sustaining importance to the child's self-esteem and coping ability and, in this sense, good educational experience may be preferred to therapeutic intervention in the narrow sense of the word. Unfortunately, intensive psychotherapy and family therapy, which are often badly needed, are hardly available in most schools. Under favorable circumstances, when a relationship of mutual trust and respect exists, psychiatrists may use their special knowledge as advisers to school boards and principals and thereby assist them in shaping educational policy.

Educational settings in which psychiatrists function well are the mental health clinics in institutions of higher learning; because they assist the professional elite, which is of crucial importance in industrial countries, they are of special significance. Clements C. Fry, a pioneer in this field, developed a model psychiatric clinic as a part of the university health service at Yale University. Similar clinics, providing very useful services, now exist in many universities and colleges.[78] There can be little doubt that in these clinics many young men and women, who otherwise would have foundered, received effective help in steering through the often dramatic crises of late adolescence and young adulthood. Many students need help in finding and expressing their identities, in assuming adult responsibility and independence, in facing authority, and in weathering storms of rebellion and impulsive solutions to problems. Often, such an identity is achieved only after a moratorium, an absence for a year or more from college, which is aided, at times, by psychotherapy, at times by life experience, or both. The task of the college psychiatrist is not only to administer psychotherapy, but to aid in the development of an atmosphere in colleges that is conducive to emotional growth. Such a contribution can be made only by intimate and trusting cooperation between the faculty, administration, and the mental health division of colleges and universities.[18]

Psychiatric Services in Industry and Business

Industrial psychiatry has been a neglected field. Psychologists have shown a greater interest in occupational problems than psychiatrists and have carried on most of the "clinical" work in the field. Practically all the research concerned with such problems in industry as difficulties of planning, management, organization and control as well as frustration and alienation of the individual employer or employee has been done by behavioral scientists. Since the forties, schools of business administration are teaching the science of management based on theoretical considerations, extensive field work, and considerable experimentation.[5] Milestones in this development were Max Weber's theories of bureaucracy, the basic work by George Frederick Taylor in human engineering and the classic Hawthorne experiments at the Western Electric Company demonstrating that industrial output depends on information and motivation.[69] Sophisticated mathematical models, pioneered by Herbert Simon and the work of computers, have permitted new advances in the analysis of communication and decision making in business and industrial organizations.[71]

Experts on management are divided in their approaches. The school of scientific management takes a hard-line approach, emphasizing the importance of structural elements in the organization. The human relations school favors a soft-line approach, stressing the human element and its significance for efficient performance. The structural school assumes an intermediate position. Naturally psychiatrists favor—more in words than in practice—a soft-line approach in management.

Some psychiatrists, including the authors, have felt that industry and business have shown overconfidence in the use of psychometric tests and paper-and-pencil tests as clinical and industrial psychologists, widely and often uncritically, have employed them. Clinical and dynamic approaches, on the other hand, have been neglected, but there has been a growing concern with unconscious motivation, especially as it affects opinion change. Social psychologists have also accumulated considerable knowledge of group dynamics. Fused with an analytic point of view, such information is very pertinent for any administrator.[65]

Only a handful of psychiatrists occupy full-time positions in industry and business; some two hundred, or two per cent of all psychiatrists in the United States, have devoted part of their time to this kind of work. In this country, psychiatrists have been retained by management and, with rare exceptions, not by labor unions. A split in loyalty between the individual patient and the occupational organization that employs the psychiatrist poses a serious problem for the therapist; this may have something to do with the lack of popularity of this particular subspecialty among psychiatrists. It is also likely that the accent on extreme pathology, characteristic of a more ancient psychiatry, has discouraged industrialists and businessmen from seeking psychiatrists as consultants. One sign of fresh interest is the development of a few training centers for occupational psychiatry or the courses in group dynamics in which psychiatrists have begun to participate.

The functions of the occupational psychiatrist include diagnostic and therapeutic services for the individual employee and consultation with the employer, and possibly also with such employee organizations as unions. The former activities are identical with those in general psychiatric practice, with the qualification that the occupational psychiatrist, working in a mental hygiene clinic maintained by his organization, may perforce reflect the special problems of the occupational organization in his referrals. Important special problems are absenteeism, alcoholism, accidents, and also the deleterious, alienating effects of boring, monotonous, highly mechanical, routinized work. In the role of consultants to management, psychiatrists must deal primarily with distortions of communications and difficulties in human relations, which occur in any organization, such as impaired morale, the facilitating and disruptive role of clique formations, and the problems of leadership.[47] Some attention has been focused on special problems of persons in executive positions: high incidence of tension, depression, paranoid attitudes, psychosomatic syndromes and alcoholism. With the increase of the life-span, retirement has become an important problem. James S. Tyhurst has pointed to typical aspects of this problem: the denial of retirement and loss of an active occupation, and turmoil, anxiety and depression when such denial cannot be maintained.[76]

Another problem that should attract the attention of psychiatry and the social sciences is that of leisure; in an era in which man can rely increasingly on machines and electronic devices, the appropriate use of leisure time has become a major concern for social planners. It is conceivable that in due time psychiatrists and social psychologists will be able to make sound recommendations for problems arising from increased leisure. E. B. Klein mentioned to us that psychiatrists could profitably study extreme "leisure" in some of their own hospitals.

Military Psychiatry

Military psychiatry is the occupational psychiatry of the armed forces. In a world armed to the teeth, this subspecialty is necessarily important. Because of the numbers of people involved and the intrinsic control over data, this field has become an important laboratory for social psychiatry. Modern military psychiatry relies more heavily on the utilization of the social environment for therapeutic purposes than civilian psychiatry. Psychiatrists were first used, though to a limited extent, in World War I; in World War II, psychiatrists played a very significant role, particularly in the armed forces of the United States and Great Britain.[54] Under the leadership of such psychiatrists as J. Rees in Great Britain and W. C. Menninger, F. J. Braceland, and J. M. Murray in the United States, a larger number of physicians were trained in psychiatry; and after the war there was a sharp rise in the prestige of psychiatry in the United States. Among the outstanding studies of military psychiatry in the wake of World War II was Douglas Bond's monograph analyzing the unconscious motivations and fears of combat pilots.[9] His conclusion, that unconscious motivations determine to a large extent success or failure of flying personnel, offended some military leaders (because airmen must not have conscious or unconscious fears!). One of the significant therapeutic contributions of World War II psychiatry was the development of narcotherapy for soldiers suffering from combat fatigue by Roy R. Grinker and John P. Spiegel.[32]

The military psychiatrist diagnoses and treats disorders that, in many ways, are identical with psychiatric disorders in civilian life; however, military life presents certain problems that make military psychiatry a special type of pursuit. In peacetime, armed forces are huge bureaucratic organizations similar to other governmental organizations, but even then the specific tradition, morale, and task orientation of the armed forces gives military psychiatry a particular flavor. In war, particularly for combat personnel, there are, of course, unique aspects and stresses centering around the basic urge to attack and also to protect one's own life and the lives of others. New problems, such as the particular stresses encountered in extended submarine cruises and in supersonic and space flights,[70] are emerging.

In the United States during World War II, 850,000 men were rejected for service for psychiatric reasons, and 45 per cent of all medical discharges were based on psychiatric disorders. A follow-up study of war neuroses, carried out by N. A. Brill and G. W. Beebee, was highly revealing of procedures and mistakes in psychiatric selection and discharge of military personnel; apparently the large-scale rejections and discharges represented a very lavish use of manpower.[10] In general, psychiatrists in the military have used for selection short clinical interviews, which have been found surprisingly but evidently effective in screening out extreme disorders.[80] There has been a heavy reliance on objective tests, especially in the evaluation of aptitudes; however, such tests contribute relatively little to the speedy detection of behavior disorders. During World War II, there were no universal standards for the clinical assessment of draftees. Once a recruit was accepted, he passed through a rather elaborate testing program, in which psychologists were involved for the most part. In the past, one of the principles guiding armed forces medicine was that of declaring a soldier fit or unfit for duty; if unfit, and the disorder was considered lasting or severe, he had to be hospitalized or discharged. From a psychiatric standpoint, such guidelines were inappropriate or, at best, applicable only for very severe disorders such as the major psychoses. The concept of limited duty for neuroses, and even for symptoms like syncope and diseases like epilepsy, is much more appropriate, and this point of view has gradually begun to enter military medical thinking. Today, many servicemen with psychiatric disorders remain on duty and are treated in mental health clinics. A major impetus toward such reorientation came from the introduction of social psychiatric methods into army psychiatry by Colonel A. Glass[30] and David McK. Rioch.[68] Military psychiatrists developed the principle of utilization of combat soldiers with mild psychiatric disorders and blocked the traditional procedure of hasty evacuation and discharge. The result was a much more effective use of mental health workers and a more efficient application of military manpower in general. Absence without leave, inefficiency, disciplinary problems, and alcoholism are prominent in military psychiatry and have been dealt with more recently in a relatively enlightened way.

Therapy of combat neuroses was briefly discussed in a section on traumatic neuroses in Chapter 10. There can be no doubt that the older techniques of an uncovering psychotherapy with military personnel suffering from combat neuroses were improved by stressing three points: (1) The adjustment and military effectiveness of an individual in combat is largely a function of morale and leadership in the group. (2) Many breakdowns can be prevented by bolstering group morale and cohesiveness. (3) If soldiers develop combat reactions, they should not be evacuated but treated as close to the combat area as possible, where short-term psychotherapeutic methods are enhanced by sedating and tranquilizing drugs and maximal use of the total therapeutic impact of the group.[36] Such treatment requires the employment of division psychiatrists, as well as the close cooperation of line officers with psychiatrists, a policy that originated during the latter part of World War II in the United States Army.

Psychiatry and Esthetics

As Ernest Havemann writes, today there are more psychiatrists in Broadway plays and movies than warm-hearted Irish cops, Bowery drunks, and comic housemaids.[36] Cartoons of psychiatrists have invaded the sophisticated pages of the *New Yorker*, down-to-earth comic strips, and even popular texts on psychiatry.[63] The spice of the stories of confessional and exposé magazines is festooned with psychiatric jargon. Such "true stories," concocted not too skillfully and with but a minimum of psychiatric knowledge, are neither artistic nor scientific and stand in contrast to great literature. The work of literary geniuses reflects a deep and immediate knowledge of behavior; there is never the feeling of imitation or contrived application of psychiatric constructs but of a creative and intuitive grasp of the material. The most moving presentations of human psychological and social problems have not come from scientists but from creative writers and artists. It is remarkable indeed that one finds in William Shakespeare's plays virtually everything we know today of the dynamics of abnormal behavior; and they were written at a time when physicians and scientists were caught in the follies of a most uncritical belief in witchcraft. What was true for a Sophocles, Molière and Johann Wolfgang von Goethe, for August Strindberg and Dostoevski, and also for a Johann Nestroy and Mark Twain, and a great many other poets and creative writers is equally true for those great contemporary authors whose knowledge of Freud quietly enhances rather than distorts their views of man and his behavior.

Apart from the direct impact of modern psychiatry and psychology in literature, painting, and sculpture, there are certain genuine contributions of modern psychiatry to art and literature by psychiatrists who have been interested in the creative process in the sciences and arts. Several pathographies of famous artists and writers have been published, and the impact of psychoanalysis and psychiatry on literary and art criticism has been considerable. Freud had a strong interest in literature, sculpture, and painting and set the pace and tone of later investigations with his analytic studies of Jensen's Gravida,[19] of creative writing and daydreaming,[20] of an infantile reminiscence of Leonardo da Vinci,[21] and his study of Dostoevski and parricide.[25] He saw artistic creation as a sublimation of aggressive and sexual drives. Many analysts such as Ernest Jones, Ernst Kris, Erik Erikson, and others have followed Freud's example. Carl G. Jung, through his deep understanding of symbolism, had a definite appeal for artists. Kubie wrote fairly extensively about the creative process in arts and sciences, relating it to preconscious forces in contrast to unconscious forces, which are responsible for neurotic acts.[44] A classical work is Hans Prinzhorn's study in which he described form and content of the pictorial art of the insane and also related them to art in childhood and prehistoric times.[61] Karl Jaspers wrote two well-known pathographies about Strindberg and Vincent Van Gogh; the latter is probably the most frequently studied insane artist.[38] Of recent studies, Jean Delay's on André Gide is outstanding; it earned Delay one of the great scientific honors France has to bestow: membership in the *Academie de France*.[12]

Freud was less concerned with solving the riddle of the essence of art than with understanding the relationship of artistic productions to unconscious conflicts of the artist. The real artist can utilize his psychological problems to convey with great emotional impact a genuine and general insight to other human beings; the ordinary mortal, whether disturbed or normal, has neither the ability nor the drive to do this. One should remember that many creative geniuses were not only highly disturbed but were also, though not always, productive during their worst periods. Others however were relatively well balanced; certainly neurosis is no prerequisite for creativity. Psychoanalytic and psychiatric theories must not be misused to explain art and literature. We must be cognizant that appreciation of motivations is not identical with expertise in esthetics, in literary craft or scholarship, and that artistic as well as scientific creativity still are elusive and challenging problems.[73]

Psychiatry and Its Relationship to Religion and Philosophy

Cooperation between psychiatrists and clergymen has become another significant endeavor, particularly in the United States. This interest seems to stem from three needs: (1) a practical need of ministers to acquaint themselves with modern psychotherapeutic techniques; (2) the common concern of theologians and psychiatrists with the human "soul" and destiny; and (3) the need of psychiatrists and psychologists to understand religious experience. There is a wide range of opinion about whether psychiatry, in particular, psychoanalytic psychiatry, is compatible with religion. This is a facet of the larger question, whether or not science and religion are compatible, an issue that obviously goes beyond the limits of this book. The fact is that some prominent psychiatrists have been agnostics; others, devout believers. Freud viewed religion as a collective neurosis; he felt that religion inhibits thinking and a rigorous orientation to reality and held that ethics based on religion are on shaky ground.[24] Yet other analysts did not find it incompatible with their professional views to be religious. In clinical psychiatry, this issue is rarely argued. Some theologians, particularly fundamentalists of various denominations, have attacked psychoanalysis and dynamic psychiatry viciously and declared it to be heretical and antireligious. Many modern clergymen, however, have approved of dynamic psychiatry and have attempted to interpret its implications for theological issues.

Psychiatrists and the clergy are the two professional groups most frequently called upon to help persons with psychological troubles. Clergymen bring to this task little in the way of scientific techniques but much in old traditions, long experience, and the advantage of operating under the powerful auspices of the church and ultimately of their God. They have special privileges; they can seek out those whom they want to help, and they are not dependent on direct financial rewards for their services. Their services, however, are by no means free; like medical missionaries, they perform humane services that ultimately aid their creed. The addition of psychotherapy will help to modernize the techniques of the clergy, but it still remains to be seen how scientific psychotherapeutic methods mix with the approach of traditional religion. Another area concerns certain theoretical issues of interest to theologians, philosophers, psychiatrists, psychoanalysts and other behavioral scientists alike. At bottom, members of these professions are interested in the existence and essence of man. Theologians like Søren A. Kierkegaard[42] and Paul Tillich[75] have been concerned with the problems of anxiety and guilt, and an interchange of information may be helpful.

A third area of mutual interest is the religious experience itself. Since the time of William James, it has been clear that religious experience merits careful scientific study. The reality of such experience cannot be challenged; rather, the problem is to apprehend it, and the plea for a sympathetic understanding of religion makes sense. More knowledge is needed about the psychology of religion and metaphysical systems and beliefs. Investigators need not be either negatively critical nor defensively supporting, but should aim at understanding the function of religion and philosophy in the life of an individual and the specific nature of the religious experience. They should explore the mystical element scientifically and bring some clarity to a uniquely human endeavor. Psychiatrists, with their considerable and specific knowledge of the irrational, are specifically equipped to contribute to such a task.[4]

Discussions of the relationship between religion and psychiatry deal primarily with the Western religions. Certain aspects of Zen Buddhism have intrigued psychoanalysts like Erich Fromm and Karen Horney; some topics of Buddhist teaching, such as the unity of the I and the world, the emphasis on feeling rather than on thinking, are clearly relevant for dynamic psychiatry. Even certain techniques of Zen training, such as the use of insoluble riddles (*koans*), are reminiscent of some modern psychotherapeutic practices.[77]

Although Freud consistently denied that psychoanalysis is a closed philosophical system, or *Weltanschauung*,[27] Freud's statement was challenged by Fromm[29] and defended by Herbert Marcuse.[51] It cannot be denied that, in its applications in therapy or in education, certain values are favored over others, such as the value of growth over inertia and destructiveness, or a preference for the rational over the irrational.[64] These propositions are admirable maxims and compatible with any endeavor to help people to be vital and not spiritually impoverished. Perhaps one could say, as the earthy Johann Nestroy put it, that it is better to be healthy and rich than to be sick and poor. Apart from such broad recommendations, however, psychiatry and psychoanalysis are empirical sciences and leave off where philosophy begins. Yet this does not deny the need for a sound orientation to problems of human existence; psychiatry is indebted for such attempts to Martin Heidegger, Karl Jaspers, Jean-Paul Sartre, and many others and needs an orientation to the ultimate problem as much as other professional disciplines concerned with basic human problems.

Community Psychiatry

The theoretical roots of social psychiatry reach back to the turn of the century, but the history of community psychiatry is very short. In American psychiatry, the child psychiatrists William Healey and Augusta Bronner practiced first what could be termed community psychiatry by paying due attention to psychosocial factors in the diagnosis and treatment of juvenile delinquency. The movement did not gain impetus until World War II, when a large number of American psychiatrists were impressed with the potential of what dynamic psychotherapy could achieve, and also with the fact that such psychotherapy could reach only few patients. We have already mentioned the work of A. M. Querido, who became aware of how easily hospitals and clinics become overloaded and can function properly only if adequate techniques for screening and treating of prospective admissions by home-visiting emergency teams are set up.[46] This led Querido to develop extensive services within the community. Erich Lindemann, in his study of mental problems of Wellesley, Massachusetts,[49] gave community psychiatry a sound basis by exploring the concepts of crisis detection and intervention and the use of psychiatrists as consultants to the care-taking professions consisting of general practitioners of medicine, lawyers, clergymen, teachers, and welfare workers. Gerald Caplan refined and developed these concepts in his thoughtful application of principles of preventive psychiatry to problems in a community.[11]

The most important stimulus for the development of community psychiatry has come from public health. Modern psychiatrists are not only concerned with helping individual patients but are also involved with the problems of behavior disorders of populations—of communities, of countries. In dealing with mass aspects of disease, psychiatry joined forces with the specialty of public health. Psychiatrists have learned much from public-health experts, and public-health experts have agreed with psychiatrists that the mental health problem is a paramount problem of public health. The application of a philosophy of public health to the problem of behavior disorders is pertinent; public health is not satisfied merely with a program of treatment; its ultimate aim is prevention based on identification of disease carriers and hosts, the study of the spread of disease, the elimination of the noxious agent, the increase of the patient's resistance to it, and the change of environmental conditions which facilitate disease. Psychiatry has developed a similar rationale. In turn, public-health men have become cognizant that psychosocial and cultural factors are contributory to the pathogenesis of all disease. Planning of treatment for populations makes it necessary to know about the epidemiology of behavior disorders, but we are far from a definitive knowledge of incidence and prevalence of behavior disorders. Indeed, there is little agreement about what a psychiatric case is. In order to estimate needs for treatment, it will be necessary to define a case in different cultural and social contexts: for the poor and the affluent, for the illiterate, and for the educated. In the meantime, it will be necessary to organize psychiatric services, perforce on the basis of limited information. Such organization will also differ depending whether it is set up in industrial or rural areas, in advanced, or in developing countries.

In the technological civilization of modern communities and countries, the organization of such mental health services is becoming very complex.[45] A mental health department of a large industrial city or state is an elaborate organization; to administer and coordinate its services requires leadership skills of a high order. Such a department has to coordinate the services of large hospitals and clinics, whose staffs include mental health workers of many professions. It has to relate these groups to the care-taking professions and their functions in welfare agencies, schools, courts, churches, and a host of special agencies. To provide the best possible services, the mental health department must educate citizens in how to use these services. Finally, to provide and develop these service functions, the department must inform the people and their leaders about present and future mental health needs and induce them to seek and provide appropriate legislation and funds to carry out the mental health needs.

The blueprint for the functions of a modern organization of mental health services and their philosophy, "Action for Mental Health" is an important and timely study in which a team of experts under the leadership of Jack Ewalt[1] outlined existing shortcomings in psychiatric services, training, and research in our communities and point to new trends and possible developments. Some of these developments are, in the United States, within practical reach after a message by President John F. Kennedy and subsequent appropriation of funds.[55] The tasks of community psychiatry are diagnosis, therapy, rehabilitation, and prevention, as well as mental health education of the citizens of the community. These are, of course, the traditional tasks of psychiatry. Indeed, we believe that community psychiatry does not represent a revolution, but rather a significant and rapid evolution of practices. What is special and what is different, then, in community psychiatry? In general terms, we might say that good community psychiatry ought to be synonymous with good, realistic clinical psychiatry. It attempts to start earlier with detection and prevention, persist longer with therapy and rehabilitation, and coordinate its efforts more effectively by creating an interlocking system of experts and agencies. Community psychiatry aims to provide comprehensive and saturated care, as long as the patient needs it, in a defined catchment area. Of course, saturation is a utopian ideal and at best can only be approximated. The efforts of community psychiatry can be described as being more extensive than intensive. For obvious reasons, relatively little time can be spent with the individual patient. Group and milieu and drug therapies are more prominent in community psychiatry than individual psychotherapy. The focus of community psychiatry, as of all other psychiatry, of course, is the patient; however, by studying and treating the patient, the modern community psychiatrist has become intensely aware of the interpersonal and cultural factors that determine the patient's behavior and aid or hinder his recovery. He has learned to appreciate the impact of families, peer groups, of interactions in schools and jobs, and even tries actively to modify noxious factors in the patient's immediate environment.

As troublesome behavior is more prevalent in the lower socioeconomic and marginal groups, community psychiatrists are especially confronted with the serious social problems of such economically and educationally deprived populations. To remedy these evils, however, requires massive social action, exceeding by far whatever mental health workers can do.

A number of rather different institutions and a number of programs have been described as community mental health centers.[6,31] The nucleus of a typical community oriented program is still a psychiatric hospital, although we call it a mental health center today. It is, however, a different hospital from psychiatric institutions of the past. It is small, or at least divided into autonomous units related to districts of the community; beds are relatively unimportant because patients are not sick in the ordinary sense of the word. The outpatient facilities are most important. The mental health center is an active hospital; a therapeutic community, which uses all modern treatment methods; drug therapies, milieu therapies, group and family treatment have become particularly important in such centers. The turnover is relatively fast; in many of these centers the average stay is less than two months. If possible, patients are not hospitalized around the clock but stay in the center as day, or night, patients. Thus, the tie to the community is not as easily broken as in the traditional institution. The decision of who qualifies as a day, or night, patient is based less on diagnosis than on the availability of family and community resources to the patient. The transitional character of the institution is further strengthened by the fact that the boundary between inpatient and outpatient is more fluid; transfers of patients from one unit to another (if possible, retaining the same mental health worker) are more easily made. More important, the barriers between community and hospital are less formidable.

The accent on early detection has led to active intervention in crises and emergencies. For the proper functioning of a community, it is important that its emergencies are well handled. To trundle a disturbed person in a police car to the traditional public mental hospital is, in most cases, a very poor solution. Community psychiatry is now using emergency teams who are ready to see the patient in his home setting rather than to wait for his appearance in an emergency room. In some cases, these teams can prevent hospitalization or merely reduce it to a few days and even hours in an emergency unit.

Planning for discharge from inpatient services starts with the admission of the patient. One of the most important concepts of community psychiatry is sustained responsibility of patient care after the formal discharge from the institution, in outpatient clinics or by the home-treatment division of the mental health center. Continued care may be provided directly by the mental health workers of the center, but in many cases these mental health workers will help only in a consulting capacity. Many patients will be treated by visiting nurses, nonpsychiatric professional workers in schools and social agencies.[59] Some patients will benefit from the care in halfway houses, which are slowly developing, and in patient clubs, which provide, when living with the family is not indicated, shelter, minimal professional supervision and the opportunity to live and work in the community. Many patients will give each other aid in such facilities. Vocational and educational rehabilitation is playing an increasing role in such a comprehensive program.

The work of community psychiatry does not end with patient care but is hopefully directed toward prevention by spotting social stresses in the family and in the institutions of the community and removing or modifying these stresses before damage occurs or before it is irreparable. This is community psychiatry's most difficult and most challenging job. We have successfully and competently improved the environment of our hospitals and made them more therapeutic. We have described the beginnings of such work in families, schools, businesses, industry, and the armed forces. As long as the patient is the primary target of our efforts, we are on relatively secure ground. When we begin to treat ill-functioning organizations, we venture into the unknown. If we were so omniscient, mental health institutions and organizations would be superior to any others, and marriages, families of mental health workers, and the methods of rearing their own children ought to be shining examples to everybody else. We can hardly point to such achievements at this time. It follows that we are wary of some of our colleagues who make fantastic claims and advocate sweeping, ambitious but inadequate "action," which is not based on sound knowledge. This does not mean that we are opposed to applied research, to experimentation and bold ideas. Indeed, we are convinced that the new community psychiatry has encouraged us to make our contribution to the attack on some of the great social and political problems of mankind;[79] it points to new and almost utopian goals. To move toward the goals of a "great society" will require enormous vision and resources and manpower. It will require considerable reorientation in training and serious examination of the appropriate numbers of trainees, their professional affiliations, and—importantly—their quality. Most of all, it will demand not less, as some believe, but rather a great deal more of basic and clinical research. This is a task of the future.

NOTES

1. *Action for Mental Health: Final Report of the Joint Commission on Mental Illness and Health* (New York: Basic Books, 1961).
2. Theodor W. Adorno, E. Frenkel-Brunswick, D. J. Levinson, and N. R. Sanford, *The Authoritarian Personality* (New York: Harper, 1950).
3. August Aichhorn, *Wayward Youth* (New York: Viking, 1953).
4. Kenneth E. Appel, John W. Higgins, Mortimer Ostow, and Eilhard von

Domarus, "Religion," in Silvano Arieti, ed., *The American Handbook of Psychiatry* (New York: Basic Books, 1959), Vol. II, pp. 1777.

5. Chris Argyris, *Personality and Organization* (New York: Harper, 1957).
6. Leopold Bellak, ed., *Handbook of Community Psychiatry and Community Mental Health* (New York: Grune & Stratton, 1964).
7. Viola M. Bernard, "Education for Community Psychiatry in a University Medical Center," in Leopold Bellak, ed., *Handbook for Community Psychiatry and Community Mental Health* (New York: Grune & Stratton, 1964).
8. Bruno Bettelheim, *Love Is Not Enough* (Glencoe, Ill.: The Free Press, 1950).
9. Douglas D. Bond, *Love and Fear of Flying* (New York: International Universities Press, 1952).
10. Norman A. Brill and G. W. Beebee. *A Follow-up Study of War Neuroses* (Washington, D.C.: United States Government Printing Office, 1955).
11. Gerald Caplan, *Principles of Preventive Psychiatry* (New York: Basic Books, 1964).
12. Jean Delay, *La Jeunesse d'André Gide*, 2 vols. (Paris: Gallimard, 1956).
13. J. Louise Despert, *Children of Divorce* (Garden City: Doubleday and Co., 1953).
14. Henry Dicks, "Clinical Studies in Marriage and the Family: A Symposium on Methods. I. Experiences with Marital Tensions Seen in the Psychological Clinic," *British Journal of Medical Psychology* 26 (1953), 181.
15. Leonard J. Duhl and R. L. Leopold, "Some Contributions of Psychoanalysis to Social Psychiatry" presented to the Academy of Psychoanalysis, New York: December 1964.
16. Émile Durkheim, *Suicide* (Glencoe, Ill.: The Free Press, 1951).
17. Erik H. Erikson, *Identity and the Life Cycle* (New York: International Universities Press, 1959).
18. Dana L. Farnsworth, "Social and Emotional Development of Students in College and University, *Mental Hygiene*, 43 (1959), parts 1 and 2, 358.
19. Sigmund Freud, "Delusions and Dreams in Jensen's Gravida" [1907], *Standard Edition* (London: Hogarth Press, 1959), Vol. IX.
20. Sigmund Freud, "On Creative Writers and Day Dreaming" [1908], *Standard Edition* (London: Hogarth Press, 1959), Vol. IX.
21. Sigmund Freud, "Leonardo da Vinci and a Memory of His Childhood" [1910], *Standard Edition* (London: Hogarth Press, 1957), Vol. XI.
22. Sigmund Freud, "Totem and Taboo" [1912–13], *Standard Edition*, (London: Hogarth Press, 1961), Vol. XIII.
23. Sigmund Freud, "Group Psychology and the Analysis of the Ego" [1921], *Standard Edition* (London: Hogarth Press, 1961), Vol. XVIII.
24. Sigmund Freud, "The Future of an Illusion" [1927], *Standard Edition* (London: Hogarth Press, 1961), Vol. XXI.
25. Sigmund Freud, "Dostoievski and Parricide" [1928], *Standard Edition* (London: Hogarth Press, 1961), Vol. XXI.

26. Sigmund Freud, "Civilization and Its Discontents" [1930] *Standard Edition* (London: Hogarth Press, 1961), Vol. XXI.
27. Sigmund Freud, "New Introductory Lectures on Psychoanalysis" [1933], *Standard Edition* (London: Hogarth Press, 1961), Vol. XXII.
28. Erich Fromm, *The Sane Society* (New York: Rinehart, 1955).
29. Erich Fromm, *Sigmund Freud's Mission* (New York: Harper, 1958).
30. Albert J. Glass, "Observations upon the Epidemiology of Mental Illness in Troops during Warfare," in *Symposium on Preventive and Social Psychiatry* (Washington, D.C.: Walter Reed Army Institute of Research, 1952).
31. Raymond Glasscote, David Sanders, H. M. Forstenzer, and A. R. Foley, *The Community Mental Health Center* (Washington, D.C.: Joint Information Service of the American Psychiatric Association, 1964).
32. Roy R. Grinker and John P. Spiegel, *Men under Stress* (Philadelphia: Blakiston, 1945).
33. Jay Haley, "Marriage Therapy," *Archives of General Psychiatry,* 8 (1963), 213.
34. F. Gentry Harris, *Stress in Combat and in Other Military Situations* (Oxford: Mental Health Research Fund, 1956).
35. Irving D. Harris, *Educational Blocks to Learning* (Glencoe, Ill.: The Free Press, 1961).
36. Ernest Havemann, *The Age of Psychology* (New York: Simon & Schuster, 1957).
37. August B. Hollingshead and Fredrick C. Redlich, *Social Class and Mental Illness* (New York: John Wiley, 1958).
38. Karl Jaspers, *Strindbergh und Van Gogh* (Berlin: Springer, 1926).
39. Maxwell Jones, *The Therapeutic Community* (New York: Basic Books, 1953).
40. Abram Kardiner, *The Individual and His Society* (New York: Columbia University Press, 1939).
41. Abram Kardiner and Lionel Ovesey, *The Mark of Oppression* (New York: Norton, 1951).
42. Søren A. Kierkegaard, *The Concept of Dread,* English translation (Princeton: Princeton University Press, 1942).
43. Lawrence S. Kubic, "Psychoanalysis and Marriage," in Victor W. Eisenstein, ed., *Neurotic Interaction in Marriage* (New York: Basic Books, 1956).
44. Lawrence S. Kubie, *Neurotic Distortion of the Creative Process* (Lawrence, Kansas: The University of Kansas Press, 1958).
45. Paul V. Lemkau, "Mental Hygiene," in Silvano Arieti, ed., *American Handbook of Psychiatry* (New York: Basic Books, 1959), Vol. II, pp. 1948.
46. Paul V. Lemkau and N. Crocetti, "The Amsterdam Municipal Service," *American Journal of Psychiatry,* 117 (1961), 779.
47. Harry Levinson, *Emotional Health in the World of Work* (New York: Harper and Row, 1964).
48. Harold I. Lief, "What Your Doctor Probably Doesn't Know about Sex." *Harper's* 229 (December 1964), 92.

49. Erich Lindemann, "Mental Health—Fundamental to a Dynamic Epidemiology of Health," in Iago Galdston, ed., *Epidemiology of Health* (New York: Health Education Council, 1953).
50. Rudolph M. Loewenstein, *Christians and Jews: A Psychoanalytic Study* (New York: International Universities Press, 1951).
51. Herbert Marcuse, *Eros and Civilization* (Boston: Beacon Press, 1955).
52. William H. Masters, "The Sexual Response Cycle of the Human Female," *Western Journal of Surgery, Obstetrics and Gynecology*, 68 (1960), 57.
53. William H. Masters, "The Sexual Response of the Human Male," *Western Journal of Surgery, Obstetrics and Gynecology*, 71 (1963), 85.
54. William C. Menninger, *Psychiatry in a Troubled World* (New York: Macmillan, 1948).
55. Message from the President of the United States Relative to Mental Illness and Mental Retardation, *American Journal of Psychiatry*, 120 (1964), 729.
56. M. F. Ashley Montague, "Marriage—a Cultural Perspective," in Victor W. Eisenstein, ed., *Neurotic Interaction in Marriage* (New York: Basic Books, 1956).
57. H. B. M. Murphy, *Flight and Resettlement* (UNESCO Publications, 1955).
58. A. S. Neill, *Summerhill: A Radical Approach to Child Rearing* (New York: Hart Publishing, 1960).
59. Beulah Parker, *Psychiatric Consultation for Non-psychiatric Professional Workers* (U. S. Department of Health, Education and Welfare Monograph, 1958), No. 53.
60. Talcott Parsons, *Social Structure and Personality* (New York: Free Press of Glencoe, 1964).
61. Hans Prinzhorn, *Die Bildnerei der Geisteskranken* (Berlin: Springer, 1923).
62. Fritz Redl, "The Concept of a Therapeutic Milieu," *American Journal of Orthopsychiatry*, 29 (1958), 721.
63. Fredrick C. Redlich and June Bingham, *The Inside Story* (New York: Alfred A. Knopf, 1953).
64. Fredrick C. Redlich, "Die Psychoanalyse und das Wertproblem," *Psyche*, 9 (1959), 481.
65. K. A. Rice, *Learning for Leadership* (London: Tavistock Publications, 1965).
66. David Riesman, *The Lonely Crowd* (New Haven: Yale University Press, 1950).
67. Frank Riesman, Jerome Cohen, and Arthur Pearl, eds., *Mental Health of the Poor* (New York: Free Press of Glencoe, 1964).
68. David McK. Rioch, "Preface," *Symposium on Preventive and Social Psychiatry* (Washington, D. C.: Walter Reed Army Medical Center, 1957; U. S. Government Printing Office, 1958).
69. Fritz Jules Roethlisberger and William John Dickson, *Management and the Worker* (Cambridge: Harvard University Press, 1940).
70. George E. Ruff and E. Z. Levy, "Psychiatric Research in Space Medicine," *American Journal of Psychiatry*, 115 (1959), 793.
71. Herbert A. Simon, Models of Man (New York: Wiley, 1957).

72. Albert J. Solnit and M. H. Stark, "Pediatric Management of School Learning Problems of Underachievement," *New England Journal of Medicine*, 26 (1959), 988.
73. Morris I. Stein and Shirley J. Heinze, *Creativity and the Individual* (Glencoe, Illinois: Free Press, 1960).
74. Harry Stack Sullivan, *Fusion of Psychiatry and Social Science* (New York: Norton, 1964).
75. Paul Tillich, *The Courage to Be* (New Haven: Yale University Press, 1952).
76. James S. Tyhurst, "Retirement," *Research Publication, Association for Research in Nervous and Mental Disease*, 35 (1956), 237.
77. Alan Watts, *Psychotherapy East and West* (New York: Pantheon, 1961).
78. Bryant M. Wedge, ed., *Psychosocial Problems of College Men* (New Haven: Yale University Press, 1958).
79. Bryant M. Wedge, "Social Psychiatry and Political Behavior," *Bulletin Menninger Clinic*, 28 (1964), 53.
80. Cecil L. Wittson and W. A. Hunt, "The Predictive Value of the Brief Psychiatric Interview," *American Journal of Psychiatry*, 107 (1951), 582.

NAME INDEX

SUBJECT INDEX